The American Drug Scene

An Anthology

James A. Inciardi
University of Delaware

Karen McElrath
University of Miami

Roxbury Publishing Company

Library of Congress Cataloging-in-Publication Data

The American drug scene: an anthology/[edited by] James A. Inciardi, Karen McElrath.
   p. cm.
   Includes bibliographical references and index.
   ISBN 0-935732-61-6
   1. Drug abuse—United States. I. Inciardi, James A., 1939- II. McElrath, Karen, 1959- .
HV5825.A696 1994
362.29'12'0973—dc20   94-21133
                                                                       CIP

THE AMERICAN DRUG SCENE: AN ANTHOLOGY

Publisher and Editor: Claude Teweles
Supervising Editor: Dawn VanDercreek
Copy Editors: Anton Diether, Joyce Rappaport, Dawn VanDercreek,
   and Sacha A. Howells
Cover Design: Marnie Deacon
Typography: Synergistic Data Systems

Printed on acid-free paper in the United States of America

This paper meets the standards for recycling of the Environmental Protection Agency

Manufactured in the United States of America

ISBN 0-935732-61-6

Roxbury Publishing Company
P.O. Box 491044
Los Angeles, California 90049-9044
(213) 653-1068

Table of Contents

Preface   ix

About the Contributors   x

Introduction   xii

Part I
Perspectives on Drug Use and Addiction

Introduction   1

1. Why People Take Drugs   3
   Andrew Weil

   Weil suggests that drug use results from the natural desire of
   people to alter their levels of consciousness.

2. Doorway to Excess   12
   Harvey Milkman and Stanley Sunderwirth

   A neurobiological view of drug addiction.

3. A Sociological Theory of Drug Addiction   23
   Alfred R. Lindesmith

   Lindesmith argues that opiate addiction results from the conscious awareness that continued drug use is necessary to prevent the pain associated with opiate withdrawal.

4. The Use of Marijuana for Pleasure: A Replication
   of Howard S. Becker's Study of Marijuana Use   34
   *Michael L. Hirsch, Randall W. Conforti,
   and Carolyn J. Graney*

   Howard Becker believed that deriving pleasure from marijuana
   is a learned process. He suggested also that marijuana users
   progress through a series of stages. Hirsch and his colleagues
   test Becker's theory in their study of marijuana users, many of
   whom are college students.

Part II
Legal Drugs

Introduction   43

5. A Brief History of Alcohol   45
   Harvey A. Siegal and James A. Inciardi

   A capsulized history of the likely origins of alcohol use and its
   early evolution.

6. Alcohol, Sex, and Aggression   50
   Jack H. Mendelson and Nancy K. Mello
   An examination of the relationships between alcohol, male fer-
   tility, and sexual potency, and between alcohol and aggression.

7. Who Profits from Tobacco Sales to Children?   57
   Joseph R. DiFranza and Joe B. Tye
   The authors estimate sales of tobacco to youth and present data
   on the profits from these sales for tobacco companies and state
   and federal governments.

8. High Anxiety   63
   Consumer Reports
   A critical look at the addictive nature of some types of tranquil-
   izers and sleeping pills.

9. Anabolic Steroids: An Ethnographic Approach   71
   Paul J. Goldstein
   Goldstein describes patterns of the illicit use of anabolic ster-
   oids and their distribution.

Part III
Marijuana

Introduction   85

10. Marijuana: Assassin of Youth   88
    Harry J. Anslinger and Courtney Ryley Cooper
    Anslinger and Cooper argue against marijuana use in the 1930s,
    noting the harmful effects of the drug.

11. Cannabis Retail Markets in Amsterdam   94
    Dirk J. Korf
    A description of Amsterdam coffeeshops that cater to users of
    marijuana and hashish.

12. Marijuana: The Forbidden Medicine   100
    Lester Grinspoon and James Bakalar
    The authors report on the medical benefits of marijuana.

13. Are There Dangers to Marijuana?   106
    Marc A. Schuckit
    Schuckit offers several negative effects for users of marijuana.

Part IV
Narcotics

Introduction   109

14. Becoming a Heroin Addict   111
    Dan Waldorf
    Waldorf describes the social setting that surrounds the initial
    use of heroin.

15. Taking Care of Business—The Heroin Addict's
Life on the Street   121
Edward Preble and John J. Casey

Preble and Casey describe the daily activities of heroin users,
suggesting that use of the drug creates a sense of purpose in
users' lives.

16. Difficulties in Taking Care of Business   133
Marsha Rosenbaum

A description of the relationship of the addict couple.

17. Chasing the Dragon   144
Marc A. Schuckit

Schuckit describes opiate users who inhale vapors and compares this group to individuals who use heroin intravenously.

18. Nonaddictive Opiate Use   147
Norman E. Zinberg

An analysis of the social setting as it relates to controlled heroin
use.

Part V
Cocaine

Introduction   159

19. Cocaine: Recreational Use and Intoxication   162
Ronald K. Siegel

Siegel examines five categories of cocaine use: experimental,
social-recreational, circumstantial-situational, intensified, and
compulsive.

20. Survival Sex: Inner-City Women and Crack-Cocaine   172
*H. Virginia McCoy, Christine Miles,
and James A. Inciardi*

A description of sex-for-crack exchanges among women users.

21. How Women and Men Get Cocaine: Sex-Role Stereotypes
and Acquisition Patterns   178
Patricia J. Morningstar and Dale D. Chitwood

The authors compare sex-role stereotypes with reported behaviors among male and female cocaine users.

Part VI
Hallucinogenic Drugs

Introduction   187

22. Ethnographic Notes on Ecstasy Use Among Professionals   189
*Marsha Rosenbaum, Patricia Morgan,
and Jerome E. Beck*

Rosenbaum and her colleagues examine patterns of Ecstasy use among working professionals, noting that stressful lifestyles contribute to drug usage among these individuals.

23. Misuse and Legend in the 'Toad Licking' Phenomenon   194
Thomas Lyttle

The author describes the alarmist views by media, law-enforcement officials, and drug-treatment experts regarding the alleged toad-licking craze.

24. The Dusting of America: The Image of Phencyclidine (PCP) in the Popular Media   204
John P. Morgan and Doreen Kagan

A review of the history of PCP in the American drug scene, focusing on its negative image.

25. 'More than Medical Significance':
LSD and American Psychiatry 1953-1966   214
John R. Neill

A description of the changing views of LSD among psychiatrists.

Part VII
Drugs and Crime

Introduction   221

26. The Drugs-Crime Connection   224
*David N. Nurco, Timothy W. Kinlock,
and Thomas E. Hanlon*

A methodological critique of various studies that explore the links between drug use and crime.

27. Heroin Use and Street Crime   237
James A. Inciardi

Inciardi's study suggests that the relationship between drugs and crime is much more complex than previously thought.

28. Kids, Crack, and Crime   245
James A. Inciardi and Anne E. Pottieger

The relationship among crack-cocaine use, drug trafficking, and street crime among serious delinquents.

29. The Drugs/Violence Nexus: A Tripartite Conceptual Framework   255
Paul J. Goldstein

Goldstein addresses three methods by which drug use and violence are connected: psychopharmacological, economic-compulsive, and systemic.

Part VIII
AIDS and Drug Use

Introduction   265

30. Kickin' Down to the Street Doc: Shooting Galleries in the
    San Francisco Bay Area   268
    Sheigla Murphy and Dan Waldorf

    A description of formal and informal urban drug-shooting ha-
    vens and their purposes.

31. The Risk of Exposure to HIV-Contaminated
    Needles and Syringes in Shooting Galleries   277
    James A. Inciardi, J. Bryan Page, Duane C. McBride,
    Dale D. Chitwood, Clyde B. McCoy, H. Virginia McCoy,
    and Edward Trapido

    The authors investigate behaviors of injection drug users who
    frequent shooting galleries, estimating the probability for their
    exposure to HIV-contaminated needles.

32. Needle Access as an AIDS-Prevention Strategy
    for IV Drug Users: A Research Perspective   284
    Merrill Singer, Ray Irizarry, and Jean J. Schensul

    A description of needle-exchange programs, their benefits, and
    suggestions to improve community support for such programs.

Part IX
Treatment

Introduction   299

33. The Therapeutic Community for Substance Abuse:
    Perspective and Approach   301
    George De Leon

    A description of the methods by which therapeutic communi-
    ties operate.

34. Methadone Maintenance: A Theoretical Perspective   309
    Vincent P. Dole and Marie Nyswander

    Dole and Nyswander report findings from their early study of
    heroin users treated with methadone maintenance.

35. Alcoholics Anonymous   314
    Karen McElrath

    A brief overview of the history, philosophy, organization, and
    program components of Alcoholics Anonymous.

Part X
Policy

Introduction   319

36. Drug Prohibition in the United States: Costs,
    Consequences, and Alternatives   322
    Ethan A. Nadelmann

    Nadelmann offers several reasons for the failure of the "War on
    Drugs," suggesting that legalization of certain drugs is the bet-
    ter alternative.

37. Against the Legalization of Drugs   336
    James Q. Wilson

    Wilson argues against the legalization of heroin and cocaine,
    claiming that drug availability affects consumption and that
    counter-arguments should not be based on comparisons be-
    tween illegal narcotics and legal alcohol.

38. Hawks Ascendant: The Punitive Trend of American Drug Policy   345
    Peter Reuter

    Reuter discusses three alternative views for addressing the ille-
    gal drug problem: the supply-side perspective, the treatment-
    based prohibition perspective, and the legalization perspective.

Subject Index   365

Preface

If anything has been learned about drug use in the United States, it is an awareness that the problem is both dynamic and continually shifting and changing. There are fads, fashions, and even rages in the drugs of abuse. Heroin, marijuana, cocaine, LSD, and many other drugs have all had their periods of currency. While one substance may be considered the drug of choice for a few months, the popularity of others may endure for years or even a generation or more. Drug "epidemics" (periods during which there are many new users) come and go as well. For example, the United States experienced an epidemic of cocaine use during the 1880s and 1890s, followed by a decline early in the twentieth century, then a re-emergence two decades ago. Several heroin epidemics occurred during the second half of this century, and the current crack-cocaine epidemic began in the mid-1980s.

The tenor and direction of drug-control policies tend to shift as well. Although major changes in drug policy have been infrequent, intermittent anti-drug fads and fashions often arise during periodic "wars on drugs." Such initiatives as "zero tolerance," asset forfeiture, mandatory minimum sentences for small-time traffickers, compulsory treatment for drug-involved offenders, and numerous others have experienced periods of acceptance and disfavor. And, not surprisingly, the public, political, and ideological reactions to the drug policies of White House incumbents have been abundant, ardent, and enduring.

The materials in *The American Drug Scene* were selected and organized to reflect the changing patterns, problems, perspectives, and policies that are defining and redefining drug use in the United States. In the articles to follow, as well as in the introductory commentaries, the information presented is both historical and contemporary, theoretical and descriptive, dispassionate and spirited. We hope that readers will find the material both interesting and instructive.

Appreciation is extended to the following colleagues whose comments and suggestions at various early stages were most helpful in developing this anthology: Howard Abadinsky, Saint Xavier University; Patricia A. Adler, University of Colorado, Boulder; Ronald L. Akers, University of Florida; Bruce L. Berg, Indiana University of Pennsylvania; Jay Corzine, University of Nebraska, Lincoln; Richard Dembo, University of South Florida; Patrick G. Donnelly, University of Dayton; Drew Humphries, Rutgers University; Jerome Rabow, University of California, Los Angeles; Craig Reinarman, University of California, Santa Cruz; David R. Rudy, Morehead State University; William Skinner, University of Kentucky; Richard C. Stephens, Cleveland State University; N. Prabha Unnithan, Colorado State University; and Richard A. Wright, University of Scranton. ✦

James A. Inciardi
Key Largo, Florida

Karen McElrath
Key Biscayne, Florida

About the Contributors

Harry J. Anslinger (deceased) was the first U.S. Commissioner of Narcotics and presided over the Federal Bureau of Narcotics from 1930 through 1962.

James Bakalar is a lecturer in law at Harvard Medical School and has published widely in the area of drug abuse.

Jerome E. Beck is a researcher with the Institute for Scientific Analysis in San Francisco.

John J. Casey is affiliated with the Department of Economics at Georgetown University in Washington, D.C.

Dale D. Chitwood is an associate professor in the Department of Sociology at the University of Miami in Coral Gables, Florida.

Randall W. Conforti is an associate at the Ranch Rehabilitation Service in Menomonee Falls, Wisconsin.

Courtney Ryley Cooper (deceased) was a journalist and author of such "true crime" classics as *Ten Thousand Public Enemies* (1935), *Here's to Crime* (1937), and *Designs in Scarlet* (1939).

George De Leon is the director of the Center for Therapeutic Community Research in New York City.

Joseph R. DiFranza is a physician with the Fitchburg Family Practice Residency Program at the University of Massachusetts Medical School.

Vincent P. Dole is a physician and clinician with Rockefeller University in New York City, and founder of the methadone-maintenance treatment modality for narcotics addiction.

Paul J. Goldstein is a sociologist, ethnographer, and associate professor in the School of Public Health at the University of Illinois.

Carolyn J. Graney is affiliated with the Department of Sociology at Lawrence University in Appleton, Wisconsin.

Lester Grinspoon is a professor of psychiatry at Harvard Medical School and has published widely in the area of drug abuse.

Thomas E. Hanlon is an associate research professor at the Maryland Psychiatric Research Center, Department of Psychiatry, University of Maryland School of Medicine.

Michael L. Hirsch is a faculty member in the Department of Sociology at Lawrence University in Appleton, Wisconsin.

Doreen Kagan is a researcher in the Departments of Pharmacology and Medicine at Mt. Sinai School of Medicine in New York City.

Timothy W. Kinlock is a research associate at Friends Medical Science Research Center in Baltimore, Maryland.

Dirk J. Korf is an assistant professor and senior researcher in the Criminological Institute at the University of Amsterdam.

Alfred R. Lindesmith (deceased) was a professor of sociology at Indiana University and one of the first researchers to conduct sociological studies of addiction.

Thomas Lyttle is a freelance writer and publisher of the journal *Psychedelic Monographs and Essays*.

Duane C. McBride is a professor in the Department of Behavioral Sciences and director of the Alcoholism and Drug Dependency Research Center at Andrews University in Berrien Springs, Michigan.

Clyde B. McCoy is professor and director of the Comprehensive Drug Research Center at the University of Miami School of Medicine.

H. Virginia McCoy is an associate professor in the Department of Public Health at Florida International University in Miami.

Nancy K. Mello is a professor of psychology at Harvard Medical School and has been conducting research on alcohol problems for almost three decades.

Jack H. Mendelson is a professor of psychiatry at Harvard Medical School and has been conducting research on alcohol problems for almost three decades.

Christine Miles is a research associate in the Comprehensive Drug Research Center at the University of Miami School of Medicine.

John P. Morgan is a physician affiliated with the Sophie Davis School of Biomedical Education at the City University of New York.

Patricia Morgan is affiliated with the University of California at Berkeley.

Patricia J. Morningstar is a researcher and ethnographer who has been conducting studies of cocaine use since the early 1970s.

Sheigla Murphy is an ethnographer with the Institute for Scientific Analysis in San Francisco.

Ethan A. Nadelmann is an assistant professor of politics and public affairs in the Department of Politics and the Woodrow Wilson School of Public and International Affairs at Princeton University, and Chairman of the Princeton Working Group on the Future of Drug Use and Alternatives to Drug Prohibition.

John R. Neill is an associate professor of psychiatry at the University of Kentucky College of Medicine in Lexington.

David N. Nurco is a research professor in the Department of Psychiatry at the University of Maryland School of Medicine.

Marie Nyswander (deceased) was a physician and clinician with Rockefeller University in New York City, and co-founder of the methadone-maintenance treatment modality for narcotics addiction.

J. Bryan Page is an associate professor in the Department of Anthropology at the university of Miami in Coral Gables, Florida.

Anne E. Pottieger is a sociologist and senior scientist in the Center for Drug and Alcohol Studies at the University of Delaware.

Edward Preble (deceased) was an anthropologist and ethnographer with Manhattan State Hospital and spent much of his career conducting street studies of the New York City drug scene.

Peter Reuter is the co-director of the Drug Policy Research Center at the RAND Corporation.

Marsha Rosenbaum is a sociologist and ethnographer at the Institute for Scientific Analysis in San Francisco and the author of the classic work *Women on Heroin* (1981)

Marc A. Schuckit is a professor of psychiatry at the University of California School of Medicine, and director of the Alcoholism Research Center at the San Diego Veterans Administration Hospital.

Harvey A. Siegal is a sociologist and ethnographer, and professor and director of Substance Abuse Intervention Programs at Wright State University School of Medicine in Dayton, Ohio.

Ronald K. Siegel is a psychopharmacologist and associate research professor at UCLA.

Edward Trapido is the associate director of the Sylvester Comprehensive Cancer Research Center at the University of Miami School of Medicine.

Joe B. Tye is an MBA affiliated with the Baystate Medical Center in Springfield, Massachusetts.

Dan Waldorf is a sociologist and ethnographer with the Institute for Scientific Analysis in San Francisco and author of the classic work *Careers in Dope* (1973).

Andrew Weil is a graduate of Harvard Medical College, a research associate in ethnopharmacology at the Harvard Botanical Museum, and an adjunct professor of addiction studies at the University of Arizona.

James Q. Wilson is the Collins professor of management and public policy at UCLA.

Norman E. Zinberg is a clinical professor of psychiatry at Harvard Medical School and is best known for his classic work *Drug, Set, and Setting* (1984). ✦

Introduction

The American drug scene has a long and enduring history. To begin with, the drinking of alcohol to excess is centuries old. In *The Life and Times of the Late Demon Rum*, the celebrated American social historian and biographer J.C. Furnas suggested that alcohol came to the Colonies with the first English and Dutch settlers, and that the drinking of "spirits" and "strong waters" dates back to the first days of the emerging American republic. Tradition had taught that rum, gin, and brandy were nutritious and healthful. Distilled spirits were viewed as foods that supplemented a limited and monotonous diet; as medications that could cure colds, fevers, snakebites, and broken legs; and as relaxants that would relieve depression, reduce tension, and enable hard-working laborers to enjoy a moment of happy, frivolous camaraderie. By the early 1700s, nearly all Americans of every occupation and social class drank alcoholic beverages in quantity, sometimes to the point of intoxication. By the end of the eighteenth century, the daily per-capita drinking of Americans was almost a half pint of hard liquor.

The use of other drugs for the enhancement of pleasure and performance or for the alteration of mood also dates back several centuries. Perhaps it all began with Thomas Dover, who developed a form of medicinal opium sold as *Dover's Powder*. Introduced in England in 1709 and several years later in the Colonies, it contained one ounce each of opium, ipecac (the dried root of a tropical creeping plant), and licorice combined with saltpeter, tartar, and wine. The attraction of Dover's Powder was in the euphoric and anesthetic properties of opium. For thousands of years, opium had been a popular narcotic. A derivative of the *Oriental poppy* (Papaver somniferum L.), it was called the "plant of joy" some 4,000 years ago in what has been called the "Fertile Crescent" of Mesopotamia.

The introduction of Dover's Powder in the Colonies apparently started a trend. By the latter part of the eighteenth century, medications containing opium were readily available throughout urban and rural America. They were sold over-the-counter in pharmacies, grocery and general stores, at traveling medicine shows, and through the mail. They were marketed under such labels as *Ayer's Cherry Pectoral*, *Mrs. Winslow's Soothing Syrup*, *McMunn's Elixir*, *Godfrey's Cordial*, *Scott's Emulsion*, and *Dover's Powder*. Many of these remedies were seductively advertised as "painkillers," "cough mixtures," "soothing syrups," "consumption cures," and "women's friends." Others were promoted for the treatment of such varied ailments as diarrhea, dysentery, colds, fever, teething, cholera, rheumatism, pelvic disorders, athlete's foot, and even baldness and cancer. The drugs were produced from imported opium, as well as from the white opium poppies that were grown legally in the New England states, Florida and Louisiana, the West and Southwest, and, during the Civil War, the Confederate States of America.

For thousands of years, opium had been the only known product of the Oriental poppy. In 1803, however, a young German pharmacist, Frederick Serturner, isolated the chief alkaloid of opium. Serturner had hit upon *morphine*, which he so named after Morpheus, the Greek god of dreams. The discovery was to have profound effects on both medicine and society; for morphine was, and still is, the greatest single pain reliever the world has ever known. With the invention of the hypodermic syringe, the use of morphine by injection in military medicine during the Civil War and the Franco-Prussian War granted the procedure legitimacy and familiarity to both physicians and the public. Furthermore, hypodermic medication had its pragmatic aspects—it brought quick local relief, its dosage could be regulated, and it was effective when oral medication was impractical. The regimen, however, was used promiscuously. Many physicians were anxious to illustrate their ability to quell the pains suffered by their patients, who in turn expected instant relief from any discomfort.

Beyond opium and morphine, the over-the-counter medicine industry branched out even further—to cocaine in the 1880s and heroin in the late 1890s. By the close of the nineteenth century, it was estimated that millions of Americans were addicted to over-the-counter medications. Agitation had already begun for controls over the manufacture and distribution of products containing cocaine, opium, and their various derivatives. One result was the passage of the Pure Food and Drug Act in 1906, which prohibited the interstate transportation of adulterated or misbranded food and drugs. The act brought about the decline of over-the-counter medications because, henceforth, the proportions of alcohol, opium, morphine, heroin, cocaine, and a number of other substances in each preparation had to be indicated. As a result, most of these remedies lost their appeal.

The Pure Food and Drug Act merely imposed standards for quality, packaging, and labeling; it did not actually outlaw the use of cocaine and opiate drugs. Public Law No. 47, 63rd Congress [H.R. 1967], more popularly known as the Harrison Act, sponsored by New York Representative Francis Burton Harrison and passed in 1914, ultimately served that end. The new legislation also went a long way toward altering public and criminal-justice responses to drug use in the United States for generations to come. The Harrison Act required all people who imported, manufactured, produced, compounded, sold, dispensed, or otherwise distributed cocaine and opiate drugs to register with the Treasury Department, pay special taxes, and keep records of all transactions. As such, the act was a revenue code designed to exercise some measure of public control over drugs rather than to penalize all users of narcotics in the United States. In effect, however, penalization is specifically what occurred. Although subcultures and criminal cultures of drug users already existed well prior to the passage of the Harrison Act, the legislation served to expand their membership. Since then, "drug use" has generally been viewed not only as a social problem in the United States, but a criminal problem as well.

From the 1920s through the 1990s, there have been many drugs of abuse—heroin, cocaine, crack, LSD, PCP, Ecstasy, the amphetamines and methamphetamines, and numerous others—all of which are discussed in the sections that follow. In addition to the many papers and articles describing these drugs, their patterns of use, and their impact on society, other topics are covered, including the linkages between drug use and crime, the AIDS/drug connection, treatment initiatives, and alternative drug-control policies.

Before proceeding further, however, it is important that readers gain an understanding of the basic drug-related terms which are frequently used in this book and whose meanings are often taken for granted. The following is a short glossary of the most important definitions:

A. Basic Drug Groups

Psychoactive drugs: drugs that alter perception and consciousness, including analgesics, depressants, stimulants, and hallucinogens.

Analgesics: drugs used for the relief of varying degrees of pain without rendering the user unconscious. There are both *narcotic* and *non-narcotic* varieties of analgesics.

Depressants: drugs that act on and lessen the activity of the central nervous system (CNS), diminishing or arresting vital functions.

Sedatives: CNS depressant drugs that produce calm and relaxation. Alcohol, barbiturates and related compounds, and minor tranquilizers are sedative drugs.

Hypnotics: CNS depressant drugs that produce sleep. Barbiturates, methaqualone, and chloral hydrate are hypnotic drugs. As such, a number of drugs are both sedatives *and* hypnotics.

Stimulants: drugs that stimulate the central nervous system and increase the activity of the brain and spinal cord. Amphetamines and cocaine are CNS stimulant drugs.

Hallucinogens: drugs that act on the central nervous system, producing mood and perceptual changes that vary from sensory illusions to hallucinations. Sometimes referred to as "psychedelics," hallucinogenic drugs include marijuana, hashish, LSD, PCP, and psilocybin.

B. Dependency Terms

Addiction: drug craving accompanied by a physical dependence which motivates continuing usage, resulting in tolerance to a drug's effects and a syndrome of identifiable symptoms when the drug is abruptly withdrawn. Narcotics, barbiturates, and cocaine are all addicting drugs.

Tolerance: a state of acquired resistance to some or all of the effects of a drug. Tolerance develops after the repeated use of certain drugs, resulting in a need to increase the dosage to obtain the original effects.

Cross-tolerance: among certain pharmacologically related drugs, tolerance to the effects of one will carry over to most or all others. For example, a person who has become tolerant to the euphoric effects of secobarbital is likely tolerant to those of all other short-acting barbiturates.

Cross-addiction: also referred to as *cross-dependence*, a situation in which dependence between drugs of the same pharmacological group is mutual and interchangeable. For example, persons addicted to heroin can use methadone or some other narcotic in place of the heroin without experiencing withdrawal symptoms.

Withdrawal: the reactions and behaviors that ensue if a dependent user abruptly ceases intake of a drug.

Detoxification: the removal of physical dependency.

C. Drug Reactions

Potentiation: the ability of one drug to increase the activity of another drug when the two are taken simultaneously. This can be expressed mathematically as $a + b = A$. For example, aspirin (a) plus caffeine (b) increases the potency of the aspirin (A).

Synergism: similar to potentiation, a situation in which two or more drugs are taken together and the combined action dramatically increases the normal effects of each drug. A synergistic effect can be expressed mathematically as $1 + 1 = 5$ and typically occurs with mixtures of alcohol and barbiturates.

Antagonism: a situation in which two drugs taken together have opposite effects on the body. An antagonistic reaction can be expressed mathematically as $1 + 1 = 0$ and typically occurs with certain mixtures of depressants and stimulants.

Idiosyncracy: an abnormal or peculiar response to a drug, such as excitation from a depressant or sedation from a stimulant.

Side effect: any effect other than one the drug was intended to produce, such as stomach upset from aspirin.

D. Routes of Drug Administration

Intravenous (IV): injected into the vein.

Intramuscular (IM): injected into the muscle.

Cutaneous: absorbed through the skin.

Subcutaneous: inserted under the skin.

Insufflation (inhalation): drawn into the lungs through the nose or mouth.

Oral: swallowed and absorbed through the stomach.

Vaginal: absorbed through vaginal tissues.

Anal: absorbed through rectal tissues.

Sub-lingual: absorbed through the tissues under the tongue. ✦

Part I

Perspectives on Drug Use and Addiction

Why do people take drugs? For the enhancement of pleasure or performance? To relieve anxiety or boredom? As an escape from reality? To suppress feelings of sorrow, inadequacy, guilt, or other emotional pain? Likely all of these reasons, and many more. In fact, there may be as many reasons for taking drugs as there are people who use them. Moreover, theories are legion, so much so that one publication of the National Institute on Drug Abuse devoted its entire 488 pages to outlining the major views.

Although many early explanations of substance abuse considered it to be a "moral weakness," a number of investigators have described drug users as maladjusted, hostile, immature, dependent, manipulative, and narcissistic individuals, suggesting that drug use is just one more symptom of their disordered personalities. Others suggest that since drug use is an integral part of the general culture that surrounds the user, it is learned behavior. And there are other explanations: the bad-habit theory, disruptive-environment theory, cognitive-control theory, social-deviance theory, biological-rhythm theory, subcultural theory, social-neurobiological theory, and many more.

Quite popular for many years was the theory of the "addiction-prone personality," elucidated by Dr. Kenneth Chapman of the United States Public Health Service several decades ago:

> . . . the typical addict is emotionally unstable and immature, often seeking pleasure and excitement outside of the conventional realms. Unable to adapt comfortably to the pressures and tensions in today's speedy world, he may become either an extremely dependent individual or turn into a hostile "lone wolf" incapable of attaching deep feelings toward anyone. In his discomfort, he may suffer pain—real or imaginary. The ordinary human being has nor-

mal defense machinery with which to meet life's disappointments, frustrations, and conflicts. But the potential addict lacks enough of this inner strength to conquer his emotional problems and the anxiety they create. In a moment of stress, he may be introduced to narcotics as a "sure-fire" answer to his needs. Experiencing relief from his pain, or an unreal flight from his problems, or a puffed-up sense of power and control regarding them, he is well on the road toward making narcotics his way of life.

Stated differently, when "stable" people are introduced to drugs, they will discard them spontaneously before becoming dependent. Those who have "addiction-prone personalities," because of psychoses, psychopathic or psychoneurotic disorders, or predispositions toward mental dysfunctioning, "become transformed into the typical addict."

For a number of contemporary theorists, drug use is related to a more basic need for *pleasure*, plain and simple. For example, there is extensive physiological, neurological, and anthropological evidence to suggest that we are members of a species that has been honed for pleasure. Nearly all people want and enjoy pleasure, and the pursuit of drugs—whether caffeine, nicotine, alcohol, opium, heroin, marijuana, or cocaine—seems to be universal and inescapable. It is found across time and across cultures (and species). The process of evolution has, for whatever reasons, resulted in a human neurophysiology that responds both vividly and avidly to a variety of common substances. The brain has pleasure centers—receptor sites and cortical cells—that react to "rewarding" dosages of many substances. Or as University of California pharmacologist Larry Stein explained it in 1989:

> The fact that *cells* respond to a reward shows just how deeply embedded in the design of the brain this

reinforcement mechanism is. . . . Dopamine and the opioid peptides are transmitters in very powerful control systems based on a certain chemistry. . . . Along come poppy seeds and coca leaves that have chemicals very similar to these central systems. They go right in, do not pass GO. To say that cocaine or amphetamines, or heroin or morphine, should be highly appealing is an understatement.

Regardless of the theory put forth, it would appear that drug users are of four basic types—*experimenters*, *social-recreational users*, *involved users*, and *dysfunctional abusers*.

The *experimenters* are by far the largest group of drug users (not including alcohol users). They most frequently try one or more drugs in a social setting, but the drug does not play a significant role in their lives. They use their drug of choice experimentally because their social group relates the drug's effects as being pleasurable. Experimenters do not seek out a drug but may use it when someone presents it to them in an appropriate setting. In this situation, they may smoke marijuana or "snort" cocaine once or twice because the drug does something *to* them. As a University of Delaware senior commented about his first cocaine experience:

I generally don't use drugs, except maybe a little grass now and then. My only experience with coke was a few weeks ago in the dormitory. My roommate came in with a couple of other guys and started getting high on it. They kept trying to get me to do some, and finally I snorted some just for the heck of it. When I did, it was quite a blast at first, from my head all the way down, and then I felt like I was floating. After, I felt a little weird. . . . It was good.

Social-recreational users differ from experimenters primarily in terms of frequency and continuity of consumption. For example, they may use drugs when they are at a party and someone presents the opportunity. Drugs still do not play a significant role in these users' lives. They still do not actively seek out drugs but use them only because it does something to them—it makes them feel good. A 28-year-old Miami woman related:

Partying can be even more fun with a few lines of coke. I never have any of my own, but usually I'll tie in with some guy who does. We'll get a little stoned, and maybe go to bed. It's all in good fun. . . . Another time, I was on a double date and this guy had some good *toot*. We drove up to Orlando and went into Disney World. Do you know what it's like

goin' through the haunted mansion stoned like that? It's a whole different trip. . . .

The great majority of alcohol use occurs in a social-recreational context.

For *involved users*, a major transition has taken place since their social-recreational use of drugs. As users become "involved" with a particular drug, they also become drug seekers. Their drug of choice becomes significant to their lives. Although they are still quite able to function—in school, on the job, or as a parent or spouse—their proficiency in many areas begins to decline markedly. Personal and social functioning tends to be inversely related to the amount of time that involved users spend on using drugs. They still have control over their behavior, but their use of the drug occurs with increasing frequency for some adaptive reason; their drug does something *for* them.

Involved users are of many types. Some use drugs to deal with an unbearable work situation, indulging in controlled amounts several times a day. Others use drugs to enhance performance or bolster their self-esteem. And still a third group regularly use drugs to deal with stress, anxiety, or nagging boredom. As one involved cocaine user, a self-employed accountant, put it:

I seem to be always uptight these days with almost everything I do. Everybody seems to always want something—my clients, my wife, the bank, the world. . . . A few *lines* [of cocaine] every two-three hours gets me through the day—through the tax returns, the tension at home, the bills, sex, whatever. Without the coke I'd probably have to be put away somewhere. . . .

The *dysfunctional abusers* are what have become known as "cokeheads," "alcoholics," and "addicts." For them, drugs have become the significant part of their lives. They are personally and socially dysfunctional and spend all of their time involved in drug-seeking, drug-taking, and other related activities. Moreover, they no longer have control over their drug use.

In the four selections that follow, a variety of perspectives on drug use and addiction are presented, ranging from the "natural mind" view of Andrew Weil and the sociological work of Alfred R. Lindesmith, to the more psychological and neurobiological explanations of Harvey Milkman and Stanley Sunderwirth. ✦

1. *Why People Take Drugs*

Andrew Weil

Andrew Weil, a graduate of Harvard Medical College, believes that people of all cultures are born with the desire to periodically alter their consciousness. He suggests that this desire can be observed in children at very young ages; but because adults frown upon these actions, children learn to suppress or conceal their urges through socialization. According to Dr. Weil, the use of alcohol and other drugs is a natural expression of our innate desires to experience different states of consciousness. He describes his own experiences with mescaline as well as those of others who have used the drug. Finally, he notes the importance of "set" and "setting," suggesting that these two factors may have a greater influence on an individual's drug experience than the drug itself.

The use of drugs to alter consciousness is nothing new. It has been a feature of human life in all places on the earth and in all ages of history. In fact, to my knowledge, the only people lacking a traditional intoxicant are the Eskimos, who had the misfortune to be unable to grow anything and had to wait for white men to bring them alcohol. Alcohol, of course, has always been the most commonly used drug, simply because it does not take much effort to discover that the consumption of fermented juices produces interesting variations from ordinary consciousness.

The ubiquity of drug use is so striking that it must represent a basic human appetite. Yet, many Americans seem to feel that the contemporary drug scene is something new, something qualitatively different from what has gone before. This attitude is peculiar, because all that is really happening is a change in drug preference. There is no evidence that a greater percentage of Americans are taking drugs, only that younger Americans are coming to prefer illegal drugs, like marijuana and hallucinogens, to alcohol. Therefore, people who insist that everyone is suddenly taking drugs must not see alcohol in the category of drugs. Evidence that this is precisely the case is abundant, and it provides another example of how emotional biases lead us to formulate unhelpful conceptions. Drug taking is bad. We drink alcohol. Therefore, alcohol is not a drug. It is, instead, a "pick-me-up," a "thirst quencher," a "social lubricant," "an indispensable accompaniment to fine food," and a variety of other euphemisms. Or, if it is a drug, at least it is not one of those bad drugs that the hippies use.

This attitude is quite prevalent in the adult population of America, and it is an unhelpful formulation for several reasons. In the first place, alcohol is very much a drug by any criterion and causes significant alterations of nervous functioning, regardless of what euphemistic guise it appears in. In fact, of all the drugs being used in our society, alcohol has the strongest claim to the label *drug*, in view of the prominence of its long-term physical effects. In addition, thinking of alcohol as something other than a drug leads us to frame wrong hypotheses about what is going on in America. We are spending much time, money, and intellectual energy trying to find out why people are taking drugs; but, in fact, what we are doing is trying to find out why some people are taking some drugs that we disapprove of. No useful answers can come out of that sort of inquiry; the question is improperly phrased.

Of course, many theories have been put forward. People are taking drugs to escape, to rebel against parents and other authorities, in response to tensions over foreign wars or domestic crises, in imitation of their elders, and so on and so on. No doubt, these considerations do operate on some level (for instance, they may shape the forms of illegal drug use by young people), but they are totally inadequate to explain the universality of drug use by human beings. To come up with a valid explanation, we simply must suspend our value judgments about kinds of drugs and admit (however painful it might be) that the glass of beer on a hot afternoon and the bottle of wine with a fine meal are no different in kind from the joint of marijuana or the snort of cocaine; nor is the evening devoted to cocktails essentially different from the day devoted to mescaline. All are examples of the same phenomenon: the use of chemical agents to induce alterations in consciousness. What is the meaning of this universal phenomenon?

It is my belief that the desire to alter consciousness periodically is an innate, normal drive analogous to hunger or the sexual drive. Note that I do not say "desire to alter consciousness by means of chemical agents." Drugs are merely one means of satisfying this drive; there are many others, and I will discuss them in due course. In postulating an inborn drive of this sort, I am not advancing a proposition to be proved or disproved but simply a model to be tried out for usefulness in simplifying our understanding of our observations. The model I propose is consistent with observable evidence. In particular, the omnipresence of the phenomenon argues that we are dealing not with something socially or culturally based, but rather with a biological characteristic of the species. Furthermore, the need for periods of non-ordinary consciousness begins to be expressed at ages far too young for it to have much to do with social conditioning. Anyone who watches very young children without revealing his presence will find them regularly practicing techniques that induce striking changes in mental states. Three- and four-year-olds, for example, commonly whirl themselves into vertiginous stupors. They hyperventilate and have other children squeeze them around the chest until they faint. They also choke each other to produce loss of consciousness.

To my knowledge these practices appear spontaneously among children of all societies, and I suspect they have done so throughout history as well. It is most interesting that children quickly learn to keep this sort of play out of sight of grownups, who instinctively try to stop them. The sight of a child being throttled into unconsciousness scares the parent, but the child seems to have a wonderful time; at least, he goes right off and does it again. Psychologists have paid remarkably little attention to these activities of all children. Some Freudians have noted them and called them "sexual equivalents," suggesting that they are somehow related to the experience of orgasm. But merely labeling a phenomenon does not automatically increase our ability to describe, predict, or influence it; besides, our understanding of sexual experience is too primitive to help us much.

Growing children engage in extensive experimentation with mental states, usually in the direction of loss of waking consciousness. Many of them discover that the transition zone between waking and sleep offers many possibilities for unusual sensations, such as hallucinations and out-of-the-body experiences, and they look forward to this period each night. (And yet, falling asleep becomes suddenly frightening at a later age, possibly when the ego sense has developed more fully. We will return to this point in a moment.) It is only a matter of time before children find out that similar experiences may be obtained chemically; many of them learn it before the age of five. The most common

route to this knowledge is the discovery that inhalation of the fumes of volatile solvents in household products induces experiences similar to those caused by whirling or fainting. An alternate route is introduction to general anesthesia in connection with a childhood operation—an experience that invariably becomes one of the most vivid early memories.

By the time most American children enter school, they have already explored a variety of altered states of consciousness and usually know that chemical substances are one doorway to this fascinating realm. They also know that it is a forbidden realm, in that grownups will always attempt to stop them from going there if they catch them at it. But, as I have said, the desire to repeat these experiences is not mere whim; it looks like a real drive arising from the neurophysiological structure of the human brain. What, then, happens to it as the child becomes more and more involved in the process of socialization? In most cases, it goes underground. Children learn very quickly that they must pursue anti-social behavior patterns if they wish to continue to alter consciousness regularly. Hence, the secret meetings in cloakrooms, garages, and playground corners where they can continue to whirl, choke each other, and, perhaps, sniff cleaning fluids or gasoline.

As the growing child's sense of self is reinforced more and more by parents, school, and society at large, the drive to alter consciousness may go underground in the individual as well. That is, its indulgence becomes a very private matter, much like masturbation. Furthermore, in view of the overwhelming social pressure against such indulgence and the strangeness of the experiences from the point of view of normal, ego-centered consciousness, many children become quite frightened of episodes of non-ordinary awareness and very unwilling to admit their occurrence. The development of this kind of fear may account for the change from looking forward to falling asleep to being afraid of it; in many cases, it leads to repression of memories of the experiences.

Yet, co-existing with these emotional attitudes is always the underlying need to satisfy an inner drive. In this regard, the Freudian analogy to sexual experience seems highly pertinent. Like the cyclic urge to relieve sexual tension (which probably begins to be felt at much lower ages than many think), the urge to suspend ordinary awareness arises spontaneously from within, builds to a peak, finds relief, and dissipates—all in accordance with its own intrinsic rhythm. The form of the appearance and course of this desire is identical to that of sexual desire. And the pleasure, in both cases, arises from relief of accumulated tension. Both experiences are thus self-validating; their worth is obvious in their own terms, and it is not necessary to justify them by reference to anything else. In other words, episodes of sexual release and episodes of suspension of ordinary consciousness feel good; they satisfy an inner need. Why they should feel good is another sort of question, which I will try to answer toward the end of this chapter. In the meantime, it will be useful to keep in mind the analogy between sexual experience and the experience of altered consciousness (and the possibility that the former is a special case of the latter rather than the reverse).

Despite the accompaniment of fear and guilt, experiences of non-ordinary consciousness persist into adolescence and adult life, although awareness of them may diminish. If one takes the trouble to ask people if they have ever had strange experiences at the point of falling asleep, many adults will admit to hallucinations and feelings of being out of their bodies. Significantly, most will do this with a great sense of relief at being able to tell someone else about it and at learning that such experiences do not mark them as psychologically disturbed. One woman who listened to a lecture I gave came up to me afterward and said, "I never knew other people had things like that. You don't know how much better I feel." The fear and guilt that reveal themselves in statements of this sort doubtless develop at early ages and probably are the source of the very social attitudes that engender more fear and guilt in the next generation. The process is curiously circular and self-perpetuating.

There is one more step in the development of adult attitudes toward consciousness alteration. At some point (rather late, I suspect), children learn that social support exists for one method of doing it—namely, the use of alcohol—and that if they are patient, they will be allowed to try it. Until recently, most persons who reached adulthood in our society were content to drink alcohol if they wished to continue to have experiences of this sort by means of chemicals. Now, however, many young people are discovering that other chemicals may be preferable. After all, this is what drug users themselves say: that certain illegal substances give better highs than alcohol. This is a serious claim, worthy of serious consideration.

At this point, I would like to summarize the main ideas I have presented so far and then illustrate them with personal examples. We seem to be born with a drive to experience episodes of altered consciousness. This drive expresses itself at very early ages in all children in activities designed to cause loss or major disturbance of ordinary awareness. To an outside, adult observer, these practices seem perverse and even dangerous, but in most cases adults have simply forgotten their own identical experiences as children. As children grow, they explore many ways of inducing similar changes in consciousness and usually discover chemical methods before they enter school. Overwhelming social pressures against public indulgence of this need force children to pursue anti-social, secretive behavior patterns in their explorations of consciousness. In addition, the development of a strong ego sense in this social context often leads to fear and guilt about the desire for periods of altered awareness. Consequently, many youngsters come to indulge this desire in private or to repress it. Finally, older children come to understand that social support is available for chemical satisfaction of this need by means of alcohol. Today's youth, in their continuing experimentation with methods of changing awareness, have come across a variety of other chemicals which they prefer to alcohol. Thus, use of illegal drugs is nothing more than a logical continuation of a developmental sequence going back to early childhood. It cannot be isolated as a unique phenomenon of adolescence, of contemporary America, of cities, or of any particular social or economic class.

I feel confident about this developmental scheme for two reasons. First, I have seen it clearly in the histories of many hundreds of drug users I have interviewed and known. Second, I have experienced it myself. I was an avid whirler and could spend hours collapsed on the ground with the world spinning around—this despite the obvious unpleasant side effects of nausea, dizziness, and sheer exhaustion (the only aspects of the experience visible to grownups). From my point of view, these effects were incidental to a state of consciousness that was extraordinarily fascinating—more interesting than any other state except the one I entered at the verge of sleep. I soon found out that my spinning made grownups upset; I learned to do it with other neighborhood children in out-of-the-way locations, and I kept it up until I was nine or ten. At about the age of four, like most members of my generation, I had my tonsils out, and the experience of ether anesthesia (administered by the old-fashioned open-drop method) remains one of my strongest memories of early life. It was frightening, intensely interesting, and intimately bound up with my thoughts about death. Some years later, I discovered that a particular brand of cleaning fluid in the basement of my house gave me a similar experience, and I sniffed it many times, often in the company of others my age. I could not have explained what I was doing to anyone; the experience was interesting rather than pleasant, and I knew it was important to me to explore its territory.

Alcohol was not forbidden in my home; I was even allowed occasional sips of cocktails or after-dinner cordials. Because I never liked the taste of alcohol, I was unable to understand why grownups drank it so often. I never connected it with my own chemical experiences. I did not discover a real alcohol high until I was a senior in high school; then, at age sixteen, it suddenly became clear to me what alcohol was—another method, apparently a powerful one, of entering that interesting realm of consciousness. Soon, I fell into a pattern of weekend drinking parties, at which everybody consumed alcohol in order to get drunk. These highs were enjoyable for a time, but once their novelty wore off, I indulged in them for purely social reasons. Before long, I began to find the objective, physical effects of alcohol unpleasant and hard to ignore. I hardly knew of the existence of illegal drugs and would not have considered trying them. To me, marijuana was a narcotic used by criminals, and I had no idea why anyone would take amphetamines or opiates.

In the summer of 1960, just before I entered Harvard College as a freshman, I read an article in the Philadelphia *Evening Bulletin* about the death of a student at a southern California college, supposedly from an overdose of mescaline. He had been taking it "to get inspiration for papers in a creative-writing course." A paragraph from a recent paper was quoted—a visionary description of "galaxies of exploding colors." Mescaline was identified as an experimental drug, largely unknown, said to produce visions. My curiosity was aroused at once, and I resolved to devote my ingenuity to getting and trying mescaline.

At Harvard, excessive weekend consumption of alcohol by students and faculty was the rule rather than the exception, and I went along with the majority, even though the experience of being high on alcohol had long since ceased being interesting to me in my explorations of consciousness. Use of illegal drugs was non-existent except in a very submerged underground. I read everything I could find in scientific journals about mescaline, then came across Aldous Huxley's famous essay, *The Doors of Perception*. The little book convinced me that my intuitions about mescaline as something to be checked out were right. For example, I read:

> . . . [mescaline] changes the quality of consciousness more profoundly and yet is less toxic than any other substance in the pharmacologist's repertory.[1]

And:

> . . . it had always seemed to me possible that, through hypnosis, for example, or autohypnosis, by means of systematic meditation, or else by taking the appropriate drug, I might so change my ordinary mode of consciousness as to be able to know, from the inside, what the visionary, the medium, the mystic were talking about.[2]

Huxley made a convincing case that mescaline was the appropriate drug. Coincidentally, he appeared at the Massachusetts Institute of Technology that fall to give a series of Saturday lectures on visionary experience that were broadcast on the Harvard radio station. I listened carefully to Huxley's thesis that altered states of consciousness included the highest forms of human experience and that chemicals like mescaline were the most direct means of access.

> That humanity at large will ever be able to dispense with Artificial Paradises seems very unlikely. Most men and women lead lives at the worst so painful, at the best so monotonous, poor, and limited, that the urge to escape, the longing to transcend themselves, if only for a few moments, is and has always been one of the principal appetites of the soul. Art and religion, carnivals and saturnalia, dancing and listening to oratory—all these have served, in H. G. Wells' phrase, as Doors in the Wall. And for private, for everyday use, there have always been chemical intoxicants. All the vegetable sedatives and narcotics, all the euphorics that grow on trees, the hallucinogens that ripen in berries or can be squeezed from roots—all, without exception, have been known and systematically used by human beings from time immemorial. And to these natural modifiers of consciousness, modern science has added its quota of synthetics. . . .[3]

As a project for David Riesman's course on American society, I began to write a long study of psychoactive drugs and social attitudes toward them. An instructor in the course suggested that I look up a psychologist, Timothy Leary, who, he thought, was actually doing research with hallucinogens.

I first talked with Leary in his tiny office in the Center for Personality Research on Divinity Avenue. He spoke with sincerity, conviction, and enthusiasm about the potential of drugs like LSD, psilocybin, and mescaline. He envisioned a graduate seminar based on regular consumption of hallucinogens, alternating with intensive periods of analysis to identify and apply the insights gained while high. He predicted that within ten years everyone would be using the drugs "from kindergarten children on up." And he did not anticipate strong opposition by society. I asked whether I could be a subject in his psilocybin studies. He said no, he was sorry, but he had promised the university administration not to use undergraduates. He encouraged me to try to get mescaline, which he thought would be possible.

It took two months and only moderate ingenuity to obtain legally a supply of mescaline from an American chemical firm. Then seven other undergraduates and I began taking mescaline and evaluating our experiences with great care. A dozen experiences I had with the drug in 1961 (in half-gram doses) were highly varied. Most were nothing more than intensifications of preexisting moods with prominent periods of euphoria. Only a small percentage of the time did the sensory changes (such as constant motion of boundary lines and surfaces or vivid imagery seen with the eyes closed) seem worth paying much attention to. In a few instances, great intellectual clarity developed at the peak of the experience, and insights were gained that have had lasting importance. After a dozen trips (we called them "sessions"), I was able to see that much of the mescaline experience was not really so wonderful: the prolonged wakefulness, for example, and the strong stimulation of the sympathetic nervous system with resultant dilated eyes, cold extremities, and stomach butterflies. Yet, its potential for showing one good ways of interpreting one's own mind seemed enormous. Why was that potential realized so irregularly?

During the year that our drug ring operated out of Claverly Hall, I had a chance to watch perhaps thirty mescaline experiences of other undergraduates, and, again, what was most striking was the variability of these sessions. All of the experiences were mostly pleasant, with no bad reactions, but no two were alike, even in the same person. What we were seeing was also being noted by Leary and Alpert in their continuing studies with psilocybin. They gave the drug to large numbers of intellectuals, artists, alcoholics, prisoners, addicts, and graduate students; reported that the vast majority of the experiences were positive; and pointed out the importance of "set" and "setting" in determining the subject's reaction. Set is a person's expectations of what a drug will do to him, considered in the context of his whole personality. Setting is the environment, both physical and social, in which a drug is taken. Leary and Alpert were the first investigators of the hallucinogens to insist on the importance of these two variables. Without them, we are unable to explain simply why the drug varies so unpredictably in its psychic effects from person to person and from time to time in the same person. With these variables, the observations become suddenly clear; hence, the usefulness of the concept of set and setting.

I will discuss this concept and its implications when I talk about marijuana. At this point, I will merely note that the combined effects of set and setting can easily overshadow the pharmacological effects of a drug, as stated in a pharmacology text. One can arrange set and setting so that a dose of an amphetamine will produce sedation or a dose of a barbiturate, stimulation. The first time I tried mescaline, my set included so much anxiety (a roomful of people sat around watching to see what would happen) that I felt nothing whatever for four hours after swallowing the dose and, thereafter, only strong physical effects. There were simply no psychic effects to speak of. This phenomenon has been reported often with marijuana (which I did not try until two years later) and is of great significance, for it argues that the *experience* associated with use of a drug may not be as causally related to the drug as it appears to be.

It is not my purpose here to recount my drug experiences. I write of them to indicate that the route to mescaline, for me and others, was a highly logical one traceable back to earliest childhood. My desire to try mescaline, once I had learned of its existence, was as natural as my desire to whirl myself into dizziness, hallucinate while falling asleep, sniff cleaning fluid, or get drunk in high school. I did not take mescaline because I went to Harvard, met Timothy Leary, rebelled against my parents, was motivated, or sought escape from reality. I took it because I was a normal American teenager whose curiosity had survived thirteen years of American education. And it is instructive to note that the way mescaline first came to my attention was through a scare story in a newspaper describing a fatal reaction to the drug (a most improbable event, as it turns out).

Now, when I say that people take drugs in response to an innate drive to alter consciousness, I do not make any judgment about the taking of drugs. The drive itself must not be equated with the forms of its expression. Clearly, much drug taking in our country is negative in the sense that it is ultimately destructive to the individual and, therefore, to society. But this obvious fact says nothing about the intrinsic goodness or badness of altered states of consciousness or the need to experience them. Given the negativity of much drug use, it seems to me there are two possibilities to consider: (1) altered states of consciousness are inherently undesirable (in which case, presumably, the drive to experience them should be thwarted); or (2) altered states of consciousness are neither desirable nor undesirable of themselves but can take bad forms (in which case the drive to experience them should be channeled in some "proper" direction). Do we have enough evidence to make an intelligent choice between these possibilities?

Primarily, we need more information about altered states of consciousness. Altered from what? is a good first question. The answer is: from ordinary waking consciousness, which is "normal" only in the strict sense of "statistically most frequent"; there is no connotation of "good," "worthwhile," or "healthy." Sleep and daydreaming are examples of altered states of consciousness, as are trance, hypnosis, meditation, general anesthesia, delirium, psychosis, mystic rapture, and the various chemical "highs." If we turn to psychology or medicine for an understanding of these states, we encounter a curious problem; Western scientists who study the mind tend to study the objective correlates of consciousness rather than consciousness itself. In fact, because consciousness is non-material, there has been great reluctance to accord it the reality of a laboratory phenomenon; psychologists, therefore, do not study consciousness directly, only indirectly, as by monitoring the physiological responses or brain waves of a person in a hypnotic trance or in meditation. Non-material things are considered inaccessible to direct investigation, if not altogether unreal. Consequently, there has been no serious attempt to study altered states of consciousness as such.

In the East, psychological science has taken a very different turn. Subjective states are considered more directly available for investigation than objective phenomena, which, after all, can only be perceived through our subjective states. Accordingly, an experiential science of consciousness has developed in the Orient, of which yoga is a magnificent example. It is a science as brilliantly articulated as Western conceptions of neurophysiology, but no attempt has been made to correlate it carefully with the physical realities of the nervous system as demonstrated by the West.

Therefore, Eastern science should be helpful in understanding altered states of consciousness, but it must always be checked against empirical knowledge of the objective nervous system. Now, one of the puzzling and unifying features of altered states of consciousness is their relative absence of physical correlates. For example, there are really no significant physiological differences between a hypnotized person and an unhypnotized person, or even any way of telling them apart, if the hypnotized subject is given appropriate suggestions for his behavior. As we shall see, the same holds true for the person high on marijuana—he is not readily distinguishable from one who is not high. Consequently, research as we know it in the West really cannot get much of a foothold in this area, and the scientific literature is dreadfully inadequate.

Nevertheless, I think it is possible to come to some useful conclusions about altered states of consciousness from what we can observe in ourselves and others. An immediate suggestion is that these states form some sort of continuum, in view of how much they have in common with each other. For example, trance, whether spontaneous or induced by a hypnotist, is simply an extension of the daydreaming state, in which awareness is focused and often directed inward rather than outward. Except for its voluntary and purposeful character, meditation is not easily distinguished from trance. Masters of meditation in Zen Buddhism warn their students to ignore *makyo*, sensory distortions that frequently resemble the visions of mystics or the hallucinations of schizophrenics. In other words, there is much cross-phenomenology among these states of consciousness, and, interestingly enough, being high on drugs has many of these same features, regardless of what drug induces the high.

The sense of physical lightness and timelessness so often reported by drug users is quite common in trance, meditation, and mystic rapture, for instance. Great ease of access to unconscious memories is also common in these states. Hypnotic subjects capable of sustaining deep trances can be "age regressed"—for example, made to reexperience their tenth birthday party. In deepest trances, awareness of present reality is obliterated, and the subject is amnesic for the experience when he returns to normal consciousness. In lighter trances, age-regressed subjects often have a sense of dual reality—the simultaneous experience of reliving the tenth birthday party, while also sitting with the hypnotist. Exactly the same experience is commonly reported by users of marijuana, who often find themselves spontaneously reliving unconscious memories as present realities; I have had this sense of dual reality myself on a number of occasions when I have been high on marijuana in settings that encouraged introspective reverie.

I want to underline the idea that these states form a continuum beginning in familiar territory. When we watch a movie and become oblivious to everything except the screen, we are in a light trance, in which the scope of our awareness has diminished but the intensity of it has increased. In the Oriental scientific literature, analogies are often drawn between consciousness and light: intensity increases, as scope decreases. In simple forms of concentration, like movie-watching or daydreaming, we do not become aware of the power of focused awareness, but we are doing nothing qualitatively different from persons in states of much more intensely focused consciousness where unusual phenomena are the rule. For example, total anesthesia sufficient for major surgery can occur in deep trance; what appears to happen is that the scope of awareness diminishes so much that the pain arising from the body falls outside it. The conscious experience of this state is that "the pain is there, but it's happening to someone else." (Patients given morphine sometimes report the same experience.) I have myself seen a woman have a baby by Caesarean section with no medication; hypnosis alone was used to induce anesthesia, and she remained conscious, alert, in no discomfort throughout the operation.

I have also seen yogis demonstrate kinds of control of their involuntary nervous systems that my medical education led me to believe were impossible. One that I met could make his heart go into an irregular pattern of beating called fibrillation at will and stop it at will. Such men ascribe their successes in this area solely to powers of concentration developed during regular periods of meditation. There is no need, I think, to point out the tremendous implications of these observations. Because we are unable to modify consciously the operations of a major division of our nervous system (the autonomic system), we are prey to many kinds of illnesses we can do nothing much about (cardiovascular diseases, for example). The possibility that one can learn to influence directly such "involuntary" functions as heart rate, blood pressure, blood flow to internal organs, endocrine secretions, and perhaps even cellular processes by conscious use of the autonomic nervous system, is the most exciting frontier of modern medicine. If, by meditation, a man can learn to regulate blood flow to his skin (I have seen a yogi produce a ten-degree-Fahrenheit temperature difference between right and left hands within one minute of getting a signal; the warmer hand was engorged with blood and dark red, the cooler hand was pale), there is no reason why he could not also learn to shut off blood flow to a tumor in his body and thus kill it.

Another chief characteristic of all these states is a major change in the sense of ego, that is, in awareness of oneself as a distinct entity. Thus, when we catch ourselves daydreaming, we wonder where we were for the past few minutes. Now, it is most interesting that many systems of mind development and many religions encourage their adherents to learn to "forget" themselves in precisely this sense. For example, in Zen archery (an application of Zen technique that can be used as a spiritual exercise) the meditating archer obliterates the distinction between himself and the bow; hitting the bull's eye with the arrow then becomes no more difficult than reaching out and touching it, and the shot is always a bull's eye. D. T. Suzuki, who brought Zen to the attention of the West, has written of this process: "The archer ceases to be conscious of himself as the one who is engaged in hitting the bull's eye which confronts him."[4] In fact, the ability to forget oneself as the doer seems to be the essence of mastery of any skill. And since the observing ego is the center of normal waking consciousness, the essence of mastery of any skill is the ability to forsake this kind of consciousness at will.

Furthermore, mystics from all religious traditions testify that this same loss of sense of self is an essential aspect of the highest of human experiences—an assertion the Christian might associate with Jesus' words: "Whoever loses his life for my sake will gain it."[5] In higher forms of yogic or Buddhist meditation, the aim is to focus consciousness on a single object or thought and then to erase all notion of anyone doing the meditation. Patanjali, the ancient writer who first codified and recorded the principles of the much more ancient science of yoga, wrote of *samadhi* (the highest state of consciousness envisioned in yoga): "When alone, the object of contemplation remains and one's own form is annihilated, this is known as *samadhi*."[6] *Samadhi* is a real experience that has been attained by many.

It is noteworthy that most of the world's highest religious and philosophic thought originated in altered states of consciousness in individuals (Gautama, Paul, Mohammed, etc.). It is also noteworthy that creative genius has long been observed to correlate with psychosis, and that intuitive genius is often associated with daydreaming, meditation, dreaming, and other non-ordinary modes of consciousness.

What conclusions can we draw from all this information? At the least, it would seem, altered states of consciousness have great potential for strongly positive psychic development. They appear to be the ways to more effective and fuller use of the nervous system, to development of creative and intellectual faculties, and to attainment of certain kinds of thought that have been deemed exalted by all who have experienced them.

So there is much logic in our being born with a drive to experiment with other ways of experiencing our perceptions, in particular to get away periodically from ordinary, ego-centered consciousness. It may even be a key factor in the present evolution of the human nervous system. But our immediate concern is the anxiety certain expressions of this drive are provoking in our own land, and we are trying to decide what to make of altered states of consciousness. Clearly, they are potentially valuable to us, not inherently undesirable, as in our first hypothesis. They are also not abnormal, in that they grade into states all of us have experienced. Therefore, to attempt to thwart this drive would probably be impossible and might be dangerous. True, it exposes the organism to certain risks, but ultimately it can confer psychic superiority. To try to thwart its expression in individuals and in society might be psychologically crippling for people and evolutionarily suicidal for the species. I would not want to see

us tamper with something so closely related to our curiosity, our creativity, our intuition, and our highest aspirations.

If the drive to alter consciousness is potentially valuable and the states of altered consciousness are potentially valuable, then something must be channeling that drive in wrong directions for it to have negative manifestations in our society. By the way, I do not equate all drug taking with negative manifestations of the drive to alter consciousness. Drug use becomes negative or abusive only when it poses a serious threat to health or to social or psychological functioning. Failure to distinguish drug use from drug abuse—another unhelpful conception arising from emotional bias—has become quite popular, especially in federal government propaganda. The National Institute of Mental Health continues to label every person who smokes marijuana an abuser of the drug, thus creating an insoluble marijuana problem of enormous proportions. Professional legal and medical groups also contribute to this way of thinking. In fact, the American Medical Association has gone so far as to define drug abuse as any use of a "drug of abuse" without professional supervision—an illustration of the peculiar logic necessary to justify conceptions based on emotional rather than rational considerations.

Certainly, much drug use is undesirable, despite the claims of drug enthusiasts, although this problem seems to me much less disturbing than the loss to individuals and to society of the potential benefits of consciousness alteration in positive directions. But let us not get ahead of ourselves. Our inquiry in this chapter is directed to the question of why people take drugs. I have tried to demonstrate that people take drugs because they are means of satisfying an inner need for experiencing other modes of consciousness and that whether the drugs are legal or illegal is an unimportant consideration. To answer the question most succinctly: people take drugs because they work.

Or, at least, they seem to.

✳ ✳ ✳

Andrew Weil, "Why People Take Drugs," from *The Natural Mind*. Copyright © 1972, 1986 by Andrew Weil. Reprinted by permission of Houghton Mifflin Co. All rights reserved.

For Discussion

If drug use can result from the natural desire to alter one's consciousness, why do we punish drug offenders for something over which they have little control?

Notes

1. Aldous Huxley, *The Doors of Perception* (New York: Perennial Library, 1970), pp. 9-10.

2. *Ibid.*, p. 14.

3. *Ibid.*, pp. 62-63.

4. D. T. Suzuki, Introduction to *Zen in the Art of Archery* by Eugen Herrigel (New York: Vintage Books, 1971), p. 10.

5. Matthew 16:26; compare Luke 10:24.

6. Patanjali, *Yoga Aphorisms* III:3, quoted by James Hewitt in *A Practical Guide to Yoga* (New York: Funk and Wagnalls, 1968), p. 146. Further commentary on this aphorism may be found in *How to Know God: The Yoga Aphorisms of Patanjali*, translated by Swami Prabhavananda and Christopher Isherwood (New York: Signet Books, 1969), pp. 122-123. ✦

2. *Doorway to Excess*

Harvey Milkman
AND
Stanley Sunderwirth

The term "addiction" seems to have a variety of meanings. In "Doorway to Excess," the authors describe the phenomenon of addiction and examine the changing definitions of the term. Their particular point of view is a biosocial perspective in which addictive behaviors are socially constructed through biochemical changes. Findings from their studies suggest that drug use is related to stress reduction and an individual's particular drug of choice is related to his or her personality.

> . . . some to dance, some to make bonfires, each man to what sport and revels his addiction leads him.
>
> —*Othello*, Act II, Scene 2

The Broad Scope of Addiction

In the drama of human excess, experience is the protagonist, and drugs or activities are merely supporting actors. We are compelled by repetitious urges to become energized, to relax, to imagine those three citadels of consciousness are the beacons of compulsive behavior.

Recognition that the term *addiction* should transcend drug abuse has emerged from the problem of categorizing so-called non-addictive and addictive drugs. By the late 1960s, it became clear that some people could become compulsively involved with marijuana and LSD, substances that seemed to have a relatively low potential for physical dependency. Meanwhile, it was quietly discovered that some users could maintain relatively casual relationships with opium derivatives, such as heroin or codeine, customarily associated with rapidly increased tolerance and severe discomfort upon discontinuance.

Gradually, addiction came to imply psychological need, over and above the traditional constructs of physical demand and distress upon withdrawal. Those who displayed alcohol-related behavior problems—irrespective of whether they were physically dependent—were increasingly regarded as alcoholic. Certainly, alcoholism has psychological and social characteristics far more subtle than the seizures or hallucinations often associated with hospital-based recovery programs.

By the early 1970s, the concept of addiction was further extended to include non-intoxicating substances, so that smoking and eating were widely accepted as addictive behaviors. Compulsion, loss of control, and continuation, despite harmful consequences, became new criteria for the determination of addiction. Furthermore, the notion of a drug of choice suggested that some individuals would become harmfully involved with only some substances, depending on their specific needs. This implied that, despite the inherent pleasure-inducing properties of certain drugs, only a proportion of those who experimented would slip into a pattern of compulsive use. Moreover, not only did people react differently to the same drug, but the same person might display entirely different patterns of use or abuse at various times of life. Some users might shift from cocaine abuse to heroin; or from marijuana and LSD to heavy consumption of alcohol and cocaine.

In the 1980s, cigarette smoking and overeating have been universally acknowledged as major threats to physical well-being; yet, millions of people attest to their inability to control these behaviors and regard themselves as addicts. Parallels have been drawn between traditionally held ideas about drug involvement and a host of pleasure-fueled activities far removed from the compulsive intake of food or drugs. It has become regular practice for people to describe themselves as "addicted" to seemingly harmless activities like aerobics or watching MTV. Media-construed syndromes, such as "chocoholism," "workaholism," or "Dungeons and Dragoholism" have suddenly appeared, along with a plethora of biologically oriented explanations for these behaviors. Phenylethylamine, found in chocolate, is rumored to be the chemical of love, and endorphins, our internal opiates, are proposed as the special rewards for runners who push beyond the "wall." Television, magazines, and newspapers have all jumped on the bandwagon of a commonalities approach to habitual behaviors.

An impressive assembly of researchers, writers, and theoreticians have contributed the professional underpinning to media's obsession with addiction. The addictive personality is described by various scientific reports as impulsive, rule-breaking, nonconformist, and depressed. Youngsters who later develop compulsive problem behaviors often experience difficulty in school and in their family relationships. Auto accidents, fighting, truancy, delinquency, and vicious struggles with parents are common. Perhaps the entire spectrum of anti-social behavior patterns provides some relief to unfortunate juveniles who encounter familial inadequacy, poverty, bereavement, or geographic instability.

It is unnecessary to develop separate sets of principles to explain how drug use and other compulsive behaviors gain control over human life. Drugs, food, sex, gambling, and aggressive episodes all give prompt, salient, and short-lasting relief to the people who indulge in them. In addition to sharing pleasure-inducing properties, both substance use and other mood-altering activities tend to produce an initial state of euphoria which is then followed by a negative emotional state; that is, a high followed by a low. This post-euphoric discomfort gives further impetus to repetition of the rewarding activity. The old "hair of the dog" remedy of drinking to relieve hangover symptoms is consistent with this idea.

Abraham Wikler has developed a two-stage model for the origins and progression of narcotics addiction which is applicable to other compulsions as well. In the *acquisition* phase, the novice begins and continues a potentially compulsive activity because of pleasurable sensations brought about through the experience. The environment where the desired feeling occurs becomes associated with a "rush," or sense of well-being. The pleasure setting becomes a composite of cues that stimulate craving for the need-satisfying activity. The alcoholic, for example, who has previously enjoyed the euphoria brought on by drink cannot resist temptation when fate delivers him or her to the neighborhood bar or an old friend's New Year's Eve party. The human body eventually adapts to most novel stimulation by reducing the potency of its effect. The user or performer soon needs more of the mood-altering activity, in order to experience similar alterations in feeling. The addicted climber must increasingly seek out more difficult cliffs, and the hooked sky diver compulsively finds more challenging and frightening drops.

In the *maintenance* stage of addiction, a person is no longer motivated by any sense of pleasure from the need-gratifying behavior. Rather, the repetitive activity now serves only to relieve the sense of despair and physical discomfort that is felt when the mood-altering action or substance is not present. The user can only "break even" by performing his or her tension-relieving activity. Without it, the addict suffers from a devastating combination of physical dependence and an even more complicated and stressful environment. The compulsive meditator, for example, increasingly seeks out quiescent relaxation to escape from stress that builds around increasing social isolation and decreased productivity at home and at work.

Loss of control and progressive deterioration of social, economic, or health functions have emerged as the familiar course of human compulsion. Treatment techniques for a variety of habitual problem behaviors have thus become increasingly modeled after widely publicized drug and alcohol intervention approaches. In juvenile crime prevention, for example, Scared Straight! is a technique that parallels the Synanon Game for drug addicts. High-risk juveniles are systematically exposed to severe baiting and verbal confrontation by a group of convicts at various phases of their rehabilitation. Gamblers Anonymous, Overeaters Anonymous, and Sexaholics Anonymous are contemporary treatment organizations that rely heavily on the twelve-step recovery process originally developed by Alcoholics Anonymous. For example, the sex addict who accepts treatment subscribes to a dictum only slightly modified from the first of the Alcoholics Anonymous Twelve Steps: "We admitted that we were powerless over lust [alcohol]—that our lives had become unmanageable."

The person who regards himself or herself as "sexaholic" acknowledges that he or she has lost control over sex and no longer has the power of choice. Sex has become an addiction, just as drinking is for the alcoholic who can no longer control his or her consumption. For the married sexaholic, sobriety means having sex only with the spouse. Any form of lust, including sex with oneself or with other partners, is considered progressively destructive. For the unmarried sexaholic, sexual sobriety involves freedom from lust and sex of any kind.

The contemporary emphasis on viewing each instance of human compulsion as a separate diagnostic entity has led to enormous conceptual redundancy and economic waste in our prevention and service-delivery systems. In many ways, the noun "sexaholic" could be replaced by any other human activity, in which we are prone to excess. The essential Alcoholics Anonymous message for self-help remains the same: stop the behavior! Go to meetings! Get a sponsor! Ask for help!

Biochemistry: The Gateway to Excess

Addiction is evident when one becomes progressively unable to control the beginning or end of a need-fulfilling activity. Yet, below the surface of this descriptive formulation are more profound explanatory links. The seemingly unrelated ramblings about "newly discovered" addictions which have been reported in countless media presentations are actually connected by a biochemical thread. The 1974 discovery of enkephalins by John Hughes and Hans Kosterlitz set the stage for a higher level of conceptualization regarding human compulsion. Enkephalins and related compounds called endorphins are pain-killing molecules that are produced naturally in the brain. These potent, mood-altering chemicals bear striking structural similarity to opiates and appear to behave in similar ways. The realization that the brain can produce its own opiates has led to a reexamination of the biochemical mechanisms of human behavior. In the past decade, thousands of scientific treatises have explored relationships between thoughts, feelings, behavior, and brain chemistry.

Advances in scientific understanding of the mechanisms of neurotransmission have led to a significant departure from the increasingly archaic spiritual and moralistic definitions of addiction. It has become obvious that individuals can change their brain chemistry through immersion in salient mood-altering activities, as well as through ingesting intoxicating substances. Imagine the rush (altered brain chemistry) of first leaping and then free-falling from an airplane at an altitude of 13,000 feet. Recognizing that danger-seeking may involve a compulsive alteration in brain chemistry, we are inescapably led to redefine addiction.

Addiction: Self-Induced Changes in Neurotransmission that Result in Behavior Problems

This new definition encompasses a multi-disciplinary understanding of compulsive problem behaviors that involves the concepts of personal responsibility (the behaviors are self-induced); biochemical effects (the body's neurotransmission changes); and social reactions (society absorbs the costs and consequences of problem behaviors).

In the past, advocates for mind-altering substances have rationalized drug use in terms of "mind expansion" or "spiritual discovery." Peyotism is currently practiced in the United States by several thousand members of the Native American Church. This group believes that ingestion of the hallucinogenic buds of the peyote plant will serve as an antidote for alcoholism and as a conduit to spiritual healing. Scientifically, these alterations of perceptual reality are the result of self-imposed changes in the delicate electrochemical balance of the brain. The schism between science and the heart is perhaps most evident as when a "flower child" resists the notion that his or her cherished drug experiments are simply mucking up or crudely interfering with natural brain functions.

Compulsive problem behavior is solely the responsibility of the brain, which may be described as the most complete entity in the universe. Its fifty billion or so nerve cells, called neurons, communicate with each other through trillions of interconnections. This "talking" is referred to as neurotransmission, and its language is chemistry. More specifically, neurotransmission is the way in which signals or impulses are sent from one neuron to another. From a purely biochemical standpoint, neurotransmission controls all emotion, perceptions, and bodily functions. In essence, this process is responsible for all thoughts and actions. If we should lose a hand or a foot, we are still recognized as the same person, but if our synaptic chemistry changes dramatically, we seem to possess altogether different personalities. The often frightening hallucinations and bizarre delusions of those with schizophrenia are poignant examples of this phenomenon.

The brain's neurons are composed of three basic parts: the soma, or cell body; the axon, which carries impulses away from the soma; and the dendrites, which receive impulses from other neurons. The soma acts as a small computer. It must decide from a "discussion" with a multitude of surrounding neurons whether to "fire" and send the impulse to the axon, or to remain dormant. Since this is the soma's only decision, and it is made very quickly, we may think of the soma as a "fast idiot." As with pregnancy, firing either occurs or it does not, in accord with the "all or nothing" principle. There are no weak or strong impulses; all impulses are of the same magnitude. The intensity of feeling is determined by the *frequency* of neuronal firing, rather than by the strength of the electrochemical jolt.

One of the more interesting facts about the brain is that it is not hard-wired. That is, unlike the telephone system, the brain has no physical contacts among its trillions of interconnecting neurons. Each nerve cell is physically separated from the fifty billion other collaborating brain units by a small space called a synapse. When the soma fires, the impulse travels down the long fiber of the axon to the synapse separating the axon of one neuron from the dendrites of another. The impulse is carried across the synapse to the receiving neuron by small molecules that are released into the synapse. These molecules, known as neurotransmitters, move across the synapse and attach themselves to sites known as receptors, which are embedded in the membrane of the postsynaptic terminals of the dendrites. The receptors are tailor-made to receive only neurotransmitters that have a shape that complements that of the receptor. This relationship between neurotransmitter and receptor is very much like a lock and key. Just as only a key with the correct shape will work in a given lock, only those neurotransmitters with the right shape will activate the specific receptors designed for them.

If a sufficient number of receptors on the postsynaptic membrane become occupied by neurotransmitters, there is a change in the electrical balance of this membrane that results in a transfer of the impulse from the presynaptic neuron to the postsynaptic neuron. The impulse then travels to the soma of the postsynaptic neuron, where it is combined with inputs from many other synaptic junctions. The soma of the postsynaptic neuron must now make its own "decision" of whether to fire, based upon the multitude of synaptic inputs.

Just as it is possible to put keys of slightly different shapes into a given lock, it is possible to introduce into the synapse molecules with shapes similar to neurotransmitters that will attach to the receptor sites. However, these pseudo-neurotransmitters (chemical prostitutes) do not change the electrical balance of the postsynaptic membrane and, in fact, block the receptor sites from receiving neurotransmitters that transfer the nerve impulse. The blocking of the receptor sites with phony neurotransmitters is much like putting a Ford key in a Mercury ignition. The key will fit but will not turn the switch and, in fact, will prevent inserting the Mercury key that would turn the motor on. Introduction of man-made chemicals that block certain receptor sites is the basis for the chemical treatment of schizophrenia. A drug (for example, Haldol) occupies receptor sites on the postsynaptic membrane, normally occupied by the neurotransmitter dopamine. The electrical balance of the cell membrane remains intact, and the impulse cannot be transferred to adjacent cells. This reduces the overactive neurotransmission usually associated with schizophrenia.

When an impulse has been transmitted to the postsynaptic neuron, the electrical balance of that neuron must be restored, before it can receive the

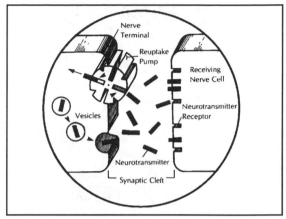

Figure 1. Ordinary Action in the Brain

Typically, cells communicate with chemicals called neurotransmitters. The supply of the transmitters is kept in balance by the ability of the transmitting cell to reabsorb—scientifically called "reuptake"—some of the chemical in the synaptic cleft.
Source: *Reprinted from Scientific American by The New York Times, March 22, 1983.*

next impulse. This balance is restored through the release of neurotransmitters from the postsynaptic receptor sites. Released neurotransmitters may be reabsorbed and safely stored in the synaptic vesicles of the presynaptic terminal, where they are protected from destruction and may be reused as needed. However, a number of interesting things can happen to the neurotransmitters before they reach the safe hiding place of the synaptic vesicle. If cocaine is ingested, this tends to prevent the neurotransmitters from being recycled into the presynaptic terminal, resulting in an excess of neurotransmitters in the synapse. Since more neurotransmitters are available for attachment to receptor sites, more receptor sites will be occupied, with a resultant increase in the rate of neurotransmission and thus the state of arousal. This, of course, is why the individual ingested cocaine in the first place.

The more rapid the neurotransmission in particular parts of the brain, the more intense is the feeling. Both substances (such as cocaine) and activities (such as skydiving) have the ability to alter neurotransmission and, therefore, change the way we feel about ourselves and the outside world. That activities can dramatically affect our mood is illustrated by a sensationalized example:

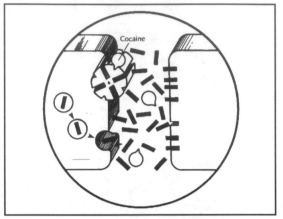

Figure 2. Cocaine in the Brain

Cocaine slips into the reuptake pump, inhibiting its ability to balance the amount of neurotransmitters traveling between cells. This can result in an overstimulation of the receiving cells. Some have linked that interaction to euphoria.
Source: *Scientific American. The New York Times, March 22, 1983.*

You are sitting alone in your room, feeling sorry for yourself because of the loss of a close relationship. All of a sudden, out of nowhere, there appears a full-grown, person-eating Bengal tiger, obviously looking for her meal. Your depression instantly disappears in a rush of rapidly accelerating neurotransmission. You grasp a chair and thrust it menacingly toward the ferocious beast, while shrieking obscenities at the top of your lungs. You run as fast as your legs will carry you.

This highly arousing situation has obviously provoked powerful alterations in your brain chemistry. As if you had ingested a strong dose of cocaine or amphetamine, your neurotransmission is so fast that relaxation or sleep is out of the question, and your depression is nowhere in sight. In a similar manner, activities can evoke sensations of relaxation that correspond to decreases in neurotransmission. The distress and agitation caused by a shouting match with your spouse can be diminished through an orgy of eating.

People may repeat certain behaviors to bring about alterations in neurotransmission consistent with their characteristic ways of dealing with stress. That is, the person who actively confronts fear or tension repeatedly seeks out risk-taking activities or stimulant drugs in order to increase neurotransmission. The person who is prone to passive withdrawal seeks out activities or drugs that lower neurotransmission.

In today's chemical society, people are more likely to reach for drugs than to engage in activities that alter neurotransmission. However, regardless of whether we choose activities or substances, the possibility of addiction always lurks in the convolutions of our brains, where all compulsion originates. Biochemically, addiction results from neuronal adaptation to repeated and salient attempts to alter "normal" levels of neurotransmission. For example, the person who seems to thrive on becoming energized attempts to raise neurotransmission above the "normal" or baseline level. Unfortunately, he or she is confronted with enzymatic changes in the brain that counter the desired rise in neurotransmission.

In the acquisition phase of an arousal addiction, a person is able, almost at will, to alter his or her neurotransmission by engaging in activities or drug use. As has been said, however, "It is not nice to fool Mother Nature"; that is, it is not wise to synthetically alter the balance of the human brain. A corollary is: "You can't fool Mother Nature for very long." Repeated mind-altering episodes of the same intensity soon bring about changes in the amount of protein molecules (enzymes) required for neurotransmitter-induced reactions to occur. These enzymatic changes result in the need for higher doses of activities or drugs for the person to reach the level of subjective arousal experienced at the beginning of the addictive process.

In the maintenance phase of addiction, brain chemistry is so altered that the addict compulsively attempts to maintain a level of neurotransmission that will reduce the imbalance and suffering induced by enzymatic changes. Enzymatic changes occur *slowly*, and the time required to attain dependency (reach the maintenance phase) varies from person to person. Also, brain-enzyme levels that have been gradually altered do not immediately return to normal, even though the activity responsible for the changes has ceased. For this reason, the stopping or reducing of compulsive stimulation is often followed by a subjective experience of depression, or "crash." This is because enzyme levels have slowly adapted to counter the repetitive elevation in neurotransmission, brought about through activities that are suddenly eliminated. The brain's altered and more slowly responding enzyme levels remain constant for the immediate future. Hence, the maintenance-phase addict who goes "cold turkey" suffers biochemical withdrawal—whether habituated to cocaine or rock climbing.

In a similar manner, activities that lower the brain's neurotransmission are countered by enzyme changes that hold neurotransmission at a normal level. In the end, Mother Nature wins again. The addict must choose between attempting to maintain an acceptable level of neurotransmission by increasing sedation—through drugs or activities—or "kick" the habit. Cessation introduces a dramatic state of agitated discomfort, because the substance or activity responsible for lowered neurotransmission has been removed, while the powerful enzymatic changes that battled to raise the level of neurotransmission remain present.

Pick Your Parents Carefully

A genetic component is known to exist in addictive behavior. Behavior geneticists have studied heritable factors in such diverse phenomena as schizophrenia, criminality, and cigarette smoking. These forms of behavior, and virtually all other addictions that have been studied, seem to be influenced by both genetic and environmental factors. Behavioral geneticist Gerald McClearn of Pennsylvania State University suggests that the enzyme produced by a given gene might influence hormones and neurotransmitters in a way that contributes to the development of a personality potentially more susceptible than most to external influences, such as peer-group pressure. A genetic predisposition of this type may ultimately become an important determinant of how an individual lives his life. Yet, identical twins, who possess exactly the same genetic make-up, do not always develop similar patterns of behavioral excess. We must look at individual differences in experience to understand more completely the origins and progression of addiction. It is not nature *or* nurture but nature *and* nurture that seem to influence many behavioral traits. As one man has said, "The frightening part about heredity and environment is that we parents provide both."

More than 140 research studies indicate an increased incidence of alcoholism in families where one or more members had been diagnosed as alcoholic. In general, these studies show that the children, male or female, of an alcoholic father or mother have two to four times the probability of becoming alcoholic than is the population norm. Relatively little has been done to study the role of genetic factors in other compulsive problem behaviors. The studies that have attempted such assessments of eating disorders and cigarette smoking find that, although inheritance is a significant factor, human compulsion answers heavily to the social setting in which it may or may not occur.

The genetic basis of alcoholism has been traced to the deficiency of an enzyme (aldehyde dehydrogenase) necessary for the body's disposal of alcohol. The relationship between genetics and enzymatic susceptibility is as follows. Enzymes are the proteins in our body responsible for the breakdown or metabolism of drugs. They bring about a change (usually an increase) in the speed of bodily processes. Any aberration or alteration in those enzymes involved in the metabolism of alcohol or drugs is reflected in the way the body disposes of the drug. The enzymes' dysfunctional response to the addict's chosen drug is at the core of the concept of inherited addictive disease.

The relationship between enzymes and parentally transmitted genes is schematized below.

Parents ➡ DNA ➡ RNA ➡ Enzymes

Enzymes are formed from a template of ribonucleic acid (RNA), which in turn is generated from a template of deoxyribonucleic acid (DNA). DNA is the genetic material that we inherit from our parents. If they should provide us with defective DNA, this would be reflected in faulty enzyme systems. For this reason, besides abstinence, a most effective way to avoid addiction is to "pick your parents carefully."

Patching Yourself from Without

Given that we may voluntarily alter our neurotransmission to achieve a desired feeling, why do only some of us become compulsively involved in this pursuit? After all, most people can have a drink or occasionally rage at the race track without going off the deep end. Most addictionologists—even those who disagree about other matters of causation and treatment—agree that low self-regard is a crucial factor in all forms of addiction. The chronic absence of good feelings about oneself provokes a dependence on mood-changing activity. Manifest or masked, feelings of low self-worth are basic to most dysfunctional lifestyles.

One way of coping with disquieting factors is to immerse oneself in an activity that is incompatible with serious self-evaluation. The climber, clinging to a mountain face with only a rope, pitons, and a tenuous foothold, has few moments to spare on self-derogation. The risk taker may figuratively bridge the crevasse of his or her sense of inadequacy by temporary surrender to something outside the self. A 32-year-old male cocaine user reported a particularly vivid dream that illustrates this point:

> I recall seeing my personality as a huge concave surface. It looked like a great ceramic bowl with irregularly spaced craters on an otherwise smooth surface. Somehow, I could patch the holes with an ultrafine putty made of cocaine paste. The new, shimmering surface appeared nearly unmarred.

The user's drug or activity of choice often depends on his or her style of coping with troubled feelings about the self. In a research study at Bellevue Psychiatric Hospital in New York, Harvey Milkman and William A. Frosch found a striking relationship between personality and drug of choice. Those who prefer heroin usually cope with stress through relaxation and isolation. In sharp contrast, amphetamine users are likely to confront a hostile or threatening environment with physical or intellectual activity. Clinical observations of people who use hallucinogens, such as LSD, confirm that they characteristically rely on imagery, daydreaming, and altered thought processes to reduce tension. The examples shown in Table 1 illustrate differences between compulsive users of heroin, amphetamine, and LSD in their management of self-esteem.

The key that opens the doorway to excess for the preaddict is the good feeling that he or she learns to create, and repeatedly recreate, through self-determined activity. Unaccustomed to the wine of success, the novice experiences as a godsend any involvement that provides escape from the increasing sense of despair borne of repeated failures in the "straight world." He or she not only delights in a reprieve from tension, but experiences elevated feelings of self-worth for having discovered the ability to produce a pleasurable sensation. In *The Road to H*, Isidor Chein and his collaborators describe the addict's infatuation with self-determined mood change:

> In [heroin] addicts with strong craving . . . it is in large measure a psychic consequence of achieving a state of relaxation and relief from tension or distress through one's own activities, not through a physician's recommendation or prescription, but through an esoteric, illegal, and dangerous nostrum. We can observe an analogous phenomenon in people who win the Irish Sweepstakes; win on dice, cards, horses, or numbers; or even in persons who park in no-parking zones without getting a traffic ticket. They feel important, worthwhile, and interesting; they feel a sense of pride and accomplishment. Such an illusory achievement is an important psychic phenomenon, particularly important when it stands out by contrast with the remainder of a person's life.

The Beacons of Compulsion

After studying the life histories of drug abusers, we have seen that drugs of choice are harmonious with an individual's usual means of coping with stress. The discovery of a need-fulfilling drug is usually a serendipitous event; the novice becomes infatuated because of the immediate reduction of stress achieved through the experience. Incipient addicts usually experience behavioral compulsion and loss of control before ever ingesting a psychoactive substance. Juvenile delinquency, persistent and vicious family struggles, and inability to adequately cope with everyday demands are common childhood precursors to drug abuse. Heroin users often show histories of passivity, alternating with uncontrolled rage; stimulant users describe multiple episodes of life-threatening impulsiveness; those who rely on hallucinogens report that they regularly avoided problems through fantasy during prolonged periods of their childhood.

We repeatedly pursue three avenues of experience as antidotes for psychic pain. These preferred styles of coping—satiation, arousal, and fantasy—seem to have their origins in the first years of life. Childhood experiences, combined with genetic predisposition, are the foundations of adult compulsion. The drug group of choice—depressants, stimulants, or hallucinogens—is the one that best fits the individual's characteristic way of coping with stress or feelings of unworthiness.

Table 1

Use of Various Drugs to Regulate Self-Esteem

Heroin	Amphetamine	LSD
How do you feel about yourself generally?		
Lousy. I don't like myself.	I think I'm all right, y'know.	I feel like a voyager in an awesome adventure.
What about your looks, do you think you're good-looking?		
I don't like them and I don't know why.	I think they're all right. I'm satisfied. Yeah, I think I'm good-looking.	Sometimes, I feel like an alien, like I'm a gorgeous being from another planet.
How do you compare with others your age?		
Right now, I know I don't compare well. I can't control my desire for drugs. I can't do what I want to do . . . I can't be a man, I am not doing anything.	I don't think I'm as mature, serious, or business-minded as a 25-year-old should be. As a man, I'm all right. I'm big and strong, and I try to be kind. I love women and I dig kids.	I don't compare myself to others. I just think about how I'm dealing with my own karma, so I can improve my chances now and in a future life.
What do you believe that other people think of you?		
That I'm a cop-out; some people would say degenerate.	I think others like me a great deal. They really do not say it, but I know they do. I make friends easily, and people smile and they embrace me and make me feel like I'm not rejected.	They think I'm on a path of spiritual discovery. That I am in touch with some cosmic force that they would like to understand.
What kind of person would you like to be?		
I'd just be average and get along, say middle-class. I want to be able to work and be middle-class. I don't have goals of making a million or anything, just make a living.	I would like to be free of drugs. I would like to not even have to put a grape pop in my mouth, if I didn't want to. Right now, I'm taking vitamin D and taking grape ice pops. I'm playing with kids. I bought a yo-yo yesterday. I'm laughing a lot and enjoying life.	I would like to be in flow with the forces of the universe . . . to experience oneness with people and nature . . . to merge with the cosmos.

Note: *Adapted from H. Milkman and W. Frosch. "On the preferential abuse of heroin and amphetamines."* The Journal of Nervous and Mental Disease *156:4, 242-48 (1973).*

People do not become addicted to drugs or mood-altering activities as such, but rather to the satiation, arousal, or fantasy experiences that can be achieved through them.

Addicts whose basic motivation is satiation, for example, are likely to binge on food or television watching, or to choose depressant drugs, such as heroin. Psychologically, they are trying to shut down negative feelings, by reducing stimulation from the internal or external world. The life of the satiation type of addict bears striking similarity to that of a child during the first year of life. The mouth and skin are the primary receptors of experience, and feelings of well-being depend almost completely on food and warmth. Harvard Medical School's Edward J. Khantzian and Howard Shaffer suggest that depressants provide a pharmacologic defense against the user's own aggressive drives. Binge eating or excessive television watching may fulfill the same adaptive role by helping people quiet strong hostile impulses. On a biochemical level, the effect of satiation activities may be similar to that of opiates. Growing dependence on behaviors, such as overeating and watching television, may be analogous, though more subtle, versions of opiate addiction.

While satiation addicts try to avoid stimulation and confrontation, others actively seek it. The behavior associated with the arousal mode of gratification includes crime, gambling, risk taking, and use of stimulant drugs, such as amphetamines or cocaine. These addicts seek to feel active and potent in the face of an environment that they view as overwhelmingly dehumanizing. They are often boastful about their artistic talent, intellectual skill, and sexual or physical prowess. Their vast expenditures of mental and physical energy are designed to deny underlying fears of helplessness. This posture is reminiscent of two- and three-year-olds coping with the world of giants in which they live. Asked, "Who is biggest or toughest?" they often reply, "I can beat up Daddy." They protect themselves through the defense of magical denial: "I am really not helpless and vulnerable; I am powerful and feared."

The third type of addict, who uses fantasy as the preferred way of dealing with the world, favors repetitive activation of what some researchers refer to as right-hemisphere thinking. Thoughts become dreamlike with rapidly shifting imagery and illogical relations between time and space. This style of coping often includes preoccupation with day or night dreams, compulsive artistic expression, or various forms of mystical experience, sometimes expressed as a quest for the feeling of oneness or cosmic unity. People who rely on this style partially overcome their fears by creating fantasies, in which they are effective and important. They may travel with extraterrestrials, encounter the "Grim Reaper," or have their body entered by a supernatural entity.

These addicts favor hallucinogens, such as LSD, mushrooms containing psilocybin, or peyote. Interestingly, the two basic types of chemical molecules—variations of indole and phenylethylamine—present in nearly all hallucinogens are also found in many compounds that occur naturally as neurotransmitters. For example, dopamine and norepinephrine have the basic phenylethylamine structure, whereas serotonin has the indole structure. The fantasy aspects of some artistic, romantic, or spiritual activities may be brought about by conversion of the brain's own indole or phenylethylamine compounds into hallucinogenic variations of these chemicals.

Limbic Sensation and Cortical Content

In addition to producing different patterns of neurotransmission, the three types of addiction seem to involve different parts of the brain. Mood shifts appear to be influenced by the limbic system, located near the middle of the brain. This system is associated with emotions and with sexual, feeding, and aggressive responses. As arousal decreases, moods may downshift from relaxation to tranquility and finally to a state of blissful satiation. Conversely, increases in arousal are accompanied by changes in experience from ordinary alertness through creativity and ultimately manic states.

While the limbic system appears to play a major role in pleasurable sensations connected with al-

tered levels of arousal, the convoluted outer brain, known as the cerebral cortex, is an important determinant of mental content. Excessive activity in the cortex of the right hemisphere may help explain the uncontrolled imagery found in the fantasies of cocaine users, mystics, and schizophrenics. Similar cortical activity in the left hemisphere may be responsible for feelings of superreality that some individuals report during high-risk activities, such as rock climbing and sky diving, which require an accurate and logical appraisal of one's options.

Society and the Deviant Career

Differences in neurotransmission, influences from the limbic and cortical systems, and the effects of various brain enzymes all interact with powerful social forces that can push susceptible individuals toward activities that have a high dependency potential. Computer games, public lotteries, and telephone escorts are just a few examples of widely available escapes from routine existence. Advertising plays on the human quest for effortless, impersonal reduction of stress. There is an implicit promise that participation in activities with high dependence potential will diminish the discrepancy between actual self-concept and ideal self-concept. Tobacco and alcohol propaganda provide the most blatant examples of this phenomenon. A visual, ego-ideal fantasy is provided in association with the product, often accompanied by a verbal suggestion for indulgence: "Come to X-Brand country." In this context of promoted immediacy, the individual moves through a network of social interactions that may influence his or her reliance on particular channels of behavioral excess.

In the earliest phase of preaddict development, a child may possess a subtle yet identifiable characteristic that steers him or her in the direction of addiction. Consider the two-year-old who enjoys his or her first taste of beer, or the young boy whose nickname is "Lucky" or "Romeo." The young person may be valued conditionally, so that parental affection depends on performance of expected behaviors. Further channelization occurs when an early sense of low self-worth is relieved through rewards associated with a specific activity. The dejected child may begin to feel potent on attaining external reinforcers, such as drugs, money, or sex.

Although parental role models and styles of child rearing are viewed as important contributors to future coping patterns, adolescent adjustment is inextricably bound to peer influence. According to

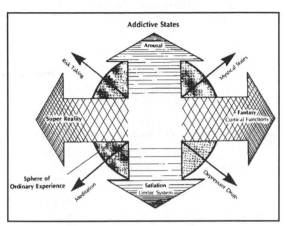

Figure 3. Addictive States

While the brain's limbic state appears to play a major role in the pleasurable sensations of addiction, the cerebral cortex influences mental content. Its right hemisphere may be involved in fantasy experiences, such as those achieved through LSD or other imagination-oriented activities. The heightened sense of reality experienced during compulsive risk taking or work may be linked to activity in the left hemisphere.

Denise Kandel of Columbia University, the most reliable finding in drug research is the strong relation between one person's drug use and concurrent use by friends. The strength of the adolescent's motive toward peer conformity is symbolized by the flamboyant dress rituals among punks.

If a person's channelization toward problem behaviors continues into early adulthood, opportunities for success diminish as he or she is increasingly imprisoned, both socially and personally, within a deviant role. The adolescent reaches a point of no return when the social and personal costs of changing life-styles seem to outweigh the benefits. Imagine the difficulty of a seventeen-year-old school dropout and long-standing street-gang member suddenly attempting to become an athlete or college student. Eventually, the young addict is labeled by those around him or her as a member of a deviant subgroup, such as alcoholic, obese, or criminal. This stigmatization tends to further decrease the addict's sense of self-worth. A youngster may begin to enact socially expected roles, such as being irresponsible, non-conforming, or impulse-ridden. The stereotyped individual thus becomes further engulfed in a pattern that restricts his or her life opportunities. As the addict now drifts from stable family and love relationships, social settings are increasingly selected because of their potential for immediate gratification. The bar, sex parlor, discotheque, or video arcade may become important islands of alienated comfort.

The addictive progression often culminates in dramatic conflict with the environment. Heightened environmental demands and repeated personal failures require increasingly severe efforts to recoup self-esteem through excessive activity. The downward spiral of functioning may lead to a variety of social-service interventions, including hospitalization, incarceration, or both, often occurring on a cyclical basis. What social scientists have labeled as relapse may simply reflect another episode in the naturally oscillating course of the addict's futile struggle to regain control.

The process of becoming addicted may be conceptualized as a "deviant career." Novices advance through a series of social stages, as they progress to full status in their offbeat professions. The ripple effect from being labeled or stigmatized as a type of addict—fatty, junkie, alcoholic, and so on—may last throughout a person's lifetime.

Multiple Disciplines: The Cutting Edge

Considering the complex biological, psychological, and social forces that promote behavioral excess, it is not surprising that those who attempt treatment for their compulsions usually fail. From 60 to 80 percent of all addicts who attempt abstinence relapse within six months. It can be excruciatingly difficult to overcome renegade biological processes that are further encouraged by powerful social and psychological influences. Yet, it can be done.

Biologically, the question is: can the human brain gain control over inherited impulses that were appropriate for prehistoric man but are inappropriate in the twentieth century? We know that activities that lead to compulsive lifestyles are self-induced and are under both cortical and limbic system control. We also know that the cerebral cortex, the center of thought and memory in homo sapiens, is much larger in humans than in other animals. With this great reasoning capacity, we should be able to exercise more control over the basic emotions directed by the lower brain centers. A multi-disciplinary understanding of addiction should provide the conflict-solving abilities of our cortex with the power it needs to control our lives more success-fully.

The term *dharma* is used in Hindu philosophy to describe a person's free will or ability to control *karma*, that which an individual brings into the world when born. In today's terms, we may look at dharma as cortical control and karma as the inner brain inheritance. Clearly, humankind has the ability to exercise dharma over karma: we need not be slaves to our compulsive behavior.

* * *

Harvey Milkman and Stanley Sunderwirth, "Doorway to Excess," from *Craving for Ecstasy: The Consciousness and Chemistry of Escape*. Reprinted with the permission of Lexington Books, an imprint of Macmillan, Inc. Copyright © 1987 by Lexington Books.

For Discussion

1. If drug use can be explained in part by neurobiological factors, why do we punish drug offenders for behaviors over which they have little control?

2. Discuss the conflict between neurobiological factors of addiction and homo sapiens' ability to exercise control over the basic emotions directed by the lower brain centers. After reading this chapter, do you think addicts deserve the stigma society places on them? ✦

3. A Sociological Theory of Drug Addiction[1]

Alfred R. Lindesmith

Various theories have been developed to explain drug use and addiction. Current explanations are grounded in the sociological, psychological, or biological sciences. Some theories are interdisciplinary in that they seek to combine two or more of these perspectives. Regardless of where they originate, theories of addiction are important in that they contribute to our understanding of the causal factors that lead to drug dependence. If we are able to identify the causal processes, we are in a better position to develop social policies and treatment initiatives that can serve addicts more effectively.

In this essay, dating back to 1938, the late Alfred R. Lindesmith criticizes the psychiatric explanation of opiate addiction. Psychiatrists, he argues, attach moral labels (e.g., "psychopaths") to addicts and assume that the continued use of opiates results from the addict's need to "escape from life." Although Lindesmith recognizes that users experience euphoria during their early stages of narcotics use, he disagrees with psychiatrists' assertions that the continuous use of opiate drugs is always for the sake of a "high." His sociological theory assumes that opiate addiction results from the conscious awareness that continued drug use is necessary to eliminate or prevent the pain associated with opiate withdrawal. Addicts do not use opiates to escape from life; rather, they do so to avoid withdrawal.

The problem of drug addiction has been an important one in this country for several decades and has proved to be a difficult one to handle from a theoretical, as well as from a therapeutic, standpoint. In spite of more than a half-century of experimentation with "cures," the drug addict has continued to relapse and thereby aroused the wonder and ire of those who have attempted to treat him. It has frequently been said that the drug user cannot be cured "if he doesn't want to be cured"; but this appears to beg the question, for it is the very essence of addiction that the victim desires to use the drug—and also, at the same time, desires to be free

of it. An indication of the strength of the addict's attachment to his drug is furnished by the fact that when the Japanese government in 1929 permitted unregistered opium-smokers in Formosa to register and gave them the choice of applying for either a cure or a license, only thirty out of approximately twenty-five thousand asked for the cure.[2]

Current explanations of the drug habit appear to center about a few general conceptions and modes of approach, none of which have led to convincing results. Psychiatrists have often regarded the use of opiates as an escape from life and have viewed addicts as defective persons seeking to compensate for, or avoid, their inferiorities and mental conflicts.[3] As would be expected, addicts have been labeled as "psychopaths," with the assumption that the attachment of this ambiguous label in some mysterious way explained the phenomenon. Various statements, as to the percentage of defective persons among addicts, have not been accompanied by any comparison with the percentage of defective persons in the general, non-addicted population. In fact, the need or desirability of this sort of comparison does not seem to have occurred to the majority of these writers.

This point of view contrasts the "psychopath," who is assumed to be susceptible to addiction, with "normal" persons, who are presumed by implication to be immune, or, if they accidentally become addicted, they are said to quit and remain free. No evidence has been produced, however, which indicates that any but an exceedingly small percentage of addicts ever remain free of the drug for long periods of years,[4] and no "normal" person has ever been shown to be immune to the subtle influence of the drug. It appears from an examination of the literature that all "normal" persons who have been foolhardy enough to imagine themselves immune and have consequently experimented upon themselves and taken the drug steadily for any length of time, have become addicts, or "junkers," as they usually style themselves.[5] The contention that any type of person can be readily cured of the drug habit in a permanent sense is without any support in terms of actual evidence. We have found that narcotic agents and others who are in close contact with the actual problem, ordinarily acquire a wholesome fear of the drug and do not delude themselves concerning their own capacity to resist its influence.

A French medical student,[6] in the course of writing a thesis on morphine, decided to experiment upon himself. For five consecutive days, he took an injection each evening at about nine o'clock. He reported that after three or four injections he began to desire the next ones, and that it cost him a decided effort to refrain from using it the sixth night. He managed to carry out his plan, but clearly implied that, if he had continued the experiment for a short time longer, he believed that he would have become addicted. The addict, in his opinion, is un homme perdu, who is rarely able ever again to retain his freedom. This account constitutes an interesting document for the individual who believes that he or anyone else is immune to addiction by reason of a superabundance of will-power or because of an absence of psychopathy. In 1894, Mattison advised the physician as follows:

> Let him not be blinded by an underestimate of the poppy's power to ensnare. Let him not be deluded by an over-confidence in his own strength to resist; for along this line, history has repeated itself with sorrowful frequency, and—as my experience will well attest—on these two treacherous rocks hundreds of promising lives have gone awreck.[7]

Sir William Willcox states:

> We know people who say: "I am a man, and one having a strong will. Morphine or heroin will not affect me; I can take it as long as I like without becoming an addict." I have known people—sometimes medical men—who have made that boast, and without exception they have come to grief.[8]

The conception of opiates as affording an escape from life also does not appear to be satisfactory or correct in view of the well-known fact that the addict invariably claims that all the drug does is to cause him to feel "normal." It is generally conceded that the euphoria associated with the use of opiates is highly transitory in character, and, while it is true that during the initial few weeks of use the drug may cause pleasure in some cases and may function as a means of escape, still, when addiction is established, this no longer holds true. The drug addict, who is supposed to derive some mysterious and uncanny pleasure from the drug, not only fails to do so as a rule but is also keenly aware of the curse of addiction and struggles to escape it. Far from being freed from his problems, he is actually one of the most obviously worried and miserable creatures in our society.

Finally, we may call attention to the fact that the current conception of the addict as a "psychopath," escaping from his own defects by the use of the drug, has the serious defect of being admittedly inapplicable to a certain percentage of cases. L. Kolb, for example, finds that 86 percent of the addicts included in a study of his had defects antedating and presumably, explaining the addiction. One may, therefore, inquire how addiction is to be explained in the other 14 percent of the cases. Are these persons addicts, because they are free from defects? The assumption is sometimes made that those in whom defects cannot be found have secret defects which explain the addiction. Such an assumption obviously places the whole matter beyond the realm of actual research. Moreover, one may ask, who among us does not have defects of one kind or another, secret or obvious?

In general, it appears that the conception of the drug addict as a defective psychopath prior to addiction is more in the nature of an attempt to place blame than it is an explanation of the matter. It is easy and cheap to designate as "inferior" or "weak" or "psychopathic" persons whose vices are different from our own and whom we consequently do not understand.[9] Similarly, the "causes" of addiction as they are often advanced—"curiosity," "bad associates," and the "willingness to try anything once"—suffer from the same moralistic taint. Undoubtedly, these same factors "cause" venereal disease; yet, science has ceased to be concerned with them. In the case of drug addiction, we still are more interested in proving that it is the addict's "own fault" that he is an addict than we are in understanding the mechanisms of addiction.

It was noted long ago that not all persons, to whom opiate drugs were administered for sufficiently long periods of time to produce the withdrawal symptoms, became addicts. It frequently occurs in medical practice that severe and chronic pain makes the regular administration of opiates a necessity.[10] Some of the persons who are so treated show no signs of the typical reactions of addicts and may even be totally ignorant of what they are being given. Others to whom the drug is administered in this way return to it when it has been withdrawn, and become confirmed addicts. This fact caused German and French students of the problem to adopt distinct terms for the two conditions—those who received the drug for therapeutic reasons and who showed none of the symptoms of the typical "craving" of addicts were spoken of as cases of "chronic morphine poisoning," or "morphinism"; whereas, addicts in the ordinarily accepted sense of the word were called "morphinomanes" or, in German, Morphiumsüchtiger.[11] Attempts have been made to introduce such a usage in this country, though without success, and it is consequently awkward to try to refer to these two conditions. In this paper, the term "habituated" will be used to refer to the development of the mere physiological tolerance; whereas, the term "addiction" will be reserved for application to cases in which there is added to the physiological or pharmacological tolerance a psychic addiction, which is marked by the appearance of an imperious desire for the drug and leads to the development of the other characteristic modes of behavior of the drug addict, as he is known in our society. For persons who are merely habituated to the drug without being addicted, there is no need for special conceptual treatment any more than persons who have had operations need to be set off as a distinct class. Once the drug has been removed, these persons show no craving for it or any tendency to resume its use, unless, perhaps, the disease for which the opiate was originally given reappears.

Any explanation of the causation of drug addiction must attempt to account for this fact, that not all persons who are given opiates become addicts. What are the factors which cause one man to escape, while the next, under what appear to be the same physiological conditions, becomes an incurable addict? Obviously, the factor of the patient's knowledge of what he is being given is an important one, for clearly, if he is ignorant of the name of the drug, he will be unable to ask for it or consciously to desire it. The recognition of the importance of keeping the patient in ignorance of what drugs he is being given is quite general. Various devices which serve this end, such as giving the drug orally rather than hypodermically, keeping it out of the hands of the patient and permitting no self-administration, mixing the dosage of opiates with other drugs whose effects are not so pleasant and which serve to disguise the effects of the opiate, etc., have been advocated and have become more or less routine practice. But in some cases, individuals who are fully aware that they are receiving morphine (or some other opium alkaloid) may also not become addicted, even after prolonged administration.[12] Other factors, besides ignorance of the drug administered, must therefore operate to prevent the occurrence of addiction in such cases. What seems to account for this variability—and this is the crux of the theory being advanced—is not the knowledge of the drug administered, but the knowledge of the

true significance of the withdrawal symptoms when they appear and the use of the drug thereafter for the consciously understood motive of avoiding these symptoms.[13] As far as can be determined, there is no account in the literature of anyone's ever having experienced the full severity of the withdrawal symptoms in complete knowledge of their connection with the absence of the opiate drug, who has not also become an addict. Addiction begins when the person suffering from withdrawal symptoms realizes that a dose of the drug will dissipate all his discomfort and misery. If he then tries it out and actually feels the almost magical relief that is afforded, he is on the way to confirmed addiction. The desire for the drug, and the impression that it is necessary, apparently become fixed with almost incredible rapidity, once this process of using the drug to avoid the abstinence symptoms has begun. Among confirmed addicts, it appears to be the general rule also that those who have the greatest difficulty in obtaining regular supplies of narcotics ("boot and shoe dope fiends") are precisely those who develop the most intense craving for it and use it to excess when the opportunity presents itself. In other words, deprivation is the essential factor both in the origin of the craving and in its growth.

In order to prove the correctness of the theory advanced, it is necessary to consider, first, its applicability to the general run of cases—that is, to determine whether or not addicts become addicted in any other way than through the experience with withdrawal—and whether there are non-addicts, in whom all of the conditions or causes of addiction have occurred without actually producing addiction. We do not have the space here to go into an extended analysis and explanation of any large number of cases. We can only state that, from our analysis of the cases that have come to our attention, both directly and in the literature, it appears to be true without exception that addicts do, in fact, become addicted in this manner and that addiction does invariably follow whenever the drug is used for the conscious purpose of alleviating withdrawal distress. That this is the case is strikingly brought out by the addict's own argot. The term "hooked" is used by drug users to indicate the fact that a person has used the drug long enough so that, if he attempts to quit, withdrawal distress will force him to want to go on using the drug. At the same time, "to be hooked" means to be addicted, and anyone who has ever been "hooked" is forever after classified by himself, as well as by other addicts, as belonging to the in-group, as an addict, a "user" or "junker," regardless of whether he is using the drug at the moment or not.[14] Similarly, a person who has not been "hooked," regardless of whether he is using the drug or not, is not classified as an addict.[15] It is a contradiction in terms of addict argot, therefore, to speak of "a junker who has never been hooked" or of an individual who has been "hooked" without becoming an addict. Addict argot admits no exceptions to this rule. We found that drug users invariably regard any query about a hypothetical addict who has not been compelled to use the drug by the withdrawal distress, or about a hypothetical non-addict who has, as incomprehensible nonsense. To them, it is self-evident that to be "hooked" and to be an addict are synonymous.[16]

As we have indicated, our own experience is in entire accord with this view of the addict, as it is crystallized in his vernacular. In addition, we have found certain types of cases which bear more directly upon the theory and which offer conclusive and, we may say, experimental verification of the theory. It is upon cases of this type which we wish to concentrate our attention.

Crucial instances which strongly corroborate the hypothesis are those cases, in which the same person has first become habituated to the use of the drug over a period of time and then had the drug withdrawn without becoming addicted; and then, later in life, under other circumstances, become a confirmed addict. Erwin Strauss[17] records the case of a woman

> who received morphine injections twice daily for six months, from February to July of 1907, on account of gall stones. After her operation in July, the drug was removed and the patient did not become an addict[18] but went about her duties as before, until 1916, nine years later, when her only son was killed at the Front. She was prostrated by her grief and, after intense anguish and thoughts of suicide, she thought of the morphine which had been administered to her nine years before. She began to use it, found it helpful, and soon was addicted. *What is particularly noteworthy is that, when asked if she had suffered any withdrawal symptoms when the drug was withdrawn the first time in 1907, she stated that she could not recall any.* [Italics are mine.]

Another case of the same kind was interviewed by the writer.

A man, Dr. H., was given morphine regularly for a considerable period of time when he underwent three operations for appendicitis with complications. He was not expected to live. As he recovered, the dosage of morphine was gradually reduced and completely withdrawn without any difficulty. Although the patient suffered some discomfort during the process and knew that he had been receiving morphine, he attributed this discomfort to the processes of convalescence. Dr. H. had had occasion to see drug addicts in his medical practice and had always felt a horror of addiction and had sometimes thought he would rather shoot himself than be one. This attitude of horror remained unaltered during the hospital experience just related. Several years later, Dr. H. contracted gall-stone trouble and was told that an operation would be necessary. Opiates were administered, and Dr. H., who wished to avoid another operation at all costs, administered opiates to himself, hoping that the operation might not be necessary. He began to use the drug for pains of less and less significance, until he found himself using it every day. He became apprehensive during this process, but reasoned with himself that there was nothing to be alarmed about, inasmuch as drug addiction was certainly not the horrible thing it was supposed to be and he was certain that he would have no difficulty in quitting. His horror of addiction disappeared. When he attempted to quit, he found that it was more difficult than he had supposed. He, of course, noticed the regular recurrence of the withdrawal illness and *then realized in retrospect that he had experienced the same symptoms, without recognizing them, several years before.* [Italics are mine.]

A third case of the same kind is briefly mentioned by Dansauer and Rieth,[19] and two others have come to the attention of the writer. Obviously, the number of instances in which a coincidence of this kind is likely to occur is very small, but those that have been found, unequivocally and without exception, indicate that, if morphine is withdrawn carefully, without the patient's recognizing or noticing the symptoms of abstinence, no craving for the drug develops. The typical phenomena which signalize addiction, such as the tendency to increase the dose inordinately, to exhibit and feel a powerful desire to obtain the drug at any cost, and to be unhappy without it—these phenomena do not put in their appearance, until the patient has discovered that there are withdrawal symptoms of a persistent severe character and has used the drug for a time, solely or chiefly to prevent these symptoms from appearing. In the argot of the addict, when this has occurred, the person is "hooked"; he "has a habit." If he quits before it occurs or if he resolutely refrains from using the drug to alleviate the abstinence symptoms the first time he experiences them, he may still escape. If the symptoms occur in their full intensity, however, the impulse to seek relief in the drug, when it is known that only the drug will give relief, is irresistible—especially since the patient is not likely to realize that the danger of addiction is present. He thinks only of the fact that he can obtain relief from those terrible symptoms, which, to the uninitiated, may be genuinely terrifying.

As an illustration of the process of the establishment of addiction which we are attempting to isolate, another case of a man who became addicted in medical practice may be cited.

> Mr. G. was severely lacerated and internally injured as the result of an accident. He spent thirteen weeks in a hospital, during which time he received frequent doses of morphine, some hypodermically and some orally. He paid no attention to what it was that was being used on him and felt no effects of any unusual character, except that the medicine to some extent relieved him of pain. He was discharged from the hospital and, after several hours, began to develop considerable discomfort and irritability and the other symptoms of morphine withdrawal. He had no idea what was the matter. In about twelve hours, he was violently nauseated and, during his first night at home, called his family physician in at two o'clock in the morning, fearing that he was about to die. The physician also was not certain what was wrong, but gave him some mild sedatives and attempted to encourage him. The violence of the symptoms increased during the next day, to such an extent that Mr. G. began to wish that he would die. During the course of the second night, the family physician decided that he was perhaps suffering from withdrawal of opiates and gave Mr. G. an injection of morphine to find out. The effect was immediate; in about twenty minutes, Mr. G. fell asleep and slept on in perfect comfort for many hours. He still did not know what he had been given, but when he woke up the next day the doctor told him and said, "Now we are going to have a time getting you off!" The dosage was reduced and in a week or two the drug was entirely removed, but Mr. G., during this short time,

had become addicted. After the drug had been removed for a few days, he bought himself a hypodermic syringe and began to use it by himself.[20]

It may seem surprising, at first glance, that many addicts do not know what is wrong with them the first time that the abstinence symptoms occur. This is not difficult to understand when one realizes that many persons seem to think that withdrawal symptoms are purely imaginative or hysterical in character. Even in spite of the occurrence of these symptoms in animals, which have been subjected to the prolonged administration of opiates, and in spite of their occurrence in patients who have no idea what opiates are or that they have been given any, students of drug addiction have sometimes asserted that these symptoms have no physiological basis. In view of this belief among the instructed, it is easy to understand the layman who believes the same thing when he begins to experiment with the drug. Furthermore, there is nothing whatever in the initial effects of the drug to furnish the slightest clue as to what happens later. As the use of the drug is continued, in the same proportion that tolerance appears, and the positive effects diminish, the withdrawal symptoms increase, until they obtrude themselves upon the attention of the individual, and finally become dominant. In most cases of confirmed addiction, the drug appears to serve almost no other function than that of preventing the appearance of these symptoms.

One of the most difficult features of addiction to account for, by means of any explanation of the drug habit in terms of the positive effects, or euphoria, supposed to be produced by it, is the fact that during the initial period of use there takes place a gradual reversal of effect, so that the effects of the drug upon an addict are not only not the same as their effects upon a non-addicted person, but they are actually, in many respects, the precise opposite.[21] This is true both of the physiological and of the psychological effects. The initial dose causes one to feel other than normal; whereas in the case of the addict, the usual dose causes him to feel normal when he would feel below normal without it. The euphoria initially produced by the drug has often been emphasized as a causative factor, but inasmuch as this euphoria, or "kick," disappears in addiction, the continuation of the drug habit cannot be explained in this way.[22] Moreover, when administered therapeutically to allay pain, there is often absolutely no euphoria produced even in the initial period, and the patient may nevertheless become addicted. In fact, it is possible for a person to be unconscious during the entire initial stage when tolerance is established and still become addicted, as a consideration of the implications of the case of Mr. G. shows. It is this reversal of effect which accounts at one and the same time for the seductive aspect of opiates, as well as for their insidiousness. As they cease to produce pleasure, they become a necessity and produce pain if removed. The euphoria produced by the drug at first makes it easy to become addicted, but does not account for the continuance of the habit when the euphoria is gone. A theory which makes the withdrawal distress central in addiction takes account of this reversal of effects.

It follows, if one believes that the drug habit is to be accounted for on the basis of the extraordinary or uncanny state of mind it is sometimes supposed to produce, that addicts should be able to recognize such effects immediately and easily. It is a notorious fact, however, and one that baffles the addicts, as well as those who study them, that under certain conditions the drug user may be completely deceived for varying periods of time into believing that he is receiving opiates, when he actually is not, or that he is not receiving any when, as a matter of fact, he is. We shall not elaborate this point any more than to call attention to the fact that it has been put into practice as a principle in a number of gradual reduction cures, wherein, without the addict's knowledge, the amount of the drug was gradually reduced and finally withdrawn entirely, while injections of water or a saline solution were continued.[23] Then, when the addict had been free of opiates for several days, or a week, or even more, he was told that he had not been getting any of his drug for some time and usually discharged, sometimes in the vain hope that this experience might prove to him that it was only his "imagination" which led him to think he needed his drug! The fact that such a thing is possible is evidence that the direct positive effects per se are not sufficiently extraordinary to make addiction intelligible.

The tendency of the addict to relapse may be readily explained in terms of the viewpoint outlined as arising from the impression that is made upon him when he observes the remarkable and immediate effects the drug has in dissipating unpleasant physical or mental states. What the addict misses when he is off the drug is not so much the hypothetical euphoria as the element of control. On the drug, he could regulate his feeling tone; when he is

not using it, it appears to him that he is the passive victim of his environment or of his changing moods. During the initial period of use, the only effects of an injection to which attention is paid are ordinarily the immediate ones lasting but a few minutes or, at most, a half-hour or an hour or so. This episodic significance of injections changes into a continuous twenty-four-hour-a-day sense of dependence upon the drug only after the addict has learned from the recurrence of the beginnings of withdrawal symptoms, as the effects of each shot wore off, that the drug was necessary to the continuance of his well-being. He learns to attribute effects to the "stuff," which are in part imaginary—or rather, projections of the need for it which he feels. When he is off, every vicissitude of life tends to remind him of his drug, and he misses the supporting and sustaining sense of its presence. And so, the ordinary pleasures of life are dulled, something seems to be amiss, and the unhappy addict eventually relapses—either deliberately or otherwise. If he does not relapse, it appears that he nevertheless remains susceptible to it for long periods of years. Cases of relapse after as long as ten or more years of abstinence are recorded.[24]

The thesis of the paper is that addiction to opiate drugs is essentially based upon the abstinence symptoms which occur when the effects of the drug are beginning to wear off rather than upon any positive effects or uncanny or extraordinarily pleasurable state of mind erroneously supposed to be produced by the drug in continued use. Addiction is established in the first instance in a process involving

1. The interpretation of the withdrawal symptoms as being caused by the absence of opiates,[25] followed by

2. The use of the drug for the consciously understood purpose of alleviating these symptoms or of keeping them suppressed.

As a result of this process there is established in the addict the typical desire for the drug, a constant sense of dependence upon it, and the other attendant features of addiction. The attitudes which arise in this experience persist when the drug has been removed and predispose toward relapse. When the point is reached at which withdrawal symptoms intrude themselves upon the attention of the individual and compel him to go on using the drug, he also has forced upon him the unwelcome definition of himself as a "dope fiend." He realizes then what the craving for drugs means and, applying to his own conduct the symbols which the group applies to it, he is compelled to readjust his conception of himself to the implications of this collective viewpoint. He struggles against the habit and then eventually accepts his fate and becomes "just another junker." Obviously, when the withdrawal distress has entered into the conscious motives of the person, and he realizes that he must anticipate the recurrence of these terrible symptoms, if he does not assure himself of a supply of the drug, and when the definition of self as an addict has occurred, the drug user becomes ripe for assimilation into the culture of drug addiction, as it exists chiefly in our underworld.

The proposed theory has advantages and implications beyond those already mentioned. It is applicable in form to all cases and, as indicated, an extensive exploration of the literature, as well as many interviews with addicts, has so far failed to uncover a single negative case, even of a hearsay type. Moreover, it harmonizes and rationalizes various aspects of the habit which have often been regarded as paradoxical or contradictory in character—as, for example, the fact that addicts claim they do not obtain pleasure from the drug, the initial reversal of effects, and the strange tendency of addicts to relapse when, from a medical standpoint, they appear to be cured.

A number of further implications of the point of view presented seem to have important bearings on certain theories of social psychology and of sociology. Thus, students of the writings of George H. Mead will notice that the hypothesis follows the lines of his theory of the "significant symbols" and its role in human life. According to the view presented, the physiological effects of the drug do not become effective in influencing the psychic and social life of the person, until he has applied to them the "significant symbols" (or perhaps, in Durkheimian language, "collective representations") which are employed by the group to describe the nature of these effects. Addiction, in other words, appears as a process which goes on, on the level of "significant symbols"—it is, in other words, peculiar to man living in organized society in communication with his fellows.[26]

This theory rationalizes and explains the reasons for the ordinary rules-of-thumb employed in the therapeutic administration of morphine to prevent addiction. Some of these rules and practices include (1) keeping the patient in ignorance of the drug being used, (2) mixing other drugs with different and less pleasing effects with the opiate, (3) varying the mode of administration and disguising the drug in various kinds of medicines. The significance of these practices appears to be that they prevent the patient from attributing to morphine the effects which it in fact produces—in other words, they prevent the patient from applying certain collective symbols to his own subjective states, prevent the whole experience from being associated with the patient's preconceptions of drug addiction, and so prevent addiction.

The proposed hypothesis has the further advantage of being essentially experimental in character, in the sense that it is open to disproof, as, for example, by anyone who doubts it and is willing or foolhardy enough to experiment on himself with the drug. As has been indicated, the writer has been unable to find any record in the literature of an experiment of this character which, prolonged enough to be a test—that is, which lasted long enough so that the withdrawal distress upon stoppage of the drug was pronounced—did not result in addiction. This appears to constitute an exception to what is often assumed to be true of knowledge in the field of the social sciences—namely, that it confers, *ipso facto*, the ability to control. It is in accord with the well-known fact that addiction to narcotic drugs is peculiarly prevalent in those legitimate professions in which theoretical knowledge of these drugs is most general—that is, in the medical and allied professions.

A further significant implication of the viewpoint presented is that it offers a means of relating phenomena of a purely physiological variety to cultural or sociological phenomena. The interpretation of withdrawal distress, which we have emphasized as a basic factor in the beginning of addiction, is, it should be emphasized, a cultural pattern, a social interpretation present in a formulated fashion in the social milieu exactly like other knowledge or beliefs. When the organic disturbances produced by the withdrawal of the drug intrude themselves upon the attention of a person, they impede his functioning and assume the nature of a problem, demanding some sort of rationalization and treatment. The culture of the group supplies this rationalization by defining the situation for the individual and, in so doing, introduces into the motives and conceptions which determine his conduct other factors which lead to addiction whenever the drug is continued beyond the point at which this insight occurs.

Finally, we should like to emphasize again the methodological implications of the study. A great deal of argumentation has taken place in sociology on the matter of methodology—whether universal generalizations are possible or not, concerning the role of statistical generalizations and of quantification generally, and concerning the so-called case method. Most of these arguments have tended to take place on an abstract level; whereas, it would seem that in the final analysis, they can be settled only in terms of actual results of research. We, therefore, regard it as significant that the theory advanced in this study is not quantitative in form, nor is it a purely intuitive generalization which is not subject to proof, but that it is experimental in form, in spite of the fact that it is based upon the analysis of data secured largely in personal interviews. It is, moreover, stated in universal form and is, therefore, not dependent upon or relative to a particular culture or a particular time. As such, it provides the possibility of its own continuous reconstruction and refinement, in terms of more extended experience and of more elaborated instances. In other words, it provides a place for the exceptional or crucial case, which George H. Mead has described as the "growing point of science."[27]

Comment

The writer does not state whether his study relates to any one form of drug addiction, but it seems he is concerned chiefly, if not solely, with morphine addiction. At least, he discusses addiction in which withdrawal symptoms are prominent, and so his theory does not seem to apply to types of addiction, such as cocaine, hasheesh, and others, in which withdrawal symptoms are absent or of a minor nature.

It is stated that "addiction begins when the person suffering from withdrawal symptoms realizes that a dose of the drug will dissipate all his discomfort and misery." And, furthermore: "If he fails to realize the connection between the distress and the opiate, he escapes addiction." How often does this occur? Conceivably, in some patients who have received such drugs to alleviate pain or as sedatives. But we presume that the author does not intend to suggest that many drug addicts are established in the course of medical treatment. Apart from such cases, may we not consider that an individual who persists in securing drugs and administering them

to himself, until he is likely to suffer withdrawal symptoms of any degree, is in fact already an addict? And that withdrawal symptoms are then a complication in the course of drug addiction, dependent on the fact that tolerance for the drug has been acquired? But that does not explain why the individual became an addict, although it might be offered as a reason for the difficulty in giving up the addiction, if he so desires or is requested. We would again recall the forms of drug addiction, in which there are few or no withdrawal symptoms.

The cases quoted by the author as crucial for the corroboration of his hypothesis are not convincing. The case quoted from Strauss does not seem to lend any support to the hypothesis. This woman did not become an addict because of withdrawal symptoms, but in an effort to secure relief from a state of acute mental depression. As the case report states: "She began to use it, found it helpful, and soon was addicted." When it is stated that persons may relapse "after as long as ten or more years of abstinence," then surely the renewal of addiction is not due to withdrawal symptoms.

Throughout the paper, there are several statements which call for comment. Thus, it is said that current theories of drug addiction tend to be moralistic, rather than scientific. This does not seem a correct interpretation of the many physiological and psychiatric studies on the subject. Again, references should be given for the statement—in regard to the nature of withdrawal symptoms—that "students of drug addiction have sometimes asserted that these symptoms have no physiological basis." It is stated that "the victim desires to use the drug—and also at the same time desires to be free of it." In what proportion of cases? Too often, one has found the addict seeking a "cure" with the aim of having his tolerance cut down because of financial difficulties, or because the dosage was too high for practical purposes. The author talks of "the drug," but experience with drug addicts shows so often that they have been addicted to several drugs, depending on available supplies and, after a period of abstinence through failure of supplies, would start in afresh on drugs of which they had no previous experience. What were they seeking, if not some form of satisfaction or pleasure or relief from a state of emotional distress or difficulty of life?

One cannot pass over a striking statement: "This appears to constitute an exception to what is often assumed to be true of knowledge in the field of the social sciences—namely, that it confers, *ipso facto*, the ability to control." We are reminded of the musings of one, Burns, who had knowledge but had not always the ability to control—and had knowledge of that also. Thus, in the "Unco Guid, or the Rigidly Righteous":

> One point must still be greatly dark,
> The moving why they do it;
> And just as lamely can ye mark
> How far perhaps they rue it.

Comment section by:
David Slight
Department of Psychiatry
University of Chicago

Rejoinder

A considerable portion of Dr. Slight's comments are based upon an implicit conception of method which is fundamentally different from our own. We assume, and stated in our article, that a scientific explanation must be stated in terms of factors or processes which are present in all the members of the class to which the generalization is supposed to apply. There is no evidence in Dr. Slight's comments that he has taken any account of this principle, and it is for this reason that he has failed to discuss the main issues. When he asserts, concerning the case given by Strauss, "This woman did not become an addict because of withdrawal symptoms, but in an effort to secure relief from a state of acute mental depression," he does not take into account a fact which is known to all—that many addicts begin to use the drug under circumstances which have no connection whatever with "mental distress." Some addicts, for example, first tried the drug in connection with a sex affair with a prostitute, and others first learn about the drug in medical practice. One may also ask if it would not be reasonable to suppose that the woman in this case experienced mental depression at some time during her six-month attack of disease nine years before she became an addict? Why did she not become addicted then? Dr. Slight does not touch this problem.

In the sentence beginning "Apart from such cases . . ." Dr. Slight appears to imply either that no addicts are created in medical practice or that, if they are, they should be excluded from the argument. Medical practice today does create new addicts—not many, but some. They are addicts in precisely the same sense as others are, and any generalization must include them. Concerning the latter part of this same sentence, we may say for a rather large percentage even of addicts on the street that the withdrawal symptoms are not at first understood. This was true in about 50 percent of our cases. A number of them had to have the symptoms explained to them by addicts or by doctors.

The implication that knowledge of the drug being given and of the withdrawal symptoms is irrelevant, and that the sheer brute fact of having used the drug long enough to produce withdrawal symptoms in itself constitutes addiction is directly contradicted in medical practice itself. The patient who is given morphine in hospitals is kept in ignorance of what is happening to him, and this is done for the explicit purpose of preventing addiction. Medical men quite generally maintain that this practice has, in fact, been very effective. Several decades ago, when such techniques were not as widely employed, medical practice did, in fact, create many new addicts.

The principle that an explanation must be applicable to *all*, rather than to some, of the cases is again ignored when he asks, "What are they [the addicts] seeking if not some form of satisfaction or pleasure or relief from a state of emotional distress or difficulty in life?" This view is simply the current common-sense misconception of the problem, and it explains nothing. It entirely ignores those cases in which addiction is a consequence of the sheer accident of disease. In terms of this view, how is one to account for continued addiction in that group of addicts for whom the major "emotional distress or difficulty in life" is the addiction itself?

The questions of fact which Dr. Slight raises cause us to wonder where he obtained the information upon which he bases his statements. He is correct when he surmises that we were concerned only with opiate addiction, but he repeatedly refers to the use of other drugs and says that addicts shift readily from one drug to another, depending upon available supply. This is incorrect. Opiate addicts shift only from one opiate to another. Chicago addicts use mainly heroin, for which they may pay as much as two hundred dollars an ounce. As a consequence, they cannot afford to use other drugs, and very few do. If an addict is utterly unable to obtain an opiate, he does only one thing—he "kicks his habit"; that is, he breaks the continuity of his addiction. During abstinence, some addicts may try other drugs or drink whiskey, but that does not prove that all forms of drug-taking are alike any more than the fact that some disappointed lovers turn to drink proves that sex activity and alcoholism are alike.

* * *

Alfred R. Lindesmith, "A Sociological Theory of Drug Addiction," *American Journal of Sociology*, 43 (1938), pp. 593-613. Copyright © 1938 by The University of Chicago Press. All rights reserved. Reprinted by permission.

For Discussion

Can Lindesmith's theory apply to drug users for whom the drug of choice is not accompanied by withdrawal symptoms? Why or why not?

Notes

1. The study on which this paper is based was carried out at the University of Chicago under the direction of Dr. Herbert Blumer.

2. Report to the Council of the League of Nations by the Committee of Enquiry into the Control of Opium Smoking in the Far East, II (1930), p. 420.

3. This general view is not only widespread among psychiatrists, but is popularly held as well. The great majority of writers in medical journals on this subject assume it. It may be found elaborated in a typical form in the following articles by L. Kolb: "Pleasure and Deterioration from Narcotic Addiction," *Jour. Ment. Hyg.*, Vol. IX (October, 1925); "Drug Addiction in Relation to Crime," *ibid.*, (January, 1925); "The Struggle for Cure and the Conscious Reasons for Relapse," *Jour. Nerv. and Ment. Dis.*, Vol. LXVI July, 1927); and "Drug Addiction—A Study of Some Medical Cases," *Arch. Neurol. and Psychiat.*, Vol. XX (1928). It is also developed by Dr. Schultz in "Rep. of the Comm. on Drug Addicts to Hon. R. C. Patterson, etc.," as reported in *Amer. Jour. Psychiat.*, Vol. X (1930-31).

4. Dansauer and Rieth ("Über Morphinismus bei Kriegsbeshädigten," in *Arbeit und Gesundheit—Schriftenreihe zum Reichsorbeitsblatt*, Vol. XVI [1931]), found that 96.7 percent of 799 addicts had relapsed within five years after taking a cure. Relapse after more than ten years is sometimes mentioned. We ourselves were acquainted with an addict who stated that he had abstained for fifteen years before resuming the drug. We have never encountered or read an authentic account of any so-called cured addict who did not show by his attitudes toward the drug that the impulse to relapse was actively present.

5. It is characteristic of practically all addicts, prior to their own addiction that they do not expect or intend to become addicts.

6. L. Faucher, *Contribution d l'étude du rêve morphinique et de la morphinomanie* (Thèse de Montpellier, No. 8 [1910-11]).

7. *JAMA*, Vol. XXIII.

8. *Brit. Jour. Inebriety* XXXI, 132.

9. The aim of this paper is to present a sociological theory of opiate addiction which appears to offer possibilities for a rational and objective understanding of the problem without any element of moralization. This theory is based upon informal and intimate contact over a long period of time with approximately fifty drug addicts. The main points of the theory have been tested in the material available in the literature of the problem, and no conclusions have been drawn from case materials collected, unless these materials were clearly corroborated by case materials in the literature.

10. Dansauer and Rieth (*op. cit.*) cite two hundred and forty such cases. Many of these cases had used the drug for five or more years without becoming addicts.

11. See e.g., Levinstein, *Die Morphiumsucht* (1877); F. McKelvey Bell, "Morphinism and Morphinomania," *N.Y. Med. Jour.*, Vol. XCIII (1911); and Daniel Jouet, *Étude sur al morphinisme chronique* (Thèse de Paris [1883]).

12. The case of Dr. H., cited later in this paper, is such a case.

13. Withdrawal distress begins to appear after a few days of regular administration but does not ordinarily become severe until after two, three, or more weeks, when its severity appears to increase at an accelerated rate. In its severe form, it involves acute distress from persistent nausea, general weakness, aching joints and pains in the legs, diarrhea, and extreme insomnia. In isolated cases, death may result from abrupt withdrawal of the drug.

14. We have checked this point with addicts who had voluntarily abstained for as long as six years. They unhesitatingly declared themselves to be addicts who happened not to be using drugs at the time—i.e., "junkers" or "users" who were "off stuff."

15. A type of individual who uses the drug without being hooked, is the one who uses it, say once a week, and thus avoids the withdrawal distress. Such a person is called a "joy-popper" or "pleasure-user" and is not regarded as an addict, until he has used the drug steadily for a time, experienced withdrawal distress, and become hooked. He then permanently loses his status as a "pleasure-user" and becomes a "junker." An addict who has abstained for a time and then begins to use it a little bit now and then is not a "pleasure-user"—he is just "playing around." See D. W. Maurer's article in the April, 1936, issue of *American Speech*.

16. As the other evidence which indicates how central and how taken for granted the role of withdrawal distress in addiction is, we may mention that the addict's word "yen" refers simultaneously to withdrawal distress *and* to the desire for the drug. Also, "to feel one's habit" means to feel the withdrawal distress. Addicts call cocaine non-habit-forming, because it does not cause withdrawal distress when stopped.

17. "Zur Pathogenese des chronischen Morphinismus," *Monatschr. fur Psychiat. und Neurol.*, Vol. XLVII (1920).

18. As defined, e.g., in the *Report of the Departmental Committee on Morphine and Heroin Addiction* to the British Ministry of Health: "A person who, not requiring the continued use of a drug for the relief of the symptoms of organic disease, has acquired, as a result of repeated administration, an overwhelming desire for its continuance, and in whom withdrawal of the drug leads to definite symptoms of mental or physical distress or disorder."

19. *Op. Cit.*, p. 103.

20. Interviewed by the writer.

21. This has been partially emphasized by Erlenmeyer, as quoted by C. E. Terry and Mildred Pellens, *The Opium Problem* (1928), pp. 600 ff.; and it has been noted, in one way or another, in much of the physiological research that has been done on morphine effects.

22. The English Departmental Committee in 1926 (*op. cit.*) stated that, whatever may have been the original motive, the use of the drug is continued not so much from that original motive as "because of the craving created by the use" (quoted in Terry and Pellens, *ibid.*, pp. 164-65).

23. *Ibid.*, pp. 577 ff., quoting C. C. Wholey; *ibid.*, pp. 572 ff., quoting M. R. Dupony. A number of addicts have somewhat sheepishly admitted to us that they had been deceived in this manner for as long as ten days.

24. Rolb, "Drug Addicts—A Study of Some Medical Cases," *loc. cit.*

25. It is significant to note that this belief that withdrawal distress is caused by the absence of the opiate is not adequate or correct from the standpoint of physiological theory.

26. Very young children, the feeble-minded, and the insane would not be expected to have the necessary sophisticated conception of causality or the ability to manipulate "significant symbols" which, as we have indicated, are necessary preconditions of addiction.

Dr. Charles Schultz, in a study of 318 cases found only 14 patients, or less than 5 percent, who were "probably high-grade morons, and even these gave the impression of having their dull wits sharpened by the use of drugs" (*loc. cit.*). Regarding insanity—it has been noted that it confers immunity to addiction, and that insanity appears to occur less frequently among the blood relations of addicts than among the blood relatives of samples of the general population. O. Wuth, "Zur Erbanlage der Süchtigen," *Z. für die Ges. Neur. und Psychiat.*, CLIII (1935), pp. 495 ff.; Alexander Pilcz, "Zur Konstitution der Süchtigen," *Jahrb. für Psychiat.*, LI (1935), pp. 169 ff.; Jouet, *op. cit.*; Sceleth and Kuh, *JAMA*, LXXXII, p. 679; P. Wolff, *Deutsche medizinische Wochenschrift*, Vol. LVII, in his report on the results of a questionnaire, etc. Note the testimony by Gaupp, Bratz, and Bonhoeffer.

On the immunity of children, see R. N. Chopra et al., "Administration of Opiates to Infants in India," *Indian Med. Gaz.*, LXIX (1934), pp. 489 ff.; "Opium Habit in India," *Indian Jour. Med. Research*, Vol. XV (1927); "Drug Addiction in India and Its Treatment," *Indian Med. Gaz.*, LXX (1935), pp. 121 ff.

27. In an essay, "Scientific Method and Individual Thinker," in *Creative Intelligence* (1917). ✦

4. The Use of Marijuana for Pleasure: A Replication of Howard S. Becker's Study of Marijuana Use

Michael L. Hirsch,
Randall W. Conforti,
and
Carolyn J. Graney

Howard S. Becker was perhaps the first of many researchers to examine the sociological aspects of marijuana use. His major efforts in this regard appear in his classic work Outsiders: Studies in the Sociology of Deviance *(Free Press, 1963). Based on interviews with 50 marijuana users, Becker proposed that gleaning pleasure from marijuana smoking occurs through a learning process. Further, he noted that marijuana users progress through a series of stages. Beginners learn to master techniques (e.g., inhalation, appropriate dosage) from experienced users. Occasional users smoke marijuana intermittently; that is, when the opportunity arises. More frequent use characterizes regular users who must arrange for a steady supply of marijuana for self-use.*

In the following essay, Michael L. Hirsch, Randall W. Conforti, and Carolyn J. Graney report on an attempt to replicate Becker's original study. Their research was based on interviews with 50 marijuana users, half of whom were college undergraduates. Although they found some support for Becker's model, they also noted some discrepancies.

It seems an historic truism that the presence of drugs or drug use within a given culture engenders controversy or public debate about the relationship of drugs to the larger social order (Braudel 1979). American culture is no exception. Within recent historical memory, our culture has both criminalized and decriminalized the production and use of alcoholic beverages. We currently are involved in a debate about drug use that ranges from those who

would declare a war on the traffickers and users of materials deemed illicit, to the suggestion that drug use generally should be decriminalized (Ridding 1989; Keer 1988).

Historically, sociologists (and other social scientists) have contributed to the debate surrounding drug use. This is done not by choosing sides, but rather by providing interested parties with explorations of the relationship between social context and drug use (Conforti 1989; Yamaguchi and Kandel 1985; Seeman and Anderson 1983; Radosevich 1979; Alexander 1963). This includes understandings of how drug use is related to cultural belief systems (Room 1976; Mulford and Miller 1959), typologies of drug users (Bloomquist 1971), and conceptualizations of drug addiction (McAuliffe and Gorden 1974; Ray 1964).

In the field of sociology, the work of Howard S. Becker stands out as both the touchstone of sociologically inspired drug research (Becker 1953) and the work responsible for the development of what has come to be known as labelling theory in the study of deviance (Becker 1973, 1964). In part, Becker's work has remained relevant because of the enduring nature of the drug debate itself. Questions of individual predispositions to drug use/criminal behavior, challenged by Becker as early as 1953, have re-emerged as behavioral explanations today (e.g., Walters and White 1989). In addition, Becker's thesis that an understanding of marijuana use could be obtained by approaching the drug as an object from which individuals learn to derive pleasure is itself worthy of re-examination. The utility of such a conception is likely to extend beyond the use of marijuana to drugs such as cocaine and crack.

It is because of the explanatory power of Becker's initial approach and the needs of policy makers/drug counselors today that a re-examination of Becker's work is warranted. In doing such a re-examination, the authors have chosen as their vehicle a replication of Becker's original work. Though the value of replicative work has generally been noted (e.g., Denzin 1989; Schwartz and Jacobs 1979), attempts at replication are particularly important (and rarely attempted) when dealing with contextual models (given the fluidity of contextual reality). In what follows, recent efforts to corroborate Becker's work will be discussed. General points of confirmation will be noted, as well as extensions of his original work, reasons for these extensions, and suggestions for further research.

Method

In Becker's original research (1953), the snowball-sampling method was utilized as the means of obtaining 50 marijuana users willing to be interviewed. Snowball sampling, noted for its strength in penetrating relatively closed populations and its utility in network analysis but not for yielding representative samples (True 1989), yielded a mixed demographic sample in Becker's work. (His sample was somewhat heavily weighted toward musicians who made up approximately 112 of the subjects. In a recent phone interview Becker reported not having kept any more detailed information about his sample than what is reported above). Site selection, determined by Becker's Chicago residency, was not stated as a methodological issue in the original research.

Becker's interviews were conducted informally, with no set questionnaire format being utilized. Interviewees were asked general questions by Becker regarding their initiation to and use of the drug. They were not directed toward any specifics by Becker, as he took notes of their commentary (Becker's recollection in a recent phone interview). It is from such an informal conversational style that Becker gathered his data, and it is upon this data that Becker bases his stage theory/typology of users.

Like Becker's, our research is based upon data gathered from 50 marijuana users. Also, like Becker's, our respondents were obtained through the use of the snowball-sample method. However, whereas Becker's respondents were all derived within one municipal area (Chicago), our respondents are split between two municipal areas, Milwaukee and the Fox River Valley in Wisconsin (the respective homes of the authors).

Demographically, more information is available regarding our respondents than for Becker's. In comparison to Becker's sample, in which musicians account for 50 percent of the sample, 50 percent of our sample is made up of undergraduate students from both metropolitan areas. The remaining 25 respondents come from a wide range of social positions which include house painters, mechanics, nurses, lawyers, teachers, and middle managers. Respondents in our sample ranged in age from 18 to 44 and included 32 men and 18 women. All of our respondents were of European descent.

The greatest methodological difference between Becker's work and our own is in the interview process itself. Whereas Becker's interview process was informal in nature, we took a number of set questions into the interview. Our questions, drawn from the discussions reported by Becker, were designed to yield data similar to that which he obtained (Becker 1953, 1973). Thus, whereas Becker abstracts a "becoming-a-user pattern" from his informal interviews, we specifically questioned respondents about their earliest contacts with the drug and asked them to reconstruct chronologically their relationship to the drug. Such reconstruction was to include both behavioral and attitudinal aspects, and when such information was not forthcoming in a given interview, respondents were specifically asked to fill in omissions, if possible.

Within the format of this more formal interview procedure, several questions were included with the hope of extending Becker's original work. One advantage of replicative research in this instance was the possibility of asking questions designed to extend the research in the direction where deficiencies in the original work were suspected. In this case we questioned Becker's "becoming-a-user" pattern for what we perceived as its neglect of the period of time which preceded the point of an individual's stated willingness to try the drug. Other questions were asked about projections toward future use on the part of reporting individuals, fears they associated with the use of the drug, opinions on legalization, etc. This was information absent from Becker's original work, yet deemed of interest by our research team.

Results

Becker's Path to Pleasurable Usage and Stages of Marijuana Use

Becker's original work (1953) surrounds his belief that the use of marijuana could be constructively approached, if the drug itself was conceived of as an object from which pleasure could be derived. Unless an individual develops "a conception of the drug as an object which could be used for pleasure . . . marijuana use was considered meaningless and did not continue" (Becker 1953). Beginning his life histories of marijuana use with individuals at a "point of willingness to use the drug," Becker outlines a three-stage process through which individuals obtain a conception of the drug as an object from which pleasure may be derived. This process includes: 1) learning a technique which supplies "sufficient dosage for the effects of the drug to appear"; 2) both experiencing and recognizing the effects of the drug; and 3) learning to enjoy the effects (Becker 1953). In addition, Becker notes that, at each juncture on the way toward pleasurable use of the drug, the initiate is aided by and dependent upon the guidance of others.

In subsequent discussions of the same data, Becker (1973) utilizes the concept "career" as a way to understand behavioral patterns related to marijuana use. For Becker, a behavioral career is a ". . . sequence of movements (on the part of the individual) from one position to another" within the social milieu (Becker 1973). Here, focusing on the individual, Becker constructs a three-stage model to describe the changes an individual goes through on the path to becoming a bona fide user of the drug (Figure 1). His stages include: 1) the beginner, a person involved in initial encounters with the drug (the stage within which the above three steps are subsumed); 2) the occasional user, one whose drug use is sporadic or determined by chance; and 3) the regular user, one whose systematic (daily) use has led him or her to procure personal supplies of the drug [it is important to note that Becker views stages 1 and 2 as transitional, stage 3 seemingly the only stable use pattern] (Becker 1973).

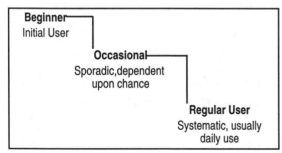

Figure 1*
*Our construction

Verification of Becker's Path and Stages of Marijuana Use

Whereas Becker begins his life histories "with the person having arrived at the point of willingness to try marijuana" (Becker 1953), we have included in our life histories the orientations individuals had to the drug before an opportunity to use the drug arose in their life. Our logic for doing so is as follows: as it seems unlikely that those who "arrived at the point of willingness to try marijuana" have reached that point by the same path, it should be of interest to those studying drug-use patterns how different people "arrive" at this same point of willingness.

Preconceptions of the Drug

One half of our respondents held what may be considered negative preconceptions about the drug, the remaining one half being split between those with neutral preconceptions (37 percent) and positive preconceptions (13 percent). Among those holding negative positions were those who recounted anti-drug instruction, knowledge of family members who had varying drug problems, and those who associated the use of marijuana with the socially undesirable. Among those holding neutral positions were those who had no real knowledge of the drug (positive or negative reports), those who held some intellectual curiosity regarding its use, and those who saw it as relatively harmless, equating its use with the use of tobacco and/or alcohol. Among those holding positive views of the drug were those who thought it was "cool" to smoke the drug, had hearsay evidence regarding its "enjoyable" effects, and had early in their lives seen people enjoying themselves with the drug.

Becoming Willing to Use the Drug

How individuals come to be willing to use the drug of course varies with their original preconceptions. For those who were positively oriented to the drug, a willingness to experiment already existed; they lacked only the opportunity. For those with neutral orientations to the drug, "willingness to use the drug" per se often didn't develop. Instead, opportunities to try the drug arose (most often in situations where peers or siblings were using it) and respondents found themselves trying the drug without any forethought regarding its use. Those with negative preconceptions went through the greatest changes on their way toward a willingness to try the drug. Among this group, two avenues were associated with the change in their orientations to the drug. For some, willingness first appeared after encounters with others who commanded their respect and who either used the drug in front of them or discussed its use with them. For others, a willingness to use the drug arose as part of a more general movement away from an unquestioned willingness to uphold the status quo.

First Encounters

All of the respondents in our study reported first-use encounters as having involved other individuals closely associated with and important to their day-to-day life activities. Of those cited as involved in initiations were close friends, boyfriends or girlfriends, family members [siblings and cousins (one person reported smoking with her mother sometime after her initial use)], classmates, and roommates. Initiation gatherings ranged from experimentation with only one other present, to contexts of larger social groupings, here parties being most often cited. It is important to note that none of our respondents spoke of initially using the drug while alone or alone with a stranger or group of strangers.

The Path to the Pleasurable Usage of Marijuana

Our respondents generally corroborate Becker's description of the elements making up the path toward the pleasurable usage of marijuana (as well as the importance others play in learning the proper use of the drug, recognition of its effects, and their enjoyment of the effects). Our research suggests that Becker's three-step presentation is simplistic. There is much to be learned by more closely examining the variance that exists between individual paths to pleasurable usage.

Experiences on the way toward pleasurable use of the drug vary a great deal. There are those who get high, perceive that they are high, and enjoy the high the first time they smoke; and those that smoke 30-40 times over the course of 2-3-year period before they get high for the first time. Although Becker (1953) states that "(T)he novice does not ordinarily get high the first time he smokes marijuana . . ." we found that 34 percent of our respondents reported getting high the first time they used the drug. The majority of these reported favorable encounters (although two reported the ill effects of nausea and vomiting; there were a few neutral reactions reported as well). An additional 32 percent reported getting high after the first 2-3 attempts, 30

percent after several attempts and the remaining 6 percent after 30-40 uses.

Our respondents' reasons for continued experimentation with the drug after the initial encounter varied in relation to the results of the first experience and the original reasons for their use of the drug. Others did not get high the first time and defined the feeling of "being high" enjoyable. An attempt to recreate that state was motivation enough to try the drug again, for those who did not get high the first time, as well as those who got high but had neutral or negative reactions. When their original willingness to try the drug was associated with a positive motivation toward its use (including those whose original preconception had been negative), this motivation continued even after the failure of the first attempt. Most had anticipated the possibility of "not getting high" their first attempt. Among this group, second and third attempts at using the drug tended to be more deliberately planned and executed than were their initial attempts. One respondent continued his experimentation by stealing small amounts of the drug from his parents' supply.

Such planned attempts by the above group were in sharp contrast to those who had neutral orientations to the drug at the time of its first use. For this group, later attempts at "getting high" proved to be much more passive and haphazard. Whereas the above mentioned group had been more likely to seek out the drug after their initial use, further experimentation by this latter group was often as unexpected as was their initial use. However, regardless of original motivations and results of initial use, once an individual's own experience with the drug proved to be favorable, continued use was predicated on the desire to re-experience pleasurable sensations.

Career Patterns of Use

In our attempt to corroborate this part of Becker's work, our respondents were asked to reconstruct chronologically their relationship to the drug, beginning with their preconceptions and moving to present use. In comparing Becker's model to our information, we find that his model is somewhat descriptive of the behavioral transitions experienced by individuals experimenting with the drug's use. As it now stands, however, his model is both sequentially incomplete and conceptually limited. Conceptual limitations become evident, as we attempt to place our respondents into his classification system.

The first sequential limitation is the most obvious; we have already discussed its absence. This is Becker's exclusion of a stage, wherein individuals develop a willingness to experiment with the drug. Given its importance to an understanding of drug use, the addition of an orientation stage to Becker's model seems to be reasonable.

Other sequential limitations, blurred with the model's conceptual limitations, become evident when we look beyond the beginner stage and attempt to place respondents into the occasional and regular use categories. Becker's criteria for placement . . . occasional use being chance usage and regular use being systematic usage with self-procuring behaviors . . . makes it difficult to place those whose occasional use is at times systematic (e.g., attending parties hoping the drug will be available), and those whose regular use is at times augmented by chance occurrence (e.g., a weekend user who happens to smoke during the week, if confronted with an unexpected opportunity). We must also ask if it is meaningful to extend the regular use category from those who systematically procure and use the drug 2-4 times per month or year to those whose systematic procurement translates into a daily use frequency of 4-9 times. Would it be at all meaningful to create an abuse/addiction category to deal with those whose use may be self-defined as problematic? If so, how would we place such a category into the current model? Also, though Becker's work suggests that both the beginner and the occasional use categories are transitional stages, the majority of our respondents seem to have maintained a use pattern which falls in between his occasional and regular use categories. How do we account for such non-transition within his framework?

It is at this point in our attempt to replicate Becker's work that we are faced with our greatest challenge. If we stay with Becker's model, we find that we are unable to categorize individuals who consider themselves to be drug abusers, who have quit using the drug, who have never used the drug and are orienting toward its use (or not orienting toward its use, for that matter), or whose patterns fall between his occasional and regular use categories. If we respond to these limitations by constructing a typology of present career use patterns, an approach that would allow for the classification of all respondents, we risk losing the temporal progression of the original model.

Discussion

A comparison of our work with Becker's reveals a general corroboration of his thesis, i.e., the utility of understanding marijuana as an object from which individuals learn to derive pleasure, as well as points of contention regarding the process through which individuals learn to derive enjoyment from the drug, and regarding his typology/stage theory of drug use patterns. We will begin our discussion with points of contention, move to points of confirmation, and conclude with suggestions regarding the direction of future research.

Points of Contention

As noted above, in his analysis of the data, Becker derives a three-step process through which individuals learn to derive pleasure from the use of marijuana. Our research leads us to question the reliability of Becker's description of this process for, as we note above, a large percentage of our respondents reported both getting high and enjoying the high at the time of their first use. As we look to explain the discrepancy between the two studies, several factors come to our attention, all of which relate to the time lapse between the original work and our replicative efforts.

First, we must recognize the existence of both the availability of technologies specifically designed to increase the drug dosage an individual is able to take in a single encounter and the availability of more powerful strains of the plant marijuana. Both the technologies for the smoking of the drug and the nature of the drug being smoked have increased the likelihood that an individual's first encounter will result in the presence of the drug's effects.

In addition to the above changes, cultural attitudes have changed to the extent that first encounters themselves may have taken place in settings that were less clandestine or anxiety-provoking than was true of the time Becker did his research. It is likely that all of these factors taken together have changed first encounters to such an extent that we may no longer rely on Becker's model to understand the reality of initial encounters.

Our next departure from Becker's work is more critical and relates to the utility of his typology/stage theory of use patterns. As noted above, Becker's typology (Figure 1) suggests that those who come to enjoy the effects of the drug progress in their use of the drug to the point of regular use. The suggestion that all marijuana smokers are or will become regular (daily) users of the drug is not corroborated by the information provided by our informants, many of whom have used the drug for years but do not fit into his regular use category. It is possible that marijuana users in Becker's time all progressed to regular use of the drug, but we find this to be unlikely. Instead, we believe it is time to abandon Becker's model altogether and consider a more recent alternative offered by Van Dijk (1972).

Van Dijk's model (Figure 2) begins with initial contact with the drug and moves through three possible stages, experimentalism, integrated use, and excessive use, toward the possibility of addiction. The advantages of such a model over Becker's relates both to the inclusion of the stated possibility of an addictive use category (the initial three categories here being equated to Becker's three stages in order) but also the possibility of stabilized intermediate use patterns. In addition, Van Dijk's model explicitly allows for the return to earlier patterns of drug use, as well as the discontinuing of drug use at any stage.

Though such a model of use is superior to Becker's in terms of its explanatory power, both models neglect that stage prior to first contact with the drug which has been pointed to in our research of user's preconceptions. If we were to amend Van Dijk's model to include such a stage (Figure 3), we would have a model which not only allows us to place all of our respondents within stated categories, but would also allow us to visualize how preconceptions influence the continuation of experimentation after initial contact with the drug.

Points of Convergence

The major point of convergence between Becker's work and our own lies in our belief in the utility of approaching marijuana as an object from which individuals must learn to derive pleasure, before drug use behavior will be evidenced. It is in the reconstruction of our respondents' relationships to the drug that we are able to gain an understanding of the motivations which led both to initial experimentation with the drug and subsequent or continued use. The explanatory power of such an approach derives from the focus upon the interactive environment, within which individuals learn to use and enjoy the drug. Such a focus argues against, then and now, theoretical positions which seek to explain drug use by positing predispositions toward drug use/criminal behavior in the individuals themselves.

Directions of Future Research

Though our review of Becker's work is not without criticisms, we believe his work has raised questions that need to be answered. First, his structural/interactive approach to understanding marijuana use does point to the normative components of the learning situation which influence drug use. What Becker does not address (nor do we in this work) is the way in which other individuals, in similar situations to those who become marijuana users, do not become users themselves. If the structural/interactive model is to gain in the power of explanation, we must be willing to explore the life worlds of both the user as well as the non-user, in an attempt to understand the move-

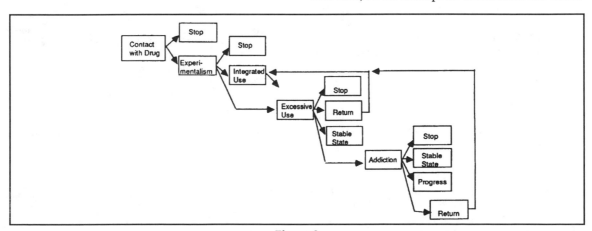

Figure 2

Van Dijk's Model

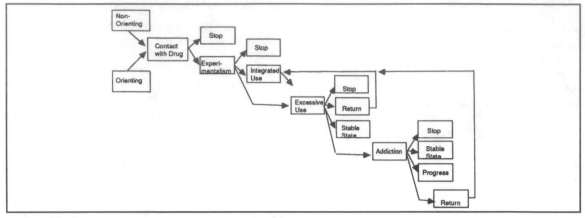

Figure 3

Revised Model

ment of some toward drug use and the continued non-use on the part of others.

Second, we believe that there is great utility in the manner of research Becker began and we have continued. We believe much could be learned, if we expanded our study of drug use by undertaking similar research of other drugs, both legal (e.g., alcohol and tobacco) and illegal (e.g., crack, cocaine, LSD, etc.). Though we may assume similar "becoming-user" patterns will hold for all drugs, differences may exist between them as well. In any event, much may be gained by just such a comparison.

Finally, we believe much could be gained by cross-cultural studies of drug use as well. In particular, it would be of interest to study the differences in drug use experience between cultures which hold the same drug to be licit and illicit. Such comparisons may yield information regarding the role cultural norms play in the regulation of drug use and, perhaps, the control of drug effects.

Conclusion

There is no doubt that Becker's work will continue to serve as a benchmark for those generally interested in drug use. Our attempt to replicate his work was motivated both by a desire to venerate an old master and a desire to continue to improve our stock of knowledge regarding drug use. In the comparative dialogue created by our replicative attempt, we have noted cultural changes that contributed to the variance between our respective results, attempted to correct what we believe to have been inadequacies in the original work, and also raised

questions which go beyond the scope of this research.

* * *

Michael L. Hirsch, Randall W. Conforti, and Carolyn J. Graney, "The Use of Marijuana for Pleasure: A Replication of Howard S. Becker's Study of Marijuana Use," Handbook of Replication Research. Copyright © 1990 by Select Press. All rights reserved. Reprinted by permission.

For Discussion

Hirsch and his colleagues expand upon Becker's theory of marijuana use. To what extent can their theory apply to other drug use?

References

Alexander, C. N., Jr. (1963). Consensus of mutual attraction in natural cliques: A study of adolescent drinkers. *The American Journal of Sociology 69*, 395-403.

Becker, H. S. (1953). Becoming a marijuana user. *The American Journal of Sociology 59*, 235-242.

Becker, H. S. (1964). *The other side*. London: The Free Press.

Becker, H. S. (1973). *Outsiders: Studies in the sociology of deviance*. New York: The Free Press.

Bloomquist, E. R. (1971). *Marijuana: The second trip*. Beverly Hills: Glencoe Press.

Braudel, F. (1981). *The structures of everyday life (Vol 1)*. New York: Harper and Row.

Conforti, R. W., and Hirsch, M. L., Graney, C. (1989). *The use of marijuana for pleasure*. Conference paper, Spring 1990 Midwest Sociology Convention. Denzin, N. K. (1989). *The research act*. Englewood Cliffs: Prentice-Hall.

Keer, P. (1988). The unspeakable is debated: Should drugs be legalized? *The New York Times*.

McAuliffe, W. E., and Gorden, R. (1974). A test of Lindesmith's theory of addiction: The frequency of euphoria among long-term addicts. *American Journal of Sociology 79*, 795-801.

Mulford, H., and Miller, D. (1959). Drinking behavior related to definitions of alcohol: A report of research in progress. *American Sociological Review 24*, 385-389.

Radosevich, M., Lanza-Kaduce, L., Akers, R. L., Krohn, M. D., et al. (1979). The sociology of adolescent drug and drinking behavior: A review of the state of the field. *Deviant Behavior 1*, 15-35.

Ray, M. B. (1964). The cycle of abstinence and relapse among heroin addicts. In H. S. Becker (ed.), *The other side* (pp. 163-178). London: The Free Press.

Ridding, A. (1989). Western panel is asking end to all curbs on drug traffic. *The New York Times.*

Room, R. (1976). Ambivalence as a sociological explanation: The case of cultural explanations of alcohol problems. *American Sociological Review 41*, 1047-1062.

Schwartz, H., and Jacobs, J. (1979). *Qualitative sociology: A method to the madness.* New York: The Free Press.

Seeman, M., and Anderson, C. S. (1983). Alienation and alcohol: The role of work, mastery, and community in drinking behavior. *American Sociological Review 48*, 60-77.

True, J. A. (1989). *Finding out: Conducting and evaluating social research.* Belmont: Wadsworth.

Van Dijk, W. K. (1972). *Complexity of the dependence problem: Interaction of biological with psychogenic and sociogenic factors. Biochemical and pharmacological aspects of drug use.* Haarlem: DeErven F. Bohn.

Walters, G. D., and White, T. (1989). The thinking criminal: A cognitive model of lifestyle criminality. *Criminal Justice Research Bulletin 4*, 1-10.

Yamaguchi, K., and Kandel, D. B. (1985). On the resolution of role incompatibility: a life event history analysis of family roles and marijuana use. *American Journal of Sociology 90*, 1284-1293. ✦

Part II

Legal Drugs

A major element in the American drug scene is the use and abuse of *legal* drugs—alcohol, tobacco, prescription stimulants and sedatives, anabolic steroids, and other substances as well—as a response to boredom, frustration, stress, and loneliness; or, as in the case of steroids, for the enhancement of physical performance. Because these drugs are legal, they are potentially available to everyone. And because alcohol and tobacco are sold over the counter with few controls, their use is widespread.

Alcohol is the most widely used drug in the United States. More than 160 million Americans, ages 12 years and above, have used alcohol at some point in their lifetimes; some 132 million have had a drink in the past year; and just over 100 million have consumed alcohol in the past month. Moreover, the annual per capita consumption of adult Americans is 2.5 gallons of pure alcohol.

Although the majority of those who use alcohol are social-recreational drinkers, problem drinking is widespread. As indicated in Table 1, the costs of drinking are staggering—well in excess of $100 billion annually. Yet, in spite of these costs, alcohol remains something of a social enigma. On the one hand, it is the worst killer drug in the United States; it causes more havoc, violence, damage, and death than all other drugs combined—legal *and* illegal. But on the other hand, when used responsibly and in moderation, it can be a relatively safe and pleasant drug for the majority. In fact, there is evidence suggesting that when used regularly in small amounts, alcohol can even be healthful and reduce blood cholesterol.

The "problem" seems not to lie with alcohol *per se*, but with its misuse. Because alcohol is legal, it is readily available to anyone deemed to be of age. Moreover, alcohol has had numerous roles—social, medical, and religious—in human cultures around the globe for thousands of years. For these reasons,

many users fail to understand that it is a dangerous drug, with a high addiction potential and the prospect of severe physical harm through overuse.

Table 1
Estimated Costs of Alcohol Abuse in 1990

Core Costs in	$ Billions
Direct	
Treatment	15.70
Health support services	1.81
Indirect	
Mortality	21.17
Reduced productivity	76.48
Lost employment	6.20
Other Related Costs	
Direct	
Motor vehicle crashes (Injuries and damages)	3.15
Crime	3.07
Social welfare	0.06
Other	4.28
Indirect	
Victims of crime	0.23
Incarceration	3.48
Motor vehicle crashes (Lost employment)	0.68
TOTAL	**$136.26**

Source: *Substance Abuse Report*, June 15, 1991, p. 3.

While the use of alcohol in moderation may be beneficial to the body, such is not the case with tobacco. Consider the numbers:

- In 1994, there were 24 million male smokers in the United States—a decrease of 4.9 million since 1965.

- In 1994, there were 22.3 million female smokers in the United States, an increase of 1.2 million since 1965.

- Each year in the United States, there are approximately 419,000 tobacco-related deaths, the great majority of which are from cardiovascular disease and lung cancer. A significant number of these deaths are among non-smokers, the result of chronic inhalation of second-hand smoke.

- 80 percent of all smokers began smoking before age 20, the average age at 14.5 years.

Like alcohol, tobacco is something of a social enigma. Cigarette smoking is considered the most important preventable cause of death in the United States, yet cigarettes are one of the most heavily advertised products. Cigarette advertising themes typically associate smoking with high-style living; healthy activities; and economic, social, and professional success. And interestingly, cigarette advertising campaigns increasingly target women, minorities, and blue-collar workers—groups that account for an increasing proportion of the cigarette-smoking population.

If cigarettes were outlawed in the United States, there would be both costs and benefits. On the positive side:

- **Longer Lives.** There is strong evidence supporting links between smoking and heart disease, lung cancer, and a shortened life span. A ban could reduce human suffering and increase life and productivity.

- **Health-Care Savings.** Studies suggest that the billions of dollars now spent each year on smoking-related diseases could be saved.

- **Less Illness.** It is generally agreed that smokers are ill more often, and remain ill longer, than nonsmokers. A ban would reduce smoking-related absenteeism, saving companies billions of dollars each year.

- **Increased Productivity.** Without cigarette breaks, smokers would gain a month's work each year.

- **Fewer Fires.** The costs from smoking-related accidental fires are considerable—in lives, lost productivity, and property damage.

On the other hand, a ban on producing, manufacturing, using, and exporting tobacco products would have numerous costs for the U.S. economy:

- **Job Losses.** The jobs of the 47,000 workers employed by the nation's tobacco companies would be at risk.

- **Reduced Tax Revenues.** In 1993, cigarette taxes generated $11.9 billion in state and federal taxes. This revenue would vanish.

- **Reduced Exports.** Tobacco generates a $4-billion trade surplus which would be lost.

- **Farm Reductions.** Tobacco farming would disappear, and the potential for replacement crops is uncertain.

The outlawing of tobacco products is unlikely. It would be unworkable, and few Americans—smokers and nonsmokers alike—support the idea. In a 1994 *Time*/CNN poll, for example, 73 percent of the adult population (smokers and nonsmokers) felt that everyone should have the right to make his or her choice whether to smoke. Interestingly, however, in terms of smoking in the workplace, 95 percent felt that it should be banned, or at least limited to special smoking areas.

The use of prescription drugs present a range of other issues and problems, both medical and social. In the selections that follow, the focus is on alcohol, tobacco, tranquilizers, and anabolic steroids. ✦

5. A Brief History of Alcohol

Harvey A. Siegal

AND

James A. Inciardi

Alcohol has had an enduring history. In the following essay, Harvey A. Siegal and James A. Inciardi contemplate the likely origins of alcohol use and its early evolution. A number of interesting facts about alcohol are also examined, including the different kinds of alcohol, the meanings of "proof" and "blood alcohol content," and how alcohol affects the body.

The desire to temporarily alter how our minds process the information brought by our senses is perhaps one of the oldest and most pervasive of humanity's wishes. In fact, some researchers have suggested that the need to do so is as powerful and permanent as the in-born drives of self preservation, hunger, and security (Weil, 1972). In its pursuit, people have, at various times and in various places subjected their bodies to beatings and mutilation, starvation and sensory deprivation; they have focused their minds solely on a single object, or let consciousness expand without direction; and they have often pursued a more direct route, changing the brain's chemistry by ingesting a chemical substance. Of all of these, the chemical that has probably been used by more of the earth's people in more places and times is one of the by-products of a simple organism's conversion of sugar and water into energy. It is ethanol, or beverage alcohol. Each year, countless millions of people experience, both positively and negatively, the effects of this domesticated drug we call alcohol.

More is known about alcohol than any other drug; yet, it staggers the imagination about how much more there remains to learn. Our experiences with this most familiar and comfortable of drugs could readily constitute a social history of civilization. We've lauded and vilified it. We've brought it into our most important religious rituals and have included it as part of our significant rites-of-passage. Conversely, we've discouraged its use; even prohibited its manufacture and sale by constitutional amendment. Wars have been fought over it and underworld empires have been built on the proceeds from its sales. It's been acclaimed as having the power to comfort and cure and is held responsible for thousands of deaths each year, billions of dollars in losses, and an incalculable amount of human suffering. All of us, in some way, have been touched or influenced by this drug, so let's take a brief look at its history.

Early History

Like many significant inventions, the specifics of alcohol's discovery is not known. We conjecture that it likely occurred during the neolithic age. Perhaps someone left wild berries, fruit, or even grapes in a vessel for a few days. When they returned, airborne yeasts had already begun fermenting the mixture. The result—which we call "wine"—undoubtedly proved to be more interesting and enjoyable than the original fruit, and, like other innovations, it did not take people long to improve their invention.

As people settled into communities and began cultivating plants and domesticating animals instead of just simply hunting and gathering their food, they found that a surplus often ensued. Surplus grains could also be fermented once the starch in them—which by itself would not ferment—could be rendered into sugar. To accomplish this, as is still done in parts of the world today, these early agriculturists found that chewing the grain somehow changes it into a fermentable mixture. We know now that the chemical responsible for this transformation—ptyalin—is found naturally in saliva. Other societies discovered that by allowing the grain to germinate, then roasting the new shoots, the fermentation process could be initiated. In this way, the beverage we know as "beer" came into being. People discovered that not only fruits, berries, and grains could be used to produce alcohol, but leaves, tubers, flowers, cacti, and even honey could be fermented as well.

These early concoctions (roughly designated as wines or beers), however, were limited in their alcoholic strength. As yeasts metabolize the sugar, carbon dioxide (which is what makes bread rise, wine bubble, or gives beer a head) and alcohol are released as by-products. When the alcoholic content of the mixture exceeded 11 percent or 12 percent the process slowed markedly as it approached 14 percent, the yeasts were rendered inactive (i.e., killed), and the process of fermentation stopped entirely. In addition to the limitation imposed by the biology of the yeasts, the alcoholic content could be affected by the producers themselves. For example, including more sugar (or fermentable material) would increase the amount of alcohol that would be produced. Whether the producers were willing to allow the yeasts the time necessary to complete the fermentation process or were too eager to consume the brew to wait, this influenced its alcohol content.

It was not until the time of the Crusades that Europeans were able to consume alcoholic beverages more potent than beer or wine. The Crusaders returned from the Holy Lands having learned a process known as distillation. To distill wine, it first would be heated. Because alcohol has a lower boiling point than water, it would vaporize first. Then, as this vapor cooled, it condensed back into liquid form. This distillate made a considerably more potent beverage. In fact, beverages of quadruple potency now became possible. These were known as "distilled spirits" or "liquors", referring to the essence of the wine.

Aqua Vitae—The Water of Life

What is this drug which has been called by some the "water of life"—*aqua vitae*, in scholastic Latin, or *ambrosia*, the nectar of the gods—and "the corruptor of youth" and the "devil's own brew" by others? Ethyl alcohol or ethanol (whose chemical formula is C_2H_5OH) is a clear, colorless liquid with little odor but a powerful burning taste. Ethanol is just one of many alcohols such as methyl (wood) and isopropyl (rubbing) alcohol. All others are poisonous and cannot be metabolized by the body.

In addition to ethanol and water, alcoholic beverages generally contain minute amounts of substances referred to as "congeners." Many of these chemicals are important to the flavor, appearance, and aroma of the beverage. Brandy, for example, is relatively rich in congeners while vodka contains relatively few.

Alcoholic beverages differ in strength. Beer generally has an alcoholic content of 5 percent; malt liquors are slightly higher. Natural wine varies in alcoholic content between 6 percent and 14 percent. Fortified wines—i.e., those that have had additional alcohol added—contain between 17 percent and 20 percent alcohol. Liquor or spirits contain approximately 40 percent ethanol. The common designation of "proof" originated centuries ago in Britain as a test for the potency of a beverage. To accomplish this test, if gun powder saturated with alcohol burned upon ignition, this was taken as "proof" that the liquor was more than half pure alcohol. In the United States, proof is calculated as being roughly twice the proportion of ethanol by unit volume of beverage; for example, an 86-proof Scotch is 43 percent alcohol.

Although the relative strengths of the beverages differ, current standard portions that are consumed actually provide the same amount of ethanol to drinker. For example, the same quantity of alcohol is consumed if someone drinks either a 12-ounce can or bottle of beer, a three- to four-ounce glass of wine, or a mixed drink made with one and one-half ounces (i.e., one shot) of distilled spirits. Thus, the claim that "I don't drink much alcohol, but I do drink a lot of beer" is simply not true.

Alcohol's Effects

Unlike most other foods, alcohol is absorbed directly into the blood stream without digestion. A small amount passes directly through the stomach lining itself; most, however, progresses on to the small intestine where it is almost entirely absorbed. The feeling of warmth that one experiences after taking a drink results from the irritating effect that alcohol has on the tissues of the mouth, esophagus (food-tube), and stomach. Alcohol does not become intoxicating until the blood carrying it reaches the brain. The rapidity with which this occurs is in large measure determined by the condition of the stomach. An empty stomach will facilitate the absorption of the alcohol, while a full stomach retards it. To some degree, the type of beverage consumed has an effect on absorption, as well. Beer, for example, contains food substances which tend to retard this absorption. Drinks which are noticeably carbonated—such as champagne—seem to "quickly go to one's head," since the carbon dioxide facilitates the passage of alcohol from the stomach to the small intestine.

Alcohol is held in the tissues of the body before it is broken down (i.e., metabolized), like any other food or chemical substance. The body metabolizes alcohol at a steady rate, with the individual being able to exercise virtually no control over the process. Therefore, a healthy man who weighs approximately 160 pounds, drinking no more than three-fourths of an ounce of distilled spirits every hour could consume more than a pint in a day's time without experiencing any marked intoxication. If the same quantity was consumed over an hour or two, however, the person would be very drunk. Today, much research is directed at finding an "anti-

A Brief History of Alcohol 47

dote" for alcohol: a chemical that would either break down the alcohol itself, or accelerate the body's metabolic process. Although several promising lines of research are underway, it will likely be many years before something is commercially available. Finally, the belief that black coffee (i.e., caffeine) is an "antidote" is without fact. What the caffeine does do, however, is to stimulate the drinker—the intoxicated person is still "drunk," but he or she may, after several cups of black coffee, feel more awake.

Ethanol is broken down (metabolized) by the liver. In experiments, animals have had their livers removed, and then were given ethyl alcohol. The alcohol remained, much like wood (methyl) alcohol, in their bodies without being metabolized and exhibited the toxic effects—such as nerve damage—brought on by unpotable alcohols. How does this process work? The liver produces and holds the enzymes responsible for alcohol metabolism. Once in the liver, alcohol combines with its enzymes. Alcohol is initially transformed into acetaldehyde, a chemical considerably more toxic than alcohol. Almost instantaneously, other enzymes convert the acetaldehyde into acetic acid (the same compound that constitutes vinegar), an essentially innocuous substance. The acetic acid is then further metabolized into carbon dioxide and water. Interestingly, one of the treatment strategies for managing alcoholism employs this metabolic process itself. In it, Disulfiram (Antabuse), a chemical which compromises the body's capacity to convert acetaldehyde to acetic acid is used as an adversive agent. By itself, Disulfiram has little effect on a patient who takes a daily dose of it. If alcohol is consumed while Disulfiram remains in the body, the produced acetaldehyde collects quickly, much to the great discomfort of the drinker. The patient is warned of this unpleasant effect, and the consequent fear of it can help increase his or her motivation to abstain from alcohol.

Alcohol does have some nutritional value. The primitive brews and concoctions were probably richer in nutritional value, especially carbohydrates, vitamins, and minerals than the highly refined beverages we consume today. Alcohol itself is a rich source of calories which are converted into energy and heat. An ounce of whiskey, for example, provides approximately 75 calories, the equivalent of a potato, an ear of corn, a slice of dark bread, or a serving of pasta. The caloric content of mixed drinks is greater, since the sweeteners of the mixer

provides additional calories. These extra calories are, of course, fattening, if the drinker does not reduce his or her intake of other foods.

The fact that alcohol provides sufficient calories for subsistence provides an additional health hazard. Many heavy drinkers express a preference to "drink their meals." While alcohol does provide calories, other nutrients, such as proteins, vitamins, and minerals vital to health and well being, are entirely lacking. These heavy drinkers often suffer from chronic malnutrition and vitamin-deficiency diseases. In fact, adult malnutrition apart from heavy drinking is extremely rare in the United States.

Alcohol exerts its most profound effects on the brain. The observable behavior produced by drinking is as much a result of the social situation in which a person drinks as it is the drinker's mood and expectations about what the drinking will do and the actual quantity of alcohol consumed. For example, after drinking the identical quantity and type of beverage one might experience euphoria or depression, while another may feel full of energy or simply wish to sleep; or a drink found initially stimulating might encourage sleep. Pharmacologically, alcohol is a central nervous system depressant drug. Currently, neuro-scientists are studying the operation of specific bio-chemical mechanisms, but some research has suggested that alcohol acts most directly on those portions of the brain which control sleep and wakefulness.

The amount of alcohol within a person is conventionally described as Blood Alcohol Content (B.A.C.). This measures the proportion of alcohol that might be found within an individual's bloodstream and can be assessed by analyzing body substances such as blood, breath, or urine. Although, as we mentioned, the effects vary by both drinking situation and the experience that the drinker has had, we can roughly expect to see some of the following occur. After two or three drinks in a short period of time, a person of about 160 lbs. will begin to feel the effects of the drug. These include feelings of euphoria, freeing of inhibitions, and perhaps impaired judgment. Such a person would have an approximate B.A.C. of 0.04 percent.

If our subject has another three drinks in a short period, his or her B.A.C. will elevate to around 0.1 percent. Now, besides affecting the higher centers of thought and judgment located in the cerebral cortex, the alcohol is beginning to act on the lower (more basic) motor areas of the brain. By law, in virtually all the states, this person would now be judged incapable of operating a motor vehicle and, if caught doing so, would be charged with Driving Under the Influence (DUI). The person would have some difficulty walking and appear to lurch somewhat; there would be noticeable decline in activities requiring fine hand-eye coordination; and one's speech would be somewhat slurred.

At higher concentrations of alcohol from 0.2 percent BAC and up (resulting from the consumption of at least 10 ounces of spirits), more of the central nervous system is affected. The drinker has difficulty coordinating even the simplest of movements and may need assistance to even walk. Emotionally, he or she appears very unstable and readily changes from rage to tears and then back again. At 0.40 percent to 0.50 percent BAC, alcohol depresses enough of the central nervous system's functions that the drinker may lapse into a coma. At concentrations of 0.60 percent BAC and above, the most basic centers of the brain—those that govern respiration—are so suppressed that death may occur.

Alcohol and Health

Abusive drinking has a profoundly negative influence on virtually every one of the body's organ systems. This negative impact occurs directly through the irritating and inflaming properties the drug has, and indirectly as an effect of alcohol's metabolism by the liver. Further, like many other drugs, tolerance (both physiologic and psychologic) to alcohol occurs. As such, one needs to drink more to achieve the desired effects. Naturally, the more one drinks, the greater the (potential and actual) damage caused by alcohol.

Alcohol irritates the lining of the stomach, which in turn causes an increase in the amount of gastric juices secreted. These irritate, inflame, and ultimately can chemically abrade the stomach's lining, causing ulcers. Alcohol can damage the small intestine itself, compromising the organ's ability to absorb nutrients, especially vitamins. Other organs that are involved in the digestive process, such as the pancreas, are damaged as well; adult-onset diabetes is typically linked to abusive drinking.

Since the liver is responsible for metabolizing the alcohol consumed, it is this organ which is most affected. Not only is the liver abused by the irritating and inflaming properties of alcohol, but, as it metabolizes the drug, proteins broadly described as "free fatty acids" are released. These settle throughout the liver and other internal organs, ultimately compromising their function by blocking blood and other vessels. The livers of alcohol abusers are characterized by fatty deposits, dead and dying tissues, and evidence of scarring. Ultimately, the organ may be so compromised that it fails entirely, and death follows.

While there is support for the notion that very moderate alcoholic consumption—i.e., never more than two glasses of wine a day—has healthful benefits, heavy drinkers have increased rates of cardiovascular problems. Heart disease is more prevalent among this group—who are more likely to be heavy cigarette smokers as well—than the general population.

Chronic abuse of alcohol can have disastrous effects on the central nervous system. Alcohol is a tolerance producing and ultimately addicting drug. For the addicted person, withdrawal distress can be life threatening. Longer term, permanent damage can include dementia, profound memory loss, the inability to learn, and impaired balance and coordination. Alcoholic people have higher rates of depression, suicide, and evidence of other mental illnesses.

Alcohol abuse is linked with automobile accidents, especially among adolescents. It is estimated that almost one-half of fatal crashes involve drinking. Other accidents, drownings, burns, and trauma are strongly associated with drinking. Drinking has been associated with violence, especially domestic violence and child abuse. Finally, when consumed by a pregnant woman, alcohol can cause profound damage to the fetus. Babies born suffering from fetal alcohol syndrome are less likely to survive, more likely to fail to thrive and manifest both physiologic and psychologic developmental problems.

Alcohol, humanity's oldest domesticated drug, is also one of its greatest enemies. In the United States, we estimate that there are almost 10 million alcohol dependent or alcoholic people and perhaps twice that proportion of "problem drinkers." We estimate that each year alcohol abuse costs our nation well in excess of one hundred billion dollars in terms of loss, health care, and decreased productivity. We do pay a large personal and societal price for this chemical comfort.

A Note on the Social History of Alcohol In the United States

Most societies have used alcohol medicinally, ritually, or recreationally. Colonial America was no exception. Beer and wine were made and universally consumed. Distilling grain into "ardent spirits" as a way of promoting the production, storage, and shipment of agricultural products was encouraged. Drunkenness seldom occurred in public and was reportedly not widespread. As the country moved from colonial to revolutionary America, the scene changed; towns grew and social-control mechanisms became more formal. Intoxication was reviled, and drunkenness was defined as a private weakness and a social ill. Thus, America's "drinking problem" began to emerge.

Shortly thereafter, the beginnings of a temperance movement appeared. Initially dominated by a New England aristocracy interested in maintaining the old social order, the movement was concerned about alcohol use at all levels of society. Calvinist temperance preachers expressed fear of the common man who, with drink, spoke profanely, engaged in infidelities, and did not work as he should. By the 1830s, the temperance movement had lost its aristocratic air and became more egalitarian (and middle class) with the inclusion of Methodist, Baptist, and Presbyterian preachers. From the Civil War until the 1890s, the movement attempted to sell the virtues of the well-regulated middle-class life to the working and lower classes. The message was simple: remain sober, work hard, and become a member of the middle class (Gusfield 1962).

At the forefront of the temperance movement in the late 1890s was the Women's Christian Temperance Union (WCTU) and its dynamic leader, Frances Willard. While leading the WCTU in its crusade to abolish drink, she was simultaneously involved in a variety of progressive social reform movements, ranging from women's suffrage to the labor unions' right to strike, to calls for universal childhood education. The WCTU, along with the Anti-Saloon League and the Methodists' Board of Temperance, spearheaded the drive that led to the passage of the Eighteenth Amendment to the U.S. Constitution. When ratified in 1920, the amendment prohibited the manufacture, sale, and transportation of intoxicating liquors (Gusfield 1962).

Prohibition was deemed successful, at first. Hospital admissions related to alcohol consumption—liver disease—declined as many people practiced abstinence. Nevertheless, heavy drinkers continued to drink, and a newly created crime—bootlegging—emerged and took hold. In fact, it is generally conceded that American organized crime was born out of the era of prohibition. By the early 1930s, abstinence was no longer the social norm. A movement to repeal the Eighteenth Amendment grew. Supporters of the repeal argued that the Eighteenth Amendment violated personal liberties, was in fact unenforceable, and created crime (R. Howland and T. Howland 1978). The noble experiment came to an end on December 5, 1933, when the Twenty-first Amendment repealed the Eighteenth. Although prohibition resulted in fewer alcohol-related illnesses, it was a miserable failure in almost every other aspect. Hoping to restore a moral order to America, its chief contribution was to foster crime and support a profound disrespect for the law.

The lessons learned from alcohol are both valuable and complex. There is, simultaneously, great good and danger in psychoactive drugs. The challenge to us all lies in learning as much about them as we can. If we choose to imbibe, we should do so in a responsible manner that will not endanger the health and well being of others or ourselves.

* * *

Harvey A. Siegal and James A. Inciardi, "A Brief History of Alcohol." Copyright © 1995 by Roxbury Publishing. All rights reserved.

References

Gusfield, J. R. 1962. Status conflicts and the changing ideologies of the American temperance movement. In *Society, Culture, and Drinking Patterns*, D. J. Pittman and C. R. Snyder (eds.), New York: John Wiley and Sons.

Howland, R. W., and T. W. Howland. 1978. 200 years of drinking in the United States. In *Drinking: Alcohol and American Society—Issues and Current Research*, J. A. Ewing and B. A. Rouse (eds.), Chicago: Nelson-Hall.

Weil, A. 1972. *The Natural Mind*. Boston: Houghton Mifflin. ✦

6. Alcohol, Sex, and Aggression

Jack H. Mendelson

AND

Nancy K. Mello

Alcohol has been said to increase sexual desire and diminish sexual performance. Further, a relationship between alcohol and aggressive behavior has also been documented. For example, alcohol is often a factor in violent crime, such as rape and assault, and plays a major role in homicide.

In the this article, researchers Jack H. Mendelson and Nancy K. Mello consider how alcohol affects male fertility, sexual potency, and aggressive behavior. They report that alcohol lowers the level and production of testosterone which, in turn, affects sexual performance and indirectly impacts on fertility and sexual desire. The authors suggest that, because hormones represent the intervening factor in the relationship between alcohol and sex, hormones might also be an important factor in explaining aggression. Mendelson and Mello also review studies which demonstrate that levels of aggression and sexual arousal increase when people believe that they have imbibed alcohol, regardless of whether alcohol was ingested.

Science has yet to discover the essential biological mechanisms that regulate the most commonplace human drives and behaviors. For example, the intricate processes that control hunger and satiation remain an enigma, despite knowledge about the requirements for good nutrition. Sleep, once thought to be a necessary restorative for weariness and fatigue, is now believed also to serve a reprogramming and information storage function. The scientific study of sexual behavior is a very recent phenomenon, and systematic investigation of aggressive behavior is just beginning. Thus, it is not surprising that the relationships between alcohol use and sex and aggression are shrouded in folklore and ignorance.

Alcohol does affect both sex and aggression. There is increasing evidence that some facets of these behaviors are regulated by the same brain hormone systems. It is now possible to measure hormone levels and trace the pattern of episodic fluctuations. Many hormones are secreted in irregular pulses or surges. The frequency and amplitude of these hormonal pulses may change as a function of some external stimulus, such as alcohol, an erotic film, or an aggressive provocation. Changes in the secretory activity of one hormone are controlled by changes in other hormones, which in turn influence the activity of still other hormones. It is difficult to conceive of a more perfectly orchestrated, intricately balanced system than this symphony of neuroendocrine hormones. Examination of the co-variation between neuroendocrine hormones, sex and aggression, and how these patterns are modulated by alcohol may someday clarify these fundamental biological processes.

Alcohol and the Biology of Sex

Sophistication in neuroendocrinology is not one of the virtues commonly attributed to Shakespeare. Yet, less than a decade ago, Macbeth was one of two citations on alcohol effects on sexual function in a leading text on pharmacology. There has been a rapid expansion of knowledge in this area in the last few years, but Shakespeare's summary remains one of the most concise and accurate:

MacDuff: What three things does drink especially provoke?

Porter: Marry, sir, nose painting, sleep, and urine. Lechery, sir, it provokes and unprovokes. It provokes the desire, but takes away the performance: therefore, much drink may be said to be an equivocator with lechery; it makes him and it mars him; it sets him on and it takes him off; it persuades him and disheartens him; makes him stand to and not stand to; in conclusion, equivocates him in a sleep and, giving him the lie, leaves him.

[Macbeth, Act II, Scene 3]

This passage describes several commonly experienced effects of alcohol intoxication, which have a clear and predictable physiological basis. "Nose painting" refers to the enlargement and reddening of the nose that occurs in some alcohol abusers, and which cartoonists often use to depict the alcoholic. This reddening and enlargement is due to increased blood flow to the nose, as well as to the skin elsewhere on the body. The sensation of warmth after alcohol consumption reflects the increased blood flow to the skin. Paradoxically, this sensation of increased warmth is actually associated with a *loss* of body heat. As peripheral blood vessels dilate, the expanded surface area releases more heat, just as large windows lose more heat than small windows. Thus, although one may feel warmer after drinking, the actual heat loss may lower body temperature. This seldom-appreciated fact can be added to the list of perils of drinking alcohol to combat an Alaskan winter's night.

The porter's observation that alcohol provokes urine is familiar even to the occasional imbiber. Alcohol does not produce more urine as the result of increased fluid volume in the body; rather, alcohol suppresses the effects of a hormone that controls urine output from the kidneys. This hormone (vasopressin) is secreted by the pituitary gland in the brain. Under ordinary conditions, vasopressin inhibits excessive urine output (diuresis). However, when alcohol suppresses the urine inhibitor vasopressin, this leads to a concomitant increase in urine output. Curiously, alcohol inhibits vasopressin, only when blood alcohol levels are rising and not when blood alcohol levels are stable or falling.

Just as the ways in which alcohol affects peripheral blood flow and urination are complex upon close examination, so too is the effect of alcohol on sex. The porter's comment succinctly summarizes alcohol's almost contradictory effects on sexual behavior. How does alcohol act to increase sexual desire but diminish sexual performance in males? The same brain structures that regulate peripheral blood flow and control urine-volume output also control the secretory patterns of hormones that influence sexual function. It has recently been discovered that alcohol directly affects these hormones and their regulatory interactions.

One important sex hormone affected by alcohol is the male hormone, testosterone. Testosterone is produced by the testes and plays an important role in human sexual development and sexual function. One of its most important functions is to permit normal development of male secondary sexual characteristics during puberty. Without testosterone, normal male hair growth and development, deepening of the voice, as well as the development of the external genitalia, will not occur. But even after puberty, testosterone remains important for male sexual function. Sufficient levels of testosterone are necessary for both sexual performance (penile erection) and for fertility.

Alcohol and Fertility

Although penile erection is necessary for ejaculation, normal fertility is dependent on the "accessory" male sexual glands. The "accessory male" sexual glands produce fluids that are necessary for the sperm cell to survive. These fluids also determine sperm motility, which affects whether or not the ejaculate reaches and fertilizes the ovum.

The fluid in which the sperm cells are discharged, the seminal fluid, contains large amounts of sugar called fructose. Fructose is the sugar ordinarily found in many fresh fruits, but in the human body this sugar is produced only by the seminal vesicles of the male. Fructose secreted into the seminal fluid provides a very potent source of energy which is necessary for sperm cell mobility. The sperm cell uses fructose as a rapidly available energy source for movement of its flagella (the tail-like appendage of the sperm cell). When testosterone levels are low, fructose production in the seminal vesicles is decreased and sperm motility is diminished. Thus, heavy alcohol consumption may not only reduce sexual potency in males, but it may also act to decrease fertility.

Alcohol and Sexual Performance

The porter in *Macbeth* comments that too much drink "makes him stand to and not stand to." The porter may have been referring to the fact that, although men can achieve an erection when heavily intoxicated, they often fail to maintain the erection. Failure to maintain penile erection can lead to severely compromised sexual function. Kinsey observed, in his early reports on male sexuality, that the most frequent cause of male impotence was alcohol abuse or a recent history of excessive alcohol intake. Although male impotence is multiply determined, recovery from alcohol-abuse problems is often accompanied by improved sexual potency.

Does alcohol affect testosterone levels in a way that adversely affects maintenance of male penile erection? Recent studies of male alcoholics have shown that alcohol directly suppresses testosterone levels. Moreover, the magnitude of fall in testosterone levels is related to the amount of alcohol consumed. The more alcohol ingested and the higher the blood alcohol levels, the lower the testosterone levels. Often abrupt cessation of drinking is followed by a rebound increase in testosterone levels. The alcoholic men studied did not have evidence of liver disease, a condition which might otherwise account for changes in testosterone levels.

Alcohol suppresses testosterone production in all men, not just in alcoholics. When healthy young adult men drank moderate amounts of alcohol in an ordinary cocktail-party setting, plasma testosterone levels fell as blood alcohol levels rose. When blood alcohol levels were highest, testosterone levels were lowest. Thus, even moderate amounts of alcohol can suppress testosterone levels, regardless of past drinking history of the individual. These findings are consistent with observations that both alcoholic men and occasional social drinkers may suffer from impotence if they drink enough alcohol before attempting sexual intercourse.

Alcohol, Sexual Desire, and Hormones

But if alcohol suppresses male testosterone levels, and thereby compromises penile erection, how can this be reconciled with Shakespeare's observation recounted by many others, that men may experience increased sexual desire during heavy intoxication? To understand this paradox, we need to consider the nature of the interaction between the brain and the testes. The brain regulates the pituitary gland, and the pituitary in turn regulates the testes. A diagram depicting the interrelationships between brain, pituitary, and testes is shown in Figure 1. Testosterone production is preceded by a sequence of changes in hormonal levels, and these hormones also may have some behavioral effects. The brain controls the production of a hormone (LHRH) that stimulates the pituitary gland to produce a second hormone (luteinizing hormone, or LH), which travels in the bloodstream to stimulate production of yet a third hormone, testosterone.

Alcohol lowers testosterone levels by a curious and complex mechanism. One component of this mechanism involves the neural regulation of testosterone production. Testosterone exerts a "feedback" effect on the brain and the pituitary which is analogous to the way in which a governor regulates the speed of an engine. When testosterone levels are high, the brain and the pituitary are signaled to reduce production of the hormones that stimulate testosterone production. When testosterone levels are low, the brain and pituitary are signaled to produce more of the hormone that stimulates testosterone production. Consequently, when testosterone levels decrease following alcohol intake, the brain

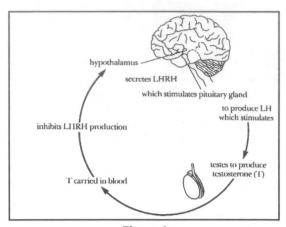

Figure 1

Hormonal relationships

and pituitary are instructed to produce more hormones that stimulate increased production of testosterone by the testes. Circulating levels of LH, the pituitary hormone that regulates testosterone production, are significantly increased when men are most intoxicated and when their testosterone levels are lowest.

The high circulating level of this pituitary hormone, LH, has a direct effect on behavior, in addition to stimulating the testes to produce testosterone. Luteinizing hormone also stimulates brain cells that have a crucial role in the regulation of both sexual and aggressive behavior. When a surge of luteinizing hormone occurs after alcohol-induced suppression of testosterone, this LH surge affects both the testes and the brain. Some scientists speculate that increased sexual desire following alcohol intake by males is related to the increase in luteinizing hormone secretion. Research shows episodic surges of LH occur at the same time that young men reported feeling sexually aroused when they were shown erotic stimuli.

It now appears that when alcohol reduces testosterone levels, this signals the brain and the pituitary to produce more luteinizing hormone. The subsequent surge in luteinizing hormone levels stimulates more testosterone production and also stimulates increased sexual desire through its direct action on the brain.

The mechanism by which alcohol reduces testosterone has only recently been clarified. The brain and the pituitary are not the primary sites of alcohol's effects on male sex hormones; rather, alcohol suppresses testosterone production in the testes. Recent studies have shown that the testes metabolize and break down alcohol in a manner similar to that which occurs in the liver. Although the liver is the prime organ for metabolizing alcohol, the testes also possess the necessary enzymes to oxidize alcohol. Thus, when men drink alcohol, some of the alcohol is broken down by the testes.

The enzymes used to metabolize alcohol in the testes are also crucial for the production of testosterone. When alcohol is metabolized in the testes, these enzymes are diverted from their normal role, and testosterone production is decreased. Researchers have recently identified the specific enzyme co-factor (a substance called NAD) that is depleted in the testes during alcohol oxidation. At present, there is no known way to administer this substance to humans to overcome the suppressive effects of alcohol on testosterone production.

Other drugs also affect male sexual behavior and testosterone levels, but through different biological mechanisms. For example, opium derivatives, such as morphine and codeine and heroin, also suppress male testosterone levels and also impair sexual function. But unlike alcohol, opiates depress rather than increase sexual desire. One reason that opiates and alcohol affect sexual desire differently is because these drugs have opposite effects on the pituitary and gonadal hormones. Unlike alcohol, opiates inhibit testosterone production by first inhibiting LH, the pituitary hormone that stimulates testosterone production. This decrease in luteinizing hormone is consistent with reports by opiate addicts that opiate drugs decrease their desire for sexual activity. Over time, opiates also decrease an addict's sexual performance or potency.

Alcohol and Male Feminization

In addition to decreasing testosterone and potency and increasing sexual desire, alcohol also has other effects on male sexuality. In 1926, an astute clinician noted that male alcoholics with liver disease developed enlargement of the breasts (gynecomastia) and shrinkage of the testes (testicular atrophy). These observations were subsequently confirmed in many clinical studies. For years, it was believed that alcohol-induced liver disease was the cause of breast enlargement and testicular atrophy. Only within the past decade has it been shown that male alcoholics whose liver function is normal can also develop testicular atrophy and gynecomastia. Thus, liver disease associated with alcoholism is not

necessary for feminization to occur in male alcoholics. Precise details of how alcohol produces severe and irreversible feminization in some male alcoholics are unknown, but prolonged suppression of testosterone levels is one important contributing factor.

Alcohol and the Biology of Aggression

It has been long known that many components of sexual and aggressive behavior are controlled by the *same* hormonal and central nervous system processes. Although alcohol intoxication is not invariably associated with aggressive behavior, brawls in a barroom differ quantitatively and qualitatively from disputes in a tea room. Since alcohol can affect sexual behavior and change hormone levels that are important in the regulation of male sexual function, this may have important implications for understanding how alcohol affects aggression.

Scientists have identified minute regions of the brain that contain nerve cells that regulate both aggressive and sexual behavior in animals. These brain cell aggregates are quite remarkable, because they can "sense" sex hormones circulating in the blood. These cells are called steroid receptors, because they can bind with the sex steroid hormones, such as testosterone. This binding affects activity of the steroid receptor cell itself and the activity of other nerve cells that these cells regulate. Certain steroid receptor cells have the remarkable capacity to convert one sex steroid hormone to a dramatically different hormone. For example, testosterone can be converted to estradiol. Testosterone is the male sex hormone, whereas estradiol is the most prominent female hormone of the estrogen family. It has been discovered that sex steroid action on the brain can affect very complex sexual behaviors, such as courting, grooming, and coitus.

The brain centers that regulate sexual activity also are important in the regulation of aggressive behaviors. The range of aggressive behaviors in animals that are affected by sex steroid action on the brain includes predatory functions necessary for survival, as well as spontaneous killing behavior, which has no known survival role.

There has been a concerted effort to discover if aggression is associated with any particular hormone. Because the regulation of any single hormone is so complexly related to many other hormones, no simple answers have emerged. Research in primates has shown that dominance hierarchies often parallel testosterone levels; i.e., the alpha male who leads the troop has higher testosterone levels than subordinates. Measurements of testosterone in primates, before and after a fight, have shown that testosterone falls after a defeat and increases after a victory. Fascinating as these observations are, there are also many exceptions which prevent any definite conclusions about the role of a hormone in aggression.

Consider a familiar example. Male animals are castrated to decrease sexual behavior, and there is usually also a striking decrease in aggressive behavior. Castration, as well as alcohol, lowers testosterone levels. Most pet owners know that castration or spaying of a male dog or cat produces these changes in general behavior. Animals that were aggressive or predatory tend to become gentle and docile. In man, castration was once used to produce eunuchs valued as asexual guardians of the harem. Their relative docility or aggressivity is not a matter of scientific record.

The astute reader will notice an apparent contradiction. If alcohol intoxication is often associated with increased aggression and lower testosterone, but decreased testosterone in turn seems related to docility, how can these be reconciled? This is one of the many unresolved questions about the interactions between alcohol, behavior, and neuroendocrine hormones.

Whatever the contributing biological factors, the relationship of alcohol and aggression in humans is amply documented. It is commonly believed that drinking enhances courage and alleviates fear and apprehension in the face of danger. Although alcohol may have a salutary effect in promoting courage and aggression in certain life-threatening situations, in most instances, alcohol-related aggression is destructive to the aggressor as well as the victims.

Alcohol-related aggression in this society exacts an enormous toll. Over 50 percent of highway fatalities are associated with alcohol abuse or alcoholism. Studies of alcohol effects on driving behavior have consistently demonstrated that alcohol impairs skill and judgment. However, these effects on performance may not be the most crucial consequences of alcohol intoxication on driving behavior. There is increasing evidence that alcohol intoxication is associated with a great increase in risk-taking and overt aggression while driving. The ordinarily courteous and conservative driver may become quarrelsome and drive aggressively after drinking. Recent police statistics indicate that intoxicated individuals, involved in minor accidents, frequently leave their vehicles and verbally or physically attack the other driver.

Another example of alcohol-induced aggression is the high incidence of homicide associated with alcohol abuse. It is estimated that a large proportion of perpetrators (and victims) of homicide were drinking heavily before commission of a crime. In societies where male drinking and macho behavior is condoned, the vast majority of all homicides occur in the context of heavy drinking. Less dramatic, but more frequent, is the common observation that intoxicated males in barroom settings frequently become quarrelsome and aggressive. Alcohol intoxication in the social drinker or sustained inebriation in an alcoholic is often accompanied by the enhanced probability of the emergence of aggression and belligerence.

Although the evidence is far from complete, the data suggest that alcohol may directly alter the biological mediators of sex and aggression through its actions on the brain, the pituitary, and the gonads. But biology alone does not determine human behavior, and expectations about alcohol's effects can also influence sexuality and aggression.

Alcohol and Expectancy

The power of expectations about alcohol effects has long been appreciated by those bartenders who "water the drink" to increase their profit margin. The diluted alcohol may be just as satisfying to the customer as an unadulterated drink and far more satisfying for the balance sheets. Social scientists have also made a convincing case for the importance of expectations about alcohol on subsequent behaviors. One dramatic example is the finding that people who believed they were given alcohol acted more aggressively than people who believed they were given tonic (an alcohol placebo). Expectations changed behavior independently of whether the subjects had actually received alcohol or not.

In a model study of the influence of expectancy about alcohol's effects on aggression, 48 people were told they would receive alcohol and another 48 people were told they would receive tonic. In fact, half of the people in *each* group were given alcohol and the other half were not. The measure of "aggression" was the intensity and duration of electric shocks administered to a person in another room in the context of a "teaching exercise." People who expected alcohol administered longer and more intense shocks than people who expected to consume tonic, regardless of the actual alcohol content of their beverage. Those who expected tonic, and actually received alcohol, were indistinguishable from those who expected and also received tonic. The expect-tonic, receive-alcohol group were also less aggressive than those who expected alcohol and actually received tonic. No subject could taste the difference between vodka and the tonic placebo at a rate better than chance. Consequently, expectancy rather than any drug discrimination factors appeared to influence the expression of aggression.

If the belief that alcohol has been consumed is just as effective as alcohol itself in increasing aggressive behavior in social drinkers, this strongly suggests that other aspects of intoxication are modulated by expectation. It is often argued that alcohol may provide an acceptable excuse for aggression and other deviant behaviors that are usually considered unacceptable. Alcohol intoxication is often "blamed" for a variety of types of asocial acting out, when, in fact, it may merely set the stage.

Alcohol is commonly believed to increase sexual arousal, and this expectation may be as significant a factor in reports of sexual feelings as the hormonal accompaniments. This possibility was examined in a study similar to the study of alcohol, aggression, and expectancy. Sexual stimuli were erotic films. Half of the subjects, all of whom were men, were told they would receive alcohol and half were told they would receive tonic; whereas, in fact, half of the alcohol-expectancy group received tonic and half of the tonic-expectancy group received alcohol. Physiological indices of sexual arousal involved a measure of penile erection, i.e., the tumescence of the penis. Although the dose of alcohol was too low to affect penile erection directly, subjects who believed they had been given alcohol showed significantly more sexual arousal than subjects who believed they had consumed tonic. Similar results were obtained when subjects listened to tape recordings of erotic narratives. Again, those who believed they had consumed alcohol became more sexually aroused than subjects who believed they had been given tonic.

When subjects were asked to rate the relative stimulating effects of erotic slides, those who believed they had consumed alcohol rated the slides as more sexually stimulating, whether they had actually consumed tonic or alcohol. Several studies have now confirmed the general finding that men who believed they had drunk alcohol became significantly more aroused by erotic stimuli than those who believed they had drunk tonic, regardless of the actual content of their drinks. Moreover, men's reports of sexual arousal and penile tumescence were usually positively correlated.

Sexual responsivity in women is affected differently by low doses of alcohol. In women, unlike men, very low doses of alcohol have been shown to *reduce* a physiological measure of arousal, vaginal pressure pulse scores. However, women's reports of sexual arousal increased with increasing alcohol dosage. In one study, women were given four different doses of alcohol in random order and were shown an erotic and a neutral film in each weekly session.

Women were asked to rate the extent to which films were sexually arousing and enjoyable, and were also monitored for their physiological responses through measurement of vaginal pulse pressure. Subjective reports of sexual arousal increased with increasing intoxication, whereas physiological measures of arousal declined. The lowest dose of alcohol (.05 gm/kg) was essentially a placebo, since it yielded no measurable blood alcohol level. Physiologically measured sexual stimulation increased during the erotic film but not during the control film when a non-alcohol placebo was given.

This apparent dissociation between sexual arousal and physiological responsivity is interesting and suggests that alcohol's alleged aphrodisiacal powers are complex indeed. To the extent that sexual gratification may be related to vaginal pulse pressure, traditional sophomoric advice to male seducers may not apply to women today. "Liquor" may not be "quicker" from the women's vantage point.

Alternatively, the apocryphal sophomores' approach to low-budget seduction may, in fact, be effective. The prototypical fraternity Don Juan reports, "We drank vodka with the orange juice, but gave the girls plain orange juice. Of course, they thought they were getting vodka with orange juice, and we were able to save money and get them drunk at the same time." Thus may chauvinism and penury combine to exploit the role of expectancy in the effects of alcohol intoxication—a strategy sanctioned, to some extent, by the dispassionate data of social science. However, since biological studies clearly show that alcohol impairs male sexual performance, diluted alcohol plus expectancy may be the best formula after all. Empirical studies of seduction (success or failure) and sexual performance and gratification under alcohol and placebo control conditions are not yet available. Candy cannot be dismissed out of hand!

We are just beginning to appreciate the complex changes in behavior that a simple molecule, such as alcohol, can produce. Why humans seek these changes remains a fascinating question. It is likely that prehistoric man accidentally discovered that alcohol enhanced sexual desire and simultaneously enhanced aggression. Perhaps this chance occurrence in some way facilitated acquisition of a mate and subsequent procreation. Transmutation of such primitive behavioral processes to contemporary behaviors associated with sex and aggression is subtle and extraordinarily complicated. Yet, if alcohol does produce changes in very basic biological drives, perhaps some individuals abuse alcohol to enhance such effects. The mood states associated with alcohol intoxication are even more ephemeral, and their possible relation to biological processes remains a mystery.

Alcohol and Female Sexuality

Except for the brief review of studies on alcohol and expectancy, the female half of the sexual equation has been blatantly ignored in the foregoing discussion. This omission reflects the information currently available rather than deliberate neglect. Sadly, research on alcoholism and alcohol effects has tended to ignore women until very recently. It has been generally assumed that conclusions drawn from studies of men apply equally to women. This may be true for some basic physiological functions, such as gastrointestinal and liver function, but the applicability to behavioral dimensions is not known.

Questions about alcohol and female sexuality have been avoided with the assiduousness of a Victorian matron. But scientific chauvinism is not entirely at fault. Study of the effects of alcohol and other drugs on sexuality in men provoked congressional displeasure as recently as 1976. A Midwestern congressman, running for re-election, declared that studies of drug effects on sexual arousal were "offensive to the sensibilities of most Americans" (*Congressional Record*, April 13, 1976, H 3299). He persuaded his congressional colleagues to stop federal funding for a research project in his home dis-

trict that addressed these issues. Special legislation was enacted as a rider to the House Appropriations Bill. Politics and prudery combined to publicize the congressman's carefully orchestrated pronouncements of outrage, and he was re-elected. So, less is known than might have been about the effects of alcohol on male or female sexuality. Only a few intrepid investigators have pursued this line of research, while endeavoring to evade the unwelcome attention of their local golden fleecers.

Although evaluation of the effects of alcohol on pituitary and gonadal hormones is far less likely to excite prurient or political interest, this area also has been neglected until very recently. Preliminary data from studies in women and in female primates suggest that single episodes of intoxication do not suppress either luteinizing hormone or estradiol. Estradiol is the female gonadal hormone equivalent to testosterone, the male gonadal hormone, and the pathways for biosynthesis are very similar for both. Although the generality of these findings remains to be established, it now appears that acute alcohol intoxication has less severe hormonal consequences for women than for men. However, chronic alcohol abuse may have equally serious effects in men and women, as inferred from the clinical literature. Alcoholism in women is associated with a number of disorders of reproductive function, ranging from complete cessation of menses to structural damage to the ovaries. These disorders are discussed more fully in Chapter 13 on alcohol and health. The importance of learning about alcohol's effects on female procreative function and sexuality is obvious.

✳ ✳ ✳

Jack H. Mendelson and Nancy K. Mello, "Alcohol, Sex and Aggression," from *Alcohol Abuse in America*. Copyright © 1985 by Bio-Behavioral Research Corporation. Reprinted by permission of Little, Brown, and Company.

For Discussion

The authors make no mention of lowered inhibitions that result from use of alcohol. Could sexual desire result more from lowered inhibitions than from hormonal changes? ✦

7. Who Profits from Tobacco Sales to Children?

Joseph R. DiFranza

AND

Joe B. Tye

The vast body of research on cigarettes and other tobacco products demonstrates that smoking is linked with various cancers and diseases of the lungs and heart. Pregnant women who smoke risk the health of the fetus; infants born to women who smoke during pregnancy often have lower than average birth weights. Smokeless tobacco carries its own risks—cancers of the mouth and gums. Most research indicates that prevalence rates for cigarette smoking have decreased since the 1970s; yet an alarming number of youths today are regular smokers. In this article, Joseph R. DiFranza and Joe B. Tye estimate the annual sales of tobacco to youth, which produce huge profits for tobacco companies. Further, children who smoke and continue to do so into adulthood produce greater returns for the tobacco companies. State and federal governments also benefit from tax revenues generated from tobacco sales to youth. The authors, suggesting that more funds be allocated for prevention, outline methods for improving the enforcement of illegal tobacco sales.

Although tobacco's victims range in age from the unborn to the elderly, the addiction that fosters tobacco use can be considered a childhood disease. According to a survey of high-school seniors, the average age for the first use of cigarettes is 13 years.[1] To protect children from tobacco, 43 states and the District of Columbia have enacted legislation that outlaws the sale of tobacco to children.[2,3] In addition, more than a dozen states have outlawed the possession of tobacco by children.[2] Unfortunately, these laws have been largely ignored by the tobacco industry and its retail distributors and, until very recently, by law enforcement and public health officials as well.[4]

The ease with which children can illegally purchase tobacco products has been previously documented.[3,5] Initial efforts at reducing sales of tobacco to children enlisted community support to encourage tobacco retailers to voluntarily comply with existing state laws. However, despite community support, without enforcement, violations of the laws remain widespread.[5]

The purpose of this analysis is twofold. First, we estimate the quantity of tobacco purchased by American youth; the monetary value of these sales, including the tax revenues collected by state and federal governments; and the profits realized by the tobacco industry from this largely illegal activity. Second, we briefly describe the implementation of some effective enforcement methods by health department and law enforcement officials that have resulted in a dramatic decline in illegal sales of tobacco to children in their communities.

Table 1
Estimated Number of Daily Smokers Aged 8 to 17 Years, Conservative Method

Age,y	No.	Dropout Rate,%	Students			Dropouts			Total No.of Smokers
			No.	%Smoking	No. of Smokers	No.	%Smoking	No. of Smokers	
8-10	10,447,000	...	...	...	...	...	...	...	58,780*
11	3,482,000	0.8	3,454,000	1.5	51,810	27,860	25	6,964	58,780
12-13	6,964,000	0.8	6,908,000	5.7	393,800	55,710	50	27,860	421,700
14-15	6,964,000	2.4	6,797,000	13.1	890,400	167,100	75	125,400	1,016,000
16-17	6,964,000	7.7	6,428,000	19.75	1,270,000	536,200	75	402,200	1,672,000
Total	34,820,000**	...	...	...	...	...	...	...	3,277,000**

*See text for explanation.
**Columns do not add because of rounding.

Analysis

Two estimates, one conservative and one comprehensive, were made of cigarette consumption by children under 18 years of age, and an average of the two was used in further computations. To this average for cigarette consumption, we added an estimate of smokeless-tobacco use. Finally, tax revenues and profits derived from these sales were computed. The following analysis details the various assumptions underlying our calculations of these estimates of cigarette and smokeless-tobacco consumption.

The conservative estimate of cigarette sales included only children who smoke daily. Estimates of the numbers of youngsters in each of four age strata, 11 to 17 years, were obtained from U.S. Bureau of the Census population projections for 1989 (Table 1).[6] Children under 11 years of age are considered separately below. Children enrolled in school were considered separately from school dropouts because smoking rates for these two groups differ dramatically.[7] Figures for school enrollment were also obtained from census data.[6]

Table 2
Estimated Annual Consumption of Daily Smokers Aged 8 to 17 Years, Conservative Method

Age,y	No. of Daily Smokers	No. of Cigarettes per Day	No. of Packs per Year
8-11	103,700	4.00	7,578,000
12-17	2,781,000	13.73	697,400,000
Total	2,885,000*	...	705,000,000'

*Columns do not add because of rounding.

Retrospective data on the age of initiation of daily smoking from a survey of high-school seniors were used to estimate the prevalence of daily smoking among students in the various age strata.[8] This was done by summing the percentages of students who had initiated smoking at younger ages. According to this survey, 20.8 percent of high-school seniors had at one time initiated daily cigarette use, but, at the time of the survey, only 18.1 percent were still daily smokers, a discrepancy of 13 percent. To take this discrepancy into account, high-school seniors who had once been daily smokers, but were not daily smokers at the time of the survey, were excluded by reducing the estimated prevalence for each age category by 13 percent.

In a survey of young children, the number of smokers aged 8 to 10 years was greater than the number of smokers who were 11 years of age.[9] However, for the purpose of our conservative estimate, it was assumed that the number of smokers under 11 years old equaled the number of 11-year-old smokers.

Data on the cigarette consumption of daily smokers 12 to 17 years old are available from a number of surveys.[2,10-13] Unfortunately, many surveys collect consumption data in strata (e.g., greater or less than half a pack per day), making it difficult to accurately and precisely estimate average consumption. Using data from a 1979 telephone survey,[10] Warner[14] estimated the average consumption of 12- to 17-year-old smokers to be 16.0 cigarettes per day. Results from two Gallup telephone surveys were an average consumption of 12 cigarettes per day in 1985 and 13.73 in 1986 for Canadian youth aged 12 to 17 years.[11,12] The cost of cigarettes is much higher in Canada, and, to the degree to which higher prices discourage children from smoking, one might expect Canadian youth to smoke less than their American peers.[14] We chose the middle and most recent of these three figures, 13.73, for our conservative calculation (Table 2). Another study of Canadian youth was used to provide an estimate of the average cigarette consumption by daily smokers under the age of 12 years of 4 cigarettes per day.[9]

The smoking rate among older school dropouts was estimated by Pirie et al.[7] to be 75 percent. It was assumed for this analysis that the rate among dropouts 11 years old and under is 25 percent and for those 12 to 13 years, 50 percent. However, the actual smoking rate in this group may be higher because of the strong association between smoking and social deviance.

It was assumed that there are 20 cigarettes to a pack with an average retail price of 129.5 cents per pack.[15] Annual cigarette sales to children under 18 years of age are estimated by this method to be $913 million.

The calculation of our comprehensive estimate (Tables 3 and 4) parallels that for the conservative estimate with the following exceptions. The same data on age of initiation[8] were used, but the adjustment for the 13 percent of previously daily smokers who no longer smoked daily was not made. Two factors suggest that these data on age of initiation are too conservative. First, the data were gathered retrospectively from the high-school class of 1988, and there is evidence of a recent increase in tobacco use among younger teenagers.[16] Second, it has been shown that in retrospective surveys people tend to recall starting to smoke at an older age than was actually the case.[17]

Table 3
Estimated Number of Daily Smokers Aged 6 to 17 Year, Comprehensive Method

| Age,y | No. | Dropout Rate,% | Students | | | Dropouts | | | Total No.of Smokers |
			No.	%Smoking	No. of Smokers	No.	%Smoking	No. of Smokers	
8-10	10,447,000	...	...	...	...	...	...	...	51,870*
11	3,482,000	0.8	3,454,000	1.3	44,900	27,860	25	6964	51,870
12-13	6,964,000	0.8	6,908,000	5.0	345,400	55,710	50	27,860	373,300
14-15	6,964,000	2.4	6,797,000	11.4	774,800	167,100	75	125,400	900,200
16-17	6,964,000	7.7	6,428,000	17.2	1,106,000	536,200	75	402,200	1,508,000
Total	34,820,000**	...	...	...	...	...	...	...	2,885,000**

*See text for explanation.
**Columns do not add because of rounding.

Estimates were made of the number of youth who smoke regularly but not every day. Among high-school seniors, the prevalence of less-than-daily smokers is 0.586 that of the daily smokers.[8] From the Canadian study, it is clear that the proportion of smokers who do not smoke every day increases with younger age groups.[9] For this calculation, it was assumed that the proportion of less-than-daily to daily smokers was 0.586 for ages 12 to 17 years. For children under 12 years, a proportion of less-than-daily to daily smokers of 3.35 was derived from the Canadian study.[9] The cigarette consumption rates for those who smoke less than daily are estimated on the basis of Canadian survey data for those age groups.[9]

Self-reports of cigarette consumption reliably underestimate actual consumption, accounting for only 72 percent of the cigarettes sold in this country.[18] The self-reported consumption rates for children were, therefore, multiplied by a factor of 1.39 to correct for this underreporting.

Our comprehensive calculation gives an estimate of cigarette consumption by youths under 18 years of age of 1.19 billion packs per year, accounting for sales revenues of $1.54 billion.

It is probably reasonable to assume that actual cigarette sales to youths fall somewhere between our two estimates. An average of our two calculations places annual cigarette sales to youths under age 18 at 947 million packs and revenues at $1.23 billion. In 1988, the federal government collected taxes on the sale of 28,562,000,000 packs of cigarettes.[15] Cigarettes consumed by children under 18 years old, therefore, represent 3.3 percent of all cigarette sales. This estimate is similar to one from Canada, where sales to children accounted for 3.6 percent of total sales.[19]

Chewing Tobacco and Snuff

In 1986, it was estimated that 1.7 million boys aged 12 to 17 years had used smokeless tobacco within the previous year.[20] Of these, 0.5 million use it at least weekly. If the 1.2 million boys who use smokeless tobacco less than weekly are excluded, and it is assumed that those who use it every week consume only one pack or can per week, at a cost of $1.25 per unit, sales of smokeless tobacco to children under 18 years would total $32,500,000 per year. Adding these revenues to those from cigarettes results in annual revenues of $1.26 billion from tobacco sales to children.

Tax Revenue

At 16 cents per pack, the 947 million packs sold to children under 18 years of age each year generate $152 million in federal tax revenue.

Cigarettes are taxed in every state, with rates varying from 2 cents per pack in North Carolina to 38 cents in Minnesota, for a national average of 18.3 cents per pack.[15] State tax revenues from the sale of cigarettes to children under 18 total approximately $173 million annually.

City and county taxes account for only 2 percent of all cigarette taxes[15] and were, therefore, excluded from this analysis.

In 1988, a total of 29 states also taxed chewing tobacco and snuff. Congress repealed the federal excise tax on smokeless tobacco in 1965.[21] It is not possible to estimate with any reliability the taxes paid by children on these forms of tobacco, because summary statistics are not available. In any case, the amount is not substantial, as 98.8 percent of all tobacco taxes paid in 1988 were for cigarettes.[15]

Table 4
Estimaed Annual Consumption of All Smokers Aged 8 to 17 Years, Comprehensive Method

Age,y	Smoking Category	No. of Smokers	No. of Cigarettes per Day		No. of Packs per Year
			Self-Reported Rate	Adusted Rate	
8-11	<Daily	393,800	0.20	0.278	1,999,000
8-11	Daily	117,600	4.00	5.560	11,940,000
12-17	<Daily	1,822,000	2.00	2.780	92,500,000
12-17	Daily	3,109,000	13.73	19.080	1,083,000,000
Total	...	5,442,400*	...	...	1,190,000,000*

*Columns do not add because of rounding.

Tobacco Industry Income and Profits

To estimate the revenues and profits to the cigarette manufacturers derived from the sale of tobacco to children, the most recent annual reports were obtained from each of the six major tobacco companies. Five reports represented 1988; the RJR Nabisco report was for 1987. Together, these companies account for approximately 98 percent of domestic tobacco sales. From largest to smallest in terms of tobacco sales, these are Philip Morris, RJR Nabisco, Brown and Williamson, Lorillard, American Brands, and Liggett and Meyers. Together, they reported operating incomes of $6.7 billion from sales of tobacco products, totaling $21.3 billion (an operating margin of 31 percent). If sales to children account for 3.3 percent of cigarette sales, these six companies share an annual $703 million in revenues and $221 million in profits from the sale of cigarettes to children.

Children who become addicted to nicotine frequently become lifelong customers of the tobacco companies. Each child who becomes addicted can, therefore, be considered an "investment" that will pay dividends into the future. Among smokers born since 1935, almost half started before the age of 18 years,[2] and, among 24-year-old smokers, 68 percent indicate that they began smoking prior to age 18.[17] It seems reasonable to conclude that approximately half of all tobacco-industry profits, $3.35 billion annually, represent the long-term profits from childhood addiction to nicotine. With the trend to earlier age of initiation, such that 90 percent of new smokers now start by the age of 19 years,[17] the proportion of tobacco-industry profits derived directly or indirectly from childhood addiction to nicotine may approach 90 percent.

Comment

In this analysis of cigarette use by children, we have estimated the profits to the tobacco industry and the tax revenues to state and federal governments. We believe our estimate of $1.23 billion in cigarette sales to children under 18 years is close to the mark. Warner[14] estimated the annual consumption of children aged 12 to 17 years to be 19.1 billion cigarettes in 1982. Assuming a price of 129.5 cents per pack of 20, this equals sales of $1.25 billion dollars.

The sale of tobacco to children is illegal in 43 states and the District of Columbia. Since we estimate that more than 3 percent ($221 million in 1988) of tobacco-company profits derive from this activity, we suggest a 3-percent "illegal drug-profits tax" levied on tobacco-industry profits to recover these funds, so that they might be used to prevent nicotine addiction among children. A precedent for this type of tax exists in the "windfall-profits tax" levied on the oil industry in response to accusations of price gouging during the energy crisis of the 1970s.

The $152 million the federal government receives annually from the sale of tobacco to children could also be earmarked for prevention. Federal expenditures for all activities related to smoking and health, including both prevention and research, totaled less than $40 million in 1986.[2] By comparison, every 9 days, children pay federal cigarette taxes equivalent to the entire budget for the Office of Smoking and Health ($3.5 million), the only federal agency devoted solely to smoking.[2]

Much more can be done to end the profiteering from tobacco sales to children. As recently as 1 year ago, it could be said that almost no effort was being made to enforce the state laws that prohibit the sale of tobacco to minors.[17] Fortunately, this is no longer true, with a variety of enforcement efforts under way in several states.

In all states, law enforcement officials have the authority to enforce state laws that restrict the distribution of tobacco to minors. In those states where restrictions on tobacco sales are public health laws, local boards of health may also have the authority to enforce existing laws, as well as issue stricter regulations of their own. Model legislation is available from the American Medical Association and STAT (Stop Teen-age Addiction to Tobacco).[22,23]

Almost all current state laws regarding the distribution of tobacco to children are inadequate, because they lack several provisions that are required to make enforcement practical. These laws were summarized recently.[2,3] Enforcement is now occurring almost exclusively in communities that have adopted more restrictive model ordinances or regulations. Details vary from community to community, but the following features are common: (1) decriminalizing the offense, by making it a civil, rather than a criminal, offense to allow for ticketing as the means of enforcement; (2) provision for some form of "sting" operation to allow for effective enforcement with minimal expenditure of community resources; (3) local licensing of tobacco vendors; (4) meaningful penalties, including substantial monetary fines and license revocation; and (5) bans or restrictions on vending machines and the distribution of free samples.

The typical operation involves a health inspector or police officer who makes the rounds of local retailers accompanied by an underaged volunteer. If the youth is illegally sold tobacco, the official issues a ticket. Penalties involve either a fine or a suspension of the tobacco retail license, the severity of each dependent on the number of prior violations. In those communities where the law is being enforced, there has been a dramatic reduction in the number of retailers who illegally sell children tobacco (*Chicago Sun-Times.* December 30, 1989:16).

The government's "war on drugs" has failed to target the one drug that kills more people than all others combined: nicotine. In a tragic cycle, the 390,000 adult smokers killed each year by tobacco are replaced by children who begin smoking by the thousands each day.[2] The power to break this vicious cycle lies with government: at least a dozen of concerned communities have demonstrated that laws prohibiting the sale of tobacco to minors can be effectively enforced with minimal effort and expense. In every state, new laws must be adopted to make enforcement practical, and local officials must commit themselves to the small effort that enforcement requires. Rather than profit from the tragedy of childhood nicotine addiction, government should declare war on the illegal sale to children of this potentially lethal drug.

* * *

Joseph R. DiFranza and Joe B. Tye, "Who Profits from Tobacco Sales to Children?" *Journal of the American Medical Association*, 263 (May 23/30,

1990), pp. 2784-2787. Copyright © 1990 by American Medical Association. All rights reserved. Reprinted by permission.

For Discussion

Why does the government fail to regulate more closely tobacco sales to youth?

Notes

1. Johnston, L. D., O'Malley, P. M., Bachman, J. G. *Use of Licit and Illicit Drugs by America's High School Students: 1975-1984*. Rockville, MD: National Institute on Drug Abuse; 1986.

2. *Reducing the Health Consequences of Smoking: 25 Years of Progress*. Rockville, MD: U.S. Dept. of Health and Human Services; 1989:302-313. A report of the Surgeon General. Publication (CDC) 89-8411.

3. DiFranza, J. R., Norwood, B. D., Garner, D. W., Tye, J. B. Legislative effort to protect children from tobacco. *JAMA*. 1987; 267:3387-3389.

4. Kirn, T. F. Laws ban minors' tobacco purchases, but enforcement is another matter. *JAMA*. 1987; 257:3323-3324.

5. Altman, D. G. Foster, V., Rasenick-Douss, L., Tye, J. B. Reducing the illegal sale of cigarettes to minors. *JAMA*. 1989; 261:80-83.

6. *Statistical Abstract of the United States 1988*. 108th ed. Washington, DC: U.S. Dept of Commerce, Bureau of the Census; 1988:15.

7. Pirie, P. L., Murray, D. M., Luepker, R. V. Smoking prevalence in a cohort of adolescents, including absentees, dropouts, and transfers. *Am J Public Health*. 1988; 78:176-178.

8. Johnston, L. D., O'Malley, P. M., Bachman, J. G. *Drug Use, Drinking, and Smoking: National Survey Results From High School, College, and Young Adults Populations 1975-1988*. Rockville, MD: National Institute on Drug Abuse; 1989. Dept. of Health and Human Services publication (ADM) 89-1638.

9. Brown, K. S., Cherry, W. H., Forbes, W. F. *The 1978 Survey of the Smoking Habits of Canadian School Children*. Toronto: The Canadian Home and School and Parent-Teacher Federation; 1978.

10. Green, D. E. *Teenage Smoking: Immediate and Long-term Patterns*. Washington, DC: National Institute of Education; 1979.

11. Canadian Gallup Poll, Ltd. *A Summary Report on Tobacco, Alcohol, and Marijuana Use and Norms Among Young People in Canada, Year 3*. Ottawa: Health and Welfare Canada; 1985.

12. Canadian Gallup Poll, Ltd. *A Summary Report on Tobacco, Alcohol, and Marijuana Use and Norms Among Young People in Canada, Year 4*. Ottawa: Health and Welfare Canada; 1986.

13. National Institute on Drug Abuse. *National Adolescent Student Health Survey*. Rockville, MD: National Clearinghouse for Alcohol and Drug Information; 1989.

14. Warner, K. E. Smoking and health implications of a change in the federal cigarette excise tax. *JAMA*. 1986; 256:1028-1032.

15. *The Tax Burden on Tobacco*. Washington, DC: The Tobacco Institute; 1988:23.

16. *The Gallup Youth Survey: Teen Smoking Still a Matter of Concern*. Princeton, NJ: George H. Gallup International Institute; February 15, 1989.

17. Kandel, D. B., Logan, J. A. Patterns of drug use from adolescence to young adulthood, I: Periods of risk for initiation, continued use, and discontinuation. *Am J Public Health*. 1984; 74:660-666.

18. Hatziandreu, E. J., Pierce, J. P., Fiore, M. C., et al. The reliability of self-reported cigarette consumption in the United States. *Am J Public Health*. 1989; 79:1020-1023.

19. Millar, W. J., Peterson, J. *Tobacco Use by Youth in the Canadian Arctic*. Ottawa: Health and Welfare Canada, Government of the Northwest Territories; 1989.

20. *The Health Consequences of Using Smokeless Tobacco*. Bethesda, MD: U.S. Dept. of Health and Human Services; 1986:15. A report of the advisory committee to the Surgeon General. National Institutes of Health publication 86-2874.

21. Connolly, G. N., Winn, D. M., Hecht, S. S., et al. The reemergence of smokeless tobacco. *N Engl J Med*. 1986; 314:1020-1027.

22. *Model Legislation on the Enforcement of Laws to Restrict Children's Access to Tobacco*. Chicago, IL: American Medical Association; 1987. AMA Proceedings No. 193.

23. STAT. *Tobacco Youth Reporter*. Autumn 1989; 4:6. ✦

8. High Anxiety

CONSUMER REPORTS

Sedatives have long been used for reducing anxiety. Though they are legal, the great majority of these drugs are addictive when used repeatedly and in high doses. Their addictive properties appear to be both physical and psychological. Heavy users experience painful withdrawal symptoms during periods of abstinence. Moreover, in some cases withdrawal can be life-threatening if not done with medical supervision. And further, combining alcohol with sedatives can result in overdose, coma, and even death.

"High Anxiety" addresses the addictive nature of tranquilizers, among the more popular of sedative drugs. Xanax is a common prescription tranquilizer, yet its negative effects are noteworthy. The drug's popularity seems to have resulted from intensive advertising and marketing strategies. Its initial acceptance stemmed from the negative attention given to Valium; yet the article suggests that Xanax is even more addictive than Valium. Other problems are noted as well, including the fact that Xanax is often prescribed by physicians who may be unaware of the adverse effects of the drug.

The woman we'll call Rachel G.—now age 31—had experienced attacks of anxiety since she was a child. But those occasional incidents did not prevent her from marrying and taking a responsible job at an East Coast biotechnology company. Then, in late 1990 and early 1991, her life took a stressful turn. There was turmoil at the lab where she worked, her mother fell seriously ill, her grandmother committed suicide, and her marriage deteriorated. In early April of 1991, after a confrontation with her boss, she had a full-blown panic attack.

"I broke into a cold sweat," she recalls. "My heart was palpitating. I swore I was having a heart attack. I was scared that I was dying. . . . I couldn't walk. I couldn't even move." The attacks went on for two days.

Rachel G. went to a psychologist for help, and simultaneously asked her regular internist for a pill to ease her suffering. Her physician prescribed Xanax (alprazolam). That was no surprise. In 1990, Xanax had become the only drug ever approved by the U.S. Food and Drug Administration for the treatment of panic disorder—repeated, intense bouts of anxiety that can make life almost unbearable.

The drug gave her some relief, but she felt it wasn't really solving her problem. After about three months on Xanax, she tried to cut her dose in half. Within 48 hours, she recalled, "I couldn't sleep. My heart was racing, and I was getting dizzy spells." Only going back up to an intermediate dose would suppress the withdrawal symptoms.

In February 1992, Rachel G. began having frightening thoughts of killing herself. She visited a psychiatrist who prescribed Tofranil (imipramine), an antidepressant that also works against panic. Today, she is doing well, still taking imipramine—and also Xanax. Though she feels the Xanax is no longer helping her, she can't bring herself to try to quit. "I know I'm going to have to experience the withdrawal symptoms," she says, "and those are the exact symptoms that I went on it to escape from in the first place."

Rachel G.'s problem is far from unusual. Xanax is not only the most common treatment for panic attacks, but also the drug most often prescribed for run-of-the-mill anxiety—the kind that anyone might experience during a rough period in life. It is now the nation's largest-selling psychiatric drug; more than that, it is the fifth most frequently prescribed drug in the U.S.

Even if you've never taken Xanax yourself, you almost certainly know someone who has. Yet the risks are significant. Anyone who takes Xanax for an extended period—even as little as a few weeks—risks developing a stubborn dependency on the drug.

Xanax is just the latest in a long line of tranquilizers that have promised to deliver psychiatry's holy grail: relief from anxiety with no significant side effects. And like the pills that came before it, Xanax has fallen short. As psychiatrists and their patients are discovering, Xanax does have some serious drawbacks—even more that the drugs it was supposed to improve on.

Like the sleeping pill Halcion (triazolam), its closest chemical relative, Xanax demonstrates that no pill can deliver peace of mind without a price. It also raises a troubling question: How did such a flawed drug become a pharmacological superstar?

The selling of Xanax has been fueled by a vigorous promotional campaign. The drug's manufacturer, the Upjohn Co., has made Xanax highly visible in the medical community by promoting it as a uniquely effective drug for panic disorder. But Xanax does not represent a remarkable treatment advance so much as a marketing coup. In fact, it is little different from other, related tranquilizers— members of the drug family known as benzodiazepines, which have held an uneasy place in American culture for three decades.

Beyond Valium

Though the word "benzodiazepine" is meaningless to most people, the trade names of the drugs in this family are almost as familiar as Kleenex or NutraSweet. The first drug in this category, Librium (chlordiazepoxide), came on the market in 1960; Valium (diazepam) came along three years later.

In 1979, a survey showed that 11 percent of Americans were taking antianxiety drugs, mostly benzodiazepines. The figure has dropped only slightly since then.

That was also the year the hazards of these drugs gained national attention through hearings held by Senator Edward Kennedy. As the hearings made clear, Valium and similar drugs caused two major problems: Physical dependency and sedation. People on benzodiazepines often found that they couldn't stop taking the drugs, and that they couldn't function well while they were on them. The drugs accumulated in the body; over time, they made the user more and more sluggish, drowsy, and forgetful.

Ironically, while the Kennedy hearings offered frightening testimony on Valium, they also set the stage for the arrival of its successor, Xanax. Introduced in 1981, Xanax was hailed as the first of a new chemical class of benzodiazepines that were completely eliminated from the body in less than half a day. Since Xanax didn't accumulate, the hope was that it wouldn't make people increasingly drowsy or slow them down as they continued to take it.

In addition to this chemical advantage, Xanax gave Upjohn a marketing edge. The patent on Valium expired in 1984, just as sales of Xanax were beginning to build. As generic competitors undercut Valium's sales, the drug's manufacturer promoted it less actively, and sales of Valium dropped further. Upjohn took advantage of the opportunity. By 1986, Xanax had overtaken Valium as the most widely prescribed benzodiazepine. By 1987, it reached fourth place on the national sales list of all prescription drugs. And in 1991, Xanax accounted for almost one fifth of Upjohn's worldwide sales.

The trouble is, Xanax has now turned out to be more addictive than Valium itself.

Stuck on Xanax

All benzodiazepines produce physical dependency if you take them long enough. Over time, it seems, the brain "learns" to expect a certain level of the drug. If the drug is removed, the brain reacts with agitation, sleeplessness, and anxiety—the symptoms that led people to take the drug in the first place. Frequently, these symptoms are worse than the original ones, a phenomenon known as the "rebound" effect. In addition, abrupt withdrawal from the drugs can cause muscle cramps and twitches, impaired concentration, and occasionally even seizures.

Unlike people who are addicted to cocaine and heroin, users of benzodiazepines don't develop a psychological craving for the drugs, or escalate the doses they take over time. But they do have a true physical dependency, and their withdrawal symptoms make the benzodiazepines extremely difficult to kick.

A number of clinical studies have found that Xanax and other benzodiazepines that are eliminated rapidly from the body produce a quicker, more severe rebound effect than drugs like Valium that are eliminated more slowly. Some people who take Xanax three times a day, a standard schedule for panic disorder, find that they even have symptoms as the drug wears off between one dose and the next.

In one major study, Dr. Karl Rickels and his colleagues at the University of Pennsylvania took 47 anxious patients who had been on benzodiazepines for a year or more and tried to take them off their medication. Fully 57 percent of the patients on Xanax and similar drugs simply could not stop taking them—but only 27 percent of the people on drugs like Valium were that physically dependent.

Other studies have produced similar results. A Yale study of patients who had taken Xanax in a four-month treatment program for panic attacks found that most of those who were still using the drug two years later had shifted to a lower dose— but only 30 percent had been able to quit the drug entirely. Similarly, a study of long-term Xanax users done at Toronto's Addiction Research Foundation found that two-thirds had tried to stop using the drug and failed.

The experience of individual doctors underscores the problem. In 1988, researchers at the

Johns Hopkins School of Medicine interviewed 31 American physicians who specialized in helping people withdraw from the benzodiazepines. Asked which drugs were especially hard for patients to give up, 84 percent of the doctors specifically mentioned Xanax, while only 29 percent cited Valium. Even under the best of circumstances, clinicians have found that, to get people off Xanax, they must reduce the dose in tiny steps—a process that often takes months.

An 'Eraser' for the Mind?

The fact that so many people try so hard to quit Xanax—as difficult as that is to do—shows that it is not an entirely pleasant drug to take. One woman we spoke with, a 41-year-old technical writer in San Francisco, started taking Xanax to deal with bouts of anxiety that made her feel "like I was going headlong toward some frightening and dangerous unknown." After taking Xanax for 14 months, she decided to stop because, as she puts it, "It made me too stupid. I just couldn't function professionally. People would say things to me, and I'd be in a sort of fog and not be able to respond appropriately." (She ultimately succeeded in quitting, but had to go through a very difficult withdrawal process—even though she was taking a low dose, one her psychiatrist told her would not cause dependency.)

A 1990 report by the American Psychiatric Association backs up this woman's experience. It found that the benzodiazepines tend to impair memory: a person on one of these drugs may have difficulty retaining new information.

Clinicians report the same problem. "One patient of mine, a physician who took Xanax, described it as 'a big eraser'. It sort of wipes out people's attention to things," says Dr. Robert J. Gladstone, a psychiatrist in Carlisle, Mass. "I think all benzodiazepines cause memory lapses, especially in the elderly," says Dr. Stuart Yudofsky, chairman of the Department of Psychiatry at Baylor College of Medicine in Houston.

Yudofsky also refers to evidence that the drugs impair coordination. And in his own experience, he says, patients who have used benzodiazepines for years have often suffered falls and head injuries.

Xanax can also have the paradoxical effect of causing rage and hostility rather than tranquility. While this is relatively rare, it's another reason for caution in using a drug that many people will be all but unable to quit.

Despite the risks, benzodiazepines have one clear use: They can be helpful for people in crisis who need short-term anxiety relief. "They're appropriate for what are called adjustment reactions," says Dr. Peter Tyrer, a professor of psychiatry at St. Mary's Hospital Medical School in London and a longtime benzodiazepine researcher. "For example,

---

All Purpose Prescriptions:
Who Takes Xanax, and Why?

Xanax presents a paradox: It is a powerful psychiatric drug, but it is most often prescribed for people who have no psychiatric diagnosis at all. While many of those people may be suffering from a serious problem with anxiety that is never recorded on a diagnostic chart, others may simply be people who ask their doctors for some relief from stress.

We analyzed data from the 1990 National Ambulatory Medical Care Survey, a representative sample of doctor's visits conducted periodically by the U.S. Government. Our analysis shows that the drug is prescribed by a wide range of different kinds of doctors, for people with a wide range of conditions—a situation that increases the odds of misuse.

Xanax is usually prescribed by physicians in general practice. In the 1990 study, only 30 percent of Xanax prescriptions were written by psychiatrists, whereas nearly half were written by family, general and internal-medicine practitioners. (Various other specialists wrote the rest.)

Of all Xanax prescriptions, only 28 percent were written for people who were diagnosed with clinical anxiety or panic attacks. Another 21 percent were for people diagnosed with depression, a condition for which the use of Xanax is still controversial. The rest were generally written for people who had no diagnosed psychiatric problem at all, although they did have a variety of medical diagnoses, the most frequent being high blood pressure. The statistics are similar to those obtained in another large national survey: IMS America, a private organization that monitors drug sales, found that only about one fourth of all benzodiazepines prescribed in 1989 were given for anxiety-related conditions.

Many of those Xanax prescriptions may have been written appropriately for people suffering from short-term anxiety triggered by a medical problem. But the data, combined with the huge sales volume of Xanax, suggest that the drug may often be prescribed as an all-purpose stress reliever. The FDA-approved package insert (which can be requested from the pharmacist) states specifically that Xanax should not be given simply to help people deal with the "stress of everyday life," and that the drug should be given only as a short-term treatment for clear symptoms of anxiety, or as a treatment for full-blown anxiety or panic disorders. ℞

if someone has been in a car accident and is nervous afterward when he goes out into the street, he could take Xanax for a short time after that."

The problem, though, is that many people who start taking tranquilizers for the short term end up staying on them over the long haul. "For anxiety, in general, these medications tend to be used much too long and in too high doses," says Dr. Yudofsky. "People get on a drug, the reason for taking it passes, but they're maintained on it week after week, year after year. That's misuse." Even Upjohn, in its own labeling for Xanax, cautions that the drug has never been established as effective for use over more than four months.

Pushing the Panic Button

The people most at risk for becoming dependent on Xanax are those with panic disorder, because they are prescribed high doses of the drug for an extended period of time to deal with their chronic panic attacks. Since they suffer from severe or disabling anxiety, they might find dependency an acceptable price to pay for effective relief. But even though Upjohn built Xanax's reputation on studies of people with panic attacks, it's not at all clear how much they were really helped.

A panic attack is intense anxiety in a concentrated dose. Victims with a severe case may suffer several full-scale attacks a day, during which their hearts race and they hyperventilate, sweat, tremble, and feel a profound sense of terror. According to the largest, most thorough survey of psychiatric problems, conducted in the 1980s by the National Institute of Mental Health (NIMH), between 4 and 7 percent of Americans have panic attacks that are frequent enough to be considered a panic disorder. The majority of people with panic disorder also have a related condition, agoraphobia—a term now used to describe a fear of ordinary activities, such as driving a car or shopping at the supermarket, that can leave the sufferer housebound.

By the early 1980s, researchers had begun to recognize that at least some types of benzodiazepines, in addition to easing ordinary anxiety, could also stop panic attacks. Upjohn proceeded to spend lavishly on studies to see whether Xanax could be used to treat panic disorder, and enlisted highly respected consultants in the effort. "The most senior psychiatrists in the world were . . . flooded with offers of consultancies [from Upjohn]," recalls Dr. Isaac Marks, a professor of experimental psychopharmacology at the University of London's Institute of Psychiatry.

In fact, the research could just as well have been done with another benzodiazepine—one called lorazepam (Ativan)—that is also cleared from the body quickly, and has also been shown to stop panic attacks. But this drug has not been under patent protection for years—and since it has not had the

---

High Notoriety:
Halcion and Prozac

Though Xanax is the best-selling psychiatric drug in the U.S., it's not the most notorious. Vying for that distinction are Prozac, a drug for depressions, and Halcion, a benzodiazepine sold as a sleeping pill.

Both Halcion and Prozac have been reported to induce irrational behavior, including outbursts of murderous violence and suicide attempts. (Halcion was even blamed by some observers for President Bush's illness on his trip to Japan.) Lawsuits have been brought against their manufacturers, seeking damages for cases of suicide and assault committed by people taking the drugs, The accusations against both drugs prompted the U.S. Food and Drug Administration to ask expert committees to look at them more closely. Here's an update.

Prozac *(Fluoxetine)*

Introduced in 1987 by the Eli Lilly Co., Prozac rocketed up the pharmaceutical best-seller list on the strength of Lilly's strenuous promotional efforts, its evident effectiveness against mild depression, and its relative absence of side effects. Overlooked in the initial enthusiasm for the drug, however, was the lack of evidence that Prozac worked well against *major* depres-

sion, a prolonged, serious psychiatric disorder that puts victims at high risk of suicide.

In any event, Prozac's honeymoon ended three years ago, when a psychiatrist published a report on six chronically depressed patients who developed obsessive, violent suicidal thoughts after starting on the drug. The psychiatrist did emphasize that these six patients had unusually severe cases of depression; they had not responded to any other treatments and five had had suicidal thoughts, though less severe ones, before they ever took Prozac. But those distinctions disappeared in the uproar that followed.

The FDA review panel, convened late in 1991, concluded that people taking Prozac did not seem to have any more suicidal or violent thoughts that patients on other antidepressants (though the panel recommended further monitoring of the drug, just in case). In the panel's view, the suicidal thinking some patients experienced was caused by the depression itself, not the drug.

Psychiatrists point out that patients can react "paradoxically" to almost any powerful drug, including Prozac, and therefore should be monitored closely—especially early in treatment, when they're getting used to the new drug. Meanwhile, Prozac remains the nation's best-selling antidepressant. ➧

profit potential that Xanax has, it has not been aggressively tested and promoted. Today, a bottle of 100 one-milligram Xanax tablets costs $72.55, according to the Red Book, a standard drug price guide. The same amount of generic lorazepam in a therapeutically equivalent dose costs as little as $3.75.

Upjohn's major study on panic was a two-phase project called the Cross-National Panic Study. Phase One, conducted in the U.S., Canada, and Australia, involved more than 500 subjects with severe panic attacks; half received Xanax and half, a look-alike placebo. Phase Two, conducted in North and South America and Europe, enrolled 1122 subjects to compare Xanax not only with a placebo, but also with imipramine, an antidepressant from a different chemical class that also blocks panic attacks (even though it has never received formal FDA approval for this use). At the time, the two studies were among the largest ever done on psychiatric drugs.

Well before the results were published, Upjohn used the research to promote its drug. The company sponsored conferences and symposiums on drug treatment for panic and anxiety, and then invited it consultants to speak at them—a strategy now used by many large pharmaceutical companies (see "Pushing Drugs to Doctors," *Consumer Reports*, February 1992). Many of those meetings were then written up in Upjohn-sponsored supplements to scientific journals, sent to thousands of psychiatrists in the U.S. and abroad.

When the Phase One results were finally published, they made a huge splash: Four articles on the study consumed the better part of the May 1988 issue of the *Archives of General Psychiatry*, the most prestigious psychiatric journal in the U.S. By that time, however, the international psychiatric community had already been hearing about Xanax as a treatment for panic for several years. Upjohn's publicity had made psychiatrists—and, later, general-practice physicians—more aware of Xanax than they were of other, similar drugs. It almost certainly was responsible for the rapid growth of Xanax as a drug for all sorts of anxiety problems, not just panic disorder.

"The Cross-National Study was the best advertising ever done," says Dr. Rickels of the University of Pennsylvania. "Upjohn sold millions of doses of this drug before they even got it approved for panic."

No Panacea for Panic

Since receiving FDA approval to market Xanax for panic disorder, Upjohn has been using data from Phase One of the Cross-National Study in ads for the drug—including ads in journals for general-practice physicians. These doctors are likely to be unfamiliar with the actual results of the study, and to take Upjohn's word for what it showed. But despite the ads' claims, the study produced highly ambiguous results.

In the first four weeks of the eight-week study, Xanax looked much better than placebo treatment. By the fourth week, 50 percent of patients taking Xanax were completely free of panic attacks, versus 28 percent of those on an inactive placebo.

Halcion *(Triazolam)*

Though marketed as a sleeping pill, not an antianxiety drug, Halcion is actually Xanax's close chemical cousin. Like Xanax, Halcion is a benzodiazepine that's eliminated from the body very rapidly, meaning you can take it to get to sleep at night without being drowsy the next day. Upjohn started marketing Halcion in 1982; by 1987, the peak of its popularity, it was the 18th largest-selling prescription drug and the largest-selling sleeping pill in the U.S.

The disadvantages of Halcion eventually made themselves known. People who used it for any length of time found that, when they tried to stop, they experienced "rebound" insomnia worse than the original. There were also reports that Halcion seemed to make some people hostile or paranoid. The FDA was worried, and analyzed the thousands of voluntary reports of adverse reactions to Halcion the agency had received from doctors. Halcion indeed was linked to more hostility reactions than any other sleeping pill, relative to the numbers prescribed.

Another troublesome side effect also emerged: Some people who took even small doses experienced a bizarre reaction called anterograde amnesia. The day after they took Halcion to get to sleep they were up and about, apparently functioning normally. But later, they would have absolutely no memory of their actions. In 1991, Halcion was banned in the United Kingdom.

An FDA advisory committee decided, in May of 1992, to let Halcion stay on the U.S. market. But the panel agreed that the original recommended dose of 0.5 milligrams a day was too high, especially for elderly people; a lower dose of 0.25 milligrams was less likely to cause side effects (though it could also make the drug less effective). The committee also recommended strengthening the package insert's warnings on rebound insomnia and hostility reactions.

While the controversy over Prozac didn't seem to affect its upward sales trajectory, Halcion's sales have suffered. By 1991 it had fallen to 38th place. And last November, in a widely publicized case, a Dallas jury decided Halcion had been partly responsible for driving a man to murder—a decision that may damage the drug's reputation even more. ℞

Many of Upjohn's ads for Xanax quote results from this midpoint of the study. But the drug's effectiveness was much less clear by the study's end. A look at the people who stayed in the study for the full eight weeks shows a remarkable picture: At the end of the study, there was no significant difference in the average number of panic attacks—or in functioning in work, home and social life—between the people who had been taking Xanax and those who were taking placebos.

In addition, the Phase One study showed clearly how severe the "rebound" effect of Xanax withdrawal is. At the two study locations in Canada, 109 patients who had completed the eight weeks of treatment were observed as the dose of the drug (or placebo) was tapered down over a month's time. The Xanax group had averaged only 1.7 panic attacks a week—and the placebo group, 2.1 attacks a week—at the end of the eight-week treatment phase. But just two weeks after they stopped medication entirely, patients in the Xanax group were back up to 6.8 attacks a week—slightly worse off than they had been at the beginning of the study. By contrast, two weeks after the patients on placebo discontinued their "drug," they averaged only 1.8 panic attacks a week.

The findings are complicated by the Phase One study's greatest flaw: About 10 percent of the people on Xanax, and half of those on placebo, dropped out between the fourth and the eighth week. At the time they left the study the dropouts from the placebo group had more symptoms than people taking Xanax—a fact that would suggest the drug was doing some good. But many people on placebo may have been suffering from withdrawal symptoms, since many had been taking benzodiazepines just *before* they entered the study. There's also no way to tell whether they would have felt better by the end of the eight-week study if they had stuck it out, as other people in the group taking placebos did.

The finding of the Phase Two study were similar to Phase One's, except they also demonstrated that the antidepressant drug imipramine worked as well as Xanax. At the end of the eight weeks, 78 percent of people taking Xanax were panic-free, compared with 81 percent of those on imipramine and 75 percent of the people on placebo—virtually identical numbers.

Upjohn researchers and their supporters believe Xanax came out the clear winner in the studies. They point out that it acts much more quickly than imipramine and is easier to take. Imipramine is one of a class of antidepressants that can cause a range of unpleasant side effects, including sedation, dry mouth, severe constipation, blurred vision, weight gain, and impotence.

But other psychiatrists focus on the fact that people taking placebos did nearly as well as those on Xanax by the end of the study—and avoided the rebound effect that plagued people on the real drug.

Short-Term Psychotherapy:
Relief Without Drugs

People with serious anxiety—including those with panic attacks—don't need to choose between a life of tranquilizers and a life under severe stress. The past decade has seen the development of a new type of nondrug treatment called cognitive-behavioral therapy. While it doesn't give the immediate relief of a drug like Xanax, it does produce results quickly—and may be the most helpful approach over the long term.

Cognitive-behavioral therapists believe that many people, perhaps even most, have panic symptoms at one time or another—a stressful situation, for example, may trigger a racing heartbeat or rapid breathing. These symptoms usually pass quickly, and most people never give them a second thought. But a few people overreact intensely when they experience panic symptoms; they misinterpret them as symptoms of impending insanity or death.

"They tend to catastrophize their symptoms," explains Dr. Robert Liberman, who treats panic-attack patients at the UCLA Neuropsychiatric Institute. "Anyone might feel dizzy getting suddenly out of a chair. A person vulnerable to panic might exaggerate that feeling, leading to sustained feelings of panic."

Cognitive-behavioral therapy works by teaching panic victims a new way of thinking about their physical symptoms. "The therapies consciously induce panic sensations—spinning patients on a chair to get dizzy, or having them run up and down stairs to get out of breath," Liberman says. "Even when their heart is pounding, and they're short of breath and dizzy, they learn that nothing terrible happens and that these sensations naturally subside."

This technique and variations on it have been studied at a number of centers, with consistent results: After an average of a dozen weekly sessions, patients have few or no panic symptoms. More important, they maintain their improvement for a year or more.

Dr. David Barlow and his colleagues at the Center for Stress and Anxiety Disorders in Albany conducted one such study, comparing cognitive-behavioral therapy with Xanax and placebo over 15 weeks. The Xanax and behavior-therapy groups experienced roughly equivalent declines in general anxiety. But two weeks after the study ended, 87 percent of the behavior-therapy patients were completely free of panic attacks, while half of those in the Xanax group were still having attacks, even though almost all were still on the drug. Late in 1991, cognitive-behavioral therapy was endorsed by an expert panel convened by the National Institutes of Health to evaluate treatments for panic disorder. ➡

That suggests that for many people, the mere act of visiting a doctor might have been reassuring enough to produce a measurable decrease in symptoms. It also suggests that nondrug treatment could help many other panic sufferers learn how to control their symptoms.

The same may be true for people who have more generalized anxiety—a form of chronic, excessive worrying, combined with physical and emotional symptoms, that affects about 4 percent of Americans, according to NIMH estimates. Xanax itself, surprisingly, has never been tested as a long-term treatment for such chronic anxiety disorders. But Dr. David Barlow, a clinical psychologist who directs the Center for Stress and Anxiety Disorders of the State University of New York at Albany, points out that the benzodiazepines in general have not proved effective for treating these problems—except to offer temporary relief of symptoms.

Barlow reviewed two decades' worth of studies that used benzodiazepines to treat chronic anxiety. He observed that patients in the "control" groups for these studies—that is, patients who received inactive placebo pills—generally improved over time. In many cases, their anxiety decreased as much as that of the people who were on the real drugs. This suggests that chronic anxiety waxes and wanes over time, and that drugs may have little effect after their initial benefit.

Recommendations

If anxiety is an inevitable part of the human condition, then the wish for a magic potion to banish anxiety is probably a timeless human desire. In our own time, drug companies have marketed one tranquilizer after another, each one supposedly safer and more effective than the one before. But tranquilizers—in particular, the benzodiazepines—are still powerful, potentially dangerous drugs, subject to abuse and misuse.

Given the hazards and their widespread use, we still know surprisingly little about the risks and benefits of long-term benzodiazepine use—and too little in particular about Xanax, now the leader of the pack.

No one knows how many people are physically dependent on Xanax and how they may be affected by it. But here are some warning signs. A recent FDA analysis of reports of adverse reactions to drugs, which physicians send to the agency voluntarily, showed a number of cases in which the drug seemed to cause bouts of rage and hostility. Those side effects were rare, and were much less common with Xanax than with Halcion. But they were six times more common with Xanax than with Ativan, relative to each drug's sales. And Ativan's suspected side effects have been cited in a pending British class-action lawsuit against its manufacturer.

Consumers Union believes that more information is necessary to determine the frequency of side effects from Xanax—not only its effects on mood, but its potential for impairing memory and causing other cognitive problems. Careful surveillance of the drug's clinical use could do much to resolve these questions.

In the meantime, if you or a loved one has a serious problem with anxiety, you need to understand your options clearly.

If you're not normally an anxious person, but are going through a particularly difficult time—a divorce or the death of a parent, for instance—you may be able to handle your anxiety with no professional help, or perhaps with a few visits to a psycho-

Short-term therapy for depression had similarly positive results in a study conducted over the past decade by the National Institute of Mental Health. For people with mild to moderate depression, both cognitive therapy and a form of short-term treatment called interpersonal psychotherapy worked as well as drug treatment (in this case, imipramine). For patients with severe depression, drug treatment worked slightly better than either kind of therapy.

Despite the evident advantages of cognitive-behavioral therapy, it is still less accessible to most people than drug treatments. Relatively few psychologists and psychiatrists are trained in this form of therapy. Most health-insurance plans reimburse poorly for psychotherapy. And without the kind of expensive publicity that the drug companies can put behind their products, nondrug approaches have received less attention than they deserve.

Not everyone is a good candidate for cognitive-behavioral therapy. "You have to have someone who is highly motivated, and some people having prolonged and frequent panic attacks are just not able to endure the pain," says Dr. John Pecknold, a McGill University psychiatrist who participated in Upjohn's Xanax study.

Nevertheless, CU's medical consultants believe psychiatrists and their patients should more frequently consider this kind of short-term therapy as a treatment for anxiety and other psychological problems. These focused, effective methods entail less risk and offer better long-term results than drug therapy generally produces. They may also have the potential to be highly cost-effective. One recent study, for example, found even a single therapy session helped many people with panic attacks to overcome the problem. ℞

therapist to talk about the immediate stress. According to Dr. Yudofsky of Baylor, exercise, dietary changes (such as giving up caffeine), and other life-style changes can also help keep anxiety in check.

It can also be useful, and appropriate, to take Xanax or another benzodiazepine to cope with acute stress—as long as you take the drug carefully. If your doctor prescribes one of these drugs, take it at the lowest dose possible and for the shortest time possible. Remember that even a few weeks of daily Xanax use can lead to dependency.

If you're suffering from panic disorder, agoraphobia, or chronic anxiety, you have a serious problem that requires professional evaluation and treatment by a psychiatrist or psychologist. It's not clear, however, that drug treatment should be your first option. CU's medical consultants recommend seeing a mental-health professional who is familiar with cognitive-behavioral therapy (described below) before resorting to tranquilizers. Our consultants who have experience in both drug and nondrug therapy generally try the nondrug approaches first.

Whatever your problem is, you should avoid Xanax and its chemical cousins if you have any history of alcohol abuse or previous problems with other benzodiazepines. Those factors in your personal history make it more likely that you will become dependent on the drug. Alternative forms of drug therapy may be less risky. Antidepressants like imipramine can block panic attacks as effectively as Xanax can. For people with chronic anxiety who do not have panic attacks, a drug called BuSpar (buspirone) can frequently reduce anxiety and does not

cause the sedation or physical dependency produced by the benzodiazepines.

Finally, if your physician does prescribe Xanax or another benzodiazepine, question him or her closely about how long you are expected to take the medication and exactly how you are to withdraw from it. While on the medication, use extreme caution when driving, since these drugs can impair coordination. Do not exceed the prescribed dose, and do not drink alcohol while on the drug. (The interaction can be disastrous; at the least, it can worsen the slurred speech, poor coordination, drowsiness, and mental slowness that often stem from use of benzodiazepines.) Inform your doctor immediately of any unexpected side effects, such as feelings of rage or agitation. And seriously consider trying some sort of psychotherapy to gain insight into your problem.

* * *

"High Anxiety." Copyright © 1993 by Consumers Union of U.S., Inc., Yonkers, NY 10703-1057. Reprinted by permission from *Consumer Reports*, January 1993.

For Discussion

1. Should the Food and Drug Administration be more or less regulatory concerning drug approval? Why?

2. Xanax and Valium have been prescribed to far greater numbers of women than men. Why?

3. Should general practitioners be permitted to prescribe Xanax and other sedatives? Why or why not? ✦

9. Anabolic Steroids: An Ethnographic Approach

Paul J. Goldstein

For the most part, the illegal use of anabolic steroids is related to the nature of athletic competition. Many team and individual sports require that participants be at a continuous peak performance. Anabolic steroids affect tissue development and produce muscle mass which may temporarily improve athletic performance. But the dangers of steroids are well documented. Users may become quite aggressive and prone to violent behavior. Continued use has been linked with tissue and organ damage, as well as various cancers.

In the following [article] Paul J. Goldstein describes patterns of illicit anabolic steroid use. His research was based on observations and interviews with individuals who frequent fitness centers in New York City. Addressing the reasons for using steroids, Goldstein describes the physical and psychological effects of these drugs. He raises the concern that needle sharing among steroid users is a method of HIV transmission and discusses the potentially lethal effects of combining steroids with other drugs.

The intent of this [article] is to make two sorts of contributions. The first is conceptual—to provide a sociological framework and a substance-abuse perspective from which the emergent social problem of anabolic steroid misuse may be viewed. The second contribution is to present some preliminary empirical findings from participant observation research that was done in health clubs and gyms in the New York City area. As part of this effort, interviews were conducted with bodybuilders, personal trainers (PTs), and gym staff.

The poor quality of available data on the use and effects of anabolic steroids and their frequent contradictory nature is consistently bemoaned. There is clearly a need to advance beyond anecdotes, rumors, and locker-room gossip. Yet, it is important to realize that reports of such "gossip" provide an insight into the manner in which users perceive anabolic steroids, their motivations for use, and both their functional and dysfunctional experiences with these substances.

The approach employed herein is part of a methodological tradition common to the study of drug abuse. It focuses on understanding users' interpretations of the etiology and meaning of drug abuse within their own sociocultural environment. This tradition, with its roots in phenomenology, is usually called qualitative methodology, or ethnography. Its primary focus is on users' perceptions of meaning and the contexts of initiation and sustaining of drug-abusing behavior (McBride and Clayton 1985).

Data about the nature and scope of anabolic steroid use are difficult to collect and becoming more so, owing to recent upgrading of penalties for both steroid possession and sale. The Anti-Drug Abuse Act of 1988 upgraded federal penalties in this area. Some states had preceded the federal government in this regard, e.g., California; others have followed suit since the federal legislation; others are considering doing so. For example, Georgia has recently upgraded penalties for steroid trafficking to a third-degree felony status. This has reportedly made steroid users and traffickers in that state more reluctant to talk to researchers. According to one social scientist who had been interviewing high school and college steroid users, mainly football players, many participants in competitive athletics will no longer discuss their steroid experiences with outsiders, because they are afraid of being turned in (John R. Fuller, personal communication, January 1989).

The key informants, or "guides," who have been introducing me into various health clubs and gyms in New York City and Long Island all cautioned me against publicly declaring any special interest in steroids. I was told that everybody would just "clam up" if they learned that was my primary interest. I have been presenting myself simply as a sociologist interested in the workout and fitness world.

There are three principal areas in which information about steroid use and distribution must be generated: epidemiology, distribution, and consequences.

Epidemiology

Some sources provide a rough indication of the extent of steroid use. The Mayo Clinic estimated more than 1 million regular steroid users in America (Couzens 1988). It has been suggested that as many as 96 percent of professional football players may have taken steroids (Jacobson 1988; Schuckit

1988). It has also been suggested that between 80 and 99 percent of male bodybuilders have taken steroids (Schuckit 1988; Hecht 1984; Lee 1985). There has been talk of increasing steroid use among female bodybuilders, as the trend in that sport has moved away from the goal of obtaining a "dancer's physique" towards increasing muscularity (Lee 1985).

Buckley and colleagues (1988) found that 6.6 percent of a national sample of 12th-grade males reported using or having used anabolic steroids. Other scattered high-school level, epidemiological information includes an unscientific survey by Miami's South Plantation High School student newspaper in 1986. It sampled 200 of the school's 2,000 pupils. Sixty-five percent knew someone who was taking steroids (Miami Herald 1988). This sort of statistic is important, because other research in the substance-abuse field has shown that having drug-using peers is one of the best predictors of drug use. Eleven percent of high-school football players in Arkansas were reported to be using anabolic steroids (Herrmann 1988). Thirty-eight percent of high-school football players surveyed in Portland, Oregon, knew where to get steroids (Charlier 1988).

Many individuals who are informed about the high-school scene stress the importance of the steroid issue. Fred Rozelle, Executive Secretary of the Florida High School Activities Association, stated that "We face a lot of problems, but we feel that the number-one concern is steroids" (Phillips and Lohrer 1989, p. 4D). Don Leggett, a Food and Drug Administration (FDA) official, said, "Bulging muscles are in. Guys want to look good at the beach. High-school kids think steroids may enhance their ability to get an athletic scholarship, play professional sports, or win the girl of their heart. Steroid use in this country has spread down to general people" (Penn 1988, p. A1). A Philadelphia physical therapist who works with athletes stated, "People think the cocaine issue is big. It's not as big as anabolic steroids. Among kids, it's epidemic" (Charlier 1988, p. A20).

Within the context of epidemiology, substance-abuse researchers have tended to emphasize the concepts of a drug-using "career" or a "natural history" of drug use. Such careers, or natural histories, may be conceptualized as having three steps:

1. Initial stage of exploration.

2. Continuing stage, in which use is regular, and the identity of the user is established.

3. Cessation from use (usually preceded by growing ambivalence towards regular use and unsuccessful attempts at detachment).

Exploration Stage

Steroid use may be viewed as a search for a competitive edge in athletics. Many athletes have a win-at-any-cost mentality. Of course, this mentality is common to areas other than athletics. The rhetoric in these other areas is remarkably similar to the steroid rhetoric. For example, I recently received a brochure for a February 1989 conference on "Achieving Excellence." The conference included seminars in financial planning, organization, innovation, and leadership skills. One of the presenters was Nancy K. Austin, author of the 1985 publication, A Passion for Excellence: The Leadership Difference. The brochure announced her presentation as follows:

> Nancy K. Austin highlights how "winners"—even those in mundane, decaying, battered, or regulated environments—create and sustain their competitive edge. They don't just do a percent or two better than the rest, they do hundreds of percentage points better. . . . This presentation will highlight those who have achieved extraordinary results under fire and how they succeeded, while others faded away.

I suspect that, if a pill or an injectable were available that was touted to guarantee such a competitive edge in business, or in grant writing, it would be used eagerly. Steroids function in this fashion with regard to athletics and body development. Of course, what happens is similar to the arms race. Those with early access to an innovation do have an edge. Soon, however, the "have nots" catch up. In the case of steroids, the word now is that everybody is doing it and competitive steroid users no longer have an edge; they must use just to stay even with their rivals.

There can be no question that there has been an escalation of muscularity in those areas in which muscularity is important. Professional athletes are bigger and stronger now than they ever were. The old cinema muscle men, like Victor Mature, look fairly puny compared to modern titans like Arnold Schwarzenegger. Charles Atlas, in his famous advertisements of three decades ago, looks like a pretty ordinary guy today. Competitive bodybuilders claim that persons who won major titles 10, or even 5 years ago, would have little chance against today's competitors. One bodybuilder claimed that today "the only way you can make even the beginnings of an amateur is by taking steroids."

The use of performance enhancers in athletic competitions are neither new nor limited to steroids. Participants in 6-day bicycle races in 1879 were alleged to have prepared as follows: the French used a mixture made from a caffeine base; the Belgians ate sugar cubes dipped in ether; others drank alcohol cordials; and sprinters used nitroglycerine (STASH 1978). In 1886, a British cyclist died from using a drug containing ephedrine, a stimulant alleged to mask fatigue and remove physiological restraints intended to prevent overexertion (STASH 1978). In remarks to the January 1984 meeting of the FDA Endocrinologic and Metabolic Drugs Advisory Committee, Thomas Murray of the Hastings Center noted that performance enhancers were popular at the turn of the century. Vin Muriani, a widely used mixture of coca leaf extract and wine, was advertised as the wine for athletes. It was reportedly used by French cyclists and by a champion lacrosse team in Peru (Hecht 1984).

A variety of other substances or techniques are employed by athletes who try to give themselves an edge on the competition. These include special dietary regimens, vitamins, bicarbonate loading (for short events), caffeine loading (for long events), and such psychological techniques as hypnosis.

Some gyms sell a wide variety of products to their clientele. A blender will mix up an Aminofuel or Carbofuel drink for $2. For an extra $1, a banana will be added. Fruit punch-like concoctions that are billed as being rich in amino acids are sold for $2. In speaking with gym regulars, it becomes clear that some persons lack the sophistication to discriminate between such products and steroids.

For young high-school athletes, getting big and strong enough to compete on the collegiate level may be vital for their future. Don Reynolds, chairman of the drug-abuse committee of Florida High School Activities Association, stated, "I think there is a lot more steroid use than we think there is. High schools is where it's at. That's where the competition for college scholarships begins" (Phillips and Lohrer 1989, p. 4D). Parents may contribute to this pressure to obtain athletic scholarships.

Steroid use should also be viewed in the context of the search for substances that increase feelings and appearances of strength. Steroid research has been likened to the search for a "superman formula" (Schuckit 1988). Stories of great strength

have intrigued our imaginations for centuries. We have television series like "The Bionic Man"; comic book superheroes like Superman and the Hulk; biblical supermen like Samson; legendary strongmen like Hercules; that staple of carnivals, the sideshow strong man; professional wrestlers; a long list of male movie stars, such as Victor Mature, Steve Reeves, and Arnold Schwarzenegger, whose muscular bodies were their main attraction for the ticket-buying public. Weight-lifting competitions are popular Olympic events. Bodybuilding contests attract large audiences and are frequently shown on cable television. Children watching Saturday morning cartoon shows aspire to the impossible-to-achieve muscularity of superheroes, such as He-Man. Popeye's spinach-eating produces the great strength that allows him to vanquish his comical opponents.

Clearly, there is something about muscular development and great strength that taps into something very basic to the male mentality. Sexual attractiveness is part of this. Young boys want to impress the girls with their muscles. One young man that I spoke to in a gym remarked that it is tough for high-school kids when a muscular guy takes their girl away. Some boys feel that they cannot compete with a guy who has a great body. It is a real incentive for them to try to develop their own bodies as fast as possible. Steroids present the promise that such aspirations can be achieved through chemistry.

In health clubs and gyms, I have observed the frustration felt by those who are working out intensely, yet who are not achieving substantial results. This frustration is intense for persons who are working out next to someone who is enjoying good results, i.e., getting bigger and stronger much more rapidly than they are. Such frustrated persons become targets of pushers who offer a short cut to physical development. Pushers may compliment persons on their successful workout regimen but stress that, if the person continues to work out at such a pace, it may take 5 or 6 more years of struggle and pain before the person will look that certain way. Of course, there is a way to get there a lot sooner. That way is, of course, the use of anabolic steroids.

Successful bodybuilders, especially competitors, are usually approached in a different fashion. Pushers of steroids may begin their sales pitch to successful bodybuilders by saying such things as the following:

1. "You're looking good, but you look unfinished. You need something in order to get that finished look."

2. "You look good enough to enter a competition. But you don't look good enough to win. You'll need something else for that."

However, a former steroid user and PT who has worked with adolescents cautions against attributing most steroid use to competitive bodybuilders or other athletes:

Forget that! I think the majority of people who use steroids don't have any idea of going into a contest. Let's not go in a direction that these steroids are being used by bodybuilders who aspire to be Mr. Universe. That's baloney. Steroids are being used mostly by men and women and young kids just for their ego.

. . . I see the kids using it today. It just blows my mind. They are using at a young age for one reason only, for their egos. Whether to get dates, whether to be part of a gang. . . . The peer pressure is enormous for strength. If you're not a rock singer, you damn well better be a muscle man.

. . . once bodybuilding hits you, it doesn't matter. Once the idea of strength and size, and feeling good about yourself and being admired and looked at, hits you, you could be from anywhere.

Users also describe a euphoric state produced by steroids. One user said, "The anabolics make you feel good mentally. They are a high."

Continuing Stage

For whatever reasons people begin steroid use, it appears that the addictive nature of the substance, the habituating effect of the workout routine itself, and the feelings of muscularity and strength that arise, create a syndrome of continued and habitual use.

Addiction is a difficult concept to operationalize. Previous research with heroin users indicated that individuals who are typically classified as heroin addicts, in fact, have patterns of use that contain many peaks and valleys, and days of non-use are frequently intermixed with days of use (Johnson et al. 1985). In other words, operational definitions of addiction, especially those employing a medical model, may be of limited value in predicting actual behavior of substance users in their environments over time.

The classic behavioral definition of addiction was that advanced by Alfred Lindesmith (1947). Essentially, he argued that persons might begin using a drug for a variety of reasons, usually involving positive feelings produced by the drug. Individuals might continue to use the drug for this reason. However, real addiction sets in when the individual experiences negative feelings, such as pain or dysphoria in the absence of the drug, attributes these negative sensations to the lack of the drug, and begins to administer the drug to ward off the negative sensations, rather than attempting to achieve a positive feeling.

A variety of knowledgeable sources, including Robert Voy, have argued that an addiction syndrome exists with regard to anabolic steroids (Jacobson 1988; Schuckit 1988). Craig Whitehead, who directed the drug-rehabilitation unit of the Haight-Ashbury Clinic, stated, "The dependence many people develop on steroids is classic" (Cowart 1987a, p. 427).

The addiction syndrome that has been described to me by habitual steroid users harmonizes well with Lindesmith's definition. Users claim that steroids function to anesthetize the body. Steroids enable the user to work out intensely, without feeling pain. However, when the user stops taking steroids, muscles and joints (especially) become very sore. Old injuries or strains that were not even noticed before begin to be very painful. The ex-user cannot work out anywhere near the level that he or she did while taking steroids. It is just too painful now. Indeed, common everyday physical tasks may become difficult and painful. Psychological feelings of depression set in. If the user returns to steroids, the pain disappears. The depression disappears. One's body feels good again. One can return to one's workout regimen.

A PT whom I interviewed described some manifestations of this addictive state of mind:

I hear it all the time. I heard it just yesterday . . . three guys . . . I asked them how they're doing. They said, "Well, good. I just got back from skiing. I can't wait to get back on the stuff." That's all you hear. And another guy, "How you been?" "Good, doing all right, you know, maintaining, but in 2 weeks I got all my stuff together now, I'm going back on the stuff." These are not competitive bodybuilders.

These are just gym guys who are printers and going to school.

A steroid user described to me the manner in which steroids affect the psychology of users and function to perpetuate use:

If you never use [steroids], you use your natural inclination to drive forward. Whatever may have been your driving force, whether it was to show your father that you can succeed in life, or whether it was being insecure and needing to have assurance from the world that you can be somebody. . . . If you have that burning up so hard in you, then you can make it with that. But once you get on the steroids, you'll lose that ability to call upon self. It then controls you, and you actually lose the ability to ever do that again. There's a part of you that goes and never comes back. . . . If you do it for one little 12-week cycle, and you can manage to get off it, and you say, "This was not for me," God bless you. But if you're stuck on that stuff for a year, you're hooked for life. You're no longer a virgin . . . you're finished. You forget a lot of the innocence that you had. Or a lot of the natural drive that is in there. 'Cause this stuff gives you a new level of aggression and power that you can't achieve on your own by thinking it out on your own anymore. You just can't. You try! Like you're lifting a dumbbell, and you give up. "I ain't going to do it. I'm leaving." But you go to the gym when you're on that stuff, and everything is going good, and your levels are real built up high. . . . You take that weight, 40 pounds heavier, and you do it. Screaming! Crazy joy! Ecstasy! It is like having an orgasm. It's better. You don't have any idea what it's like. . . . It's total orgasm. Oneness. It is like a one-cell creature reproducing itself. It's just incredible. . . . The fire, the escalation of joy and excitement, the conquering of it. And it's nowhere near as exciting when you're off the stuff as when you're on it. You just feel so good that you just want to buy 20 bottles more. That's the way it is. It's crazy.

Some users say that feelings of power become so associated with steroid use that persons begin to use steroids for social situations in which they feel insecure. For example, adolescents may take steroids before going to a party because they feel nervous, and the steroids give them a sense of being able to handle the situation. In this case, the drugs address basic feelings of inadequacy. One user stated, "You get to believe in the drugs so much that if you need a crutch you will take a few extra pills."

Several factors appear inextricably linked in a steroid addiction syndrome. For example, steroid users find it almost impossible to analytically separate the drug from the workout itself. They say that one would just not exist without the other. Without the drug, there would be no workout. Without the workout, there would be no need for the drug. It should be noted that persons who do not use steroids, yet who are also committed to working out, frequently talk about the addictive nature of a workout regimen. But serious steroid use and habitual working out seem to dissolve into a unitary lifestyle. One user vividly described this reality:

You get into the vicious cycle of doing more and more and more and doing new sophisticated stuff. . . . Then, once you're on the stuff, you feel differently. See, you're on it and all of a sudden you're making the gains. . . . And you're strong. And you have no pains like you had before. You're very euphoric. You kind of feel indestructible. And nothing matters. They can steal your car. You know, so what? If you caught the guy, you would kill him. But if you didn't, all right, the car's gone. As long as the gym is open. . . . Don't steal your food. Don't steal your steroids. But you can take my car, my wife, take anything you want. That's really how you become. And you don't know it. You're in this fog.

The gym culture itself tends to perpetuate steroid use. The gym culture is very competitive. Bodybuilders are always comparing themselves to other gym regulars or to the proverbial "new guy," as to who is biggest and strongest. Persons who are getting bigger and stronger may feel puny and weak, because a gym buddy is progressing faster than they—lifting more weight or adding more lean muscle. Girls hanging around the gym gravitate towards the biggest, strongest guys. Friends exert pressure to get back on "the stuff." The grapevine is filled with gossip about who is selling what. Special "deals" may be offered. The peer pressure to continue steroid use is strong.

Cessation From Use

Steroid users that I have talked with tend to cease their use for one of two reasons. Most younger persons seem to "mature out" when they reach an age at which career, marriage, and all the trappings of conventional lifestyles become more highly valued than a macho image of great strength and size. Older, long-term steroid users tend to quit only when their health is seriously threatened. A long-term steroid user who had been a highly successful competitive bodybuilder claimed to have almost died from liver problems about 3 years ago:

> After I got sick, I had to come off it, or I never would have come off it. I would never have come off of steroids if I didn't get sick. Never! I'd still be using it today and trying to compete at 40. But I was forced. I almost died. So, you choose between that and living. You find out living is not so bad.

Distribution

Until recently, black-market sale of steroids was estimated at more than $100 million per year (Couzens 1988; Penn 1988; Kahler 1989). However, this estimate was recently upgraded to between $300 and $400 million per year by Leslie Southwick, Deputy Assistant Attorney General (1990).

It has been estimated that more than half the steroids smuggled into the United States are counterfeit, frequently bearing the names of reputable manufacturers. Most supplies are alleged to come from Mexico (Penn 1988; Kahler 1989). These counterfeits are often produced in crude, unsanitary laboratories and are of dubious purity. Counterfeit steroids are also being manufactured in this country, in makeshift laboratories that are springing up around the United States. My own sources in gyms in the New York City area have suggested that as much as 80 percent of the steroids that they encounter are counterfeit.

One clandestine laboratory, Fountain Valley Research Laboratories, Inc., located 35 miles south of Los Angeles, was shut down recently. It produced what were labeled as East German steroids. The labels read: *Eigentum Der DDR-Versenden Gesetzlich Verboten*—"Property of GDR, export prohibited." The steroids fetched $180 per bottle. "East German steroids are rated the best," said a California lawman. "Their athletes have the reputation of being better, bigger, and stronger" (Penn 1988, p. A20).

The Department of Justice has recently expressed an interest in the use and trafficking of steroids. Assistant Attorney General John Bolton stated the following:

> Not only are we concerned with the risks associated with the unprescribed use of legitimate steroids [by adolescents], risks such as upsetting the hormonal balance and stunting growth, but of equal or greater concern is the unauthorized use of illegitimate ster-

oids which have no FDA approval and are made under less than sanitary conditions. We think it's a very dangerous problem. . . . You will see a lot more prosecutions. Prosecution of steroid cases is a priority for the civil division. (Kahler 1989, p. 29)

Justice officials have reportedly obtained federal convictions or guilty pleas against 60 steroid traffickers in the 2-1/2 years preceding October 1988. About 120 more persons face charges (Penn 1988). In December 1988, former British Olympic medalist David Jenkins was sentenced to 7 years in prison, followed by 5 years probation, and was fined $75,000 for his role in arranging for a Tijuana plant, Laboratorios Milano de Mexico, to produce anabolic steroids and smuggle them across the border for distribution in the United States (Kahler 1989).

There are indications that traditional drug traffickers are involved in steroid distribution. There are also indications that they are conducting their business in the traditional ways of drug traffickers. The following account appeared in the *Wall Street Journal*:

> According to criminal charges filed in San Diego last year, when a man in Phoenix reneged on a steroid deal, his supplier sent an emissary named Leonard T. Swirda. Mr. Swirda took along an accomplice carrying a 12-inch club, a double-edged knife and leather gloves weighted with metal, says the indictment, which accuses Mr. Swirda of beating and cutting the dealer. In a separate action, Mr. Swirda last May was indicted for cocaine trafficking in Spokane, Washington. (Penn 1988, p. Al, A20)

The underground world of steroid use and trafficking is prone to the same sorts of hustles and scams that we are more used to hearing about with regard to street drugs, such as cocaine or heroin. One common hustle concerns the difference in price between generic and name-brand steroids. Brand names, of course, fetch a higher price. Inexperienced users are frequently sold generic steroids, but are charged brand-name prices.

A former steroid user, speaking of the great prevalence of bogus steroids, recalled a product called Bolasterone:

> Bolasterone. It swept the country. They made millions. Millions, these California guys. All it was, was vegetable oil, a little bit of testosterone, and liquid aspirin. And they called it Bolasterone. And they hyped it up so much. It was selling for $250 to $275 a bottle. You would do anything to get this stuff. [They

said] "Mr. Olympia used it! Secretly." I tell you, Madison Avenue could not have come up with a better campaign to sell this stuff. . . . If you had a bottle of it, I mean you could sell it for anything. . . . [It was hyped] through the grapevine. Underground. The network is incredible. From gym to gym to gym. . . . They'll say, "Did you see M.? He put on 15 pounds in a week." "What the hell is he using?" "Don't say anything. He's using Bolasterone!" "Wow. What the hell is it? Can you get it?" "Yeah, I can."

It is difficult to estimate actual costs to users because of a wide variability in patterns of use. Serious long-term users may spend as much as $200 to $400 per week on steroids and the accompanying pharmacopoeia. Since such users may go on cycles of steroid use lasting 12 to 14 weeks, each cycle can cost in the thousands of dollars. Users are generally afraid of being caught short in the middle of a cycle, and like to have all the drugs that they will be using in hand before they start their cycle.

Cycles generally begin with a few pills of this kind, a few pills of that kind during the first week; gradually the number and strength of pills is increased; then injectibles are introduced into the cycle. As the weeks go by, the number of pills and shots increase, until a plateau is reached; for example, about the ninth week of a 14-week cycle. Then users come back down the same way they went up.

Younger, or less experienced or committed users, will use considerably less. Some persons may be long-term users, but take only one injection per week. Adolescents may go on shorter cycles, perhaps only 6 weeks. Some adolescents will only use when they have the money to do so. These youngsters may take a very few pills or shots on an irregular basis.

As with most drug use, a primary way of supporting one's own steroid use is trafficking in the substance. Also, since many users do not use that much, they are able to support their steroid use by working, getting money from women, stealing from their parents, or engaging in petty theft. Competitive athletes may be supplied by coaches, promoters, or other interested parties.

Steroid use may also be supported by male friends. Older or wealthier homosexuals are frequently interested in the company of young, male bodybuilders. These homosexual liaisons may involve sexual activity or remain at the friendship level. Older bodybuilders report that this phenomenon was more common prior to the advent of AIDS than it is today.

Male bodybuilders may obtain employment for which their muscularity especially qualifies them. Some examples of these sorts of jobs include bouncers, male dancers in such clubs as Chippendales, and models.

PTs

One of the hallmarks of the sociological approach is a focus on social structure and social roles. David Matza summarized the sociological approach nicely in a discussion of delinquency:

> The distinguishing feature of sociological theory, in contrast to formulations stressing personality, lies in the prominence of the social situation. Sociology brings to the foreground the social circumstances that form the backdrop for personality theory. (Matza 1964, p. 17)

In doing ethnographic research in health clubs and gyms, I was struck by a particular social role— the PT. PTs enjoy a high status in the "workout" world. They are the cognoscenti, the knowledgeable insiders, the gurus. They instruct their clients in a wide variety of areas, including workout techniques, diet, nutritional supplements, and sometimes in the use of steroids. PTs typically work with a heterogeneous clientele that may include overweight housewives, professional football players, competitive bodybuilders, adolescents who want to look better, and simple gym habitués.

Most clients do not appear interested in ascertaining potential PTs' educational or professional credentials; they are more concerned with how PTs look. If a PT has a title, e.g., Mr. America, that seems to carry the most weight with potential clients. The title is proof of the PT's ability to condition a body; it is a real status thing to be able to say that Mr. America is one's PT. Additional status is held by PTs with ties to professional athletics. It enhances clients' status to be able to say that their PT trains football players. It is also fun to feel like an insider, e.g., to get some gossip about sports celebrities.

Individuals become PTs for a variety of reasons. The basic reason is, of course, money. PTs tend to be young men and women beginning a career in the fitness business, young athletically oriented persons who reject a 9-to-5 office existence, or older athletes who are retired from competition and who may have few marketable job skills. Health clubs pay very low wages. At one health club that I visited, the fitness director, who had 3 years experience, a bachelor's degree, and some credits towards a masters degree, made $19,000 per year. There is a need to supplement salary by taking on private clients, who will pay about $25 per hour.

Bartering is not uncommon among PTs. For example, one young female PT that I spoke with has a client who is a psychiatrist. They exchange hours of physical training for hours of therapy.

PTs' income may be erratic. Clients go in and out of phases of life dedicated to working out. Clients are usually fairly wealthy and may do lots of traveling. They may go south during the winter, cutting substantially into a PT's income.

PTs may recruit and see clients at a number of different health clubs or gyms. They may spend some mornings at this gym; some afternoons at that gym; some evenings at yet another. They may also go to client's homes. Their network of contacts tends to be far-reaching.

There appears to be a growing professionalization of the fitness field, exemplified by the growth of degree programs in physical education, biomechanics, exercise physiology, and so on. New young holders of professional certifications are in conflict with older fitness and bodybuilding trainers whose knowledge is experiential rather than learned from books.

Older PTs used their own bodies as their laboratories, experimenting with various workout routines, nutritional programs, and drugs, including steroids. The success of particular regimens was subjectively determined and also objectively determined in terms of looks, performance, and titles achieved.

I have observed conflict in health clubs between younger credentialed PTs and older non-credentialed PTs. They argue over which pieces of equipment to install and what sort of training regimens are appropriate to use. They are in competition for clients, scarce jobs, and the acceptance of their point of view, as to how the subject matter in their field should be taught. The situation may be viewed, from the standpoint of occupational sociology, as a case of developing professionalism, which poses interesting sociology-of-knowledge issues, regarding experiential vs. academic knowledge.

The prevalence of PTs is difficult to estimate. Most trainers that I spoke with were reluctant to make any quantitative estimates. The best "guesstimates" that I was able to obtain were that there are about 1,000 PTs in New York's Nassau County going to persons' homes, and about 1,500 working in clubs. The American College of Sports Medicine certifies trainers, but it appears that most trainers work without certification; and, hence, it would be difficult to ascertain how many PTs there actually are.

For comparative purposes, there are approximately 1,200 Aerobics and Fitness Association of America (AFAA)-certified aerobics instructors teaching on Long Island, which includes Nassau and Suffolk counties, according to Peg Jordan, editor of *American Fitness* magazine. However, about 50 percent of all Long Island instructors have had no professional training at all. That percentage is better than the national average, in which only an estimated 17,000 of 100,000 aerobic instructors are AFAA-certified (Hancock 1989).

PTs play an interesting role with regard to steroid use and distribution. Some may be users themselves. PTs may be motivated to use steroids, because they feel a need to look perfect. Their ability to secure and maintain clients may depend on how good they look, how good their clients perceive them as looking, and how they perceive themselves as looking.

More important, PTs, as bodybuilding gurus, have a strong influence on their clients. This influence may be exerted to encourage or discourage steroid use. Experienced PTs, because of their wide networks of contacts, may be pressured by clients to supply them with steroids. PTs may be financially motivated to supply steroids to clients that ask for them. In addition to the profit to be made from selling steroids, PTs are primarily concerned with maintaining clientele. If they do not supply steroids to a client that requests them, the client may find another PT that will supply steroids. The original PT then loses a client. One PT remarked that, for this reason, he will not train bodybuilders anymore:

> It just got to be too nuts. What with you trying to please everybody. Who wants this, who wants that, and you're watching everybody self-destruct. I couldn't take it. When you train bodybuilders, that one-to-one trainer will certainly be looked upon as the guru of many things. And certainly, it affords the trainer an opportunity to make a lot of money. But it isn't the one-to-one trainer who is the source of distribution of the stuff. Really. It occurs, and it happens, but he isn't the main. He doesn't get into it to do that.

Older PTs, especially those who are or have been steroid users themselves, express horror at the naivete with which many young persons approach the use of steroids. Many PTs feel a responsibility to coach the young person in the proper use of these substances to minimize the potential health consequences. A 57-year-old man who claimed to have taken one shot of decadurabolin per week, "forever," said that the kids today were worrying him:

[They are] . . . using so much stuff. I walk into the gym, and they're all 17 years old, and they all look like pus heads. . . . They are all puffed out with water. And they have very little muscle. Because they are just throwing crap into their bodies. They have no idea. . . . And who knows what they are doing to their insides. . . . They're stupid by taking the steroids so wrong.

A PT remarked that everyone is different, and the steroid users must be medically monitored, both while on cycles and when between cycles:

Blood tests . . . white-cell counts. We're looking to see liver, kidney problems. We are looking to see pancreatic and pituitary problems. We want to see their testosterone levels, estrogen levels, nitrogen levels. We want to see their blood-sugar level, thyroid, adrenal, and, if they have normalized, they can go back on them. If it's 4 weeks, they can go back on them. If it is 4 months, they have to keep taking the test until they're normal. If not, no sense going back on it again. The body won't react. They just keep getting worse. You do need a healthy body to keep this stuff working to the maximum.

Additional factors mentioned as important were levels of minerals, such as calcium and magnesium. Steroids are calcium-depleting.

With regards to steroids currently being used, I am told that the trend today is towards veterinary steroids. One user described this trend in the following way:

Veterinary drugs are cheaper, they come in much larger quantities, and they're much better. . . . They're more anabolic. The androgenic ones tend to build fat, hold water. . . . Race horses are the biggest users of anabolic steroids. They cannot breed a horse that's full of water and fat. Every tiny micro-ounce must be muscle, or he's not going to win a race. He cannot carry any extra weight. So, if you have ever seen a race horse up close, it's built like the greatest bodybuilders of the world. They are

ripped to the bone. And they are very muscular and thick. So, that has certainly seeped its way down . . . in the last 20 years. And a lot of the drugs they are using now are the veterinary drugs. The Winstrol-V, [and others]. . . . They come in these huge 50-cc bottles.

I don't think the veterinarians are selling them to bodybuilders. I think they're a lot more sensible than that. But it is filtering down through the veterinary market. I think maybe the distributors or the salesmen have found the market.

Consequences

Some experienced steroid users place much of the responsibility for the current problem on pharmaceutical companies and suggest that the nature and scope of health consequences are likely to increase in the future. A long-term steroid user stated the following:

Athletes that used them in the late forties, they . . . used it very sparingly, so anybody who developed a tumor here or there, it had to be very scarce. Then the fifties came, and some synthetics came in to being used. Then the sixties came, and a little more research got involved in it. Around the late sixties or early seventies, the drug companies realized there was a hell of a market here for the stuff. So, they threw some dollars into research. Now, the steroids are so sophisticated and are getting even more sophisticated. The old ones are not even available anymore. They got a whole new line. . . . The more powerful ones weren't being used, certainly not as often as today. Now, in the eighties, and going into the nineties, they are using anabolics that . . . work so fast, they are so powerful . . . I don't think the body has caught up with the dosage or the science of it all. . . . And not as many people were using it as they are today, because the sport [bodybuilding] was not as popular in the past as it is today. . . . So, 20 years from now, you're going to see a whole bunch of people dying. But you are going to have to wait 20 years.

There is a long list of health consequences that have been associated with the use of anabolic steroids. Unfortunately, good clinical documentation and elaboration, obtained through rigorously controlled experimental studies, is lacking in most areas. However, the list of commonly discussed health consequences of steroid use includes liver problems (tumors, peliosis hepatitis), kidney problems, hypertension, psychiatric problems (depression, aggression), sexual problems in males (testicular atrophy, decreased sperm production, gynecomastia), sexual problems in females (menstrual irregularities, shrinkage of breast tissue, hypertrophy of the clitoris, facial hair, deepened voice), acne, physical injuries, cholesterol difficulties, cardiovascular problems, stunted growth in adolescents, male pattern baldness, fetal damage, gallstones, and so on. Since most of these topics are covered by other chapters in this volume, I chose to focus my discussion of health consequences on only two areas that are of traditional interest to drug-abuse researchers: (1) interactions between steroids and other drugs and (2) needle sharing.

Steroids and Other Drugs

In the area of health consequences, the National Institute on Drug Abuse (NIDA) should have a special interest in interaction effects between steroids and other drugs of abuse. In this regard, experienced steroid-using bodybuilders hold a taken-for-granted prohibition against using cocaine while on a steroid cycle. They claim that there is a great danger of heart attacks if the two substances are mixed. One user stated that whenever he reads of a young athlete dying suddenly of a heart attack, he immediately suspects an interaction between steroids and cocaine.

Amphetamines may be used to help drive the workout regimen. Long-term steroid users report that, as the years go by, steroids lose their ability to provide the driving force for the workout routine. At this point, "speed" may come to be used. Under the influence of speed, bodybuilders report going "nuts," working out until totally exhausted, and then "falling out."

No one that I have spoken with reported any specific interactions between alcohol and steroids. In fact, most of the bodybuilders who shared their experiences with me were very moderate drinkers or abstainers. Interestingly, one person observed that, in his opinion, persons who have great tolerance to alcohol tend to have a great tolerance to steroids:

> Those who get drunk on a beer really get a lot of side effects real quick on steroids. Migraine headaches, bloody noses, deep acne—tremendous scarring of the face. It is funny. . . .

Experienced steroid users also report using a wide variety of other drugs along with steroids. The primary purpose of these other drugs is to cope with the side effects of the steroids. For example, in order to prevent or retard the spread of acne, antibiotics are used. Nolvadex is medicine used in the treatment of breast cancer. It is an antiestrogen. Bodybuilders may use Nolvadex during steroid cycles to keep their estrogen levels down.

When coming off a steroid cycle, human chorionic gonadotropin (HCG) and Clomid are used. HCG is a polypeptide hormone produced by the human placenta. It is derived from the urine of pregnant women. The use of exogenous hormones (steroids) tends to depress the body's natural hormone production. Heavy steroid users wish to return to normal levels of testosterone as quickly as possible when they come off a steroid cycle. They claim the body is usually sluggish and just takes too long to return to normal hormonal activity. HCG is reportedly used to simulate an estrogen buildup in the male which "shocks" the system into a more rapid recovery. Clomid, a female fertility drug, is alleged to perform the same trickery. Teslac and Halotestin are also reported to accomplish this result.

Long-term steroid users claim that there is a right way to do steroids which involves full knowledge of pharmacological "chain reactions." The above discussion has just presented a few of the substances that are commonly employed by anabolic steroid users who were interviewed in the New York City area. Some of these users maintain amazing pharmacopeias.

There are two contrary health-consequence aspects of this multiple-drug use. The first relates to the utility and dangers of this wide range of drugs being used by the most pharmacologically sophisticated steroid users. The other health-consequence aspect refers to the fact that many users are not sophisticated; they are not aware of potentially damaging side effects or the means for circumventing them. Many young men can barely afford the steroids that they are using. They see the purchase of these other substances as a low-priority item in an already strained budget. A sophisticated PT stated the following:

> These kids, of course, don't know anything about this. . . . I get the reaction from them like I have two heads. Some of them don't want to listen to it. They say, "I'm just taking my 'tes' or my Dianabol 'cause my friend is taking them." But anybody who is serious about going on them . . . and who is really interested in his health and going on a couple of cycles, will have to absorb this.

Needle Sharing

Persons using injectable steroids are prone to all the health hazards common to needle users of any substance. This includes diseases associated with bacterial infections caused by injections with non-sterile equipment. This practice may lead to localized infection problems, such as abscesses and cellulitis, or systemic problems, such as endocarditis, hepatitis, and AIDS.

A competitive bodybuilder reported that a number of his colleagues had problems when they were first learning how to inject themselves:

> A lot of people don't know how to do it. They do it eventually, because they feel they have to. Or they get a friend who learned from a friend who learned from a sister who is a nurse. That's generally how it works. And you learn how to put it in a muscle. A lot of guys have come to me that they hit a vein and they are black or blue. . . . You hit too much in the same site and you get tumors all the time. A lot of bodybuilders had to get those cut out. . . . Actually, you get huge fibroid lumps that develop from hitting the same sites.

Harold Connally, an Olympic gold medalist in the hammer throw, testified to the following before a U.S. Senate Committee in 1973:

> It was not unusual in 1968 to see athletes with their own medical kits, practically a doctor's, in which they would have syringes and all their various drugs. . . . I know any number of athletes on the '68 Olympic team who had so much scar tissue and so many puncture holes on their backsides that it was difficult to find a fresh spot to give them a new shot. (Hecht 1984, p. 14)

All competitive athletes that I have spoken with denied using dirty needles or sharing needles. As one person stated, "The guy who's selling you the needles wants you to buy 100 needles. He don't want to sell you two needles."

However, in some inner-city gyms, I did get reports that heterosexual lovers, perhaps spouses, who are working out together will sometimes share needles. It's part of the "we do everything else together, so why not this" feeling. A young woman told me that such couples decide which muscles they will work on that day, inject into that muscle, sharing the needle, and then go and do their workout.

A 1984 letter to the editor of *The New England Journal of Medicine* from six physicians at Nassau Hospital in New York described a case of AIDS in a bodybuilder using anabolic steroids. This was a 37-year-old white male who denied any history of homosexual activity. He did admit to injecting cocaine intravenously on one occasion approximately 6 months prior to hospital admission. During the 4 years before admission, the patient had injected anabolic steroids intramuscularly on a weekly basis. The needles were often shared with other bodybuilders at various gyms. The physicians state that their experience with this patient indicates that intramuscular injection of anabolic steroids through shared needles may serve as a mode for dissemination of the AIDS virus. "Because this practice appears to be common among many athletes . . . persons at risk must be warned" (Sklarek et al. 1984, p. 1701).

A recent issue of *Sports Illustrated* featured a story on Benji Ramirez, a 17-year-old boy from Ashtabula, Ohio, who was alleged to have died from steroid-related heart problems. While there appears to be some question as to both the cause of death in this case and the nature and extent of Ramirez's actual involvement with steroids, the story does contain the following account:

> Another of Ramirez's classmates . . . says that on two occasions last summer he purchased steroids from Ramirez and used them in his company. In both instances, Ramirez injected the classmate in the buttock and then injected himself. (Telander and Noden 1989, p. 78)

It is not clear from this account whether the boys shared the needle. The possibility seems to be present here and in other cases, in which naive youngsters with limited financial resources may be involved with injectable steroids.

Needs for Further Research

It is customary, and frequently gratuitous, to end a research paper with a statement of the need for future research. However, in the area of anabolic steroids, that need is clear and immediate. The following sorts of data are needed:

1. Good epidemiological data are needed regarding incidence and prevalence of steroid use in different populations.

2. Data are needed on the frequency and volume of steroid use in different populations, including data on concomitant use of other substances with steroids.

3. Data are needed regarding the consequences of increasing criminal penalties for use or possession of steroids.

4. Data are needed on the health consequences and other effects of long-term use of steroids.

5. Data are needed on the natural history of steroid use in different populations, including patterns of use and cessation associated with different stages of life.

6. Given the general trend in society towards drug testing, and the specific trend towards steroid testing in both amateur and professional athletics, data are needed on (a) what should be done when a steroid-problem area, e.g., high-school football, is identified; and (b) what should be done when a specific steroid user is identified.

7. Data are needed on the patterns of steroid distribution, and how they are similar to or different from distribution patterns associated with other substances. Of special interest in this regard is the extent to which systemic violence may be beginning to be associated with black-market steroid sales.

8. Data are needed on the cost of steroid use, and how users support their consumption.

9. Data are needed on the extent to which counterfeit steroids have penetrated the market, and the specific sorts of problems associated with these substances.

10. Data need to be generated on the extent of needle sharing among steroid users. Special attention should be paid to gay populations in this regard.

11. Data are needed on the effect of steroid use among persons with existing mental disorders.

12. The role of steroid use in sports injuries needs to be further explored.

✳ ✳ ✳

Paul J. Goldstein, "Anabolic Steroids: An Ethnographic Approach," in Geraline C. Lin and Lynda Erinoff (eds.), *Anabolic Steroid Abuse* (Rockville, MD: National Institute on Drug Abuse, 1990), pp. 74-96.

For Discussion

Should we change the nature of athletic competition in order to curb the use of anabolic steroids? If so, how? What resistance could we expect from organized athletics?

References

Buckley, W. E., Yesalis, C. E., Friedl, K. E., Anderson, W. A., Streit, A., and Wright, J. E. Estimated prevalence of anabolic steroid use among male high-school seniors. *JAMA 260*(23):3441-3445, 1988.

Chapman, F. S. Steroid edge: Real or illusion. *Washington Post*, October 18, 1988. p. 8.

Charlier, M. For teens, steroids may be bigger issue than cocaine use. *Wall Street Journal*, October 4, 1988. p. A20.

Couzens, G. S. A serious drug problem. *Newsday*, November 26, 1988. p. II, 5.

Cowart, V. Steroids in sports: After four decades, time to return these genies to the bottle? *JAMA 257*(4):421-427, 1987a.

Cowart, V. Physician-competitor's advice to colleagues: Steroid users respond to education, rehabilitation. *JAMA 257*(4):427-428, 1987b.

Hancock, L. Have body, will travel. *Long Island Monthly 2*(2):21-23, 1989.

Hecht, A. Anabolic steroids: Pumping trouble. *FDA Consumer*, September 1984. pp. 12-15.

Herrmann, M. Steroids: A vague threat. *Newsday*, October 30, 1988. pp. 36, 31.

Huapt, H. A., and Rovere, G. D. Anabolic steroids: A review of the literature. *Am J Sports Med 12*(6):469-484, 1984.

Jacobson, S. NFL is late in seeing the light. *Newsday*, November 6, 1988. pp. 9, 40.

Johnson, B. D., Goldstein, P. J., Preble, E., Schmeidler, J., Lipton, D. S., Spunt, B. J., and Miller, T. *Taking Care of Business: The Economics of Crime by Heroin Abusers*. Lexington: Lexington Books, 1985.

Kahler, K. Steroids 'mania' spawning perilous new drug traffic. *The Sunday Star Ledger* (Newark), January 8, 1989. pp. 1, 29.

Lee, B. L. Growth drug hitting black market. *The Journal*, Addiction Research Foundation *15*(9):4, 1985.

Lindesmith, A. R. *Opiate Addiction*. Evanston: Principia Press, 1947.

Mann, F. Dark side of steroids plagues former boxer. *Miami Herald*, December 27, 1988. pp. 1D, 4D.

Matza, D. *Delinquency and Drift*. New York: John Wiley, 1964.

McBride, D., and Clayton, R. C. Methodological issues in the etiology of drug abuse. *J Drug Issues 15*(4):509-529, 1985.

Miami Herald. Study: 6 percent of teen boys use steroids. December 23, 1988. pp. 1A, 7A.

Penn, S. Muscling in. *Wall Street Journal*, October 4, 1988. pp. A1, A20.

Phillips, M., and Lohrer, R. High schools are considering steroid tests. *Miami Herald*, January 14, 1989. pp. 1D, 4D.

Schuckit, M. A. Weight lifter's folly: The abuse of anabolic steroids. *Drug Abuse and Alc Newsletter 17*(8), October, 1988.

Scott, J. Use of steroids by youths widespread, study finds. *Los Angeles Times*, December 16, 1988. pp. 1, 45.

Sklarek, H. M., Mantovani, R. P., Erens, E., Heisler, D., Niederman, M. S., and Fein, A. M. AIDS in a bodybuilder using anabolic steroids. *N Engl J Med 311*(26):1701, 1984.

Southwick, L. Testimony before U.S. House of Representatives Subcommittee on Crime, May 17, 1990.

STASH Staff. *Drugs in Sports*. Educational Offprint Series #219. Madison, WI: STASH, Inc., 1978.

Strauss, R. H. Controlling the supply of anabolic steroids. *Phys Sports Med 15*(5):41, 1987.

Telanders R., and Noden, M. The death of an athlete. *Sports Illustrated 70*(8):68-78, 1989.

Toufexis, A. Shortcut to the Rambo look. *Time Magazine*, January 30, 1989. p. 78.

Wieberg, S. All quiet on drug-test front—but why? *USA Today*, December 30, 1988. p. E1. ✦

Part III
Marijuana

Marijuana is a derivative of the Indian hemp plant *Cannabis sativa L.*, an annual shrub that flourishes in most warm and temperate climates and varies in height from three to 10 feet or more. The leaves are long, narrow, and serrated, forming a fan-shaped pattern; each "fan" has anywhere from three to 15 leaves, but typically only five or seven. They are shiny and sticky, and their upper surfaces are covered with short hairs. The psychoactive preparations derivative of cannabis are three:

1. **Marijuana**, the crushed and dried twigs, leaves, and flowers.
2. **Hashish**, the resinous extract obtained by boiling in a solvent the parts of the plant that are covered with the resin or by scraping the resin from the plant.
3. **Hashoil**, the dark viscous liquid produced by a process of repeated extraction of cannabis material.

The active ingredient in cannabis is delta-9-tetra-hydro-cannabinol, or simply THC. Whereas the THC content of most marijuana ranges from 1 to 5 percent, in hashish this figure can be as high as 15 to 20 percent, and twice that for hashoil.

Cannabis products vary in both name and form in different parts of the world. In Asia, for example, there is "ganja," "charas," and "bhang." *Ganja* consists of the young leaves and flowering tops of the cultivated female plant and its resin, pressed or rolled into a sticky mass, then formed into flat or round cakes. Its color is dark green or greenish-brown, and it has a pleasant smell and characteristic taste. *Charas* is the prepared resin separated from the tops of the female plant. It is pounded and rubbed until it is a grey-white powder, then made into cakes or thin, almost transparent sheets; or it is left in dark brown lumps. *Bhang* consists of the older or more mature leaves of the plant, and is often used by boiling in water and adding butter, to make a syrup. Bhang is less potent than ganja, which, in turn, is considerably weaker than charas.

In the Middle East, the word "hashish" is usually applied to both the leaves and the resin, or a mixture of the two. In North Africa, the resin and tops, usually reduced to a coarse powder, is known as "kif" in Morocco and "takrouri" in Algeria and Tunisia; in Central and Southern Africa, "dagga" refers to the leaves and tops.

Despite these many differences in nomenclature, the subjective effects of marijuana are essentially the same, although varying in intensity depending on THC content. At social-recreational use levels, these effects include: alteration of time and space perception; a sense of euphoria, relaxation, well being, and disinhibition; dulling of attention; fragmentation of thought and impaired immediate memory; an altered sense of identity; and exaggerated laughter and increased suggestibility. At doses higher than the typical recreational levels, more pronounced distortions of thought may occur including a disrupted sense of one's own body, a sense of personal unreality, visual distortions, and sometimes hallucinations, paranoid thinking, and acute psychotic-like symptoms.

Although marijuana is one of the oldest psychoactive drugs, its use in the United States is relatively recent. At the beginning of the twentieth century, what was referred to in Mexico as marijuana (also marihuana and mariguana) began to appear in New Orleans and a number of the Texas border towns. By 1920, the use of marijuana had become visible among some members of minority groups—blacks in the South and Mexicans in the Southwest. Given the social and political climate of the period, it is not at all surprising that the use of the drug became a matter of immediate concern. The agitation for reform that had resulted in the passage of the Pure Food and Drug Act in 1906 and the Harrison Act in 1914 was still active, and the movement for national prohibition of alcohol was at its peak. Moreover, not only was marijuana an "intoxicant of blacks and wetbacks" that might have a corrupting influence on white society, but it was considered particularly dangerous because of its alien (spelled "Mexican") and un-American origins.

Through the early 1930s, state after state enacted anti-marijuana laws, usually instigated by lurid newspaper articles depicting the madness and horror attributed to the drug's use. Even the prestigious *New York Times*, with its claim of "All the News That's Fit to Print," helped to reinforce the growing body of beliefs surrounding marijuana use. In an article headlined "Mexican Family Go Insane," datelined Mexico City, July 6, 1927, the *Times* reported:

A widow and her four children have been driven insane by eating the Marijuana plant, according to doctors, who say that there is no hope of saving the children's lives and that the mother will be insane for the rest of her life.

The tragedy occurred while the body of the father, who had been killed, was still in a hospital.

The mother was without money to buy other food for the children, whose ages ranged from 3 to 15, so they gathered some herbs and vegetables growing in the yard for their dinner. Two hours after the mother and children had eaten the plants, they were stricken. Neighbors, hearing outbursts of crazed laughter, rushed to the house to find the entire family insane. Examination revealed that the narcotic Marijuana was growing among the garden vegetables.

Popular books of the era were as colorful as the press in describing marijuana and the consequences of its use. For example, a 1928 publication, aptly titled *Dope*, offered the following about "hasheesh":

And the man under the influence of hasheesh catches up his knife and runs through the streets, hacking and killing everyone he meets. No, he has no special grievance against mankind. When he is himself, he is probably a good-humored, harmless, well-meaning creature; but hasheesh is the murder drug, and it is the hasheesh which makes him pick up his knife and start to kill.

Marijuana is American hasheesh. It is made from a little weed that grows in Texas, Arizona, and Southern California. You can grow enough marijuana in a window-box to drive the whole population of the United States stark, staring, raving mad.

. . . but when you have once chosen marijuana, you have selected murder and torture and hideous cruelty to your bosom friends.

In other reports, the link between anti-marijuana sentiment and prejudice was apparent. On January 27, 1929, the *Montana Standard* reported on the progress of a bill that amended the state's general narcotic law to include marijuana:

There was fun in the House Health Committee during the week when the Marijuana bill came up for consideration. Marijuana is Mexican opium, a plant used by Mexicans and cultivated for sale by Indians. "When some beet-field peon takes a few rares of this stuff," explained Dr. Fred Fulsher of Mineral County, "he thinks he has just been elected president of Mexico so he starts to execute all of his political enemies. . . ." Everybody laughed and the bill was recommended for passage.

Although marijuana is neither Mexican opium nor a narcotic of any kind, it was perceived as such by a small group of legislators, newspaper editors, and concerned citizens who were pressuring Washington for federal legislation against the drug. Their demands were almost immediately heard by Harry J. Anslinger, the then recently installed Commissioner of the Treasury Department's Bureau of Narcotics in 1930. Although it would appear that Anslinger was an ultra-right-wing conservative who truly believed marijuana to be a threat to the future of American civilization, his biographer maintained that he was an astute government bureaucrat who viewed the marijuana issue as a mechanism for elevating himself and the Bureau of Narcotics to national prominence.

Currently, marijuana is the most widely used illegal drug in the United States, although its popularity has dropped in recent years. From 1960 through the end of the decade, for example, the number of Americans who had used marijuana at least once had grown from a few hundred thousand to an estimated 8 million. By the early 1970s, marijuana use had increased geometrically throughout all strata of society; but by the onset of the 1980s, evidence indicated that marijuana use was declining. In 1975, for example, surveys showed that some 30 million people were users. By the early 1980s, this figure had dropped to 20 million, with the most significant declines among people ages 25 and under. Perhaps the younger generation had begun to realize that although marijuana was not the "devil drug," "assassin of youth," or "weed of madness" that Harry Anslinger and his counterparts had maintained, it was not a totally innocuous substance either. Perhaps the change occurred because of the greater concern with health and physical fitness that became so much a part of American culture during the 1980s, or as an outgrowth of the anti-smoking messages that appeared daily in the media. What-

ever the reason, it was clear that youthful attitudes had changed. Over the period from 1979 through the beginning of the 1990s, the proportion of seniors in American high schools who saw "great risk" in using marijuana even once or twice, rose from 9.4 percent to 24.5 percent; while the proportion of those who had *ever* experimented with marijuana declined from 60.4 percent to 32.6 percent.

In the essays that follow, a variety of perspectives are presented—ranging from Harry J. Anslinger's "assassin of youth" viewpoint to Lester Grinspoon and James Bakalar's thoughts on "marijuana as medicine." ✦

10. Marijuana: Assassin of Youth

Harry J. Anslinger

AND

Courtney Ryley Cooper

In the 1930s, Harry J. Anslinger was appointed Commissioner of the Federal Bureau of Narcotics. The following article is one of many that he wrote describing marijuana as a "Frankenstein" drug that was stalking American youth. As a result of Anslinger's crusade, on August 2, 1937, the Marijuana Tax Act was signed into law, classifying the scraggly tramp of the vegetable world as a narcotic and placing it under essentially the same controls as the Harrison Act had done with opium and coca products.

The sprawled body of a young girl lay crushed on the sidewalk the other day after a plunge from the fifth story of a Chicago apartment house. Everyone called it suicide, but actually it was murder. The killer was a narcotic known to America as marijuana, and to history as hashish. It is a narcotic used in the form of cigarettes, comparatively new to the United States and as dangerous as a coiled rattlesnake.

How many murders, suicides, robberies, criminal assaults, holdups, burglaries, and deeds of maniacal insanity it causes each year, especially among the young, can be only conjectured. The sweeping march of its addiction has been so insidious that, in numerous communities, it thrives almost unmolested largely because of official ignorance of its effects.

Here indeed is the unknown quantity among narcotics. No one can predict its effect. No one knows, when he places a marijuana cigarette to his lips, whether he will become a philosopher, a joyous reveler in a musical heaven, a mad insensate, a calm philosopher, or a murderer.

That youth has been selected by the peddlers of this poison as an especially fertile field makes it a problem of serious concern to every man and woman in America.

There was the young girl, for instance, who leaped to her death. Her story is typical. Some time before, this girl, like others of her age who attend our high schools, had heard the whispering of a secret which has gone the rounds of American youth. It promised a new thrill, the smoking of a type of cigarette which contained a "real kick." According to the whispers, this cigarette could accomplish wonderful reactions and with no harmful aftereffects. So the adventurous girl and a group of her friends gathered in an apartment, thrilled with the idea of doing "something different" in which there was "no harm." Then a friend produced a few cigarettes of the loosely rolled "homemade" type. They were passed from one to another of the young people, each taking a few puffs.

The results were weird. Some of the party went into paroxysms of laughter; every remark, no matter how silly, seemed excruciatingly funny. Others of mediocre musical ability became almost expert; the piano dinned constantly. Still others found themselves discussing weighty problems of youth with remarkable clarity. As one youngster expressed it, he "could see through stone walls." The girl danced without fatigue, and the night of unexplainable exhilaration seemed to stretch out as though it were a year long. Time, conscience, or consequences became too trivial for consideration.

Other parties followed, in which inhibitions vanished, conventional barriers departed, all at the command of this strange cigarette with its ropy, resinous odor. Finally there came a gathering at a time when the girl was behind in her studies and greatly worried. With every puff of the smoke the feeling of despondency lessened. Everything was going to be all right—at last. The girl was "floating" now, a term given to marijuana intoxication. Suddenly, in the midst of laughter and dancing, she thought of her school problems. Instantly they were solved. Without hesitancy she walked to a window and leaped to her death. Thus can marijuana "solve" one's difficulties.

The cigarettes may have been sold by a hot tamale vendor or by a street peddler, or in a dance hall or over a lunch counter, or even from sources much nearer to the customer. The police of a Midwestern city recently accused a school janitor of having conspired with four other men, not only to peddle cigarettes to children, but even to furnish apartments where smoking parties might be held.

A Chicago mother, watching her daughter die as an indirect result of marijuana addiction, told officers that at least fifty of the girl's young friends were slaves to the narcotic. This means fifty unpredictables. They may cease its use; that is not so difficult as with some narcotics. They may continue addiction until they deteriorate mentally and become insane. Or they may turn to violent forms of crime, to suicide or to murder. Marijuana gives few warnings of what it intends to do to the human brain.

The menace of marijuana addiction is comparatively new to America. In 1931, the marijuana file of the United States Narcotic Bureau was less than two inches thick, while today the reports crowd many large cabinets. Marijuana is a weed of the Indian hemp family, known in Asia as *Cannabis Indica* and in America as *Cannabis Sativa*. Almost everyone who has spent much time in rural communities has seen it, for it is cultivated in practically every state. Growing plants by the thousands were destroyed by law-enforcement officers last year in Texas, New York, New Jersey, Mississippi, Michigan, Maryland, Louisiana, Illinois, and the attack on the weed is only beginning.

It was an unprovoked crime some years ago which brought the first realization that the age-old drug had gained a foothold in America. An entire family was murdered by a youthful addict in Florida. When officers arrived at the home they found the youth staggering about in a human slaughterhouse. With an ax he had killed his father, his mother, two brothers, and a sister. He seemed to be in a daze.

"I've had a terrible dream," he said. "People tried to hack off my arms!"

"Who were they?" an officer asked.

"I don't know. Maybe one was my uncle. They slashed me with knives and I saw blood dripping from an ax."

He had no recollection of having committed the multiple crime. The officers knew him ordinarily as a sane, rather quiet young man; now he was pitifully crazed. They sought the reason. The boy said he had been in the habit of smoking something which youthful friends called "muggles," a childish name for marijuana.

Since that tragedy there has been a race between the spread of marijuana and its suppression. Unhappily, so far, marijuana has won by many lengths. The years 1935 and 1936 saw its most rapid growth in traffic. But at least we now know what we are facing. We know its history, its effects, and its potential victims. Perhaps with the spread of this knowledge the public may be aroused sufficiently to conquer the menace. Every parent owes it to his chil-

dren to tell them of the terrible effects of marijuana to offset the enticing "private information" which these youths may have received. There must be constant enforcement and equally constant education against this enemy, which has a record of murder and terror running through the centuries.

The weed was known to the ancient Greeks and it is mentioned in Homer's *Odyssey*. Homer wrote that it made men forget their homes and turned them into swine. Ancient Egyptians used it. In the year 1090, there was founded in Persia the religious and military order of the Assassins, whose history is one of cruelty, barbarity, and murder, and for good reason. The members were confirmed users of hashish, or marijuana, and it is from the Arabic "*hashshashin*" that we have the English word "assassin." Even the term "running amok" relates to the drug, for the expression has been used to describe natives of the Malay Peninsula who, under the influence of hashish, engage in violent and bloody deeds.

Marijuana was introduced into the United States from Mexico, and swept across America with incredible speed.

It began with the whispering of vendors in the Southwest that marijuana would perform miracles for those who smoked it, giving them a feeling of physical strength and mental power, stimulation of the imagination, the ability to be "the life of the party." The peddlers preached also of the weed's capabilities as a "love potion." Youth, always adventurous, began to look into these claims and found some of them true, not knowing that this was only half the story. They were not told that addicts may often develop a delirious rage during which they are temporarily and violently insane; that this insanity may take the form of a desire for self-destruction or a persecution complex to be satisfied only by the commission of some heinous crime.

It would be well for law-enforcement officers everywhere to search for marijuana behind cases of criminal and sex assault. During the last year a young male addict was hanged in Baltimore for criminal assault on a ten-year old girl. His defense was that he was temporarily insane from smoking marijuana. In Alamosa, Colo., a degenerate brutally attacked a young girl while under the influence of the drug. In Chicago, two marijuana-smoking boys murdered a policeman.

In at least two dozen other comparatively recent cases of murder or degenerate sex attacks, many of them committed by youths, marijuana proved to be a contributing cause. Perhaps you remember the young desperado in Michigan who, a few months ago, caused a reign of terror by his career of burglaries and holdups, finally to be sent to prison for life after kidnapping a Michigan state policeman, killing him, then handcuffing him to the post of a rural mailbox. This young bandit was a marijuana fiend.

A sixteen-year old boy was arrested in California for burglary. Under the influence of marijuana he had stolen a revolver and was on the way to stage a holdup when apprehended. Then there was the nineteen-year-old addict in Columbus, Ohio, who, when police responded to a disturbance complaint, opened fire upon an officer, wounding him three times, and was himself killed by the returning fire of the police. In Ohio a gang of seven young men, all less than twenty years old, had been caught after a series of 38 holdups. An officer asked them where they got their incentive.

"We only work when we're high on 'tea,'" one explained.

"On what?"

"On tea. Oh, there are lots of names for it. Some people call it 'mu' or 'muggles' or 'Mary Weaver' or 'moocah' or 'weed' or 'reefers'-there's a million names for it."

"All of which mean marijuana?"

"Sure. Us kids got on to it in high school three or four years ago; there must have been twenty-five or thirty of us who started smoking it. The stuff was cheaper then; you could buy a whole tobacco tin of it for fifty cents. Now these peddlers will charge you all they can get, depending on how shaky you are. Usually though, it's two cigarettes for a quarter."

This boy's casual story of procurement of the drug was typical of conditions in many cities in America. He told of buying the cigarettes in dance halls, from the owners of small hamburger joints, from peddlers who appeared near high schools at dismissal time. Then there were the "booth joints" or Bar-B-Q stands, where one might obtain a cigarette and a sandwich for a quarter, and there were the shabby apartments of women who provided not only the cigarettes but rooms in which girls and boys might smoke them.

"But after you get the habit," the boy added, "you don't bother much about finding a place to smoke. I've seen as many as three or four high school kids jam into a telephone booth and take a few drags."

The officer questioned him about the gang's crimes: "Remember that filling-station attendant you robbed—how you threatened to beat his brains out?"

The youth thought hard. "I've got a sort of hazy recollection," he answered. "I'm not trying to say I wasn't there, you understand. The trouble is, with all my gang, we can't remember exactly what we've done or said. When you get to 'floating,' it's hard to keep track of things."

From the other youthful members of the gang the officer could get little information. They confessed the robberies as one would vaguely remember bad dreams.

"If I had killed somebody on one of those jobs, I'd never have known it," explained one youth. "Sometimes it was over before I realized that I'd even been out of my room."

Therein lies much of the cruelty of marijuana, especially in its attack upon youth. The young, immature brain is a thing of impulses, upon which the "unknown quantity" of the drug acts as an almost overpowering stimulant. There are numerous cases on record like that of an Atlanta boy who robbed his father's safe of thousands of dollars in jewelry and cash. Of high school age, this boy apparently had been headed for an honest, successful career. Gradually, however, his father noticed a change in him. Spells of shakiness and nervousness would be succeeded by periods when the boy would assume a grandiose manner and engage in excessive, senseless laughter, extravagant conversation, and wildly impulsive actions. When these actions finally resulted in robbery the father went at his son's problem in earnest—and found the cause of it a marijuana peddler who catered to school children. The peddler was arrested.

It is this useless destruction of youth which is so heartbreaking to all of us who labor in the field of narcotic suppression. No one can predict what may happen after the smoking of the weed. I am reminded of a Los Angeles case in which a boy of seventeen killed a policeman. They had been great friends. Patrolling his beat, the officer often stopped to talk to the young fellow, to advise him. But one day the boy surged toward the patrolman with a gun in his hand; there was a blaze of yellowish flame, and the officer fell dead.

"Why did you kill him?" the youth was asked.

"I don't know," he sobbed. "He was good to me. I was high on reefers. Suddenly I decided to shoot him."

In a small Ohio town, a few months ago, a fifteen-year-old boy was found wandering the streets, mentally deranged by marijuana. Officers learned that he had obtained the dope at a garage. "Are any other school kids getting cigarettes there?" he was asked.

"Sure. I know fifteen or twenty, maybe more. I'm only counting my friends."

The garage was raided. Three men were arrested and 18 pounds of marijuana seized.

"We'd been figuring on quitting the racket," one of the dopesters told the arresting officer. "These kids had us scared. After we'd gotten 'em on the weed, it looked like easy money for a while. Then they kept wanting more and more of it, and if we didn't have it for 'em, they'd get tough. Along toward the last, we were scared that one of 'em would get high and kill us all. There wasn't any fun in it."

Not long ago a fifteen-year-old girl ran away from her home in Muskegon, Mich., to be arrested later in company with five young men in a Detroit marijuana den. A man and his wife ran the place. How many children had smoked there will never be known. There were 60 cigarettes on hand, enough fodder for 60 murders.

A newspaper in St. Louis reported after an investigation this year that it had discovered marijuana "dens," all frequented by children of high-school age. The same sort of story came from Missouri, Ohio, Louisiana, Colorado—in fact, from coast to coast.

In Birmingham, Ala., a hot tamale salesman had pushed his cart about town for five years, and for a large part of that time he had been peddling marijuana cigarettes to students of a downtown high school. His stock of the weed, he said, came from Texas and consisted, when he was captured, of enough marijuana to manufacture hundreds of cigarettes.

In New Orleans, of 437 persons of varying ages arrested for a wide range of crimes, 125 were addicts. Of 37 murderers, 17 used marijuana, and of 193 convicted thieves, 34 were "on the weed."

One of the first places in which marijuana found a ready welcome was in a closely congested section of New York. Among those who first introduced it there were musicians, who had brought the habit northward with the surge of "hot" music demanding players of exceptional ability, especially in improvisation. Along the Mexican border and in seaport cities it had been known for some time that the musician who desired to get the "hottest" effects from his playing often turned to marijuana for aid.

One reason was that marijuana has a strangely exhilarating effect upon the musical sensibilities (Indian hemp has long been used as a component of "singing seed" for canary birds). Another reason was that strange quality of marijuana which makes a rubber band out of time, stretching it to unbelievable lengths. The musician who uses "reefers" finds that the musical beat seemingly comes to him quite slowly, thus allowing him to interpolate any number of improvised notes with comparative ease. While under the influence of marijuana, he does not realize that he is tapping the keys with a furious speed impossible for one in a normal state of mind; marijuana has stretched out the time of the music until a dozen notes may be crowded into the space normally occupied by one. Or, to quote a young musician arrested by Kansas City officers as a "muggles smoker":

"Of course I use it—I've got to. I can't play any more without it, and I know a hundred other musicians who are in the same fix. You see, when I'm 'floating,' I own my saxophone. I mean I can do anything with it. The notes seem to dance out of it—no effort at all. I don't have to worry about reading the music—I'm music-crazy. Where do I get the stuff? In almost any low-class dance hall or night spot in the United States."

Soon a song was written about the drug. Perhaps you remember:

Have you seen
That funny reefer man?
He says he swam to China;
Any time he takes a notion,
He can walk across the ocean.

It sounded funny. Dancing girls and boys pondered about "reefers" and learned through the whispers of other boys and girls that these cigarettes could make one accomplish the impossible. Sadly enough, they can—in the imagination. The boy who plans a holdup, the youth who seizes a gun and prepares for a murder, the girl who decides suddenly to elope with a boy she did not even know a few hours ago, does so with the confident belief that this is a thoroughly logical action without the slightest possibility of disastrous consequences. Command a person "high" on "mu" or "muggles" or "Mary Jane" to crawl on the floor and bark like a dog, and he will do it without a thought of the idiocy of the action. Everything, no matter how insane, becomes plausible. The underworld calls marijuana "that stuff that makes you able to jump off the tops of skyscrapers."

Reports from various sections of the country indicate that the control and sale of marijuana has not yet passed into the hands of the big gangster syndicates. The supply is so vast and grows in so many places that gangsters perhaps have found it difficult to dominate the source. A big, hardy weed, with serrated, swordlike leaves topped by bunchy small blooms supported upon a thick, stringy stalk, marijuana has been discovered in almost every state. New York police uprooted hundreds of plants growing in a vacant lot in Brooklyn. In New York State alone last year 200 tons of the growing weed were destroyed. Acres of it have been found in various communities. Patches have been revealed in back yards, behind signboards, in gardens. In many places in the West it grows wild. Wandering dopesters gather the tops from along the right of way of railroads.

An evidence of how large the traffic may be came to light last year near La Fitte, La. Neighbors of an Italian family had become amazed by wild stories told by the children of the family. They, it seemed, had suddenly become millionaires. They talked of owning inconceivable amounts of money, of automobiles they did not possess, of living in a palatial home. At last their absurd lies were reported to the police, who discovered that their parents were allowing them to smoke something that came from the tops of tall plants which their father grew on his farm. There was a raid, in which more than 500,000 marijuana plants were destroyed. This discovery led next day to another raid on a farm at Bourg, La. Here a crop of some 2,000 plants was found to be growing between rows of vegetables. The eight persons arrested confessed that their main source of income from this crop was in sales to boys and girls of high-school age.

With possibilities for such tremendous crops, grown secretly, gangdom has been hampered in its efforts to corner the profits of what has now become an enormous business. It is to be hoped that the menace of marijuana can be wiped out before it falls into the vicious protectorate of powerful members of the underworld.

But to crush this traffic we must first squarely face the facts. Unfortunately, while every state except one has laws to cope with the traffic, the powerful right arm which could support these states has been all but impotent. I refer to the United States government. There has been no national law against the growing, sale, or possession of marijuana.

As this is written a bill to give the federal government control over marijuana has been introduced in Congress by Representative Robert L. Doughton of North Carolina, Chairman of the House Ways and Means Committee. It has the backing of Secretary of the Treasury Morgenthau, who has under his supervision the various agencies of the United States Treasury Department, including the Bureau of Narcotics, through which Uncle Sam fights the dope evil. It is a revenue bill, modeled after other narcotic laws which make use of the taxing power to bring about regulation and control.

The passage of such a law, however, should not be the signal for the public to lean back, fold its hands, and decide that all danger is over. America now faces a condition in which a new, although ancient, narcotic has come to live next door to us, a narcotic that does not have to be smuggled into the country. This means a job of unceasing watchfulness by every police department and by every public-spirited civic organization. It calls for campaigns of education in every school, so that children will not be deceived by the wiles of peddlers, but will know of the insanity, the disgrace, the horror which marijuana can bring to its victim. And, above all, every citizen should keep constantly before him the real picture of the "reefer man"—not some funny fellow who, should he take the notion, could walk across the ocean, but—

In Los Angeles, Calif, a youth was walking along a downtown street after inhaling a marijuana cigarette. For many addicts, merely a portion of a "reefer" is enough to induce intoxication. Suddenly, for no reason, he decided that someone had threatened to kill him and that his life at that very moment was in danger. Wildly he looked about him. The only person in sight was an aged bootblack. Drug crazed nerve centers conjured the innocent old shoe-shiner into a destroying monster. Mad with fright, the addict hurried to his room and got a gun. He killed the old man, and then, later, babbled his grief over what had been wanton, uncontrolled murder.

"I thought someone was after me," he said. "That's the only reason I did it. I had never seen the old fellow before. Something just told me to kill him!"

That's marijuana!

* * *

For Discussion

This article was published a few years after alcohol prohibition was repealed. Is it likely that the United States government will always keep some drugs illegal? How might the government benefit from certain drug prohibitions?   ✦

11. Cannabis Retail Markets in Amsterdam

Dirk J. Korf

Hashish and marijuana are sold frequently in numerous Amsterdam coffeeshops. Dirk J. Korf provides the reasons for government tolerance of cannabis sales in this part of Western Europe, describing structural and individual factors associated with the success of such coffeeshops. Both tourists and local citizens frequent these establishments, though some residents oppose the coffeeshops selling drugs. In conclusion, the author argues that cannabis use does not necessarily increase when it is readily available, but states, "There is no simple blueprint for the one and only 'correct' drug policy." However, it may be helpful to consider policies which have worked in other countries when analyzing the drug scene in America.

The Netherlands is widely known for its tolerant drug policy. Some condemn the Dutch way of handling the drug problem, others exult at it. "Coffeeshops," as the cafes and bars which sell hashish and marijuana are called, are one of the most visible examples of Dutch drug policy. This article will be restricted to the cannabis policy, as it has been analyzed in some recent studies. Furthermore, the main focus will be on Amsterdam, where the situation is rather atypical for the country as a whole. Nevertheless, where most statements about the effects of legalization are based on assumptions and projections, a closer look at a more "extreme" situation, as it can be perceived in Amsterdam, can generate empirical knowledge on important topics in the international debate on drug policy.

Why allow dealers to sell their dope? Amsterdam has about 350 coffeeshops, where one can buy hashish and marijuana of varying quality. But how is it possible that this illegal drug can be sold so easily in a Western country? Several legal studies have recently been published on this matter.

According to Frits Rüter, Professor of Criminal Law at the University of Amsterdam, the Dutch drug law is in line with the international conventions. But legislation, as he states, ". . . is not necessarily the same as criminal justice policy" (1990).

At the 1988 conference, "Dutch Drug Policy in Western European Perspective," Advocate-General Lodewijk de Beaufort, a high-ranking official from the Public Prosecutions Department, analyzed the development from a legal point of view. He explained why an illegal drug can be so openly used and sold in a Western country that is a signatory to the 1961 Single Convention (1989).

Firstly, the 1976 Opium Act separates "cannabis products" from "drugs presenting unacceptable risks." All violations of the Opium Act are crimes, except for the possession of up to 30 grams of hashish or marijuana, which is a petty offence. De facto, it is very unusual to be arrested and prosecuted for the possession of small amounts of cannabis.

This may also be the case in many other countries, as only a small proportion of all those that use cannabis ever get arrested. In many countries, however, a relatively small proportion—although a substantial total number—of cannabis users are arrested for possession and small-scale dealing; whereas, hardly anybody would be arrested for such illicit acts in the Netherlands. This situation reflects a specific Dutch connection between legislation and criminal justice policy.

According to de Beaufort, paragraph 167 of the Dutch Code of Criminal Procedure, the "expediency principle," empowers the Public Prosecutor to refrain from starting criminal procedures "on grounds derived from the public interest." This may also apply to drugs that are classified as dangerous, and thus illegal under the Single Convention. Since the possession of small amounts of hashish or marijuana is only a petty offense, and a repressive policy toward soft drugs would lead to a dangerous overlap with the hard-drug market, such a policy would not serve the public interest. So, there are no good reasons for a structural, active investigation and prosecution of cannabis offenses.

This criminal justice policy is expressed in the Guidelines for the Investigation and Prosecution of Drug Offenses, developed by the Ministry of Justice in 1976 and published in 1980. These guidelines give top priority to production, import, export, and large-scale trafficking, and a low priority to the sale of small quantities of cannabis. The Guidelines stem from the 1970s, when hashish and marijuana were more closely associated with a subcultural lifestyle than nowadays. In those days, drugs were sold in private places, on the street, and also sometimes in youth centers, subsidized by the government or local communities. Selling hashish in such a public place was—and still is—illegal, and has been quite a controversial phenomenon for some years. Nevertheless, authorities in some cities preferred to tolerate a "house dealer" with a more visible and controllable business, instead of continuing the existence of an underground market. The expediency principle left room for such experiments. These practical experiences proved very helpful when the guidelines were being developed. According to the guidelines, the house dealer "sells hemp products with the trust and protection of the staff of a youth center, and with the exclusion of others, in that youth center." The lowest segment of the cannabis market was *de facto* legalized. However, violating certain conditions, e.g., public advertising and the sale of hard drugs, will lead to immediate action (Van Vliet, in press).

House dealers, as the Minister of Justice envisaged them in 1976—as a kind of social worker—hardly exist anymore. Hashish and marijuana are predominantly sold in commercial places, mainly the so-called coffeeshops. Nevertheless, only in exceptional cases and after deliberation by a "triangle committee," consisting of the Mayor, the local Head of the Public Prosecution Department, and the Chief of Police, can action be taken.

Field studies show that differences in policy exist throughout the country; i.e., coffeeshops are very unusual in villages and small towns (Korf et al. 1989, 1990). On the other hand, no action will be taken in most urban areas, as long as no substantial nuisance is reported (loud music, many customers, etc.), minors are not attracted, or illicit hard drugs are not being sold. These regulations vary in strictness, depending on local circumstances. This dynamic process explains why the first telephone delivery service for cannabis was immediately closed and most coffeeshops in Amsterdam cannot be recognized anymore by a marijuana leaf emblem posted at the store front (Van Vliet, in press).

The Inner City of Amsterdam

As previously stated, Amsterdam has about 350 coffeeshops, which is probably as many as in the rest of the country. The city, however, accommodates only 700,000 of the Netherlands' 15 million inhabitants. Although the prevalence of cannabis use is much higher than elsewhere in the country, this can hardly explain the disproportionate number of coffeeshops. A closer look at the local situation shows a strong concentration of more than 100 coffeeshops in the inner city. In his study, "Cannabis in Amsterdam: A Geography of Coffeeshops," the economist Adriaan Jansen, associate professor at the University of Amsterdam, describes and analyzes this phenomenon. During his three-year study, he visited many coffeeshops, usually several times. He not only registered prices and sales, but also made fascinating field observations and interviewed dealers (1989).

Only a small proportion of the population live in the center of Amsterdam, but millions of tourists and other visitors come to the Dutch capital every year. They spend much of their time in only a small part of the capital: the old inner city, with its canals, museums, shops, markets, cafes, restaurants, and sex businesses. Many of these visitors are students and young adults who provide a substantial demand for cannabis, which explains the greater supply possibilities in this area. Similar areas exist in other major European cities, such as Ramblas in Barcelona and Platzspitz in Zurich. However, availability of cannabis in these cities is less visible, certainly less safe and less easy to buy, and it is often sold by street "addicts."

Jansen, however, looks further. Why are the coffeeshops not evenly spread over this area? From an economic point of view, several kinds of competition can be observed in this "extraordinary business branch."

Price determines the first kind of competition. Originally, cannabis was sold for various reasons, but profit was certainly the least of these. Importation, wholesale vending, and distribution were not strictly separated. Consequently, the increase in the number of coffeeshops in Amsterdam led to competition. Some examples of price competition have been observed (e.g., "buy-two-pay-for-one" on Wednesday at the Bulldog), but up to now this kind of competition has not been very influential. Prices vary from approximately 4 to 15 guilders per gram, depending on the kind of hashish or marijuana sold. Wholesale prices, on the other hand, are rather stable.

A variety of types of cannabis has made for competition between dealers for some time. Nowadays, almost every coffeeshop in the inner city sells more than five kinds of hashish and more than five kinds of marijuana. Other preparations, such as "hash cake" and "space balls," can also increase the variation.

The usual price for a 3-4 gram bag of hashish or marijuana is 25 guilders. Some years ago, new coffeeshops successfully introduced quantity competition, by selling smaller bags (11.5 grams) for 10 guilders. Others started selling cannabis that was not pre-packed, so customers can buy a specific amount. Nowadays, about 10 percent of the hashish and marijuana sold in the inner city is weighed on the spot.

Choosing a good location provides a fourth kind of competition. The first coffeeshops were located in out-of-the-way places. Since an important market (demand side) comes from outside the city, new coffeeshops are located near Central Station and in tourist streets. Coffeeshops located along these routes show perfectly how ineffective price competition can be, as cannabis is about 25-50 percent more expensive here. A second market is more dependent on the local population. These coffeeshops are located at and around entertainment centers, like cinemas, theaters, and discotheques.

The fifth dimension relates to the style and atmosphere of different premises. Dimly lit coffeeshops with worn carpets, broken furniture, and the smell of incense, reminiscent of the old, hippy days, hardly exist anymore. Some still remind one of the seventies, but new customers are not readily attracted. At the other end of the spectrum, one can find "extremely normal" coffeeshops; trendily decorated, bright, with many mirrors and chrome fittings. Only the smell of hashish differentiates them from other cafes, where no alcoholic beverages are sold.

All these components may contribute to the success of a coffeeshop, but, in the inner-city location, competition is most fierce. As the majority of customers do not live in the area, coffeeshops have to be located along the tourist routes to be commercially successful, as Jansen shows in his study. During his investigations, he noted that coffeeshops in locations further away from tourist areas were less successful than those sited in busy streets, around the entertainment centers.

A *Common Neighborhood*

About one third of the coffeeshops are located within a small area of Amsterdam—the inner city. Coffeeshops here reflect the metropolitan character of Amsterdam. This, however, does not mean that they are typical of the local situation. Coffeeshops are not only unevenly spread throughout the inner city, but also throughout the city as a whole; as in some neighborhoods, one can hardly find any coffeeshops. Peer Glandorff noted this phenomenon in the course of his survey of coffeeshops in 1989.

Around his college near the Rijksmuseum—and close to Jansen's study area—he saw no coffeeshops at all, but within a few minutes walking, further away from the inner city, he found plenty of them (1989).

Although this neighborhood (called "de Pijp") has few discotheques, theaters, or cinemas, it is a lively residential and shopping area. Especially the heart of the neighborhood, the Albert Cuyp market (the focal point of the east part of de Pijp) attracts thousands of people—locals, visitors, and tourists—coming every day to buy fresh vegetables or fish, clothes, and many exotic products. The market is also a well-known meeting place for the many different ethnic groups in the city: Surinams, Turks, Moroccans, etc. During his field study in de Pijp, Glandorff registered 22 coffeeshops selling hashish or marijuana, 20 cafes selling alcohol, and 2 cafes selling alcohol as well as cannabis.

At first sight, the Glandorff study seems to be in agreement with the Jansen study, as it reports quite a lot of coffeeshops in other neighborhoods, characterized by its function as a meeting place. The Albert Cuyp market is also an important meeting place for many people. But, most surprisingly, none of the coffeeshops here are located in the market. As noted by the Belgian criminologist Martine Marechal (whose study will be reviewed later in this article), coffeeshops are mainly located in side streets, away from the busy and, in summertime, highly touristic market. The coffeeshops in de Pijp depend much more on the local customers than those in the inner city. This implies that other competition variables play a more important role and could possibly be more important than the place where coffeeshops are located.

In de Pijp, like in the city center, the locations were not equally spread over the neighborhood. This contrast is even more noticeable than in the inner city. Almost all the coffeeshops in de Pijp can be found on the east side of the canal (Boerenwetering), but hardly any on the west side. A brief examination of the socio-economic profile of de Pijp provides some explanation for this.

The east side of this area is low-status, in comparison with the west side. Although the educational level is rather high, the average income is low. This can be explained by the many students who live in de Pijp. The apartments in the northeast are rather small, the density of population is high, there are many unemployed, and there is an overrepresentation of minority groups. The southeast has a somewhat higher status than the northeast. Part of the housing has recently been renovated or rebuilt; there are more shops, restaurants, and small enterprises. The densely built northeast is where most coffeeshops can be found, but also most cafes and bars.

The other side of the canal, the northwest, is mainly residential and has a low density of population. The streets are much cleaner, housing is of a higher quality, sometimes even luxurious. Here, we find less singles and divorced, and more traditional families. There are doctors and dentists, as well as consulates. Also, some upper-level schools are located in this part of the neighborhood. Unemployment is low and the population is predominantly white, higher-middle-class. The southwest is a somewhat less quiet and less chic living area. It has some stores, banks, and even a few cafes and coffeeshops. So the overall picture of this side of the canal is very different from the east part. The west side can be characterized by a lack of street activity, higher standard of living, and a stronger traditional orientation.

Other Aspects

Where Jansen emphasizes the importance of choosing the right location in a busy tourist zone, Glandorff's study suggests that other factors influence the spacial distribution of coffeeshops over the city. In de Pijp, the presence of many visitors undoubtedly contributes to the higher concentration of coffeeshops than in other areas.

Whereas tourists (foreign and domestic) strongly influence the social and economic structure of the lowest level of the cannabis market in the inner city, in other areas local citizens play a more important and maybe even central role. From a socio-economic point of view, lower-status areas with students and unemployed indicate a higher demand (east side of de Pijp) than wealthier and more family-orientated areas (west side).

But demand as such does not automatically generate supply; the presence of many (potential) cannabis users does not guarantee the opening of coffeeshops. Opposition from residents in the neighborhood can prevent entrepreneurs from starting a coffeeshop, as has happened on many occasions in the past. An example of community opposition occurred some years ago when the Municipal Health Service opened a methadone clinic in a well-to-do area. Citizens demonstrated against the clinic, successfully mobilized the media, molested staff members, and damaged the windows and door. Similar actions occur in smaller towns, with their more traditional views, where coffeeshops are not allowed to open or are quickly closed down due to civil actions. Even in Rotterdam, the second largest city of the Netherlands, opening a coffeeshop in a busy shopping street would be a novelty but would lead to protests by "normal" businesses. Hence, coffeeshops are almost exclusively located in out-of-the-way places. When we compare both parts of de Pijp, it seems plausible that there is a stronger commitment to traditional norms and values, and more social control against subcultural lifestyles on the west side.

Across the canal, the situation is very different. The many young citizens frequently change apartments and spend much of their time in other neighborhoods. Many new immigrants are predominantly orientated towards their own ethnic groups and have their own norms, values, and beliefs (Turks, Moroccans, and Surinamese have their own stores and cafes). For both groups, young citizens and immigrants, there is not a strong need to be closely involved with the main culture in the neighborhood. This certainly does not imply a lack of social control within these groups, but it seems plausible that social control, in terms of protection of traditional lifestyles and resistance to deviance from mainstream norms, is stronger in the wealthier and family-orientated area than in the lower-status neighborhood with a transient and multi-cultural population.

So far, this article has concentrated on the demand side of the cannabis market and the social structure in de Pijp. Now, let us take a look at supply side. On the eastern side, one can not only find many more cannabis users, but small-scale dealers can rent or buy premises for a reasonable price here too. They do not need much investment to begin a coffeeshop, so it is relatively easy to start a business career. However, as is true of any new business venture, many do not make much money and some go bankrupt. Nevertheless, running a coffeeshop can be a challenge, especially for those who have difficulty breaking into the regular market; e.g., minority groups, those who are unemployed and have a low education.

For these newcomers to the economic market, running a coffeeshop could mean the first step towards a higher socio-economic position. Moreover, running a coffeeshop, even if it is not very profitable, at least provides independence. Not surprisingly, some of the coffeeshops in de Pijp are run by more idealistically than economically motivated persons. They sell "good dope for a fair price" and act more like the social worker type the Advocate General had in mind when the Guidelines for the "house dealer" were drawn up. In such a coffeeshop, the price of food and beverages will be relatively low.

A *Typical Coffeeshop*

Marechal gives a good example of the "idealistic" type of coffeeshop in de Pijp. The Kabouter (The Goblin) is a very small place. There is a football table, as in most coffeeshops. An immense aquarium against one wall. Posters in the bathroom inform clients about AIDS, those in the cafe bear a political message. The middle-aged owner is strongly attached to his place and customers.

For Martine Marechal, studying coffeeshops in de Pijp was like the discovery of another world. To her, they meant "concretization of an 'intelligent' laissez-faire, so characteristic of Dutch pragmatism" (1989). She did not study all the coffeeshops in the neighborhood, but looked at different types. Some were almost exclusively visited by Moroccans or Surinamese. The Moroccan coffeeshop reminded her of the Arab cafes in Brussels: a rather empty place, some tables and kitchen chairs, and North African paintings on the wall. The Surinam coffeeshop is dominated by an "afro" style: loud reggae music, some rastas, and tropical paintings. Most coffeeshops, however, had a mixed clientele.

From her observations, Marechal constructed a hypothetical model which reflects all the most significant elements of the coffeeshops in the neighborhood.

The Ideal Pipe is not located on a busy street. It is not big, about 50 square meters. Plants in the large front window, so individual customers cannot easily be recognized from the outside. The interior is white. Three or four customers, at a large round table near the window, discuss welfare, politics, and music. Another customer reads a magazine. A young mother with a baby takes a break from shopping and drinks a cup of coffee. Table football and two slot machines in the corner. The bar is also white and clean, the furniture is another color. Music is playing. A young white man behind the bar smokes a joint with a customer; they talk about music and discotheques. He shows the price list to those who want to buy hashish or marijuana, which he sells in pre-packed bags (10 or 25 guilders each)

or cuts and weighs to order. The bartender is a young black woman. She serves soft drinks, coffee, tea, and hot chocolate, sells sweets and rolling papers. She is also busy keeping the place clean. Most customers are white and predominantly male, but some are black. At the table in the back, a small group appears quite lethargic. They listen to the music; the joint passes without much verbal communication.

Where other countries can only theorize about decriminalization of hashish and marijuana, it is a social reality in Amsterdam. This reality, Marechal concludes, is very different from other European countries. "Instead of being rejected (as a foreigner, youth, black, unemployed, or even all at once), the hash user can define him/herself here as different." But being "alternative," she states, does not imply being part of a subculture.

Separating Markets

The three field studies reviewed (Jansen, Glandorff, Marechal) had different targets, but they all describe how fast the hash-selling coffeeshops began to resemble normal cafes. The main difference is that they seldom serve alcoholic beverages, but soft drinks, tea, and coffee instead. A coffeeshop is not only a place to buy cannabis, but also a meeting place, where one can have breakfast or lunch, play table football or billiards, read newspapers and magazines, communicate, and meet friends.

Because coffeeshops are, in the main, based on economic principles, it is in the interest of the semi-legal entrepreneur to keep the soft- and hard-drug business strictly separated. The three studies reviewed all come to the same conclusion: coffeeshops do not sell hard drugs.

Jansen characterizes the relationship between the small-scale dealers and the authorities as "a subtle form of public/private partnership," which created possibilities for a rather open and profitable business. This economic activity has had a positive influence on the successful implementation of one of the main goals set by the authorities; i.e., strict separation of soft and hard drugs. The most successful coffeeshops are those without any problems with the authorities. Asking for hard drugs in a coffeeshop, Jansen concludes, is as absurd as ordering a zebra steak in an ordinary meat store.

Conclusion

The Dutch coffeeshop experiment has not resulted in a simple blueprint for the legalization of cannabis. It does, however, illustrate a pragmatic intermediate solution: small-scale dealing is tolerated under certain conditions, although still illegal; while import, export, and large-scale dealing are actively prosecuted. This solution is very different from the supermarket scenario, where young people can buy drugs like Coca-Cola and popcorn, so favored among prohibitionists in their warnings against legalization. In fact, the coffeeshops illustrate that a democratic society is able to handle a drug problem in a less prohibitionistic, more cost-effective, and less harmful way. The Dutch coffeeshops falsify the prohibitionistic assumption that decriminalization inevitably leads to an increase in drug use. Those who believe in a repressive policy towards cannabis need better arguments, since the Dutch coffeeshops do not support their deterrent prophecies.

On the other hand, although hard drugs cannot be bought in coffeeshops, they are still available. Apparently, it is possible to split the soft- and hard-drug markets, but a decriminalized mono-cannabis market does not automatically lead to the disappearance of other illicit drugs. This is not surprising—heroin has been around for almost a century and cocaine even longer, to a greater or lesser degree. Neither a prohibitionistic nor a more tolerant approach has been able totally to eradicate these markets.

The experiment also shows that there is no simple blueprint for the one and only "correct" drug policy. Within the city of Amsterdam and, moreover, throughout the Netherlands, different forms of small-scale hashish dealing are tolerated, in agreement with the local situation. Less legal repression apparently does not imply anarchy and may mean more subtle social control, even in the interest of those who sell drugs.

* * *

For Discussion

What would be the implications if similar coffeeshops were established in the United States?

References

De Beaufort, L. A. R. J. 1989. Stratrechtelijke marktbeheersing. In Groenhuijsen, M. S., and Van Kalmthout, A. M. (eds.): *Het Nederlandse Drugbeleid in Westeuropees Perspectief.* Arnhem/NL, Gouda Quint, 69-85 (English edition: Albrecht, H. J., and Van Kalmthout, A. M. (eds.), 1989, *Drug Policy in Western Europe.* Freiburg/FRG, Max Planck Institute for Foreign and Comparative Law.)

Glandorff, P. 1989. *De ruimtelijke spreading van coffeeshops in een Amsterdams stadsdeel.* Montessorilyceum, Amsterdam/NL.

Jansen, A. C. M. 1989. *Cannabis in Amsterdam: een geogratie van hashish en marijuana.* Muiderberg/NL Coutinho (will be translated into English).

Korf, D. J. 1988. Twintig jaar softdrug-gebruik in Nederland: een terugblik vanuit prevalentiestudies. *Tijdschrift voor alcohol, drugs en andere psychotrope stoffen* (14) nr. *3,* 81-89.

Korf, D. J., et al. 1989. *Drugs op het Platteland.* Assen/NL Van Gorcum.

Korf, D. J., et al. 1990. *Gooise Geneutgen.* Amsterdam/NL ICPC.

Marechal, M. 1989. *Prohibir la prohibition; politique criminelle en matire de cannabis aux Pays Bas.* Universite Catholique, Faculte de Droit, Louvain/B.

Ruter, C. E. 1990. *The Role of Law Enforcement in Dutch Drug Policy.* Metropolink Working Paper #2, Amsterdam/NL.

Sandwijk, J. R, et al. 1988. *Het gebruik van legale en illegale drugs in Amsterdam.* ISG Amsterdam/NL. (This face-to-face household survey was repeated in Winter 1989 and Spring 1990).

Guidelines for the Investigation and Prosecution of Criminal Offenses under the Opium Act (in Dutch) *Staatscourant* (Government newspaper), July 18th, 1980. The Hague/NL Government Printing Office 1980.

Van Vliet, H. J., in press. The Uneasy Decriminalization, *Hofstra Law Review,* Hofstra University, New York/USA. ✦

12. Marijuana: The Forbidden Medicine

Lester Grinspoon
AND
James Bakalar

Marijuana is the most widely used illegal drug, but there is a growing debate as to whether marijuana should be used for medicinal purposes. Proponents argue that the drug reduces the nausea associated with cancer chemotherapy, while other evidence suggests that marijuana is an effective treatment for glaucoma. In the following article Lester Grinspoon and James Bakalar discuss the issues associated with the medical use of marijuana.

Although some states permit the use of marijuana for specific medicinal purposes, the Food and Drug Administration (FDA) has yet to approve marijuana for these purposes. Grinspoon and Bakalar explain why the FDA is not likely to take such an action. Even if it did, the authors note, physicians preferring to avoid government surveillance and interference would be hesitant to prescribe marijuana.

There is overwhelming evidence that the American people think medical marijuana should be available to them. In 1991, the Louisiana legislature voted to recognize the medical value of marijuana in the treatment of paraplegic pain and muscle spasms. In 1991, the Cambridge, Massachusetts, City Council approved a "home-rule petition" that would allow physicians to prescribe marijuana after approval by the state government. A month later, San Francisco voters approved an initiative legalizing prescription use of hemp products. City officials have said that, if state and federal authorities do not intervene, patients who receive prescriptions would be permitted to grow up to six plants on their own. In 1992, Massachusetts became the thirty-fifth state to pass legislation permitting medical use of marijuana.

Reformers have worked mainly within the present regulatory system to get marijuana approved as a legitimate medicine. It would be highly desirable if that could be accomplished, but it seems unlikely.

The established federal system for certifying drugs is designed to regulate the commercial distribution of drug-company products and to protect the public against false or misleading claims about their efficacy or safety. The term drug generally refers to a single synthetic chemical that has been developed and patented, usually by a pharmaceutical company. The sponsors submit an IND [investigational new drug] application to the Food and Drug Administration and begin testing, first for safety and then for clinical efficacy. When the studies are completed, the company asks the FDA to approve a New Drug Application (NDA). To demonstrate effectiveness, the company must present evidence from controlled studies. The standards have been tightened since the present system was established in 1962. Few NDAs that were approved in the early 1960s would be approved today on the basis of the same evidence. The average time for approval of an NDA is now three years.

The research is expensive, and its cost is borne by the pharmaceutical company, which may spend two hundred million dollars or more before a chemical appears on pharmacy shelves. The company will invest that large sum if it is reasonably sure that the chemical will succeed as a medicine and earn a profit. Marijuana will probably never be approved by this process. One reason is that it cannot be patented. Another is that it is a plant material containing many chemicals rather than a single chemical. A third reason is that marijuana is taken chiefly by smoking. No drug in the present pharmacopoeia is delivered by this route.

It is an ironic situation. More is known about marijuana than about most prescription drugs. Cannabis has been tested by millions of users for thousands of years. It is one of humanity's oldest medicines, with a remarkable record of both safety and efficacy. Yet, the FDA is legally required to classify it as a "new drug" and demand the same testing it would require for an unknown substance.

Even if whole cannabis somehow became available as a prescription drug, the DEA would classify it in the same way it now classifies synthetic THC, as a Schedule II substance with a high potential for abuse and limited medical use—the most highly restricted class of prescription drug. Restrictions on Schedule II drugs are becoming tighter. Nine states now require doctors to make out prescriptions for many of these substances in triplicate, so that one copy can be sent to a centralized computer system that tracks every transaction involving these drugs. Similar legislation is pending in other states.

Even if marijuana were available as a Schedule II drug, pharmacies would be reluctant to carry it and physicians to prescribe it. Through computer-based monitoring, the DEA could know who was receiving prescription marijuana and how much. It could hound physicians who, by its standards, prescribed cannabis too freely or for reasons it considers unacceptable. The potential for harassment would be extremely discouraging. Cannabis has many potential medical uses. Many people would undoubtedly try to persuade their doctors that they had a legitimate claim to prescription. Doctors would not want the responsibility of making such decisions if they were constantly under threat of discipline by the state. Furthermore, many physicians would not consider prescribing cannabis at all, because they are victims of the government's misinformation campaign.

For all these reasons, making marijuana available as a Schedule II drug is likely to be unworkable. That leaves the only program providing medical marijuana, the Compassionate IND. Since its inception, only about forty of the thousands of patients who might benefit from medical cannabis have been approved for a Compassionate IND; only thirteen have actually received cannabis, and their supplies are often interrupted or of poor quality. The government has now decided not to provide cannabis to anyone else in the future—not even to the patients whose INDs have already been approved. That action is cruel to the few people who might have received governmental cannabis, but in a broader perspective its effect is marginal and largely symbolic. The government could never have met every legitimate claim through this program without hiring a huge administrative staff, and convincing patients that they should tolerate endless delays instead of finding marijuana on the street.

Legislation was introduced in Maine last year which would have actually allowed citizens to defend themselves under state law against criminal charges of marijuana cultivation or possession by showing that they have a diagnosis of glaucoma or are suffering from serious nausea from cancer treatment. We favor any proposal that allows some progress towards medical marijuana use, but we are not optimistic. Because the Maine legislation threatened to bypass the federal regulatory system, a conflict would be certain to arise. The federal government is unlikely to allow its hard-won authority over drug regulation to revert to the states.

Although proposals of the kind embodied in the Maine legislation do not offer a long-term solution, they do have a use. If such proposals are adopted in several states, the federal government will face a political challenge, needed debate will ensue, and public attention will be drawn to the importance of the issue.

Before we propose a solution to the medical marijuana dilemma, we wish to examine some of the deeper reasons why so many legal and institutional obstacles have been erected against it. Drug use has been assigned to various social categories, including magic, religion, medicine, and recreation. Contemporary industrial societies try to keep these categories separate, and the separation is reflected in our institutions.

Like cannabis, most psychoactive drugs now restricted by law have had significant medical uses at some places and times. These drugs have tended to fall into disuse, as their dangers are more strongly emphasized, other treatments become available, and governments place more controls on medicine. The history of social and legal response to these drugs is riddled with hypocrisy, corruption, inadequate pharmacology, and institutional self-aggrandizement by enforcement agencies.

In the nineteenth-century United States, there were almost no government controls on drug use. The growth of capitalist entrepreneurship and the spirit of liberal individualism made that period an age of self-medication and competing medical authorities. The patent-medicine industry flowered, and many of its products contained psychoactive drugs, especially alcohol and opium. Some of the psychoactive drugs, like much strong medicine, could also be powerfully poisonous. Their dangers (as well as their effectiveness) were magnified by isolation of the active chemicals in pure form and the development of such technologies as the hypodermic syringe. Mistrust of these drugs had begun to grow by the beginning of the twentieth century. The drugs had been used freely without a careful distinction between health and other purposes—an ambiguity that now began to seem dangerous.

The rise of synthetic chemistry and bacteriology created hope for a scientific medicine based on the recognition of specific agents for specific diseases. But psychoactive drugs were not specific cures; they relieved suffering in many situations. Their powers began to seem indeterminate and uncontrollable. Taking cocaine to feel alert or opiates to relax were no longer legitimated as medical treatments.

The new restraints that began to be imposed at the turn of the century resulted from an impulse to clean up society, impose classifications, and reduce disorder. The federal government assumed control of psychoactive drugs through the Pure Food and Drug Act (1906), the Harrison Narcotics Act (1914), and the Volstead Act (1919). Although alcohol was excluded in 1933 under intense public pressure, the system has otherwise persisted, and it has been elaborated in a series of laws leading to the Comprehensive Drug Abuse Prevention and Control Act of 1970 and its successors.

Government control over non-psychoactive therapeutic drugs followed a similar trend toward centralization and restriction. Federal restrictions began with the Food, Drug, Cosmetics Act of 1938. The law was amended in 1962 to establish the NDA system, under which the federal government has the power to decide which drug will be legally available to physicians. The decision had been made that even doctors need protection from misinformed or inappropriate uses of drugs. It was entirely consistent with this view for the DEA to argue in the recent marijuana rescheduling case that even widespread approval by physicians was not enough to justify making marijuana legally available as a medicine.

The greatly increased complexity of the pharmacopoeia explains some of the changes that have occurred since the end of the nineteenth century. Free individual choice seemed justifiable when the average consumer was thought to have as good a claim as anyone to evaluate the safety and usefulness of the few available medicines. In the present situation, consumers and even physicians are no longer thought capable to make that judgment for themselves. Authoritative scientific knowledge supplies the needed basis for decisions.

This model of consumer protection is a powerful justification for government control. The principle is that in a complex society far more needs to be known than any single person can learn. Under this system, drugs with medical uses are commodities, useful as instruments for certain purposes, but only with safeguards to be supplied by manufacturers and distributors under government direction.

Medical regulations are quite properly the strictest of consumer-protection laws, because the dangers involved can be so great. But even this control system is considered inadequate for psychoactive drugs. Something more than consumer protection is involved when the laws criminalize even the consumer and require a vast police bureaucracy for their enforcement. We do not fine or jail the patients of someone who practices medicine without a license or the customers of a manufacturer who disobeys consumer-protection laws; yet, mere possession of cannabis and other illicit psychoactive drugs is a federal crime. The metaphor of war is rarely invoked in the name of consumer protection but constantly used in the assault on psychoactive drugs. The reason is that laws controlling these drugs are ultimately aimed not at consumer protection but at containing what is believed to be a threat to the social fabric and moral order. Psychoactive drug use evokes the image of a plague or epidemic possibly more often and more powerfully than any other social problems. That image suggests a moral crusade that is also a public health campaign. The imagery of disease has tremendous social potency; it eliminates most moral and political doubts. Stopping an epidemic of typhoid presents no moral problems, so why should stopping an epidemic of drug abuse? Concerns about individual freedom become irrelevant.

But causes are difficult to distinguish from symptoms in such issues as public tranquility or productivity, and individual values differ. As a result, public consensus is weak. Drugs are culturally charged symbols. Repressed anxieties may be displaced onto drug users as a form of scapegoating. Marijuana was seen as a catalyst of the anti-establishment movement of the 1960s. Millions of people simply do not acknowledge the moral authority of the marijuana laws. Some are ambivalent, some are hypocritical, and some are openly or secretly in resistance. The government insists on viewing marijuana as a threat to society, but the very need to use the rhetoric of war may be a sign that the issue is not settled.

Moral consensus about the evil of cannabis is uncertain and shallow. We pretend that eliminating drug traffic is like eliminating slavery or piracy, or like eradicating smallpox or malaria. No one would suggest that we legalize piracy or give up the effort to eradicate infectious diseases. Yet, even conservative authorities like the economist Milton Friedman and the editors of the *Economist* have suggested legalizing marijuana. The people who tell their stories do not conceal their bitter resentment of laws that render them criminals. They have come to doubt that the "authorities" understand much about either the deleterious or the useful properties of this drug.

The undercurrent of ambivalence and resistance in public attitudes toward the marijuana laws leaves room for the possibility of change, especially since the costs of prohibition are also high and rising. The arrest of more than 300,000 people a year on marijuana charges contributes to the clogging of courts and the overcrowding of prisons. Federal, state, and local governments now spend nearly ten billion dollars a year on drug enforcement and hundreds of millions more to house and feed drug dealers and users in local, state, and federal prisons. A third of federal prisoners are now confined on drug charges, many of them on marijuana charges. Drugs enter the United States at a growing rate despite the war effort, which only inflates prices and keeps the trade lucrative. Crime and violence are now produced by the black market in drugs as they were produced by the black market in alcohol in the 1920s.

There are also costs more difficult to quantify. One of them is lost credibility of government. Young people who discover that the authorities have been lying about cannabis become cynical about their pronouncements on other drugs and disdainful of their commitment to justice. Another frightful cost of prohibition is the erosion of civil liberties. The use of informers and unwarranted searches and seizures are becoming more common. It is increasingly clear that our society cannot be both drug-free and free.

It is also clear that the realities of human need are incompatible with a legal distinction between medicine and other uses of cannabis. Marijuana use simply does not conform to the conceptual boundaries established by twentieth-century institutions.

In many cases, what lay people do in prescribing marijuana for themselves is not very different from what physicians do when they supply prescriptions. Consider the following case: a 92-year-old woman with severe congestive heart failure, hypothyroidism and cerebral artery insufficiency (among other maladies) complained of insomnia. Her doctor was reluctant to add one more medicine to the eight she was already receiving in the form of twenty-five pills a day, so he suggested that she drink a glass of wine at bedtime—not a conventional solution, but one that was fairly safe and proved effective. Here, the doctor was acting like a nineteenth-century physician in treating alcohol as a therapeutic substance. In the nineteenth century, he could have recommended a cannabis tincture for the same purpose. Today, alas, that is impossible, although marijuana might in some cases be safer and more effective.

Marijuana is also used in a quasi-medicinal way to enhance creativity and productivity. A common problem in the treatment of manic-depression with lithium is the complaint of patients that the medication robs them of creativity, vitality, and enjoyment of life—one reason so many of them stop taking it, despite the risks. Mild mood elevation (hypomania) often enhances creative thinking. Curiously, this is also a common feature of cannabis intoxication. In the following account, a 42-year-old health professional explains how she uses marijuana both to enhance creativity and to make continued use of lithium possible—another situation in which medical and non-medical uses are impossible to separate.

In my late twenties, while pursuing an undergraduate degree in the medical sciences, I began to experience the debilitating effects of manic-depression. At the age of thirty-four, I realized that I had to face up to my problem, sought treatment, and recovered with the help of lithium and psychotherapy. Since then I have faithfully taken lithium and have stayed in remission while continuing to grow personally and professionally.

Marijuana has also played an important part in my recovery and continued remission. I started using it regularly in my middle twenties, at about the time I entered college. In my late twenties, I moved away from the college community and no longer had access to marijuana. Within a few weeks, I realized how helpful it had been in relieving some symptoms of my mood disorder. During episodes of hypomania, I feel unpleasant tension in all my skeletal muscles; marijuana relaxed those muscles more effectively and with fewer side effects than alcohol. Luckily, I was able to gain access to marijuana again and resumed using it, taking two or three puffs two or three times a day.

My psychiatrist asked me to stop using marijuana and gave me a prescription for Xanax (alprazolam) instead. To maintain control, I took as little as I could, just as I had done with marijuana. Xanax worked, but it had undesirable side effects, such as dry mouth and sedation. I continued to use marijuana as well, although I now smoked it only once or twice a week. I stopped using Xanax as soon as the lithium took effect.

After my recovery I returned to school and earned an advanced degree in my medical profession. By now, I was noticing that lithium prevented not only hypomanic mood swings but also the state of consciousness associated with creativity. I feared losing my creativity for both personal and professional reasons. I pursue artistic hobbies for relaxation, and my work also benefits greatly from creative insights—for example, recognition of meaningful patterns in diverse data or new perspectives on obstinate problems. For that reason, I continue to use marijuana moderately. I smoke it from a small pipe; usually two or three puffs last me three to four hours. Marijuana allows me to attain the creative state of mind that is so precious to me without having to stop taking lithium and risk a relapse. I also continue to find it useful as a muscle relaxant, especially in treating menstrual cramps.

A scientist reports on the contribution of cannabis to his work:

As a scientist, I have spent years training the analytical side of my mind. I have learned to be suspicious of my data, to look for ways to test the reasonableness of my results and arrive at the same conclusions by alternative means. It is an active process of mental discipline.

What I have sometimes neglected is an awareness of the wider significance of my work and the sense of wonder that led me into the field to begin with. Often I have been unable to see an answer that lies before me. Part of the blame lies in the very training that enables me to do complicated analytical work. I ignore apparent distractions that sometimes hold the key to a solution. It is a human habit to go over old ground repeatedly, seeing what you believe to be there, rather than what is actually there (the reason people cannot proofread their own writing). I get high for short periods to remedy this problem. It allows me to turn off the rational side of my mind and think creatively. It temporarily cancels the limiting effects of my training and allows me to see my work in a different light.

It would be inefficient to follow up these new ideas while high, because I am too easily distracted. Instead, I enjoy the relaxation and keep notebooks recording my thoughts. Both the relaxation and the observation of otherwise overlooked details have been valuable contributions to my work.

Another scientist who has found cannabis useful tells his story:

I am a 40-year-old geologist who studies the surfaces of planets at a NASA research center. I began

smoking marijuana in high school. Since then, I have used it for self-exploration, and for pleasure, including enhanced appreciation of sex, music, art, and conversation. But cannabis has done more than that for me; it has actually helped me to acquire a professionally useful skill.

Planetary geologists rely on images of landforms and surface markings radioed back from spacecraft. Landforms cannot be understood unless they are perceived in three dimensions by means of stereo images—paired photographs taken from slightly different angles to mimic depth perception.

Most people use mechanical devices to judge depth from stereo photos. The machinery needed to view stereo images of planetary surfaces is particularly awkward and time-consuming to use. A few fortunate people can see three dimensions in stereo photographs without mechanical aids—a skill every planetary geologist would like to have.

When I was an undergraduate, a friend tried for months without success to teach me this skill, and I became convinced that people who said they possessed it were deluding themselves. But one evening, we smoked some especially potent marijuana, purely for pleasure. I amused myself by looking at a pair of stereo photographs that had been left in the room. Suddenly, the two pictures merged into a single three-dimensional view. It was like a gift from God. Overjoyed, I looked at other stereo pairs and discovered that I could perceive depth in them as well. I spent the rest of the evening gazing at stereo pairs. The next day, when the immediate marijuana effects had passed, I found that I retained the ability.

I believe my experience illustrates how marijuana can overcome deep conditioning, initiated immediately after birth, that locks us into perceiving reality in very narrowly defined ways. Marijuana shares with its stronger psychedelic brethren the power to cleanse the doors of perception and make the world seem as new. Its help in catalyzing the acquisition of a skill useful in my work is only one of the many blessings and insights it has provided.

The criminalization of marijuana use in general and the policies that make marijuana legally unavailable as a medicine are two problems with the same cause and the same solution. Marijuana is caught in a dual web of regulations—those that control prescription drugs in general and the special criminal laws that control psychoactive substances. These laws strangle its medical potential. The only way out is to cut the knot by giving cannabis the same status as alcohol—legalizing it for all uses and removing it entirely from the medical and criminal control systems.

Opponents of medical marijuana sometimes say that its advocates are insincere and are only using medicine as a wedge to open the way for recreational use. Anyone who has studied the history of desperate efforts to obtain legal marijuana for suffering people knows that this is false. The attitude falsely ascribed to advocates of medical marijuana is actually a mirror image of the government's attitude. The government is unwilling to admit that marijuana can be a safe and effective medicine because of a stubborn commitment to wild exaggeration of its dangers. Far from believing that medical availability of marijuana would open the way to other uses, we take the view that free availability of cannabis may be the only way to make its judicious medical use possible. Marijuana should be available for use in much the same way alcohol is now available. Cannabis conclusively lost its medical status

as an almost incidental effect of the Marijuana Tax Act of 1937, which was designed to prevent "recreational" use. The full potential of this remarkable substance, including its full medical potential, will be realized only when we end that regime of prohibition established two generations ago.

* * *

Lester Grinspoon and James Bakalar, "Marijuana: The Forbidden Medicine." Yale University Press, June, 1993. Copyright © 1993 by Lester Grinspoon and James Bakalar. All rights reserved. Reprinted by permission.

For Discussion

Discuss the problems created by a system of prescription drug approval which is motivated by potential for profit. What should be done in the case of substances which occur naturally and can't be patented? Who should pay for extensive testing of these substances? ✦

13. Are There Dangers to Marijuana?

Marc A. Schuckit

Within the context of widespread marijuana use in the United States, Dr. Marc A. Schuckit reviews anecdotal and scientific evidence on the consequences of marijuana use. He points out that marijuana affects coordination and judgment, and that users who operate motor vehicles after ingesting the drug pose a risk to themselves and others. Because of the tar and carcinogens in marijuana smoke, users also place themselves at risk for cancer. Further, marijuana increases the heart rate, decreases testosterone production in men, can affect the fetus when used by pregnant women, and can have an impact on cognitive skills.

Many of us are asked to comment on the potential dangers of the cannabinols. Sometimes, requests come from parents and teachers, and others originate with friends and relatives. In any case, the questioner is often aware of some of the pleasant effects of the drug but needs additional information to help themselves and others make informed decisions about whether taking this group of drugs involves substantial risks.

Such requests reflect the long history of use of these agents in the United States, as well as the very high prevalence of Americans who have had experiences with cannabinols. While the major active ingredient in the marijuana preparations, delta-9 tetrahydrocannabinol (THC), has been used since at least 2700 B.C., its widespread application in the United States probably dates to the early 1960s. It is now taken by members of all racial and ethnic groups, with estimates that as many as 60 million Americans have used this drug on at least one occasion. This includes perhaps 70 percent or more of individuals aged 18 to 25, most of whom take THC preparations occasionally. The percentage of users probably peaked in the late 1970s, with some evidence of a small decrease by the mid-1980s, after which the use pattern appears to have leveled off. In distinction from the usual occasional pattern of intake, at least 6 million men and women in the United States smoke marijuana products daily, usually taking from one to five cigarettes per day.

The pharmacological properties of marijuana preparations have been relatively thoroughly researched. The dose of THC increases with the quality of the preparation, with the average cigarette containing between 2.5 and 5.0 mg, approximately half of which is actively absorbed. After smoking, peak blood levels are reached within approximately 20 minutes, and intoxication lasting approximately two to three hours, depending on the dose. Eating marijuana results in a higher percentage of the drug being absorbed, a longer period of intoxication, but a slower onset and less intense peak of effects. Reflecting the high fat solubility of THC, after an hour perhaps only 5 percent of the active ingredient remains in the bloodstream, with the remainder dissolved in body fat stores from which it diffuses back into the blood. THC and its metabolites have very long half-lives, approximately 50 hours or more. Thus, the combination of redistribution from fat stores plus half-lives combine to produce traces of active ingredients in urine of chronic users for perhaps two weeks or more.

The major results of intoxication are on the brain, the heart, and the lungs. Subjective feelings include euphoria, a feeling of relaxation, sleepiness, difficulty keeping track of time, hunger, and decreased social inhibitions. As the drug dose increases, memory problems become more prominent, feelings of mild paranoia or suspiciousness can develop; and at very high doses and in the context of confusion, prominent hallucinations can develop.

The feelings of euphoria and relaxation make this drug attractive to many people. The recognition that clinically significant physical addiction is not likely to occur, and comparisons with the severe and life-threatening reactions following the ingestion of other agents, such as cocaine, have contributed to a questioning of whether marijuana preparations are actually dangerous. A number of recent studies and reviews have highlighted some potentially severe problems, and these data form the basis for this issue.

Documented Drug Dangers

Reflecting its lipid solubility and wide body distribution, as well as the prominent effects this drug exerts on the brain, it is not surprising that a wide array of established and potential problems exist. Any attempt at presenting a hierarchy of the most severe to the less intense difficulties is certainly subjective. However, after re-reviewing the literature, I have formed some of my own opinions about the drug liabilities. These are described below in a rough order, ranging from the most relevant and highly established problems to those that are either less clinically obvious or more difficult to document.

Problems with Motor Performance

One of the most prominent dangers of the cannabinols involves their effect on motor performance and subsequent driving impairment. Studies of animals, observations of humans in laboratory situations, and actual driving tests given to people under the influence of marijuana all document the potential dangers of this drug. Acute impairments in reaction time, judgment, and the use of peripheral vision are obvious during the two to three hours following acute intoxication, while either driving a car or piloting an airplane on a simulator. Some of these effects appear to remain clinically relevant for at least 24 hours following intoxication, as documented on a flying simulator apparatus. There are also ample data that the motor performance deterioration observed with the cannabinols adds to any impairment observed for alcohol, making the combination of the two drugs extremely dangerous in driving or flying situations. It seems logical to conclude that the ingestion of cannabinols contributes significantly to serious injuries and deaths on the highways. Considering the long half-life of these drugs and the evidence of impairment as long as 24 hours after smoking, I consider this problem to be most prominent and potentially lethal.

Dangers to the Lungs

Recent publications have convincingly demonstrated the respiratory-system dangers associated with smoking cannabinols. Marijuana smoke contains more irritants than tobacco, with a resulting relatively high prevalence or irritation of the lining of the respiratory tract with a subsequent cough and clinically significant danger of bronchitis. This is probably related to the greater quantity of smoke particulates, tars, and noxious gases in marijuana preparations. The result is a four-fold higher level of deposition of particulate matter compared to to-

bacco, with many of these substances appearing to be carcinogens. This, along with the potential impairments in the immune system associated with cannabinols, is likely to contribute to a significantly enhanced cancer risk for smokers.

Cardiac Problems

Another major danger rests with the effects that marijuana cigarettes have upon heart functioning. No matter what mode of ingestion is used, marijuana is likely to produce an increase in heart rate, a potentially significant problem for individuals with preexisting cardiac disease. Even more impressive, however, is the five-fold increased content of carbon monoxide, with resulting production of an altered form of the red pigment in red blood cells necessary for transporting oxygen to the rest of the body, including the heart. It is this formation of carboxyhemoglobin that is felt to contribute to some of the cardiac dangers associated with tobacco smoke.

Sexual Development and Functioning

A potential problem with all of the cannabinol preparations is the manner in which they interfere with the normal pattern of sex hormones. Both animal and human studies have documented that THC impairs the release of a number of hormones from the brain. While this effect is reversible, the result is a decreased level of testosterone which implies potentially important dangers in the sexually developing adolescent male. At the same time, in women THC crosses the placenta to the developing fetus and is excreted in breast milk, with resulting potential dangers to both pregnant women and the developing baby. The combination of direct and indirect effects might contribute to a higher rate of spontaneous abortions, as well as to an increased risk for low birth-weight babies among women who regularly ingest marijuana.

Psychiatric Difficulties

Cannabinols might have important effects upon psychiatric symptoms. It makes sense that a drug that crosses so easily to the brain, and that causes such prominent changes in feeling states is likely to worsen any preexisting major state of psychiatric impairment. While this attribute has been moderately well-documented, there is at present only anecdotal information and speculation about whether heavy intake of these agents on a regular basis might actually produce anxiety, depressive, or psychotic syndromes on its own. Favoring this speculation are the recent data from a 15-year follow-up of more than 45,000 Swedish military conscripts that documented in a six-fold increased rate of schizophrenia among those men who at the time of induction had ingested marijuana products on 50 or more occasions.

Cognitive Effects

A sixth potential danger for the cannabinols rests with the possibility of cognitive or thinking impairments associated with long-term use. This item is listed rather late in the hierarchy, because large-scale, long-term studies would be required to produce incontrovertible evidence. Nonetheless, one study suggestive of cognitive impairment was recently published from a sample of regular and heavy cannabinol users in India who were first evaluated in the early 1970s and then retested with similar instruments ten years later. Compared to controls, the regular users of marijuana products demonstrated a significant decrease of performance on a number of cognitive tests, including speed and accuracy evaluations, a reaction-time test, and a visuomotor performance test. Consistent with these results is at least one recent evaluation using a very sophisticated brain-imaging technique that demonstrated brain-ventricle size increases after two to ten months of regular use in primates. While a careful review of all of the data indicates numerous studies inconsistent with the results cited above, the difficulty in definitively documenting brain damage with chronic use, along with the potential severe consequences, if such a danger actually exists, makes it important that this area of potential danger be included in this listing.

Other Potential Problems

Finally, there are preliminary data indicating a variety of other potential dangers. This includes evidence that the cannabinols might contribute to a decrease in antibody response, as well as a decrease in some white-cell reactions to infectious agents. This possible effect might contribute to the cancer dangers apparently associated with smoking marijuana products, and raises the issue of whether regular ingestion of the drug might contribute to either the risk of infection or rate of clinical deterioration associated with AIDS.

Other speculations have focused on the possible production of a feeling state associated with lack of energy and lack of motivation. There does not seem to me to be convincing evidence that what is observed is not just a reflection of preexisting factors and/or reversible residual effects of the drug. Fears have also been expressed that the cannabinols might directly or indirectly increase the risk for misuse of other and more acutely disturbing drugs (a common-sense assumption that is very difficult to confirm).

Some Conclusions

The cannabinols produce what is usually perceived as a pleasant and moderately intense, short-term intoxication. Because many users perceive these effects as attractive, the drug is certainly capable of producing levels of psychological dependence, where users will continue ingestion despite dangers. However, the lack of obvious physical dependence, as well as the absence of the obvious and alarming levels of acute severe problems associated with other categories of drugs, have combined to yield a level of complacency about the dangers of THC preparations. . . .

* * *

Marc A. Schuckit, "Are There Dangers to Marijuana?" *Drug Abuse & Alcoholism Newsletter, 19* (August 1990), pp. 1-4. Published by the Vista Hill Foundation, San Diego, California. Copyright © 1990 by the Vista Hill Foundation. All rights reserved. Reprinted by permission.

For Discussion

Schuckit notes several potential negative effects of marijuana use. How do these effects compare with the negative effects of tobacco smoke? Why is marijuana illegal and tobacco legal?

References

Adreasson, S. Cannabis and schizophrenia. *Lancet II*:1483-1486, 1987.

Mendhiratta, S. S., et al. Cannabis and cognitive functions. *British Journal of Addiction* 83:749-753, 1988.

Negrete, J. C. What's happening to the cannabis debate? *British Journal of Addiction* 83:359-372, 1988.

Schuckit, M. *Drug and Alcohol Abuse*, 3rd ed. New York, Plenum Press, 1989.

Wu, T. C., et al. Pulmonary hazards of smoking marijuana as compared with tobacco. *New England Journal of Medicine* 318:347-351, 1988. ✦

Part IV
Narcotics

In pharmacology, a science that focuses on the chemical nature, structure, and action of drugs, *narcotics* include the natural derivatives of *Papaver somniferum L.*—the opium poppy—having both analgesic and sedative properties, and any synthetic derivatives of similar pharmacological structure and action. Thus, the range of substances that can be properly called narcotics is quite limited and encompasses four specific groups:

Natural narcotics

- opium, derived directly from *Papaver somniferum L.*
- morphine and codeine, derived from opium

Semisynthetic narcotics

- heroin
- hydromorphone (Dilaudid)
- oxycodone (Percodan)
- etorphine
- "designer drugs"

Synthetic narcotics with high potency

- methadone (discussed below)
- meperidine (Demerol)

Synthetic narcotics with low potency

- propoxyphine (Darvon)
- pentazocine (Talwin)

There are many other narcotics, but the examples indicated are the best known. The most widely used in the drug culture are methadone and heroin. Methadone was synthesized during World War II by German chemists when supply lines for morphine were interrupted. Although chemically unlike morphine or heroin, it produces many of the same effects. Methadone was introduced in the United States in 1947 and quickly became the drug of choice in the detoxification of heroin addicts.

Since the 1960s, methadone has been in common use for the treatment of heroin addiction. Known as "methadone maintenance," the program takes advantage of methadone's unique properties as a narcotic. Like all narcotics, methadone is cross-dependent with heroin. As such, it is a substitute narcotic that prevents withdrawal. More importantly, however, methadone is orally effective, making intravenous use unnecessary. In addition, it is a longer-acting drug than heroin, with one oral dose lasting up to 24 hours. These properties have made methadone useful in the management of chronic narcotic addiction. Yet, on the other hand, methadone is also a primary drug of abuse among some narcotic addicts, resulting in a small street market for the drug. Most illegal methadone is diverted from legitimate maintenance programs by methadone patients. Hence, illegal supplies of the drug are typically available only where such programs exist.

Heroin has a somewhat longer and more curious history. In 1874, British chemist C. R. A. Wright described a number of experiments he had carried out at London's St. Mary's Hospital to determine the effect of combining various acids with morphine. Wright produced a series of new morphine-like compounds, including what became known in the scientific literature as *diacetylmorphine*. His discovery of diacetylmorphine had been the outgrowth of an enduring search for more effective substitutes for morphine. This interest stemmed not only from the painkilling qualities of opiate drugs but also from their sedative effects on the respiratory system. Wright's work, however, went for the most part unnoticed.

Some 24 years later, in 1898, pharmacologist Heinrich Dreser reported on a series of experiments he had conducted with diacetylmorphine for Friedrich Bayer and Company of Elberfeld, Germany. He noted that the drug was highly effective in the treatment of coughs, chest pains, and the discomforts associated with pneumonia and tuberculosis. Dreser's commentary received immediate notice, for it had come at a time when antibiotics were still unknown, and pneumonia and tuberculosis were among the leading causes of death. He claimed that diacetylmorphine had a stronger sedative effect on respiration than either morphine or codeine, that therapeutic relief came quickly, and that the potential for a fatal overdose was almost nil. In response to such favorable reports, Bayer and Company began marketing diacetylmorphine, under the trade name of *Heroin*—so named from the German *heroisch*, meaning heroic and powerful.

Although Bayer's Heroin was promoted as a sedative for coughs and as a chest and lung medicine, it was advocated by some as a treatment for morphine addiction. This situation seems to have arisen from three somewhat-related phenomena. The *first* was the belief that Heroin was nonaddicting. *Second*, since the drug had a greater potency than that of morphine, only small dosages were required for the desired medical effects, thus reducing the potential for the rapid onset of addiction. And *third*, at the turn of the twentieth century, the medical community did not fully understand the dynamics of cross dependence. *Cross* dependence refers to the phenomenon that among certain pharmacologically related drugs, physical dependence on one will carry over to all the others. As such, for the patient suffering from the unpleasant effects of morphine withdrawal, the administration of heroin would have the consequence of one or more doses of morphine. The dependence was maintained and withdrawal disappeared, the two combining to give the appearance of a "cure."

Given the endorsement of the medical community, with little mention of its potential dangers, heroin quickly found its way into routine medical therapeutics and over-the-counter patent medicines. However, the passage of the Pure Food and Drug Act in 1906 and the Harrison Act in 1914 restricted the availability of heroin, and the number of chronic users declined.

Although narcotics use in its various forms has been common throughout United States history, its current and most typical manifestation—the intravenous use of heroin—apparently developed during the 1930s and became widespread after 1945. Between 1950 and the early 1960s, most major cities experienced a low-level spread of heroin use, particularly among the black and other minority populations. Thereafter, use began to grow rapidly, rising to peaks in the late 1960s and then falling sharply. The pattern was so ubiquitous that it came to be regarded as "epidemic" heroin use. More recent "epidemics" occurred in 1973-1974, 1977-1978, and 1982-1983, defined as such on the basis of the numbers of new admissions to heroin-treatment facilities. Yet interestingly, no one really knew how widespread heroin use was during those years, and even today the estimates are often little more than scientific guesses.

In the 1970s, the National Institute on Drug Abuse developed what it called "heroin trend indicators," relative estimates generated from a composite of reported heroin-related deaths, hospital emergency room visits, heroin-treatment admissions, and high school and household surveys. On the basis of these data, the estimated number of heroin users in the United States for 1977 ranged from 396,000 to 510,000. Throughout the 1980s and into the 1990s, government reports were maintaining that the number of heroin users in the United States was somewhere in the vicinity of 500,000, having been at that level for about a decade and a half.

In the selections that follow, a number of perspectives on heroin are presented, including initiation into addiction, supporting a habit, heroin smoking, and nonaddictive opiate use. ✦

14. Becoming a Heroin Addict

D AN W ALDORF

Much of the research on heroin focuses on addiction and the lifestyles of heroin users. Dan Waldorf is one of the few to study initiation into heroin use, and he did so by focusing on the social setting in which a sample of working-class males first used heroin. His data were collected through participant observation and unstructured interviews with the people he was studying. Waldorf notes the importance of peer and intimate friendship groups during initiation. He attributes this to new users' lack of knowledge about drug networks and about techniques used for administering the drug.

One of the few achievements, perhaps the only one, of the propaganda efforts (one can hardly call them educational or preventive efforts) of the old Federal Bureau of Narcotics was the development of the stereotype of the drug seller and the ways in which he initiated persons into drug use and abuse. This stereotype characterized the seller as a depraved profiteer who would do anything to create new users, thus assuring a ready and eager market for his sales. The motives of the seller were pure malice and profit as he skulkingly waited for innocent and unsuspecting persons (usually children) to offer them drugs, addiction, and "eventual enslavement." In this description, all the naive victim need do was use the offered drug and he would be on a sure road to addiction.

To anyone who knew anything about drug users or addiction, this stereotype was obviously erroneous. Drug sellers do not have to tempt or entice persons to use drugs; drug users usually seek out the seller. A single use of any opiate—even of the most powerful, heroin—will not cause a person to become addicted. But this simple-minded view of the drug seller and beginning drug use lived a long time, much too long a time. As recently as 1962, the White House Conference on Drug Abuse heard serious testimony from law-enforcement officials that propounded this view. To this day, the hard line taken by police, city officials, and state legislators against drug sellers, founded upon the belief that

users and sellers are different persons, reflects this stereotype.

The reasons that this stereotype has lived so long have to do with the power of the Federal Bureau of Narcotics and the failure of scientists to specify and test the more plausible and now current theory of initial drug use, i.e., that initial use of heroin occurs in a cultural and social setting that encourages and facilitates its use.

The Federal Bureau of Narcotics had, until the late 1950s, *nearly* complete domination over all other sources of information and research about illicit drug use and addiction. A good deal of the information about narcotic addiction going to legislators and the public was unfounded scientifically and filtered through a narrow enforcement perspective. This domination was so complete they could and did arrest doctors who dared to treat addicts privately and intimidate scientists who disagreed with them or propounded other views and theories. For years, Dr. Lawrence Kolb and sociologist Alfred Lindesmith were the only persons strong enough and brave enough to stand up to their blatant propaganda. With the 1950s, the power of the Bureau declined, and by the time Bureau Chief Harry T. Anslinger retired in 1962, it had taken a back seat to scientists and people actively treating addicts as sources of information on narcotic addiction and associated activities of addicts.

Researchers and writers in the field failed because they were too often seeking single or all-inclusive causes for narcotic addiction, instead of just looking at the simple processes of initial use and addiction. Everyone was too busy with the grand theory to deal with simple processes. As a consequence, there were a number of elaborate theories which anyone and everyone disputed and few data to substantiate them. The research literature is replete with small samples, 10, 20, and 30 addicts, from which generalization is difficult; so even the best theories went begging for empirical support.

Initial Use

Information and data about initial use of heroin, or of other drugs for that matter, are still very sketchy. Few researchers have systematically investigated initial heroin use, as distinct from heroin addiction. To date, there have been only two empirical studies that deal with initial heroin use; both of these were primarily concerned with the causes of addiction and gave only passing attention to the processes of addiction (beginning use, habituation, physical addiction, detoxification, abstention, re-lapse, and so forth). Bingham Dai, in his original, classic study of 40 addicts in Chicago, found that most of his small sample acquired their information about the effects of opiates through association with other opiate users and felt certain social pressures to use the drug.[1] In a 1951 study of 22 adolescent male heroin addicts at Bellevue Hospital in New York, it was found that they were commonly introduced to heroin either by a heroin seller or by another boy who was addicted.[2]

Our data support the idea that initial heroin use is a social phenomenon; the role of other persons in the initial use of heroin is crucial. Beginning heroin use is *not* a solitary activity. Persons are initiated in a group situation among friends and acquaintances. Only 17 (4 percent) of our sample of 417 males reported that they were alone the first time they used heroin; by far the majority (96 percent) reported that they used heroin the first time with one or more persons. These other persons were almost always friends and were usually of the same sex. White persons in our sample tended to use in larger groups than did blacks and Puerto Ricans.

More often than not, the persons who initiated the men and boys of our sample into heroin use had used it previously themselves. Some were addicted, but most were not. Let me illustrate this with some quotes about the circumstances of first use:

I was at a party with about ten of my friends—both guys and girls. Someone asked me whether I would like to try some horse. I was high on alcohol at the time, so I said I was game for it. That dude who turned me on was a user, not an addict.

I was at a discotheque with these two motorcycle dudes; they hung out there. I was just starting to run with them and was with a group of four or five guys. . . . We had been drinking a little beer earlier, and one of them suggested we get some H. We left the discotheque to cop. I got off in a car—mainlined. I vomited and got stoned. After a while we all went back to the discotheque and had a good time.

The first time I used, I snorted with two friends in one of their houses. One of them had tried H before and said it was a good high, so I tried it. We were going to a dance, and I wanted to be high for the dance.

The first time I used heroin . . . I wanted to be one of the fellows. I was with my girlfriend and a friend and we got rapping about dope.

My buddy said he knew where to get some (he had used before), and so I gave him some money. We got off, but I wouldn't let my girlfriend try it.

Only a minority reported that they were initiated by persons who sold heroin, and some said that they themselves were selling heroin before they actually used it:

I knew this pusher dude. You wouldn't believe the money he had; he had a green Eldorado and the best clothes you ever saw. Well, I was on my way to meet two friends one day (they were both using heroin) an' I see this dude standing on the corner, an' he looked groovy. So I asked what it was made him look so good. He said it was smack, an' I said I wanted some. He gave it to me.

I was dealing marijuana, hash, and heroin. I had been into "smoke" [marijuana] for a long time, but I never tried heroin. I guess I got curious. I had been dealing heroin for about four months, and one day a friend asked me for some and got off (skin-popped) in front of me. Seeing him get off made me want to try it, so I did.

Use of Other Drugs Before Heroin

By the time they get to heroin, most persons have had experience with other drugs; heroin is seldom the first used. More than three out of four (77 percent) of the men we interviewed reported that they had used marijuana before heroin. Only small minorities had used barbiturates (13 percent), airplane glue (11 percent), amphetamines (6 percent), cocaine (6 percent), and LSD (5 percent) before. This high incidence of marijuana use does not mean, however, that everyone who uses marijuana (or any other drug for that matter) will become a heroin user; that is another story. Such an argument is like saying that everyone who smokes tobacco will turn to marijuana. Certainly, there is an association between tobacco use and marijuana use, but one does not either lead to or cause the other.[3]

I expect that most persons had also used alcohol by that time, but unfortunately the data collected on alcohol use are not available. Questions about it were asked in our follow-up questionnaire, which, however, has never been analyzed, because the funds for the completion of the project were curtailed.

In general, the middle-class pattern of wide experimentation with a variety of drugs, progressing from marijuana to LSD, barbiturates, and amphetamines, and then to heroin, does not apply to the majority of New York addicts. This may be the result of the accessibility of drugs on the illegal markets and the greater availability of heroin, but it may also involve differing attitudes and beliefs about the effects of drugs. Many of those with whom I spoke paid no lip service to "Timothy Leary ideologies" and were not the least bit concerned with "consciousness-expanding" drugs, such as LSD and mescaline, saying that kind of high was not for them and that LSD was "another trip," implying that it was one trip that they were not interested in taking. Curiously, only a few persons connected any "consciousness-expansion" rationales with marijuana.

There were, however, exceptions to this general rule. Young, short-term users of heroin; those under 20 years old who had used heroin for four years or less; and white users, who were more often middle-class, tended to fit the pattern of wide experimentation before heroin use more than older users and blacks did.[4]

Why Heroin?

A number of reasons are given for beginning the use of heroin. Some users cited emotional states, involving problems with families or girlfriends, but the majority fell into two categories: 38 percent said that they were curious about the effects of heroin and wanted to experience it themselves, and 36 percent said that their friends were using it and they wanted to try it also.

Obviously, persons may use heroin for a combination of reasons—psychological, social, and intellectual. One 19-year-old boy from the Bronx cited all three in his description of his first use:

> I was feeling down. I had got down [had sexual intercourse] with my older brother and was packing a lot of guilt. I didn't want my friends to know what happened. A couple of days later, I was in a basement with a buddy. He had used and was strung out. He offered me some, and I was curious to know what it was like. I skin-popped, got high [felt real comfortable] and then drowsy. I guess I was trying to prove myself to my friend; I wanted to show him and the others that I could do what they were doing.

Motives for human behavior are often complex, as the above quote suggests. At any given time, it may be difficult for an individual to account for all or even a few of the reasons for the things he does. Often, we do not know why we do things; the mo-

tives remain subconscious. Without an in-depth study of the complex motivations for beginning heroin use—no such study has been made, although there has been a lot of speculation—I believe we can safely accept what addicts have told us about the pressures of a friend's use and the intellectual motive of curiosity. Experience of other drugs, marijuana and alcohol in most cases, and some association with drug users or addicts could invoke such curiosity. Users and addicts talk among themselves and with others a great deal about the effects of heroin, comparing euphorias, qualities, and so forth. One would not have to be unduly curious to decide to experience the drug personally—particularly in the current cultural climate of drug exploration. I myself am curious to know what the effects of heroin are, particularly because addicts seem so willing to give up so much to use it. The point I wish to make is that initial use of heroin is not as clouded in complex motivations as many persons would have us believe. It is, perhaps, not unlike the beginning use of other legal and illegal drugs—alcohol, tobacco, and marijuana—all of which occur in settings in which there are certain pressures toward use.

Unlike the small-town, Southern addict described by John O'Donnell[5] and the physician addicts studied by Charles Winick,[6] only one of the men of our sample attributed his initial use of heroin to the need for relief of physical pain. This was an ingenuous Puerto Rican I met at Manhattan State Hospital.

> I was working at a paint factory at the time; it was heavy, kinda back breaking work. One Sunday I was playing ball up in Central Park, you know, I always keep busy with sports, and hurt my back sliding into third base. I was really in pain when I went to work on Monday. I could hardly stoop over. After about an hour on the job, I told the guys I was working with that I was going to have to go home. Well, one of them said, "Try some of this," pulling a cap of white powder out of his pocket. I snorted it, just a little, and felt wonderful. I couldn't believe how good I felt; I worked like a whirlwind all the rest of the day.
>
> Well, the next day he sold me some more and I used it every day for two weeks. Then I started to get sick, and that's when I found out what I had been using.

Most persons felt positive effects from heroin the first time they used it. Nearly two-thirds (63 percent) of the men in our sample reported that they felt positive effects upon first use, while another 27 percent said they felt positive effects from the second to the fifth time. Rather surprisingly, seven men (2 percent) reported that they had *never* experienced positive effects from heroin use.

More white persons in our sample reported positive effects on first use (71 percent) than blacks (64 percent) and Puerto Ricans (57 percent). This may be explained by the white men's wider exploration of other drugs before the initial use of heroin; having experienced more drugs, they may be more susceptible to the euphoric effects of heroin. The most common first-use response was nausea and vomiting, followed by a euphoria that the respondents described as being different from and more intense than that produced by other drugs. This was described by one 19-year-old in a way that leads one to think that the effect for him was one of self-actualization, an effect that gave him new vitality:

My brother was using at the time; he later became addicted too. The two of us were pretty close, closer than anyone else, and I thought a lot of him. I wanted to see what made my brother take it. Well, I found out. When I got off the first time, I felt like me. I felt alive. Before I used heroin, I was always down; I didn't have any energy. When I was high, I was something else.

Most described it as an unusually pleasant euphoria that permitted a different perspective on themselves and their world. For example, this description was given by a rather precise, but otherwise inarticulate, 20-year-old:

It was nice. It brought you into a cloud [from which] you see the world better, with a good outlook. I was like out there remote from the world.

Some said that they did not feel any positive effects with the first use, only nausea, vomiting, and headaches. In subsequent use, they did experience the euphoria, however, which suggests that, as with marijuana, some persons have to learn how to respond to the drug, how to make themselves more susceptible to its effects.

Eventual Addiction

Subsequent use and eventual addiction for the men in our sample was a slow, rather gradual process. This was discovered by calculating the mean time between the different methods of use and also the time between initial use and discovery of physi-

cal dependence. The initial method of use for the majority was "snorting," sniffing the drug through the nose. Only a very few "mainlined," injected the drug directly into a vein, the first time they used. The majority continued to snort for a while; then, either because their nasal membranes became inflamed or because they learned and desired more immediate effects, they soon began "skin-popping," injecting the drug subcutaneously. Eventually the users discovered that the euphoric effects came much faster with direct injection into a vein.

We found that the mean time between their initial use of heroin and the first time they mainlined was four months.[7] The majority (66 percent) complete the process in less than 6 months, with the more precocious getting down to the serious business of mainlining in less than a month.

As in beginning use, subsequent use during the first year usually takes place with other persons. Three out of every four (75 percent) said that they usually used heroin with others during their first year of use, while only one in ten (11 percent) reported that they usually used alone during that period.

There are a number of purely mechanical reasons for this association with other heroin users. The beginning user usually does not have a ready source of supply (a "connection") and must rely upon others to buy the drug for him. Usually, the beginner will seek out a friend who has a source who then cops for both of them. Similarly, the neophyte may not possess the "works" for injecting the drug and must rely upon others for that also. Actual injection is also something that must be learned from others; it requires considerable skill and some practice to inject oneself with the often dull needles that many use. Actually, works, although rather crudely made, are far easier to use than the standard syringe.

Although our project did not explore the specific reasons for continued use after the first use, I believe that the reason for most persons was quite simple: they enjoyed the first experiences and continued the practice. For those for whom it took longer to get a positive effect, other motives, psychological or social, may have come into play until such a time as a positive effect was experienced. This was illustrated by a close friend of mine who, during a year of intensive drug use, used heroin three times:

I used smeeck three times. I kept bugging my cousin to try some. He was a pretty heavy shooter who managed to control it and didn't get addicted. The first time, I just got sick and felt drowsy. The second time was about the same as the first. I found out what it was all about the third time; it was fantastic. I knew after that that I could never take it again; I liked it too much. I knew I wasn't getting the effect the first two times. Bernie told me I wasn't getting it. I wanted to feel what he felt.

Heroin users and addicts are right, in some respects, when they say that one should not knock heroin until one has experienced it; often the drug allows the user to manage anxieties and feelings and lets him function better. This is in addition to the usual euphoria. Admittedly, these "good effects" are induced artificially, and one can assume that they will only last as long as the drug is effective, but for some it assuages deep and real anxieties and tensions. It gives them something akin to artist Roy Litchenstein's vision of "Peace Through Chemistry," a mechanical peace.

Let me illustrate some of these "good effects" with a cross-section of answers we got to the question, "What did heroin do for you?" asked informally of a small group of residents of Hart Island:

> It gave me peace of mind. I could get away from reality and forget my complexes. Straight, I felt I couldn't relate to people, and when I used drugs [heroin] I could communicate better.

> I liked getting high. It was a good feeling. Heroin made me feel secure. I really felt protected. When I was high nothing could hurt me.

> Heroin makes you forget about your problems; makes you feel you know everything. You feel strong and healthy, not weak. You can work.

These responses were from persons in an active anti-drug environment who could not deny that heroin gave them something they enjoyed. When it offers some so much, it is no wonder that the use of the drug has, for centuries, been so hard to control.

Many persons knew before they used heroin what addiction entailed and had observed what happened to addicts and how they were treated by society. Indeed, many of the persons I interviewed during the study said that while growing up they had detested addicts and had believed that addiction was something that would never happen to them. This realization did not deter them, however, as most believed that they could control their use of heroin and not become addicted.

Not all who use heroin or opiates become addicted. Lee Robins, in an important study made in 1967 of a population of "normal" black men attending an elementary school in St. Louis, Missouri, in 1932, found that 13 percent of 221 men had tried heroin at some time in their lives and that four out of five of these (10 percent of the total sample) became addicted.[8] Some try heroin and like the effects but do not wish to risk the possible addiction. I know two such persons: one whom I mentioned earlier, and another who used opium ten times while he served in the Peace Corps in Asia. He used it out of curiosity and had no intention of using it again, although he enjoyed it. I suppose it remains to be seen if they will or will not become addicted, but I doubt that either will.

Unfortunately, none of the people in our sample were so able to control their use; all were either addicted or considered in danger of becoming addicted. However, addiction is a slower process than one would think. The average time between first use and the realization of physical addiction was 11 months. This time could be as short as three weeks and as long as six years, for that was the range of time between the two events. One could say that some persons are particularly susceptible to heroin. One man told me that, after he first used heroin, he used it every day for six years until the time he was committed by his family to treatment. He claimed that he was addicted the first time that he used it but did not experience physical withdrawal until the fourth week of use.

Patterns of Continuing and Secondary Drug Use

As we saw earlier, the middle-class pattern of drug use that begins with marijuana and LSD and progresses to barbiturates and amphetamines and, eventually, heroin use does not apply to our urban working-class addicts. The New York addict uses a wide variety of drugs other than heroin and alcohol, but most of his secondary drug use occurs after heroin use and addiction, not before.

An average of 3.4 drugs other than heroin and alcohol was used with any frequency (more than six times), with more than half (55 percent) of the sample reporting having used four or more other drugs, and more than a quarter (28 percent), six or more other drugs. Length of heroin use and the ethnicity of the user seem to be closely associated with the number of drugs used. The longer men used heroin, the more secondary drugs they reported, which suggests that long-term users may find themselves in situations where they are less selective about the drugs they use and take whatever they can get. That is to say, perhaps, that drugs tend to use them rather than the reverse. White addicts may also be "used by drugs," because they reported more drugs used than either blacks or Puerto Ricans. The mean number of secondary drugs reported by whites was 4.6, as compared to 3.2 for Puerto Ricans and 2.7 for blacks. But averages are only half the story; more than half (51 percent) of the whites reported using six or more other drugs, while only a quarter (25 percent) of the Puerto Ricans and less than one out of five (18 percent) of the blacks used that many.

After heroin, which everyone used, and marijuana, which nearly everyone used (92 percent), cocaine, barbiturates, amphetamines, and methadone were, in that order, the drugs cited most often. Two out of three (66 percent) of the sample said that they had used cocaine at least once, with nearly half (47 percent) reporting that they had used it more than six times. In the recent past, cocaine was considered by street addicts as something of a luxury because of its then high cost—$10 to $15 a cap— but recently the supply has increased considerably, and the price has dropped in New York to $5 to $7, making it more available. Cocaine, as well as being taken separately, is often taken in combination with heroin; this is called "speedballing" and is said to intensify the "rush" of drugs effects. Blacks show a certain preference for "coke"; like heroin, it is readily available in Harlem and other black communities in New York, with more than half (54 percent) the blacks reporting that they had used it more than six times.

Barbiturates and amphetamines were usually used as substitutes for heroin or in conjunction with it, and only seldom exclusively. During periods when addicts cannot get heroin, whether because they do not have the money or have lost their connections or because of a local panic when heroin becomes scarce, they may simply substitute barbiturates until such a time as they can get heroin again. Both barbiturates and amphetamines may also be used to supplement heroin when the addict's tolerance for heroin has progressed past his ability to get the dosage needed to obviate withdrawal and keep him just normal, to say nothing of getting high.

Amphetamines, including methedrine, are used often in combination with heroin; but once a person has used heroin, they are seldom used singly. Many Puerto Ricans from the *Barrio*, or East Harlem, use ampules of injectable methedrine called "bombitas," or "little bombs," to "speed" them up to go out to hustle.

Unlike the white, Southern addict described by researchers at Lexington Hospital,[9] methadone in its pill form (known commercially as dolophines and in the drug argot as "dollies") is rarely used by New York addicts as a primary drug of addiction. New York heroin users prefer the heightened euphoria of heroin or cocaine to the blunted euphoria of methadone. Frequently, dollies are used to kick or cut down on the addict's habit without his having to go to a hospital or a doctor; they permit him to control his heroin habit and to continue to feel its effects without the massive doses that are needed when tolerances are high. One-third (37 percent) of the sample reported using dollies, with a quarter (26 percent) reporting using them more than six times.

Usually white addicts were more likely than blacks and Puerto Ricans to abuse secondary drugs other than heroin and to use drugs, such as LSD, barbiturates, and amphetamines before heroin. This may be the result of the sheer availability of certain drugs. The major heroin traffic in New York City is concentrated in black and Puerto Rican neighborhoods (the black ghettoes of Central Harlem, Bedford-Stuyvesant in Brooklyn, and the South Bronx, and their Puerto Rican counterparts in East Harlem and Williamsburg). But the abuse of secondary drugs by whites may also be an expression of more severe psychological problems, as John Langrod suggests:

> Although whites are more likely than blacks and Puerto Ricans to come from intact homes, earn more money, graduate from high school, not have addicted or alcoholic relatives, or be on welfare, they are less likely to have gotten along with their families, prior to and during heroin addiction, and are less optimistic about getting along with their families upon leaving the institution. It is possible that whites, despite their favorable social circumstances, may be using drugs because of more severe emotional problems, compared to blacks and Puerto Ricans, for which drug use may be more of a social phenomenon or an escape from a genuinely oppressive social-economic reality.[10]

How Long Is a Run?

It is my impression that heroin use by addicts is much more periodic than most of the research and literature on the topic suggest. Actually there is as yet no real information about the extent or periodicity of heroin use by addicts, and our study did not deal with it either. In the absence of solid research on the topic, my impressions may offer some information on a subject that has not yet been treated in any systematic way.

I became interested in this after I observed that most addicts spend a good part of their careers in addiction in jail, and that many make occasional but real efforts to abstain from heroin use after incarceration or treatment. An addict may say that he has been addicted for 13 years, but as you delve into his history, you may learn that 6 years of that time have been spent in jail, another year in various treatment programs, and, perhaps, 6 months in actual abstention outside of an institution.[11] The actual duration of physical addiction and heroin use is often much shorter and more sporadic than one would expect from the original, superficial report. What many persons may be describing is not the length of actual physical addiction, but the length of time they have considered themselves addicts—which for many may be more a social status than a physical condition.

This periodicity of drug use is illustrated in my field report of an interview with Beverly, an attractive 22-year-old white woman who was in Manhattan Rehabilitation Center:

Beverly began the use of opiates (dilaudid) when she was 17 years old. She was initiated by an older boyfriend and used every day for 3 months after her first use (from supplies stolen from a drug store by the boyfriend). After an argument with the same boyfriend, she kicked cold turkey and left the boyfriend and her home town to travel to Michigan with another boyfriend she had gone with earlier. At that time, she was off drugs for one month.

During the trip to Michigan she became pregnant; when she returned home, she realized her condition. Shortly after this realization, she went back to opiates (morphine this time) for another two and a half months. During the third month of her pregnancy, she o.d.'d (overdosed) and went to a hospital, where she stayed 5 days and was detoxified. After the hospitalization, she went to Florida with her child's father, where she remained drug-free for 9 months. She used pills occasionally at this time.

Three months after her child's birth, she returned home and began using heroin. She used heroin for 4 months, then caught hepatitis and went to the hospital for two weeks, where she was detoxified. After this hospitalization, she stayed off all drugs for 4 months while she lived with the child's father a third time. The child's father was not a drug user.

Returning home to her family, where her two addicted brothers lived, after a fight with the boyfriend, she resumed use of heroin and barbiturates and continued to use them for 16 months. She described this period:

I tried not to let my habit get too big. I would use for 5 or 6 days then stay off for a day using barbiturates. That way I could get high and not use too much stuff. Generally, if I didn't use heroin, I would use pills or dollies.

Again, she detoxified herself, this time with dollies, and was off heroin for one month. Near the end of this period, she was arrested as an accomplice in a burglary and spent two months in jail. Rather than face the charges, she chose civil certification in the state program. At the time of the interview (December 1969), she had been in Manhattan Rehabilitation for 6 months.

At the time of the interview, 58 months had elapsed since her initiation to opiates. Two-thirds (34) of those 58 months were spent using opiates, another 8 were spent in jail and treatment, and 16 were spent opiate-free on 4 different occasions.

I expect that many addicts have similar histories, with numerous periods of abstention both in and out of institutions, but they have not been documented in any systematic way. Certainly, there are persons who use heroin for long and uninterrupted stretches, but they are those who have considerable money or are successful heroin sellers who avoid arrest and incarceration—they are not the usual street addict.

Summary

How, then, do persons become addicted? It is most certainly a combination of social events operating within a cultural milieu that encourages drug use. Despite society's disdain for certain drugs, we are a drug-taking culture. Evidence of this is all around us. Sociologist Hugh Parry found in two national samples that nearly half of the United States adult population reported the use of psychotropic drugs (sedatives, tranquilizers, and stimulants) at some time, and that one-quarter was currently (1967) using one or more such drugs.[12] The mass media bombard us with encouragements to use drugs: television and radio commercials tell us to take Compoz for our nerves, Nytol for our insomnia, and, until recently, tobacco for myriad frustrations; magazines offer us alcohol of all varieties.

Doctors prescribe miracle drugs for anything from infection to mental illness. The effects of many of these drugs are like magic—the drug may assist the body to fight off infection in a matter of hours, and former long-term psychotic patients leave hospitals, where earlier it was thought they would remain for the rest of their lives. In 1969, pharmacists in the United States filled more than 202 million prescriptions for a variety of tranquilizers, energizers, amphetamines, barbiturates, and hypnotics.[13] Nearly two out of every five were new prescriptions; the rest were refills. This figure does not include those given and used in hospitals and clinics, which would raise this total considerably.

Drug companies manufacture thousands of tons of drugs each year and spend millions of dollars a year to promote their sale and use. Pierre Garai, a medical writer, estimates:

> Three quarters of a *billion* dollars are spent yearly by some sixty drug companies to reach, persuade, cajole, pamper, outwit, and sell one of America's smallest markets, the 180,000 physicians. . . .[14]

The drug companies' object in these campaigns is to sell drugs—and they do. Henry Lennard and his associates, in their most interesting book, *Mystification and Drug Misuse*, said:

Most pharmaceutical firms have experienced substantial growth since the early 1950s. For example, in 1951, one company reported net sales of 9.5 million dollars; by 1970, this sales figure had reached 83.6 million dollars. Among the principal products of this company are central nervous [*sic.*] stimulants (amphetamines and amphetamine-barbiturate combinations) and antipsychotic agents (phenothiazine compounds). While the sale of all drugs has increased greatly for the industry as a whole, the sale of psychoactive drugs has increased to a greater extent.[15]

Medicine cabinets in most homes in the United States are a veritable cornucopia of prescription and non-prescription drugs. Drugs are a part of our everyday life and an integral part of not only the youth culture, but that of adults as well. We are a drug-taking culture.

Beginning heroin use arises in group situations and out of associations with other drug users. Before persons try heroin, they usually have taken marijuana or other drugs and are curious to experiment with still others. Often, they know heroin users or addicts personally and learn from them, in glorified terms, the effects of heroin.

The social pressures of peer groups are well-known to all of us, not only to sociologists. These pressures influence our vote, they encourage us to smoke, to drink, to overachieve, to underachieve, what have you. When the climate of the peer group (and most young people find themselves in such groups, however tightly or loosely organized) is to use or abuse illegal drugs, then this behavior is expected of each member of the group, like the one-time beer drinking of college freshmen, the street gang's recruitment of warriors for "bopping" (fighting), and the ways workmen prescribe how much work can be done on the assembly line. To resist is difficult; no one wants to be considered afraid to try drugs, a party poop, yellow, or a "rate buster."

And so, a boy or girl tries heroin, and, as with most drugs, the initial experience is a pleasing one, most especially with heroin. Using heroin once will not result in addiction. Confident of his power to control his life and destiny, the individual believes that he can control his drug use; he tries the drug again and again. In some respects, the very effect of heroin supports this confidence of the user and encourages an inviolable attitude toward life. Alexander Trocchi, in his brilliant autobiographical novel, *Cain's Book*, describes these effects in a particularly revealing way:

> The mind under heroin evades perception as it does ordinarily; one is aware only of contents. But the whole way of posing the question, of dividing the mind from what it is aware of, is fruitless. Nor is it that the objects of perception are intrusive in an electric way, as they are under mescaline or lysergic acid, nor that things strike one with more intensity or in a more enchanted or detailed way, as I have sometimes experienced under marijuana—it is that the perceiving turns inward, the eyelids droop, the blood is aware of itself, a slow phosphorescence in all the fabric of flesh and bone; it is that the organism has a sense of being intact and unbrittle and, above all, *inviolable*. For the attitude born of this

sense of inviolability, some Americans have used the word "cool."[16]

Other people, other drug users, are necessary for getting and administering the drug, and the novice returns to those who provide the drug and the information about its use. As these associations develop, the beginning user may find that he gets certain comfort in these associations, as well as in the drug. They are often people like himself, and they provide an atmosphere in which to talk about and discuss his drug experiences and, perhaps, a certain identity that he did not have before, that of a drug user.

After repeated use of heroin, usually but not necessarily over an extended period, the abuse of the drug becomes a habituation without actual physical dependence. This does not necessarily require everyday use, but perhaps some regular or habitual use, as on weekends. Jazz musicians in the 1950s called this, interestingly, an "ice cream habit."

This habituation may result from a number of psychological or sociological motives, as Isidor Chein et al. have described in their work *The Road to H.*[17] The abuser may use the drug, because it eases certain anxieties and tensions he may feel; it may allow him to feel more confident as a person, to communicate and get along with others. (More than once, male addicts have told me that they used heroin, because it helped them to talk with girls.) Some use it to manage frightening hallucinations or paranoid thoughts that otherwise would cause considerable anxiety.

It may be used, because one wants to be accepted socially by an important group in his life. He or she wants to belong, and this is one way of doing it. It is often difficult to go against the tide, to be independent of the pressures of other people. New members of nearly any social group do things to ingratiate themselves with the others, and so might a youngster use heroin to show that he wants to be a part of what's happening and do what the group is doing.

Another reason might arise out of some need to establish a social identity—to be somebody, something. Establishing oneself—acquiring an identity—is difficult in our society; there are few effective rites of passage and very few institutional mechanisms to ease one into adulthood. As a consequence, some persons never make it, never feel adequate to the task, or do so only with considerable pain and anguish. For some, the social identity of a heroin user may fill this void. It may be an identity despised by society, but it is nonetheless an identity.

Heroin use may also be part of a vocation. Drug sellers at levels above the street pusher can and do make money, and persons growing up in New York ghettos know this. If one finds a good source of drugs that have not been too often diluted, there is an opportunity to make considerable money; this, in turn, can bring desired material objects, women, and a certain status among addicts and, perhaps, the larger community.

Lastly, the habitué may use the drug as an act of rebellion against his family or society. Feeling frustrated by an overwhelming family which may not allow him to conduct his life on his own terms, or by an irrational society that inculcates a need to achieve but blocks his opportunity, he lashes out against that which frustrates him. That the action of becoming a heroin user will not result in either the desired freedom or the chance for achievement is often of little moment to the individual; he acts out of a certain desperation in the only way he knows.

Obviously, there are few pure or simple motives for becoming habituated to heroin. In the complexity of human behavior, there are also complex motives. Persons may rebel against their families and at the same time seek a vocation; they may both use heroin to ease their tensions and wish to be part of a group of people. The possible combinations of motives are innumerable.

After habituation to heroin, physical addiction soon follows. Now the abuser's need is not just psychological or social, but physical as well. Now, when he does not give himself regular and sufficient dosages, he experiences withdrawal symptoms. It is now important to avoid withdrawal sickness, which becomes, perhaps, as important a motive as any of the others he may have for using drugs. Withdrawal symptoms abate in a matter of minutes after injection of heroin—magically, the addict is well or high again, where moments before he was sick. The motives for using heroin become compounded; the physical gives reinforcement to the earlier psychological and social motives for habituation, and vice versa.

Without a steady supply of drugs, the addict may experience one or more times a day a dehabilitating cycle of being sick one moment and high the next. Most, if not all, of his actions are oriented toward seeking drugs. Soon, all of life has an overwhelming purpose and focus. Life is simplified into a single, engrossing need that must be met before consideration can be given to any of the other physical or social needs that we think are necessary for any reasonable life. Nearly all activity is focused upon the day-to-day struggle to get the drug to satisfy a single need. It is as if T. S. Eliot had been talking about addicts when, in his poem "The Love Song of J. Alfred Prufock," Prufock would like to roll the universe into a single ball. It would seem that addicts do roll their lives and the universe into such a ball, the single ball of heroin.

* * *

Dan Waldorf, "Becoming a Heroin Addict," from his book *Careers in Dope*. Copyright © 1973. Used by permission of the publisher, Prentice Hall, a Division of Simon & Schuster, Englewood Cliffs, N.J.

For Discussion

Waldorf notes the importance of intimate peer and friendship groups during drug initiation. For most adolescents and young adults the peer group is the focal point of the social network. Why then do some individuals refrain from using drugs despite use among peers?

Notes

1. Bingham Dai, *Opiate Addiction in Chicago* (Shanghai: The Commercial Press, 1937).

2. Paul Zimmering, James Toolan, Ranate Safrin, and Bernard S. Wortis, "Heroin Addiction in Adolescent Boys," in *The Journal of Nervous and Mental Disease, 114* (1951).

3. Two recent books have dealt with the relationship between marijuana and heroin use: John Kaplan, *Marijuana: The New Prohibition*, (New York: World Publishing Company, 1970) and Michael Schofield, *The Strange Case of Pot* (Halmondsworth, England: Penguin Books, 1971).

4. For a more detailed report of this data, see John Langrod, "Secondary Drug Use Among Heroin Users," in *The International Journal of the Addictions*, Vol. 5, no. 4 (1970).

5. John A. O'Donnell, *Narcotic Addicts in Kentucky* (Washington, DC: U.S. Government Printing Office, 1970).

6. Charles Winick, "Physician Addicts," in *Social Problems*, Fall (1963).

7. By far the majority of our sample mainlined—96 percent in fact; 87 percent reported that it was the usual method of use, while another 9 percent said that they mainlined occasionally.

8. Lee Robins, "Drug Use in a Normal Population of Young Negro Men," in *The American Journal of Public Health*, Vol. 57, no. 9 (1967).

9. Joseph Spira, John C. Ball, and Emily S. Cottrell, "Addictions to Methadone Among Patients at Lexington and Fort Worth," in *Public Health Reports*, Vol. 83, no. 8 (1968).

10. John Langrod, "Secondary Drug Use," p. 633.

11. While it is true that persons do occasionally use drugs in prison and treatment, they seldom become physically addicted there.

12. Hugh J. Parry, "Use of Psychotropic Drugs by U.S. Adults," in *Public Health Reports*, Vol. 83 (1968).

13. See M. Balter's address to the American Public Health Association, Houston, TX, in October 1970.

14. Quoted in S. Malitz, "Psychopharmacology: A Cultural Approach," in *Symposium: Non-Narcotic Drug Dependency and Addiction*, Proceedings of the New York County District Branch, American Psychiatric Association, March 10, 1966.

15. Henry L. Lennard and associates, *Mystification and Drug Misuse* (San Francisco: Jossey-Bass, Inc., 1971).

16. Alexander Trocchi, *Cain's Book* (New York: Grove Press, Inc., 1960).

17. For a much more extensive discussion of the motives for drug use, see this and other writings of psychologist Isidor Chein listed in the bibliography. ✦

15. Taking Care of Business—The Heroin Addict's Life on the Street

Edward Preble
AND
John J. Casey

"Taking Care of Business," one of the classic papers in the drug field, begins with a brief history of heroin use and distribution in New York City from World War I through the late 1960s. The authors note trends in price, availability, and legitimate opportunities for heroin users. The primary focus of the article, however, is the various levels of heroin distribution. Importantly, Preble and Casey dispel the widely held belief that individuals use heroin as an escape. Rather, they argue, heroin allows individuals to experience purposeful lives. The daily activities in which heroin users are involved are highly rewarding to them, particularly when legitimate opportunities are not generally available.

Introduction

This report is a description of the life and activities of lower-class heroin users in New York City in the context of their street environment. It is concerned exclusively with the heroin users living in slum areas, who comprise at least 80 percent of the city's heroin-using population. They are predominantly Negro and Puerto Rican, with some Irish, Italian, and Jewish.

It is often said that the use of heroin provides an escape for the user from his psychological problems and from the responsibilities of social and personal relationships—in short, an escape from life. Clinical descriptions of heroin addicts emphasize the passive, dependent, withdrawn, generally inadequate features of their personality structure and social adjustment. Most sociological studies of heroin users make the same point. Thus, Chein et al. (1964) reported that street-gang members are not likely to become heroin users, because they are re-

sourceful, aggressive, well-integrated boys who are "reality-oriented" in their street environment. They held that it is the passive, anxious, inadequate boy, who cannot adapt to street life, who is likely to use heroin. Similarly, Cloward and Ohlin (1960) referred to heroin users as "retreatists" and "double failures" who cannot qualify for either legitimate or illegitimate careers. Unaggressive "mamma's boys" is the usual stereotype these days for the heroin addict, both for the students of narcotic use and the public at large. Experienced researchers and workers in the narcotics field know that there is no such thing as "the heroin addict" or "the addict personality." However, most attempts to generalize—the goal of all scientific investigation—result in some version of the escape theory.

The description which follows of the activities of lower-class heroin users in their adaptation to the social and economic institutions and practices connected with the use of heroin contradicts this widely held belief. Their behavior is anything but an escape from life. They are actively engaged in meaningful activities and relationships seven days a week. The brief moments of euphoria after each administration of a small amount of heroin constitute a small fraction of their daily lives. The rest of the time they are aggressively pursuing a career that is exacting, challenging, adventurous, and rewarding. They are always on the move and must be alert, flexible, and resourceful. The surest way to identify heroin users in a slum neighborhood is to observe the way people walk. The heroin user walks with a fast, purposeful stride, as if he is late for an important appointment—indeed, he is. He is hustling (robbing or stealing), trying to sell stolen goods, avoiding the police, looking for a heroin dealer with a good bag (the street retail unit of heroin), coming back from copping (buying heroin), looking for a safe place to take the drug, or looking for someone who beat (cheated) him—among other things. He is, in short, *taking care of business*, a phrase which is so common with heroin users that they use it in response to words of greeting, such as "how you doing?" and "what's happening?" *Taking care of biz* is the common abbreviation. *Ripping and running* is an older phrase which also refers to their busy lives. For them, if not for their middle- and upper-class counterparts (a small minority of opiate addicts), the quest for heroin is the quest for a meaningful life, not an escape from life. And the meaning does not lie, primarily, in the effects of the drug on their minds and bodies; it lies in the gratification of accomplishing a series of challenging, exciting tasks, every day of the week.

Much of the life of the heroin user on the street centers around the economic institutions of heroin distribution. Therefore, this report features a description of the marketing processes for heroin, from importation to street sales. The cost of heroin today is so high and the quality so poor that the street user must become totally involved in an economic career. A description of typical economic careers of heroin users will be presented. Preceding these two sections is a brief historical account of heroin use in New York City from World War I to the present, in which it will be seen that patterns of heroin use have changed at a pace and in a direction in correspondence with the social changes of the past fifty years. Theories and explanations about heroin use, based upon observations of fifty, twenty-five, or even five years ago, are inadequate to account for the phenomenon today. It is hoped that this contemporary account of the social setting for heroin use will provide useful data for the modifications of theory and practice which should accompany any dynamic social process.

Methodology

The data on which this report is based have come from interviews with patients at the Manhattan State Hospital Drug Addiction Unit and from participant observation and interviews with individuals and groups in four lower-class communities in New York City—East Harlem, Lower East Side, Yorkville, Claremont (Bronx). The communities represent the neighborhoods of approximately 85 percent of the addict patients at Manhattan State Hospital. The anthropologist's role and approach to the heroin-using study of informants was in the tradition of Bronislaw Malinowski (1922) and William F. Whyte (1955), which, in Whyte's words, consists of "the observation of interpersonal events." Another dimension was added with the modified use of research techniques, introduced by Abraham Kardiner and his collaborators (1939) in their psychosocial studies of primitive and modern cultures. The main feature of this methodology is the life-history interview with individual subjects. Initial and subsequent contacts with the research informants occurred, in all cases, with their voluntary consent and cooperation. The anthropologist had the advantage of twelve years experience of street work and

research in the study neighborhoods, and was able to enlist the assistance of long-time acquaintances for this special project. Four major ethnic groups were represented among the approximately 150 informants: Irish, Italian, Negro, and Puerto Rican.

History of Heroin Use in New York City

The recent history of heroin use in the city can be broken down into six time periods: (1) between World War I and World War II, (2) during World War II, (3) 1947 to 1951, (4) 1951 to 1961, and (6) 1961 to the present.

1. Between World War I and World II

Prior to World War II the use of heroin was limited, for the most part, to people in the *life*—show people, entertainers, and musicians; racketeers and gangsters; thieves and pickpockets; prostitutes and pimps. The major ethnic groups represented among these users were Italian, Irish, Jewish, and Negro (mostly those associated with the entertainment life). There were also heroin users among the Chinese, who had a history of opium use. The distribution of heroin by those who controlled the market was limited mostly to these people, and there was little knowledge or publicity about it.

2. During World War II

World War II interrupted the trade routes and distributorships for illicit heroin supplies, which resulted in a five-year hiatus in heroin use.

3. 1947 to 1951

When World War II ended, there was a greatly expanded market for heroin in the increased population among Negroes from the South and among migrating Puerto Ricans who came to New York during the war in response to a manpower shortage. In 1940, the Negro population in New York City was 450,000; in 1960, it was over 1 million. In 1940, the Puerto Rican population was 70,000; in 1960, it was over 600,000. As with all new immigrants in New York, they worked at the lowest economic levels, settled in slum neighborhoods, and were the victims of unemployment, poverty, and discrimination. From 1947 to 1951, the use of heroin spread among lower-class Negro and Puerto Rican people and among other lower-class, slum-dwelling people, mainly the Irish and Italians. The increased rate of use was gradual, but steady, and did not attract much attention. Most of the users were young adults in their twenties and thirties. They were more or less circumspect in their drug consumption, which they were able to be because of the relatively low cost and high quality of the heroin.

During this period, heroin was sold in number-five capsules (the smallest capsules used for pharmaceutical products). These *caps* could be bought for about one dollar apiece, and two to six persons could get high on the contents of one capsule. Commonly, four persons would contribute one quarter each and *get down on a cap*. There was social cohesion, identification, and ritual among the users of this period. Sometimes as many as twenty people would get together and, in a party atmosphere, share the powder contents of several capsules which were emptied upon a mirror and divided into columns by means of a razor blade, one column for each participant. The mirror was passed from person to person and each one would inhale his share through the nose by means of a tapered, rolled-up dollar bill which served as a straw, and was called a *quill*. A twenty, fifty, or hundred dollar bill was used on special occasions when someone wanted to make a show of his affluence. Since heroin was so inexpensive during this time, no addict had to worry about getting his fix; someone was always willing to loan him a dollar or share a part of his drug. The social relationships among these addicts were similar to those found in a neighborhood bar, where there is a friendly mutual concern for the welfare of the regular patrons. The most important economic factor in these early post-war days of heroin use was that heroin users were able to work even at a low-paying job and still support a habit, and many of them did. Relatively little crime was committed in the interest of getting money to buy heroin. A habit could be maintained for a few dollars a day, at little social or economic cost to the community.

4. 1951 to 1957

Around 1951, heroin use started to become popular among younger people on the streets, especially among street-gang members who were tired of gang fighting and were looking for a new high. As heroin use had become more common in the latter days of the previous period, the more street-wise teenagers learned about it and prevailed upon the experienced users to introduce them to it. Contrary to popular reports, experimentation with heroin by youths usually began at their initiative and not through proselytism. The stereotype of the dope *pusher* giving out free samples of narcotics to teenagers in school yards and candy stores, in order to addict them, is one of the most misleading myths about drug use. Also, contrary to professional reports about this development, it was not the weak, withdrawn, unadaptive street boy who first started using heroin, but rather the tough, sophisticated, and respected boy, typically a street-gang leader. Later, others followed his example, either through indoctrination or emulation. By 1955, heroin use among teenagers on the street had become widespread, resulting, among other things, in the dissolution of fighting gangs. Now the hip boy on the street was not the swaggering, leather-jacketed gang member, but the boy nodding on the corner, enjoying his heroin high. He was the new hero model.

As heroin use spread among the young from 1951, the price of heroin began to rise in response to the greater demand, and the greater risks involved in selling to youths. Those who started using heroin as teenagers seldom had work experience or skills and resorted to crime in order to support their heroin use. They were less circumspect in their drug-using and criminal activity, and soon became a problem to the community, especially to those who were engaged in non-narcotic illegal activities, such as bookmaking, loan-sharking, and policy (the gambling game popular among working-class people, in which a correct selection of three numbers pays off at 50 to 1). The activities and behavior of young drug users brought attention and notoriety to the neighborhood, which jeopardized racketeer operations. It was not uncommon for a local racketeer to inform the parents of a young heroin user about his activities, hoping that they would take action.

5. 1957 to 1961

In 1957, the criminal organization, or *syndicate*, which had been mainly responsible for heroin distribution (according to law-enforcement agencies and government investigation committees), officially withdrew from the market. This resulted from two conditions: the passage of stricter federal laws that included provision for conspiracy convictions, and the related fact that illegal drug use was receiving increased attention from the public and officials, especially as a result of the increased involvement of youth with heroin. The risks had become too great, and the syndicate did not want to endanger the larger and more important sources of revenue, such as gambling and loan-sharking. However, the instruction to get out of narcotics was more honored in the breach than in the observance by certain syndicate members. Those who stayed involved in narcotics operated independently. Some made it their primary operation, while others would make only one or two big transactions a year when they needed to recoup quickly from an unexpected financial loss in some other operation. Dealing irregularly in narcotics for this purpose became known as a *fall-back*—a quick and sure way to make money. The syndicate also stayed involved indirectly through loan-shark agreements. In these transactions, large sums of money were lent to narcotic dealers for a period of one month at a fixed rate of return. No questions were asked regarding its use. By this means, the syndicate avoided some of the undesirable aspects of narcotic distribution and still participated in the profits. The official withdrawal of the syndicate from narcotics created opportunities for independent operators, which resulted in a relatively free market.

6. 1961 to the Present

The next major development in the history of heroin use in the city occurred in November 1961, when there was a critical shortage of heroin. Known as a *panic*, this development, whatever its cause, had a profound effect on the course of heroin use in the city. The panic lasted only for a few weeks. During this time, the demand for the meager supplies of heroin was so great that those who had supplies were able to double and triple their prices and further adulterate the quality, thus realizing sometimes as much as ten times their usual profit. By the time heroin became available again in good supply, the dealers had learned that inferior heroin at inflated prices could find a ready market. Since that time, the cost of heroin on the street has continued to climb, through increased prices, further adulteration, and *short counts* (misrepresentation of aggregate weight in a given unit). A few minor panics—about two a year—help bolster the market. Today, an average heroin habit costs the user about $20 a day, as compared to $2 twenty years ago. This fact is responsible for a major social disorder in the city today. It has also had important effects on the personal, social, and family relationships of the heroin users themselves. There is no longer social cohesion among addicts. The competition and struggle

necessary to support a habit has turned each one into an independent operator who looks out only for himself. Usually, addicts today will associate in pairs (partners), but only for practical purposes: in a criminal effort which requires two people (as when one acts as lookout, while the other commits a burglary), to share in the price of a bag of heroin, to assist in case of an overdose of drugs, to share the use of one set of works (the paraphernalia used to inject heroin). There is no longer a subculture of addicts, based on social cohesion and emotional identification, but rather a loose association of individuals and parallel couples. Heroin users commonly say, "I have no friends, only associates."

The economic pressures on heroin users today are so great that they prey on each other, as well as on their families and on society at large. An addict with money or drugs in his possession runs a good risk of being *taken off* (robbed) by other addicts. An addict who has been robbed or cheated by another addict usually takes his loss philosophically, summed up by the expression, "That's the name of the game." Referring to a fellow addict who had cheated him, one victim said, "He beat me today, I'll beat him tomorrow." Another addict who specializes in robbing other addicts said, "I beat them every chance I get, which is all the time." Sociability, even among partners, extends no farther than that suggested by the following excerpt: "You might be hanging out with a fellow for a long time, copping together and working as crime partners. You might beat him for a purpose. You might beat him, because maybe you bought a bag together and you know it's not going to do both any good, so you beat him for it. But then you try to go and get some money and straighten him out; make it up to him." Another informant summed up the attitude between partners this way: "I'm looking out for myself—I might be sick tomorrow; anyway, he's got something working for him that I don't know about." Sometimes, a distinction is made between a hustling partner and a crime partner (*crimey*), where it is suggested that the latter is more dependable; however, as one informant put it, "There are larceny-minded crimeys." The causes of these changes in the relationships of heroin users to each other, to family members, and to other members of the community are to be found in the economic practices of heroin distribution.

The Distribution of Heroin in New York City

Heroin contracted for in Europe at $5000 per kilo (2.2 pounds) will be sold in $5 bags on the street for about one million dollars, after having passed through at least six levels of distribution. The following description of the distribution and marketing of heroin, from the time it arrives in New York until it reaches the hands of the heroin user in the street, is a consensus derived from informants in the hospital and in the street representing different ethnic and racial groups from different parts of the city. There are many variations to the account given here at all levels of the marketing process. For example, as in the marketing of any product, a quantity purchase can be made at a lower price; and a dealer who makes a rapid turnover of the product for a wholesaler will receive higher benefits for his work. All the way down the line, the *good customer* is the key to a successful operation. He is one who buys regularly, does a good volume of business, does not ask for credit or try to buy short (offer less than the established price), and can be trusted. The following account does not include all the many variations, but can be taken as a paradigm.

Opium produced in Turkey, India, and Iran is processed into heroin in Lebanon, France, and Italy, and prepared for shipment to the East Coast of the United States. A United States importer, through a courier, can buy a kilogram of 80-percent heroin in Europe for $5,000. The quality is represented to him in terms of how many cuts it will hold (that is, how many times it can be adulterated). In earlier days, when the marketing of heroin was a more controlled operation, the word of the European seller was accepted. Now, it is customary for the importer to test it, either by means of scientific instruments, or through a reliable tester—an addict who makes experimental cuts, uses the drug, and reports on its quality. The importer, who usually never sees the heroin, sells down the line to a highly trusted customer through intermediaries. If it is a syndicate operation, he would only sell to high level, coded men, known as *captains*. These men are major distributors, referred to as *kilo connections* and, generally, as *the people*.

Major Distribution

The *kilo connection* pays $20,000 for the original kilogram (kilo, kee), and gives it a one and one cut (known as *hitting it*); that is, he makes two kilos out of one by adding the common adulterants of milk sugar, mannite (a product from the ash tree, used as a mild laxative), and quinine. The proportions of ingredients used for the cutting varies with the preferences of the cutter. One may use 5 parts milk sugar, 2 parts quinine, and 1 part mannite; while another may use 2 parts milk sugar, 3 parts quinine, and 1 part mannite. All three of these products are quickly soluble with heroin. A match lit under the cooker (bottle cap) will heat and dissolve the mixture into a clear liquid in a few seconds. The milk sugar contributes the bulk, the mannite inflates the volume—described as *fluffing* it up—and the quinine heightens the sensation of the *rush* when, upon injection into the vein, the mixture first registers on the nervous system. In the cutting procedure, the substance to be cut is placed under a fine sieve, often made from a woman's nylon stocking stretched over a coat hanger. The adulterants are sifted on top of it, then the new mixture is sifted through several more times. After the cut, the kilo connection sells down the line in kilos, half kilos, and quarter kilos, depending upon the resources of his customers. He will get approximately $10,000 per half kilo for the now adulterated heroin.

The customer of the kilo connection is known as *the connection* in its original sense, meaning that he knows *the people*, even though he is not one of them. He may also be called an *ounce man*. He is a highly trusted customer. (One common variation here is that the kilo connection may sell to a third line man, known, if a syndicate operation, as a *soldier* or *button man*. He, in turn, will make a one and one cut and sell to the connection.) Assuming that the connection buys directly from a kilo connection, he will probably give the heroin a one and one cut (make two units of each one), divide the total aggregate into ounces, and sell down the line at $700 per ounce. In addition to the adulteration, the aggregate weight of the product is reduced. Known as a *short count*, this procedure occurs at every succeeding level of distribution. At this stage, however, it is called a *good ounce*, despite the adulteration and reduced weight.

The next man is known as a *dealer in weight*, and is probably the most important figure in the line of distribution. He stands midway between the top and the bottom, and is the first one coming down the line who takes substantial risk of being apprehended by law-enforcement officers. He is also the first one who may be a heroin user himself, but usually he is not. He is commonly referred to as one who is *into something* and is respected as a big dealer who has put himself in jeopardy by, as the sayings go, *carrying a felony with him* and *doing the time*; that is, if he gets caught, he can expect a long jail sentence. It is said of him that "he let his name go," or "his name gets kicked around," meaning that his identity is known to people in the street. This man usually specializes in cut ounces. He may give a two and one cut (make three units of each one) to the good ounce from the connection and sell the resulting quantity for $500 per ounce. The aggregate weight is again reduced, and now the unit is called a *piece*, instead of an ounce. Sometimes, it is called a *street ounce* or a *vig ounce* (*vig* is an abbreviation for *vigorish*, which is the term used to designate the high interest on loans charged by loan sharks). In previous years, twenty-five- to thirty-level teaspoons were supposed to constitute an ounce; today, it is sixteen to twenty.

The next customer is known as a *street dealer*. He buys the *piece* for $500, gives it a one and one cut and makes *bundles*, which consist of twenty-five $5 bags each. He can usually get seven bundles from each piece, and he sells each bundle for $80. He may also package the heroin in *half-bundles* (ten $5 bags each), which sell for $40, or he may package in *half-loads* (fifteen $3 bags), which sell for $30 each. This man may or may not be a heroin user.

The next distributor is known as a *juggler*, who is the seller from whom the average street addict buys. He is always a user. He buys bundles for $80 each and sells the twenty-five bags at about $5 each, making just enough profit to support his own habit, day by day. He may or may not make a small cut, known as *tapping the bags*. He is referred to as someone who is "always high and always short"; that is, he always has enough heroin for his own use and is always looking for a few dollars to get enough capital to cop again. The following actual account is typical of a juggler's transactions: he has $25 and needs $5 more to buy a half-load. He meets a user he knows who has $5 and would like to buy two $3 bags; he is short $1. The juggler tells him he needs only $5 to cop, and that, if he can have his $5, he will buy a half-load and give him his two $3 bags—$1, in effect, for the use of the money. When the juggler returns, he gives the person his two bags. In the example here, the person had to wait about two hours for the juggler's return, and it was raining.

For taking the risk of getting beat for his money by the juggler, for the long wait and the discomfort of the weather, the juggler was expected to go to the *cooker* with him (share the use of some of the heroin), with the juggler putting in two bags to the other person's one bag and sharing equally in the total. The juggler had his fix and now has eleven bags left. He sells three bags for $9. From the eight bags he has left he uses two himself to get straight—not to get high, but enough to keep from getting sick so that he can finish his business. Now, he sells four bags for $12 and has three left. He needs only $7 more to cop again, so he is willing to sell the last three bags for the reduced price, and he can begin a similar cycle all over again. He may do this three or four times a day. The juggler leads a precarious life, both financially and in the risks he takes of getting robbed by fellow addicts or arrested. Most arrests for heroin sales are of the juggler. Financially, he is always struggling to stay in the black. If business is a little slow, he may start to get sick or impatient and use some of the heroin he needs to sell, in order to recop. If he does this, he is in the red and temporarily out of business. A juggler is considered to be doing well, if he has enough money left over after a transaction for cab fare to where he buys the heroin. One informant defined a juggler as a "non-hustling dope fiend who is always messing the money up."

Other Specialists

There are ancillary services provided by other specialists in the heroin-marketing process. They are known as: (1) lieutenants, (2) testers, (3) dropmen, (4) salesmen, (5) steerers, (6) taste faces, and (7) accommodators.

1. *Lieutenant:* Very often, a connection or weight dealer will have in his employ a trusted associate who handles the details of transactions with the street-level dealers. He arranges for deliveries, collects the money, and acts as an enforcer, if things go wrong. He may work for a salary or a commission, or both. Sometimes, he will be given some *weight* (part of a kilo) to sell on his own as a bonus.

2. *Tester:* Heroin dealers down the line are likely to keep a trusted addict around to test the quality of the drug for them. In return for this service, he gets all the heroin he needs and pocket money.

3. *Drop-man:* This person, often a young, dependable non-user, is used by sellers to make deliveries. He works for cash and may make as much as $500 for a drop in behalf of a top-level seller. He

may also handle the transfer of money in a transaction. He is usually a tough, intelligent, trusted street youth who is ambitious to work his way up in the criminal hierarchy.

4. *Salesman:* Sometimes, the type of person used as a drop-man will be used as a street salesman of heroin for a fairly big dealer. The use of this kind of salesman is growing, because of the unreliability of addict jugglers and the desirability of having a tough person who can be trusted and not be easily robbed and cheated by addicts. Sometimes, these boys are about 16 to 18 years old and may be going to school. Being young, they usually do not have a police record, and they attract less attention from the police. One informant summed up their attributes this way: "The police won't pay much attention to a kid, but if they do get busted (arrested) they don't talk; they want to be men . . . they (the dealers) trust a guy that don't use it, because they know the guy ain't going to beat him. They got a little gang, and nobody is going to get their stuff, because they're going to gang up on the guy. In that case, they can use a gun in a hurry. The kids that sell the stuff, they don't use it. They buy clothes or whatever they want with the money." They often sell on consignment, starting with a small advance (usually a bundle) and working up to more if they are successful.

5. *Steerer:* The steerer is one who in race-track parlance would be known as a *tout*, or in a sidewalk sales operation as a *shill*. He is one who tries to persuade users to buy a certain dealer's bag. He may work off and on by appointment with a particular dealer (always a small street dealer or juggler) in return for his daily supply of drugs. Or he may hear that a certain dealer has a good bag and, on a speculative basis, steer customers to him and then go to him later and ask to be taken care of for the service. This is known as *cracking* on a dealer. One of his more subtle selling techniques is to affect an exaggerated-looking high, and, when asked by a user where he got such a good bag, refer him to the dealer. Usually, he is a person who stays in the block all day and is supposed to know what is going on; he is, as they say, *always on the set*.

6. *Taste face:* This is a derogatory term given to one who supports his habit by renting out works—loaning the paraphernalia for injecting heroin—in return for a little money or a share of the heroin. Possession of works (hypodermic needle, eyedropper fitted with a baby's pacifier nipple, and bottle cap) is a criminal offense, and users do not want to

run the extra risk of carrying them; thus, they are willing to pay something for the service. Although they perform a useful service, these people are held in contempt by other users. Taste refers to the small amount of heroin he is given (known as a *G shot*) and face is a term applied to anyone on the street who is known as a *creep, flunky,* or *nobody*.

7. *Accommodator:* The accommodator is a user who buys at a low level—usually from a juggler—for someone new to the neighborhood who has no connections. These purchases are for small amounts bought by users from other parts of the city or the suburbs. The accommodator receives a little part of the heroin or money for his services. Sometimes, he will also cheat the buyer by misrepresenting the price or the amount, or just by not coming back. However, he has to be somewhat reliable, in order to support his habit regularly in this way. Many selling arrests by undercover narcotics police are of these low-level accommodators.

The Street Bag of Heroin

The amount of heroin in the street bag is very small. A generous estimate of the aggregate weight of a $5 bag is ninety milligrams, including the adulterants. Assuming, as in the above account, that the original kilo of 80-percent heroin is adulterated twenty-four times by the time it reaches the street, the amount of heroin would be about three milligrams. There is considerable fluctuation in the amount of heroin in the retail unit, running the range from one to fifteen milligrams, which depends mainly upon the supply available in the market. The important point is that, no matter how small the amount, heroin users are never discouraged in their efforts to get it. The consensus figure of three milligrams is a good approximation for an average over a one-year period. This is the average analgesic dosage that is used in those countries, such as England, where heroin can be prescribed in medical practice. It is a minimal amount, being considered safe for someone who does not use opiates. It is equivalent to about ten milligrams of either morphine or methadone. . . .

In controlled experiments with opiate addicts, as much as sixty milligrams of morphine have been administered four times a day (Martin, personal communication 1967). Each dosage is equivalent to about twenty milligrams of heroin, which is seven times the amount in the average street bag. In another experiment, it was found that the average heroin addict "recognized" heroin at a minimum level of about fifteen milligrams—five times the amount in the street bag (Sharoff, personal communication 1967). The average dosage of methadone used in opiate-maintenance treatment is one hundred milligrams—about ten times the amount in the street bag. One informant said of the effects of a street bag today: "All it does is turn your stomach over so that you can go out and hustle, and you had better do it fast." Heroin users who are sent to jail report that they are surprised when they do not experience serious withdrawal symptoms after the abrupt cessation of heroin use. Physicians working in the withdrawal wards of narcotic treatment centers refer to the abstinence syndrome among most of their patients today as "subclinical."

The amount of heroin in the street unit has resulted in an institution known as *chasing the bag*. In a community with a high incidence of heroin use, there will be two, three, or four competing bags on the street; that is, bags which have come down through different distributorship lines. Because of the low quality of the heroin, users want to get the best one available on a given day. The number of times it has been cut and the ingredients that were used to cut it are the main considerations. The dealer who has the best bag on the street at a given time will sell his merchandise fast and do a big volume of business. A dealer with a good bag who works hard can sell forty to fifty bundles a day. A good bag dealer can sell seventy-five to one hundred bags a day. By keeping the quality relatively high—for example by giving a one and a half cut to a quantity represented as being able to hold two cuts—he makes less profit on each unit. However, this loss can be offset by the greater volume and the reduced price he gets from his wholesaler, as a result of buying more often and in large quantities.

Those with inferior bags on the street do not have a rapid turnover, but they know that sooner or later they can sell their stock, since the demand tends to exceed the supply. There are also other factors operating in their favor. Some users are not known to the dealer of the best bag and cannot buy from him except through the mediation of someone else. This service costs the prospective buyer something and he has to weigh that consideration against the better bag. Usually, however, if he is sure that one bag is much better than another one, he will find the price to pay for the service to get it; the quality of the bag, not the money, is always the primary consideration.

Another condition favorable to the dealers of inferior bags is that a user who hustles for his drugs is too busy to be around all the time waiting for a particular bag to come on the street. He is usually pressed for time and has to take what is available. If the dealer of the good bag is out recopping, the user cannot afford to wait for what may be a long time. The dealer of an inferior bag, whose heroin moves more slowly, is reliable; that is, he is always around and can be depended upon. Even in extreme cases, where a bag is so bad that the dealer builds up a surplus because of slow business, he knows that sooner or later a temporary shortage of heroin—even for a few days—will insure his selling out. Heroin does not spoil and can be easily stored for an indefinite period.

Sometimes, the dealer of an exceptionally good bag will be approached by his competitors, and they will make a deal, whereby he agrees to leave the street on the condition that they buy their bundles from him. In such a deal, those buying the good bundles will *tap the bags* (adulterate them a little more) and put them on the street at the same price. This is one of the many variations in marketing heroin.

It is common practice for a new dealer to come on the street with a good bag and keep it that way, until he has most of the customers. Then, he will start to adulterate the heroin, knowing that his reputation will carry him for a few days; by that time, he has made a good extra profit. When he starts losing customers in large number, he can build the bag up again. Users are constantly experimenting with the products of different dealers, comparing notes with other users, and attempting to buy the best bag that is around. As one informant put it: "You keep searching. If the guy is weak and you buy from him and it's nothing, then you go to Joe or Tom. Like you get a bag over here now, you run over there about in an hour and get another bag from the other guy, and get another from this other guy after a while. You just go in a circle to see. You run in different directions." One informant said, "There are no longer dope addicts on the street, only hope addicts." A report on the street that a heroin user died of an overdose of heroin results in a customer rush on his dealer for the same bag.

Economic Careers of Heroin Users

The nature of the economic careers of heroin users on the street is epitomized in the following quote from a research informant: "I believe in work to a certain extent, if it benefits my profit; but I do believe there is more money made otherwise." Another informant, in referring to a fellow user, said: "He just got no heart to be pulling no scores. He can't steal, he don't know how to steal. You can't be an addict that way. I don't know how he's going to make it."

Virtually all heroin users in slum neighborhoods regularly commit crime, in order to support their heroin use. In addition to the crimes involving violation of the narcotic laws, which are described above, heroin users engage in almost all types of crime for gain, both against property and the person. Because of the greatly inflated price of heroin and because of its poor quality, it is impossible for a heroin user to support even a modest habit for less than $20 a day. Since the typical street user is uneducated, unskilled, and often from a minority racial group, he cannot earn enough money in the legitimate labor market to finance his drug use; he must engage in criminal activity. It is a conservative estimate that heroin users in New York City steal $1 million a day in money, goods, and property. About 70 percent of the inmates in New York City Department of Correction institutions are heroin users whose crimes were directly or indirectly connected with their heroin use.

As with non-addict criminals, addict criminals tend to specialize in certain activities, depending upon their personalities, skills, and experience. One of the myths derived from the passivity stereotype of the heroin user is that the heroin user avoids crimes of violence, such as robbery, which involves personal confrontation. This no longer seems to be the case. A 1966 New York City Police Department study of the arrests of admitted narcotic (primarily heroin) addicts for selected felonies, other than violations of narcotic laws, showed that 15.1 percent of the arrests were for robbery (New York City Police Department 1966). This compared with 12.9 percent robbery arrests of all arrests (addict and non-addict) during the same year. Murder arrests among the addicts amounted to 1 percent of the selected felonies, as compared to 1.4 percent of all arrests in the same categories. The biggest differences between addict arrests and all arrests in the seventeen felony categories selected for study were in the categories of burglary and felonious assault. Among the addicts, 40.9 percent were burglary arrests, compared to 19.7 percent of all arrests; felonious assault constituted 5.6 percent among the addicts, compared to 27.9 percent of all arrests. What these figures reveal is not that heroin users avoid crimes of violence, as compared to non-addicts, but

that they avoid crimes not involving financial gain, such as felonious assault. Where financial gain is involved, as in robbery, the risk of violence is taken by heroin users in a higher percentage of cases than with non-addicts. These statistics confirm the observations and opinions of street informants, both addict and non-addict. The high percentage of burglaries committed by heroin users is often cited as evidence that, in comparison with non-addict criminals, they prefer non-violent crime. What is overlooked here is that burglary, especially of residences, always involves the risk of personal confrontation and violence. Of the 1745 burglary arrests of admitted addicts in 1966, 975 (51 percent) were residence burglaries.

Analysis of the data from the informants for this study showed the following, with regard to principal criminal occupations, not including those connected with narcotic-laws offenses: burglar—22.7 percent, *flatfooted hustler*—12.2 percent, shoplifter—12.1 percent, robber—9.0 percent. *Flatfooted hustler* is a term used on the street for one who will commit almost any kind of crime for money, depending upon the opportunities. As one self-described flatfooted hustler put it: "I'm capable of doing most things—jostling (picking pockets), boosting (shoplifting), con games, burglary, mugging, or stick-ups; wherever I see the opportunity, that's where I'm at." The main advantage of crimes against the person is that the yield is usually money, which does not have to be sold at a discount, as does stolen property. It is easily concealed and can be exchanged directly for heroin. In the case of stolen goods and property, the person has to carry the proceeds of, say, a burglary around with him, as he looks for a direct buyer or a fence. . . . This exposes him to extra risk of apprehension. When he does find a buyer, he can only expect to get from 10 percent to 50 percent of the value, the average being about 30 percent, depending upon the item—the more expensive the item, the higher the discount.

The distribution and sales of goods and property stolen by heroin users has become a major economic institution in low-income neighborhoods. Most of the consumers are otherwise ordinary, legitimate members of the community. Housewives will wait on the stoop for specialists in stealing meat (known as *cattle rustlers*) to come by, so that they can get a ham or roast at a 60-percent discount. Owners of small grocery stores buy cartons of cigarettes stolen from the neighborhood supermarket. The owner of an automobile places an order with a heroin user for tires, and the next day he has the tires—with the wheels. During the Easter holidays, there is a great demand for clothes, with slum streets looking like the streets of the Garment District.

It has often been noted that retail stores in a slum neighborhood have higher prices than those in more affluent neighborhoods, and this has been attributed to discrimination and profiteering at the expense of poor people with little consumer education and knowledge. Although such charges have some foundation, another major cause of higher prices is the high rate of pilferage by heroin users and others from such stores, the cost of which is passed on to the consumer. One chain store operation which locates exclusively in low-income neighborhoods in New York City is reportedly in bankruptcy due to a 10 percent pilferage rate. This rate compares to about 2 percent citywide.

One economic institution that has resulted directly from the increased criminal activity among heroin users is the *grocery fence*. He is a small, local businessman, such as a candy store owner, bar owner, or beauty parlor owner, who has enough cash to buy stolen goods and property on a small scale and has a place to store them. He then sells the items to his regular customers, both for good will and a profit. He provides a service for the user in providing him with a fast outlet for his goods.

The heroin user is an important figure in the economic life of the slums. In order to support a $20-a-day habit, he has to steal goods and property worth from $50 to $100. Usually, he steals outside his neighborhood, not out of community loyalty, but because the opportunities are better in the wealthier neighborhoods; and he brings his merchandise back to the neighborhood for sale at high discounts. This results, to some extent, in a redistribution of real income from the richer to the poorer neighborhoods. Although non-addict residents in the slums may deplore the presence of heroin users, they appreciate and compete for their services as discount salesmen. The user, in turn, experiences satisfaction in being able to make this contribution to the neighborhood.

The type of criminal activity he engages in, and his success at it, determine, to a large extent, the addict's status among fellow addicts and in the community at large. The appellation of *real hustling dope fiend* (a successful burglar, robber, con man, etc.) is a mark of respect and status. Conversely, *non-hustling dope fiend* is a term of denigration applied to users who stay in the neighborhood begging for money or small tastes of heroin, renting out works, or doing small-time juggling. There are also middle-status occupations, such as *stealing copper*, where the person specializes in salvaging metal and fixtures from vacant tenement buildings and selling to the local junkman. About the only kinds of illegal activity not open to the heroin user are those connected with organized crime, such as gambling and loan sharking. Users are not considered reliable enough for work in these fields. They may be used as a lookout for a dice game or policy operation, but that is about as close as they can get to organized criminal operations.

Respite from the arduous life they lead comes to heroin users when they go to jail, to a hospital, or, for some, when they take short-time employment at resort hotels in the mountains. In the present study, it was found that 43 percent of the subjects were in some type of incarceration at any given period of time. In jail they rest, get on a healthy diet, have their medical and dental needs cared for, and engage in relaxed socialization which centers around the facts and folklore of the heroin user's life on the street.

If a user has been making good money on the street, he eventually builds up a tolerance to heroin which gets to the point where he can no longer finance the habit. He may then enter a hospital for detoxification. If he stays the medically recommended period of time—usually three weeks—he can qualify for Department of Welfare assistance, which eases the economic pressures on him when he resumes his heroin-using life on the street. More often than not, however, he will leave the hospital when his tolerance has been significantly lowered, which occurs in about a week.

Some users solve the problems of too much physical and economic pressure which build up periodically by getting temporary employment out of the city, usually in the mountain resort hotels. There are employment agencies in the Bowery and similar districts which specialize in hiring drifters, alcoholics, and drug addicts for temporary work. In the summer, there is a demand for menial laborers in the kitchens and on the grounds of resort hotels. The agencies are so eager to get help during the vacation season that they go to the street to solicit workers. Some of them provide a cheap suitcase and clothes for those who need them. One informant reported about a particular agency man this way: "He'll grab you out of the street. He'll say, 'Do you want a job, son? I'll get you a good job. You want to work up in the country and get fat? You'll eat good food and everything.'" The agency charges the worker a substantial fee, which is taken out of his first check, and makes extra money by providing private transportation at a price higher than the bus fare. The heroin user usually works through one pay period and returns to the city somewhat more healthy, with a low heroin tolerance, and with a few dollars in his pocket.

It can be seen from the account in this section that the street heroin user is an active, busy person, preoccupied primarily with the economic necessities of maintaining his real income—heroin. A research subject expressed the more mundane gratifications of his life this way:

> When I'm on the way home with the bag safely in my pocket, and I haven't been caught stealing all day, and I didn't get beat, and the cops didn't get me—I feel like a working man coming home; he's worked hard, but he knows he done something, even though I know it's not true.

Conclusions

Heroin use today by lower-class, primarily minority-group, persons does not provide for them a euphoric escape from the psychological and social problems which derive from ghetto life. On the contrary, it provides a motivation and rationale for the pursuit of a meaningful life, albeit a socially deviant one. The activities these individuals engage in, and the relationships they have in the course of their quest for heroin, are far more important than the minimal analgesic and euphoric effects of the small amount of heroin available to them. If they can be said to be addicted, it is not so much to heroin as to the entire career of a heroin user. The heroin user is, in a way, like the compulsively hard-working business executive, whose ostensible goal is the acquisition of money, but whose real satisfaction is in meeting the inordinate challenge he creates for himself. He, too, is driven by a need to find meaning in life which, because of certain deficits and impairments, he cannot find in the normal course of living. A big difference, of course, is that with the street user, the genesis of the deficits and impairments is, to a disproportional degree, in the social conditions of his life.

In the four communities where this research was conducted, the average median family income is $3500, somewhat less than that of family Welfare Department recipients. Other average population characteristics for the four communities include: public welfare recipients—four times the city rate; unemployment—two times the city rate; substandard housing—two times the city rate; no schooling—two times the city rate; median school years completed—eight years. Neither these few statistics nor an exhaustive list could portray the desperation and hopelessness of life in the slums of New York. In one short block where one of the authors worked, there was an average of one violent death a month over a period of three years—by fire, accident, homicide, and suicide. In Puerto Rican neighborhoods, sidewalk *recordatorios* (temporary shrines at the scenes of tragic deaths) are a regular feature.

Given the social conditions of the slums and their effects on family and individual development, the odds are strongly against the development of a legitimate, non-deviant career that is challenging and rewarding. The most common legitimate career is a menial job, with no future except in the periodic, statutory raises in the minimum-wage level. If anyone can be called passive in the slums, it is not the heroin user, but the one who submits to and accepts these conditions.

The career of a heroin user serves a dual purpose for the slum inhabitant; it enables him to escape, not from purposeful activity, but from the monotony of an existence severely limited by social constraints, and, at the same time, it provides a way for him to gain revenge on society for the injustices and deprivation he has experienced. His exploitation of society is carried out with emotional impunity on the grounds, for the most part illusory, that he is *sick* (needs heroin to relieve physical distress), and any action is justified in the interest of keeping himself well. He is free to act out directly his hostility and, at the same time, find gratification, both in the use of the drug and in the sense of accomplishment he gets from performing the many acts necessary to support his heroin use. Commenting on the value of narcotic-maintenance programs, where addicts are maintained legally and at no cost on a high level of opiate administration, one informant said:

> The guy feels that all the fun is out of it. You don't have to outslick the cop and other people. This is a sort of vengeance. This gives you a thrill. It's hiding from them. Where you can go in the drugstore and get a shot, you get high, but it's the same sort of

monotony. You are not getting away with anything. The thing is to hide and outslick someone. Drugs is a hell of a game; it gives you a million things to talk about.

This informant was not a newcomer to the use of heroin, but a 30-year-old veteran of fifteen years of heroin use on the street. *Soldiers of fortune* is the way another informant summed up the lives of heroin users.

Not all, but certainly a large majority, of heroin users are in the category, which is the subject of this paper. It is their activities which constitute the social problem which New York City and other urban centers face today. The ultimate solution to the problem, as with all the problems which result from social injustice, lies in the creation of legitimate opportunities for a meaningful life for those who want it. While waiting for the ultimate solution, reparative measures must be taken. There are four major approaches to the treatment and rehabilitation of heroin users: (1) drug treatment (opiate substitutes or antagonists), (2) psychotherapy, (3) existentialist-oriented group self-help (Synanon prototype), (4) educational and vocational training and placement.

To the extent that the observations and conclusions reported in this paper are valid, a treatment and rehabilitation program emphasizing educational and vocational training is indicated for the large majority of heroin users. At the Manhattan State Hospital Drug Addiction Unit, an intensive educational and vocational program, supported by psychological and social treatment methods, has been created in an effort to prepare the patient for a legitimate career which has a future and is rewarding and satisfying. The three-year program is divided into three parts: (1) eight months of education, vocational training, and therapy in the hospital; (2) one month in the night hospital, while working or taking further training in the community during the day; (3) twenty-seven months of aftercare, which includes, where needed, further education and training, vocational placement, and psychological and social counseling. With this opportunity for a comprehensive social reparation, those who have not been too severely damaged by society have a second chance for a legitimate, meaningful life.

* * *

Edward Preble and John J. Casey, Jr. "Taking Care of Business—The Heroin Addict's Life on the Street," *The International Journal of the Addictions 4* (March 1969), pp. 1-24. Copyright © 1969 by Marcel Dekker, Inc. All rights reserved. Reprinted by permission.

For Discussion

The authors argue that the daily activities in which heroin users are involved create purposeful lives among users, particularly when legitimate educational and work opportunities are limited. However, some heroin users, e.g., physicians, are employed in prestigious careers in which a sense of purpose is derived from their work. How would Preble and Casey explain heroin use among these individuals?

References

Chein, Isidor, et al. *The Road to H: Narcotics, Delinquency, and Social Policy*. New York: Basic Books, Inc., 1964.

City of New York, Police Department. Statistical Report: *Narcotics*, 1966.

Cloward, Richard A., and Ohlin, Lloyd E. *Delinquency and Opportunity*. Glencoe, IL: The Free Press, 1960.

Kardiner, Arram, et al. *The Individual and His Society*. New York: Columbia University Press, 1939.

Malinowski, Bronislaw. *Argonauts of the Western Pacific*. London: Routledge and Kegan Paul Ltd., 1922.

Martin, W. R., Personal Communication, 1967.

Sharoff, Robert, Personal Communication, 1967.

Whyte, W. F. *Street Corner Society*. Chicago: The University of Chicago Press, 1955. ✦

16. Difficulties in Taking Care of Business

M<small>ARSHA</small> R<small>OSENBAUM</small>

The great majority of heroin studies have focused on male users. Although this body of research has contributed greatly to our understanding of heroin use and addiction, it is unlikely that the findings apply fully to female users. Marsha Rosenbaum is one of the first investigators to intensively study women heroin users. In the following article, taken from her highly acclaimed book Women on Heroin, *she discusses issues that are specific to women users. Dr. Rosenbaum reports that women are more likely than men to have a partner (spouse, significant other) who also uses heroin and that the drug serves to weaken an addict couple's relationship in a number of ways. Intimacy, sexuality, and other aspects of the relationship suffer because heroin becomes the most important issue in the relationship. Furthermore, traditional sex roles are often reversed with women serving as the primary earners. Finally, women begin to feel exploited and victimized and, in turn, become resentful of male partners. Interestingly, the study found that most heroin users are also mothers and that the maternal role is central to their identity. The majority of the women contacted reported that they had ceased using heroin during pregnancy and felt disdain for women who had not done so.*

The career of the woman addict involves risk, chaos, and ultimate inundation by the world of heroin. Participating in the heroin life means relinquishing other activities and, consequently, life options not related to heroin procurement and use. The woman who becomes an addict generally had little focus and commitment in her life prior to addiction. Heroin, in fact, provides her with a needed focal point as well as excitement and (albeit involuntary at times) commitment. Although the woman's career in addiction begins with excitement and expanded options, her options begin to narrow with time. The chaos and cost of the heroin life force her into illegal work and, ultimately, into dealings with the criminal justice system. Once involved with the law, her occupational options outside the heroin life are reduced; equally if not more importantly, inundation by the heroin world threatens the life option she deems most valuable: her family.

Lovers

"When drugs come into the picture, love flies out the window."

Although heroin can provide a common focus, the nature of the heroin life ultimately undermines love relationships. In the following sections, I examine relationships gaining a focus through heroin, their eventual undermining, and finally, how undermining contributes to a narrowing of options for the woman.

Heroin as Providing a Focus

The characteristic inundation by the heroin life often provides focus in a love relationship; it is the commonality shared by a couple, the direction in their relationship, the basis of understanding between them. Heroin is not unlike a shared occupation or profession, common interest in a hobby or sport, or the joint effort and interest in building a family and raising children.

While male addicts often prefer to have spouses or old ladies who are not addicts, such is rarely the case among women. Even if they had not entered the heroin world through a man, the women interviewed in this study who were part of a love relationship usually had mates who were either addicts or ex-addicts; the couple could, therefore, be categorized as an addict-couple. Since heroin, unlike most occupations or hobbies, is a full-time endeavor, the addicted couple tends to spend a great deal of time together. Many addicted couples have virtually a 24-hour relationship, doing everything together—hustling, scoring, fixing, sleeping, and eating.

Sexuality is, however, one aspect of a love relationship that is nearly omitted in the case of the typical addict-couple.[1] Due to the effects of heroin, very often the man cannot perform sexually and/or does not care about sex. The same is true for the woman:

> When I was using heroin, I found that I had very little interest in sex. I mean, sex was something I did for money. Sex was something I had very low interest in. Unless I had a strong interest in some other person, well, even then sex was secondary. Drugs took precedence over anything else. . . . Sex

wasn't important to my old man either. I've discovered this is true of most addicts. Sex was kind of a secondary thing.

The woman is often nonorgasmic while addicted, but even if she has some sexual desire, sex is too much work to be rewarding:

But then it got to the point where you don't need to have sex. Everyone finally came to the realization that, shit, it took ten hours to have an orgasm and then it was so light, it wasn't worth the energy you had to put out. By the time you had worked up to have an orgasm, you needed to get off again on dope because you weren't that high anymore. So, you didn't get to enjoy the high, so it was just like having to put out—it was like, "forget it." Everyone just turned off.

Many women claimed that the fixing routine, particularly when their partner "hit" them (administered the heroin), replaced intercourse.

Sex is not important. Your body doesn't feel any desire for sex, and to me, dope seems to take the place of sex. So, my husband hits me. It takes the place of sex subconsciously.

The sensuality and sharing aspects of doing heroin together are another replacement for sexual intercourse. As this woman put it:

My interest in sex wasn't as great because I just felt like fixing was such a . . . I just felt so good. And there's a kind of an affinity between you and your old man when you are fixing together. That you are on the same high, you both feel the same way. It's a very secure kind of feeling that I didn't need to enhance by fucking.

Above all, sexual intercourse is missed by neither partner. Consequently, the couple who genuinely cares for each other is platonically involved in all activities and tends to develop a brother-sisterlike partnership where there is interdependency with regard to earning money and often protection for the woman.[2] The partnership between addicts can become a habit, just like their joint addiction to heroin:

I don't know. I think that if the man and the woman are both strung out—if they don't really have a relationship, it's just a habit. They're shooting partners, they're crime partners, and that's about it. I think that if they were both to clean up, they'd realize that habit.

Drugs gradually come to replace all other aspects of the addict couple's relationship, so that even an otherwise expired relationship can remain intact. Just as heroin often masks physiological disease symptoms, it can cover up those aspects of a love relationship that would be intolerable without heroin. It is only when one or both "cleans up" that they realize their relationship has been based exclusively on heroin; as one woman explained:

We stuck together when we were using, but when I got on methadone and he wasn't on it, it seemed like I was kind of out of the picture. Like he'd go in the bathroom and fix his drugs, and I just didn't feel like we were communicating. He was doing one thing and I was doing another.

Heroin as Undermining

Although a partnership can be ideal for the addict-couple, drugs ultimately undermine relationships in three ways: heroin becomes the focal point of the relationship and erodes other aspects of affection or mutuality; the heroin life disrupts traditional sex-role delineation to the dissatisfaction of the couple; and unscrupulousness and money problems cause nearly constant bickering.

As mentioned before, the addict high on heroin doesn't really care about the activities of people around her/him. Sexuality is impaired due to this inability to relate intensely to another person. The focus that heroin provides for the couple is strictly functional, based on mutual pursuit and use of heroin; affection and emotional attachment nearly always suffer.

Occupational options in the heroin life often allow the woman to work when the man cannot, since she has the option to prostitute (which few men have).[3] Therefore, even if the man in a relationship does not pimp his woman, she will often have to assume the responsibility of earning money for both their habits through prostitution. One woman related:

Women bear the whole brunt of the load. You can believe that. Anytime you see a woman with a man and they got a habit, you can believe she's got to carry the load because she's the one who can go out there and literally "sell her ass." A man can't do it and he sits back and waits. . . . There is very little a man can do, very little. Nowadays, all these games that used to be played—boosting, bunco, and all that—that's all passé, man. There's articles and stuff about it in every magazine from end to end. Everybody's so down on it. Unless you go into the big time and if you go in for that, you are not going to be using no stuff. You can believe what I'm telling you. But it's the woman right out there on the street, today, tonight, where I go, where I stand—she's the one taking the chances. She's the one that gets kicked in the ass.

Such an arrangement ultimately proves unsatisfactory to both partners. Thus, the second undermining aspect is the disruption of traditional sex roles that results from differential earning power in the heroin life, a situation which is not unlike those described by Rubin in working-class marriages,[4] Liebow in lower-class black marriages,[5] and Sackman in addict relationships.[6] In each case, the man begins to resent his wife's or woman's earning power, especially if it is greater than his own. As Rubin notes:

> Indeed, it is just this issue of her [the wife's] independence that is a source of conflict in some of the marriages where women work . . . in well over one third of the families, husbands complain that their working wives "are getting too independent."

As noted by Komarovsky in regard to Ivy League men, there is confusion and discomfort when "the ideological supports for the traditional sex-role differentiation in marriage are weakening, but the emotional allegiance to the modified traditional pattern is still strong."[8] The addicted man in an economically dependent situation often becomes resentful and attempts to assert his power through violence directed at his mate. As one woman related:

> I used to come home [from a day of prostitution], and he's [her spouse] laying around, waiting for me to give him the money so we can cop [buy heroin]. We'd get the stuff and he'd try to short me saying, "I've got a bigger habit," and shit like that. I just wasn't going for it. I mean, it was me that was out on the street all day while he was laying around. I'd get pissed and then he'd just blow it . . . knock me around and stuff. One time, he nearly put me in the hospital.

The woman, who usually does not like her work, resents such violence and feels doubly exploited if her man is not working. Since it is commonly assumed that the major breadwinner will have the privilege of dispensing the heroin, the woman is especially bitter if she earns the money and her man insists not only on dividing the heroin but on giving her a smaller portion!

The unscrupulousness that periodically characterizes nearly all addicts usually enters the addict-couple's relationship and becomes a third source of undermining. In times of withdrawal sickness, one addict may rip off the other's money or heroin supply or pawn the other's belongings; one addict may gain access to heroin without splitting it with the other, which is tantamount to sexual betrayal.

An unequal division of labor, heroin, and money often leads to women's resentment and bitterness; sex-role disruption can lead to men's violence. Both ultimately undermine a love relationship. There are disagreements over how money is to be earned, how heroin is to be divided, and ultimately, how money in general is to be spent. As this woman said:

> We just fought a lot about who was getting more [drugs]. Oh, I don't know, it happens with every relationship I have. We bitch about who is getting the most dope. It's what starts happening. When I left my ex-old man . . . I knew it was me who was doing the bitching because he had most of the money. Usually, whoever is making most of the money figures they are entitled to more dope. If I was making more money, I'd figure I was entitled to more of the dope. And if somebody starts bitching, things get really fucked up. So, it works both ways. It depends on who is making the most money. It's kind of hard to keep a relationship going when you are strung out. A lot of times we sat and talked about, you know, things that we want, what we should be doing and we're not doing with our money, and the reason you ran out of money is because of dope. Yeah, and you always blame it on each other. You can't blame it on the heroin, you know? [laughing] You got to blame it on each other.

Women sometimes regret what they see as their partner's excessive use of money for drugs. Occasionally, the impetus for beginning heroin use had been to get a share of the substance for which all the family money was being spent—drugs. Later, women have similar concerns over how money is spent but are more often concerned about their children and living situation. This woman said:

> Well, right now I've been really uptight with him because I feel he is spending too much money on heroin. I wish that right now we weren't using as much as we are, because he makes money and right

away wants to spend it on dope, whereas I would rather use it for other things it should be used for—the house, our kids, you know.

There is nearly constant arguing over heroin and money, and as a consequence, most relationships involving addict-couples cannot be sustained. According to one woman interviewed:

I think drugs broke my husband and I up. I think when drugs came into the picture we were still very much in love, but the drug came in and I lost a lot of respect for him 'cause I kind of straightened my act up and I see him now laying there sick and I say, "How stupid can this asshole be?" Like right now, he's staying on my couch. He hasn't got a damned penny in his pocket. He's got no respect for himself. I've lost respect for him, and I feel that as long as the two people are into shooting, they're both sick, and they're hanging onto each other for strength.

The failure of love relationships to endure within the heroin life and the deleterious effect of this life on the health and appearance of the woman addict reduce her options to fulfill a traditional marital role. Although a few men find it advantageous to have a dope fiend old lady because of her ability to prostitute and bring in money, a woman who has been in the life for a period of time is seen as undesirable to men because of her history of addiction. Similarly, women very often see relationships with addicted men as undesirable because of their past history of addiction and all the ramifications.

Many women become bitter toward men because they feel they have been exploited and battered. Some women find love relationships with other women more satisfactory. There is less violence in such relationships and more egalitarianism. As this woman says:

Men are, they get, dependent on a woman and they get used to that and they get to the point where they don't want to go out and hustle. And you not only have to carry your weight but their weight, pay the rent, buy the food, the clothes, and take care of the kid. So, after I broke up with my husband when I was 15, I had it with men. I had a lot of old ladies but not a man. A woman will hustle right along side of you, where a man will hustle at first 'til he gets hooked. And then he'll want you to make all the money, and if you don't, you'll get your ass kicked. The inability to sustain a love relationship, whether or not as a result of the woman's own bitterness and resentment, further narrows the woman's options.

Victimized and exploited by men, she may no longer desire to establish traditional marital or quasi-marital relationships with men—one of the few options that was open to her at the outset.

Mothers

I don't like the lifestyle at all. I mean, I have fun when I'm running out there, but I miss my kid too much. Like, if I didn't have my kid, I wouldn't even worry about it. It wouldn't bother me at all. I keep on doing what I'm doing 'cause I have fun. But I got my kid. He tells me, "Mama, when are you going to take me home with you for good?" Every time I hear shit like that, I just snap inside. It really breaks me up.

Seventy percent of the women interviewed in this study were mothers; they consistently expressed concern, care, and often, guilt about their role as mothers and the well-being of their children. Moreover, they seemed to have accepted social and cultural role prescriptions and saw motherhood as central to their identity and purpose.[9] Accepting the prescribed female role, even if only ideologically, has a crucial effect on the course of the woman's career in addiction. In the following paragraphs, I discuss motherhood among women addicts. Beginning with fertility, pregnancy, and birth, I examine motherhood while addicted and the increased inability to take care of the business of mothering, and finally, the realization of narrowing options.

Fertility, Pregnancy, and Birth

It has been argued both medically and experientially that heroin addiction causes amenorrhea.[10] Most women interviewed claimed that during periods of addiction, they ceased to menstruate. This claim is problematic given changes in the quality of heroin and patterns of addiction.

In terms of purity, the quality of heroin has declined. Winick estimates the decline ranges from 87 percent pure heroin in 1920 to 2 percent today.[11] The possible effect of this decline in potency is changes in bodily alternations produced by heroin. Many heroin addicts routinely take other substances in addition to heroin, and although addicted to heroin, they have relatively mild habits. The women's addiction to heroin may, therefore, cause temporary amenorrhea but cannot be relied upon to eliminate menstruation altogether.

The inflated price and relative scarcity of heroin in the San Francisco Bay area over the last three years has had a great impact on the consistency of heroin use among addicts. It is somewhat rare to find an addict—either male or female—who has lengthy runs as a pure heroin addict; instead, the typical addict is constantly cleaning up, becoming readdicted, and cleaning up, often involuntarily, depending on the availability of heroin.[12]

Changes in quality, availability, and addiction patterns effect the woman addict's fertility, but although she may occasionally miss a menstrual period, amenorrhea cannot be counted on as a form of birth control. However, amenorrhea is often assumed, and pregnancy is not detected until other signs are present.

The state of pregnancy transforms the definition of addiction from a so-called "crime without a victim"[13] to one with a very real victim—the unborn fetus. On this issue, there was more consensus among the women interviewed than on any other single aspect of addiction: They had contempt for women who remained addicted while pregnant. All but two of the women who had had children while in the heroin life claimed that they had cleaned up when they discovered they were pregnant. Those who had not explained that since they believed heroin addiction caused them to stop menstruating and, hence, ovulating, they also believed they could not become pregnant. Many had not discovered that they were pregnant until relatively late (the fourth or fifth month), and by this time, it was both too late to have a simple first-trimester abortion and too late to clean up.

The rationale for continuing heroin use is: (1) if the heroin is going to have an ill effect on the fetus, it has already done so by the fourth or fifth month; and (2) going through withdrawal late in pregnancy is more dangerous than continuing use and giving birth to an addicted baby. This attitude characterized only a few of the women interviewed, who were also able to report numerous incidences where babies were born with a heroin habit, underwent the horrors of withdrawal, and sometimes died. The reliability of the women's accounts about their own drug use during pregnancy is questionable; nevertheless, one ethic remains strong among women in the heroin world: It is not acceptable to remain addicted while pregnant, thereby risking addiction in a newborn baby. This woman's statement represented the predominant view:

I have a thing about that [being addicted while pregnant]. I won't use drugs while I'm pregnant. It's not fair to the baby. The baby didn't say he wanted to get strung out. And it'll go right to the baby. I really feel strong about that. I only did it [heroin] a few times [maybe once a month] while I was pregnant, but I wouldn't get strung out.

The infant born to an addict is often premature and suffers from the complications of all premature births. Low birth weight is also common among babies of addicts, and withdrawal symptoms are sometimes manifested.[14] A physician described newborn withdrawal:

Toward the end of the first 24 hours of life, the infant became very restless and irritable, and exhibited marked tremors and twitchings. Blood calcium was examined and found to be normal. Shortly thereafter, vomiting and diarrhea occurred accompanied by constant shrill, high pitched crying and refusal to take feedings. Accompanying these symptoms were persistent nasal stuffiness, increased sweating and a rise in temperature to slightly over 100$ F. There were several bouts of intermittent cyanosis within the first 48 hours.[15]

Giving birth while addicted is a horror. The mother often suffers toxemia and other serious complications stemming from poor prenatal care as well as addiction.[16] For the mother who is either currently addicted or has a history of addiction, childbirth can entail psychological battering by hospital staff. Many women complained that even though they were drug-free at the time of birth, the nurses treated them with intense disrespect. (The hospital setting is sometimes the woman addict's first encounter with the social stigma attached to addiction.)

The attitude of hospital staff can set up a pattern of continued failure to comply with medical prescription for proper health care. When pregnant addicts see a physician prior to delivery, they are often treated with disdain because they are addicted. Occasionally, a sympathetic physician will attempt to see them through the pregnancy, sometimes suggesting that they not attempt withdrawal in order to protect the fetus from possible death; it is more likely that the woman will be implored to clean up, lest her baby become addicted. If the woman cannot clean up, she feels that hospital personnel are disgusted with her, hence, she tends to stay away. Therefore, when she comes in contact again with the medical world at the time of delivery, she is treated with disrespect, not only because she is a heroin addict, but because she has failed to follow the standard prenatal routine of seeing a physician regularly.

The combination of psychological battering by the hospital staff and the problems of caring for a withdrawing and ill baby can serve to spiral the woman deeper into addiction. She often feels tremendous guilt over having delivered an addicted baby and generally lacks the support of family or close friends; in short, she feels she has failed at motherhood almost before it has begun.

Mothering While Addicted

The mother who can maintain a heroin habit and take care of her children is respected in the heroin world. Although all women felt that caring for their children was most important, some were better able to accomplish the joint tasks of addiction and mothering than others. The women who were best able to combine heroin and children were those whose childcare responsibilities forced them to control their drug use; in fact, a woman would occasionally indicate that she had become pregnant and had a baby in order to control her use of heroin. But for those women whose children were not born for the purpose of controlling their use and routinizing their lives, it was an accomplishment to discipline themselves, so that their children's needs were met before their own for heroin. Just as successfully combining motherhood and a career is a source of pride to the nondrugusing woman, the ability to combine responsible mothering and heroin use is a source of pride to the addicted mother. As one woman said:

> I have custody of her. The State, you know, the police, filed to take her away from me, and the Health Department said my little girl has hypergammaglobulin anemia and her shots run me $340 a month. She gets a shot a week. And the Welfare Department told the court that she was the healthiest baby they had seen in a long time. I already had her in Head Start, you know, preschool at three years old. She was already starting to read. She could count up to 50 at three. She was clean, she had clothes and food. She was always in bed by 7:30-8:00 P.M. I was always up in the morning cooking breakfast. They said even though I had a narcotic problem and from what people told them too, like days when all I had was enough money to fix, but I would make sure she was taken

care of. And if I didn't have enough money to take care of her and fix, she would be taken care of—I wouldn't. I'd go sick.

A few women were able to carve out a routine incorporating their children's needs with their own. These two women put it well:

> I get up in the morning, go and cop—oh, about getting up in the morning—luckily my daughter has adjusted her sleeping hours to mine, so I get up in the morning, get her dressed and fed and all that. And then I proceed to see who's out and who I can cop from. And I cop and I stay out, you know, like if there are any of my regular tricks, I'll stay out and try to make some money. And then I'll go back home. I get home about 5-6-7 P.M., get the baby ready for bed, feed her, fix again, and go out and make as much money as I can; make the rent money, make the food money, and make my money to fix.

The other woman notes:

> Oh, after I fixed, she'd eat, right? That wasn't nothin' but formula and a little cereal 'cause by then it would be 9:30-10:00 A.M. before she'd wake back up. Then she'd be in there [tub] when I'd bathe and she loves water. She'd want to get in there. After I had fed her, then she'd go back to sleep. Then it's time for me to do mine again. It's sad, but it's true. I go and do my thing again, and by that time, I'd get myself together as far as putting on clothes, taking my shower, washing up, whatever. After that, I'd sit and watch TV and nod.

When an addicted mother was able to establish a routine for her heroin use, she was in an optimal position to raise her children in a manner with which she felt comfortable. For the exceptional mother, combining heroin and children meant controlling her habit and competent care of her children. The woman addict who is at the top of the heroin hierarchy, such as the successful dealer or spouse of a dealer, is best able to handle childcare: She has constant access to heroin, does not have to leave her home to work, and, therefore, can be both well (not withdrawing) and available to her children.

As previously mentioned, the addict hierarchy and stratification system is fluid; the woman at the top may find herself either incarcerated or poor, sick, and hustling in the street in a very short time. Therefore, the mother who at one point can perform her childcare duties by controlling her heroin usage and organizing her life may suddenly find her world in chaos. If she is suffering withdrawal because she hasn't the money to buy drugs or drugs are not available, it is difficult for her to take care of children of any age but especially babies and small children. Thus, older children are often given the responsibility of caring for babies. As one woman related:

> I do everything I can to make her stop crying and if she still keeps crying, I just let her cry. I stick her in the other room and close the door and let her cry—turn up the TV and then she'll cry herself to sleep. The three year old, ummm, she's well; they are both excellent kids. I don't know what I did to deserve them. [She shakes her head and shrugs her shoulders.] But they are really very easy to get along with. [She says this with obvious affection.] If I say, "Mama don't feel good today" to the three year old, she'll pretty much leave me alone. She'll occupy her sister, her little sister's time, mama her, give her the bottle, rock her.

It is also likely that the woman in these circumstances will have to resort to illegal street work to support herself (prostitution, boosting, forgery). When the addict-mother has to leave her home in order to work to support her habit or even to buy drugs, she encounters the same difficulties with childcare that other working mothers do. In addition, she is usually making very little money and is often not organized enough to know how and where to look for competent childcare. Consequently, she is sometimes forced to leave small children alone while she goes out to score or hustle; as might be expected, this can result in neglect at best and tragedy at worst.[17]

The use of potent or excessive heroin can also have a deleterious effect on the woman's ability to mother: She may go on the nod and be incapable of responding to the needs of her children. In this condition, she is functionally absent. One woman discussed two of her friends:

> This girl had been using since she was 12. One source said her baby died when she was nodding and he got a hold of some of her Ritalins. He ate them and died in the hospital. I had another friend who had nine kids. Now she doesn't have any of them. One of her kids got killed while she was nodding on the couch. The kid went out in the street and got hit by a car. Turned out to be a vegetable and wound up dying.

Although addicted, the mother with money who works at home, whether as a dealer or housewife, can often control her drug use and perform her childcare tasks (often quite admirably). But the fluid nature of the heroin world can quickly change her situation. She may escape jail but still find her life in a state of chaos that, coupled with withdrawal sickness, leads to child neglect. Street work forces the woman to be away from home and children, and thus makes her unable to care for them. The psychoactive effects of heroin can produce a state of euphoria, so that the woman is not in a position to carry out routine mothering tasks because she is on the nod. The experience of the average woman in the life—that of chaos and inundation—results in a general inability to take care of the business of mothering.

Dealing with the Inability to Take Care of Business

For the woman who recognizes her own inability to parent, who cannot control her heroin use and wants a better home for her children, the move to place her children in another environment is likely to be voluntary. The woman often has family members who are willing to take the children, so they do not have to be placed in foster homes or institutions. I found this to be the case most often among black women, who had mothers, aunts, and sisters who were available. The arrangement was seen as temporary and did not have the impact and guilt that characterizes losing children to institutions. One woman recalled:

> When I used to get hooked, everything seemed gray. I didn't realize what I was doing . . . nothing around me mattered. Even my kids didn't matter to me. I brought my kids to my mother and dropped them off. I'd give her money for them and all that shit, but I was gone. It was just that fix and that was it.

Another described what she did while addicted:

> . . . she was never neglected. If she was, I would give her to his mother and tell her, "Hey, I can't handle her right now." I would never keep her if I couldn't handle her.

When a neighbor or even a landlord who is concerned or upset about children who seem ill, neglected, or both notifies the child welfare department, a social worker then calls on the family in question to survey the situation. If the child is not severely injured, guidelines are usually set for the parents. A social worker describes the procedure.

> I would get a phone call from neighbors, landlords, sometimes even relatives, complaining that the child is being neglected. Sometimes babies are left alone or unchanged. They constantly smell like urine. Occasionally, the call reports battering, but that occurs less than just general neglect. I go out to the home, look around, and try to determine how serious the problem is. With the junkies, I tell them, "Okay, you get your [welfare] check on the first and get your food stamps. Before you buy anything else, I want you to buy two weeks worth of Pampers, two weeks worth of Similac, and *then*, if you must, the heroin."

Infrequently, the addicted mother is deemed unfit by the social agency, and her children are forcibly taken away from her. Welfare agencies do not want to take children away from their mothers, but if persistent neglect or harm is evident, they do. If the woman's family is available and cooperative, the children are placed with them; if not, they are placed in foster homes or institutions. Forcible or involuntary removal of children is, of course, a more difficult emotional experience for the mother than voluntary removal.

In the areas of motherhood and the fear of losing children, women addicts differ greatly from addicted men but very closely resemble other women in the larger society. By looking at a group of women who appear wholly deviant in occupational, physical, and social realms, it is possible to understand the pervasive nature of culture; specifically, the prescribed role of the mother in our culture and society and the way in which it is assumed. Our culture and society do make specific claims about the role of mother,[18] and women addicts, who cannot be considered ideologically liberated as defined by the women's movement, tend very much to accept society's prescriptions for this role. They see themselves as primarily responsible for their children (in contrast to the responsibility that they attribute to the children's father, which is generally extremely small). They also feel that motherhood is their single claim to worthiness; it is often their greatest responsibility. Additionally, women addicts subscribe to the notion that motherhood and fulfilling its responsibilities is the core of their own femininity. Failing at this endeavor is, therefore, equivalent, not only to being irresponsible, but to failing at womanhood in general. Because removing an ad-

dict-mother's children is socially and emotionally devastating, she attempts to forestall this almost inevitable event if possible. The threat of losing her children becomes the central element of risk in the addict-mother's life.

When children are placed in alternative homes, either voluntarily or involuntarily, the woman often ceases to attempt to control her heroin habit at all. She has given up or lost her children who had provided the impetus for keeping it together. This loss can begin a further spiraling downward into the addiction life with no holds barred. As this woman said:

> My mom called up the welfare department and said she wanted the baby put in a foster home. I got the papers served on me, went to court. They made him a ward of the court and put him in a foster home. He was two years old then. That's when I went downhill all the way. I tried at first, but they wouldn't let me see the baby for two months and I couldn't handle that . . . nothin' was going right, and I just started using heavy and heavy and heavy.

Realization of Narrowing Options

The woman begins her career in drugs with relatively reduced options: In addition to having female status, she is often poor and of a racial minority; her occupational opportunities are few due to limited educational and job skill training. Therefore, motherhood is often viewed by such women as one of the more desirable options in terms of social worth, and it is one of the only viable roles for them; yet this role is likely to be seen as "given" until it is threatened.

There are several ways that motherhood can be threatened: by physical abuse, prolonged separations, rejection by the child due to disapproval for the mother's lifestyle, or by the child adopting the heroin life. Women who could bring themselves to discuss abusing their children often feared that this abuse would destroy the mother-child relationship. As this woman said:

> My son, when I first came out the penitentiary the first time, he had done something. God knows what it was, but it wasn't anything he had done. It was a little thing that provoked what I was feeling 'cause I couldn't get a fix. And I just beat him unmercifully. Just unmerciful. God, Jesus! He doesn't remember. I've never told him either. That's the one thing I've

never told him. But I've never forgotten it either. This one beating with my kid made me make a really fast decision. I sold all my furniture, packed up my clothing, and went to my grandmother's. Never once again did I try to take the responsibility of him while addicted or drinking. I don't give a damn what anybody says, I've seen it tried a thousand and one times. Addicts cannot have their children with them. I don't give a damn how together they think they are, their kids suffer. Believe me. And their loved ones suffer. Everybody suffers around them. It isn't intended to be that way, but that's the way it is. And pretty soon, those feelings are just ice cold. All you think about is that damned monkey on your back. And everything goes. No matter how they say they got it together. And I'm speaking from my own experience plus my experience I have experienced with other people while I was hooked. And I know that you cannot be addicted and be a good mother. If you are addicted, just leave. Get away from them 'cause you are going to hurt them first.

Sometimes mistreatment takes the form of housing children in a negative environment as much as physical neglect. As this woman described:

It was just too much for me, the whole thing. My house was starting to turn into a shooting gallery. People would come over, "Let me get down here, let me get down here." I only had the one little girl at the time, but she was really mimicking, you know? She'd pick up a piece of straw and pretend like it was an outfit and it just blew me away when I saw her do that and so I said, "I'm cleaning up."

Women who have been active in the heroin life and have been separated from their children feel guilty about their absence:

When my son was born and he was just a few months old is when I started getting into it again, and I was spending as little time as I could with them. If they weren't with my mother, one of my friends were taking care of them, and I just was always tripping somewhere. I mean, I'd be gone two or three days, and they'd be with the kids. I always had the kids taken care of well. I mean, I never neglected them or anything like that but, you know, I do look back and have guilt feelings about the way I just shoved my kids off.

Some women feel that the separation deprived their children of some of the advantages they could have provided:

I feel that if I didn't get strung out, they would have had their home, they probably would have gone to parochial school, they would have had so much more. They probably would have been in Girl Scouts and Boy Scouts, and they would have had a different home life. But instead, they had to get shifted to their grandparents' house; mommy was in jail, mommy was a dope fiend. I always had everything I wanted, so I feel, like in my subconscious mind, I just give my kids whatever they want because, I guess I feel bad because I deprived them of some things, which is no good. I'm not doing them any good by doing what I'm doing.

Women who have spent a good deal of time incarcerated also have a sense that they have missed important developmental stages in their children's lives:

I missed so much out of my daughter's childhood when she was growing that I wanted to have another baby because of things I missed. Like, I never saw her when she rode her bike for the first time-stupid things like that, which a lot of people wouldn't understand. Like, she lost her front teeth and grew 'em back before I got out of the penitentiary.

Possibly the most frightening part of realizing that role options are narrowing in regard to mothering is a child's maturation. Since one of the central aspects of mothering seems to be providing a role model, many women feared that when their children matured and became cognizant of their mother's drug use, they would reject her. Neglect of basic childcare, some mistreatment, and even separation could be remedied, but setting a negative example when the children were old enough to understand was not acceptable. Some women fear and wonder how they will look to the child. As this woman said:

He doesn't know. He knows that sometimes I'm very irritable and edgy. He knows that sometimes I sleep a lot from being sick or from staying up all night using. He's gotten pretty independent from it actually. I don't feel good about it, because a lot of times when I'm sick, I can't really be there for him in the way that I'd like. Or I read to him when I'm loaded and he thinks I'm tired. I'm sure he can pick up certain vibes—I'm more there in certain ways when

I'm clean than when I'm not, but he doesn't know the details. He knows we smoke weed. He's six and a half. That it's a positive drug, it's part of my value system. He knows it's illegal, and we don't talk about it but that we do it. Same with sex. But I don't share the dope thing. I don't feel bad keeping it from him. I'd feel a whole lot worse sharing it with him because there's no way he can relate to it now. Since I see it as part of my life off and on forever, I don't know whether I'm going to go on keeping it from him or someday when he's a teenager he'll put it together. It kind of freaks me because I can't accept it in myself, and I want to be a model for him.

Other women fear that their children will accept them as role models and become addicts themselves. No woman interviewed wanted her child or anyone she cared for to become addicted. As one woman put it:

The only reason why I really want to quit and the one that gives me power to quit is for the baby. Or else, I wouldn't even try it. I'd just keep going like nothin'. Shit, what the hell? Now that I have the baby, I have something to think about, 'cause when he gets older and he knows what I'm doing, I don't want him to-I don't even want him to see me do that 'cause I don't want my kid to turn out like me, no way. I'd really regret that. I'd really feel bad about that.

Conclusion

The male addict prides himself on taking care of business when he organizes his life around his heroin habit and is able to maintain himself in this routine.[19] Heroin becomes the focus of his life and takes precedence over all other endeavors. For the woman with children, however, taking care of heroin-related business cannot be her central concern. Therefore, although men and women fare similarly in the early stages of addiction, women with children have a decided disadvantage in later maintenance phases.

When the woman addict senses that she is in a position to lose her children, either psychologically or physically, she begins to take serious stock of her situation. Since motherhood is central to her feminine identity, the label of "unfit" and subsequent loss of children is tantamount to the loss of her womanhood—she often feels intense guilt and a sense of failure over this loss. In many ways, losing her children represents a greater risk than incarceration or the other threatening aspects of the heroin life. At this point in the woman's career, she realizes that her motherhood options are, indeed, being funneled and that the sacrifice she makes for heroin is getting closer to her own person, identity, and sense of self. One woman pointed out:

When you realize that you are losing your kids, your womanhood, to that monkey on your back, that's when you've gotta get out.

The realization of narrowing options provides the impetus for the attempt out of the heroin life. Knowing that she has already put her occupational options in jeopardy, the woman can gear herself toward abstinence from heroin in order to protect the remaining option of a viable family life.[20] While she still has something to lose, the one option of motherhood, she is in an optimal frame of mind for getting out of the heroin life, ending her career in addiction.

* * *

For Discussion

1. Why are women heroin users more likely than men to have partners who also use heroin?

2. Why have most studies of heroin users focused primarily on males?

Notes

1. For a discussion of this aspect of addiction see G. De Leon and H. K. Wexler, "Heroin Addiction," pp. 36-38.

2. See D. Wellisch, G. Gay, and R. McEntee, "The Easy Rider Syndrome," pp. 425-430.

3. See D. Waldorf, *Careers in Dope*, pp. 159-177.

4. See L. Rubin, *Worlds of Pain*.

5. See F. Liebow, *Tally's Corner*.

6. See B. Sackman et al., "Heroin Addiction as an Occupation," p. 2.

7. Rubin, *Worlds of Pain*, p.176.

8. M. Komarovsky, "Cultural Contradictions and Sex Roles," p. 256.

9. For discussions of the centrality of motherhood see J. Bardwick and E. Douvan, "Ambivalence"; J. Bernard, *The Future of Motherhood*; N. Chodorow, *The Reproduction of Mothering*; N. Weisstein, "Psychology Constructs the Female."

10. See G. Blinick, "Fertility of Narcotics Addicts and Effects of Addiction on the Offspring," pp. S34-S39; E. C. Gaulden et al., "Menstrual Abnormalities Associated with Heroin Addiction," pp. 155-160; R. Hertz, "Addiction, Fertility, and Preg-

nancy," pp. S40-S41; R. Wallach, "Pregnancy and Menstrual Function in Narcotics Addicts Treated with Methadone," pp. 1226-1229.

11. C. Winick, "Epidemiology of Narcotics Use."

12. See E. M. Brecher, *Licit and Illicit Drugs*; A. Lindesmith, *Addictions and Opiates*; C. Sheppard, D. Smith, and G. Gay, "The Changing Face of Heroin Addiction in the Haight-Ashbury," p. 122.

13. For an excellent discussion of crimes without victims see E. Schur, *Crimes without Victims*.

14. See G. Blinick et al., "Pregnancy in Narcotics Addicts Treated by Medical Withdrawal," pp. 997-1003; R. L. Naeye et al., "Fetal Complications of Maternal Heroin Addiction," pp. 1055-1061; J. L. Rementeria and N. N. Nunag, "Narcotic Withdrawal in Pregnancy," pp. 1052-1056; P. Rothstein and J. B. Gould, "Born with a Habit," pp. 307-321.

15. H. Schneck, "Narcotic Withdrawal Symptoms in the Newborn Infant Resulting from Maternal Addiction," p. 585.

16. For lengthy discussions of this phenomenon see Blinick, "Pregnancy in Narcotics Addicts," p.997; L. P. Finnegan, "Narcotics Dependency in Pregnancy"; and S. K. Krase, "Heroin Addiction among Pregnant Women and Their Newborn Babies," pp. 754-758.

17. With a moderate drug dose some women can function normally, even optimally. Many women reported that when using heroin they had the ability to do housework and care for their children in ways that far exceeded their nondrugged state. One woman said:

> Taking care of the baby was hell, especially if I ain't got nothin' [heroin]. I feel bad because I have to keep laying him down there and I just feed him his bottle and then after that I say, "I can't just keep doing that." So, I try to get up, but I'm not really up to playing with him or nothin'. Then, finally, when I get my fix, I seem like I'm a whole different person. I could take care of him and take care of the house and still have more time.

18. See Bernard, *The Future of Motherhood*; Chodorow, *The Reproduction of Mothering*.

19. See E. Preble and J. Casey, "Taking Care of Business," pp. 1-24.

20. See B. S. Brown et al., "In Their Own Words," pp. 635-645; M. Rosenbaum, "Sex Roles among Deviants," (Forthcoming). ✦

17. *Chasing the Dragon*

MARC A. SCHUCKIT

In the United States, the majority of heroin users administer the drug by injection. In other countries, some users prefer inhaling opium vapors; that is, "chasing the dragon." Dr. Schuckit reports that this method surfaced in England in the late 1970s. He compares chasers with intravenous heroin users, describing the similarities and differences between the groups and noting that the extent of "chasing" in the United States is unknown. Schuckit raises some questions about the risks of chasing heroin, as opposed to injecting it.

Introduction

Most drugs can be administered by multiple routes. It doesn't seem to take long for users to discover the modes of intake that appear to produce the quickest and most intense high, and to dismiss those routes that appear to be less efficient in carrying the drug into the body and then to the brain.

Heroin, for example, is not well-absorbed when taken orally. As a result, users have developed a number of alternative methods of administration, with many in western cultures settling on an IV approach as the one that gives them the greatest "high for the buck." While this may be the most economical and efficient way to take heroin, there are high risks that result in morbidity and mortality. These include an enhanced risk for infections of the heart valves, skin abscesses, the possibility of brain damage through emboli, a higher risk for hepatitis, and a substantial risk for death through AIDS.

However, in other areas of the world, alternative modes of administration of opiates predominate. In recent years, this has included the direct inhalation of opium vapors into the lungs. This form of administration, commonly called Chasing the Dragon, results in little waste of the heroin, might have less overdose potential because of the longer time needed to inhale as compared to pressing a syringe plunger, and produces a prompt onset of an intoxication.

What Is Chasing the Dragon?

There are at least three methods for inhaling heroin or opium into the lungs. The first, most common in China and related areas such as Hong Kong, involves directly smoking a pill of heroin that is burned in an opium pipe. A second approach to smoking is to mix powdered heroin with tobacco in a cigarette. Chasing is the third form.

This approach takes advantage of forms of heroin with relatively high oil contents, because these are the forms most likely to yield the ghost-like plumes of smoke used in these procedures. Chasing involves pouring an oil-rich form of heroin onto a piece of tin foil. A flame is applied directly underneath the drug, with the result that the heroin soon liquifies, and droplets distribute over the surface of the foil. This produces a vapor which is then "chased" and inhaled through a tube. While other forms of heroin can also be chased after heating on a spoon, these practices appear to be less prevalent.

This route of drug taking meets many of the desires of addicted individuals. It is a relatively efficient use of the drug with little waste, the vapor is relatively pure heroin, and the intoxication occurs almost immediately, as the heroin vapor is rapidly absorbed into the rich blood supply of the lungs, carried back to the heart, and then directly to the brain. Finally, similar to what occurs with the steps and paraphernalia used in IV ingestion, at least theoretically, the "pleasure" and/or the reinforcing effects of drug taking might be enhanced by the types of rituals that go into Chasing the Dragon. Subsequently, these rituals themselves may develop reinforcing or pleasure-giving properties.

The History of Chasing

This approach to drug taking became popular in the late 1970s in many places in Great Britain. A number of factors contributed to this development. First, it was at this point that the relatively oily southwest Asian heroin appeared on the market. Second, during the same time frame, there developed a greater awareness of the lethal consequences of IV use in the context of AIDS, fostering a search by some users for safer but still efficient ways of taking the drug in the drug-taking community. Third, the 1970s and 1980s was a time of increasing migration to Britain of individuals from Africa, India, and the Caribbean, groups who, historically, had more experience with this mode of drug taking.

How Prevalent Is Chasing the Dragon?

Surveys in different parts of Great Britain report markedly divergent results. It appears as if the prevalence of this mode of drug administration varies by country, region, and even within different areas of the same city.

Several surveys of individuals entering treatment in London in the late 1980s indicated a high prevalence of this practice. For example, a questionnaire administered to 75 heroin-dependent individuals recently admitted to a treatment program in London revealed that 80 percent had "chased" at some time during their careers. A second English study indicated that almost 50 percent of 264 heroin-dependent individuals named chasing as their usual mode of administration. This latter finding is consistent with a 1987 review of 76 heroin addicts, 42 percent of whom listed chasing as their usual pattern. In addition, even among those people whose most recent pattern of intake was IV, 20 percent or more had "chased" in the prior 30 days.

Who Is Most Likely to Be a Chaser?

These data come from several reviews of heroin addicts in Great Britain. In most of these studies, men and women who listed chasing as their usual mode of use, especially if this was the optimal choice in the prior year, were compared to individuals whose primary mode of administration was IV.

The two groups were quite similar on a number of characteristics. This included equivalent levels of heroin used per day (approximately 700 mg), indicating that chasers did not have to use higher doses of the drug to feed their habit. Chasers and IV users were also quite similar on level of education, the proportion unemployed (80 percent), and on the report of ever having spent time in prison.

Despite these similarities, there were some interesting differences between chasing and IV-using groups. First, the chasers tended to be younger (an average of 23 vs. 27 years at the time of entering treatment), a finding that probably reflects the fact that chasing was not generally used in Great Britain before the late 1970s. Thus, individuals who entered the addiction scene prior to 1979 or 1980 might have been less likely to have chasing as an option. A second difference related to levels of life stability. Fully three-quarters of chasers, but only approximately half of IV drug users, had regular sexual partners. Third, the data also revealed that the two sexes are equally represented among chasers, a finding that contrasts to IV users where males predominate. Finally, chasers were less likely to have been convicted of possession and/or dealing in opiates (20 percent vs. 43 percent), perhaps because they were less likely to have what the police usually recognize as incriminating paraphernalia.

Several of the studies attempted to determine whether chasing was just an earlier stage that led to later IV drug dependence. The data certainly indicate that the two modes of administration are not fully independent. One-half of chasers have ever used IV, including one-third in the prior year. On the other hand, in one of the samples over 85 percent of the chasers had consistently used this mode of administration for two or more years. In addition, while figures varied with the sample chosen, one-third or more of chasers appeared to never have used opiates through an IV route. Thus, while there is a great deal of crossover, one form does not inevitably lead to the other.

The final question addressed in these comparisons of IV users and chasers relates to the probability that members of the two groups will engage in needle-sharing behavior, thus markedly increasing their risk for AIDS. Of course, the substantial minority of chasers who never used IV do not expose themselves to this excessively risky behavior. In addition, at least one study indicated that those chasers who have used IV in the past were much less likely than the regular IV users to have ever shared needles; 17 percent for the chasers vs. 71 percent for the regular IV users.

In summary, there are many similarities between IV opiate users and chasers. Both have some level of legal problems, difficulties maintaining regular interpersonal relationships, and they share a high rate of unemployment. The level of physical addiction in chasers and IV drug users is probably similar, at least as gauged by the milligrams per day of heroin used. On the other hand, chasers appear to be younger, do show some evidence of greater stability, at least in interpersonal relationships, exhibit a less tumultuous legal history, at least regarding opiate-related arrests, and appear to be less likely to engage in needle sharing if they do use IV.

Are There Significant Dangers to Chasing?

In any of its forms, heavy repeated use of opiates is likely to produce both psychological and physical dependence. This makes it likely that chasers will experience the whole panoply of problems in controlling drug use, stopping intake, and in staying clean. Through any route of intake, heroin is capable of addicting a child in utero.

When all samples are taken together, it is also apparent that most (certainly not all) chasers also take IV drugs. Thus, they are more likely than the people in the general population to acquire bacterial endocarditis, potentially lethal hepatitis, and AIDS.

It is also probable that chasing carries some risks of its own. There are reports of severe constrictions of the breathing tubes (bronchospasm) with acute use of opiates through this method. Similarly, it appears likely that chasing can worsen preexisting pictures of asthma, and might actually be able to cause a repetitive asthma-like picture itself.

Some Conclusions

The route of administration of a drug can have a major impact on the patterns of problems that are likely to develop. In the recent decade, a variation of the ancient habit of opium smoking has developed and made its presence felt in Great Britain. The rate of Chasing the Dragon in that country appears to be relatively high, with a substantial minority of men and women using this mode of administration as their sole drug-use pattern.

The rate of chasing in United States populations is not known. This may reflect differences between different cultures, but might also be a consequence of many surveys not having asked the right questions.

Whether highly prevalent in the United States or not, this is an interesting phenomenon. Recognizing that this form of opiate use is rarely described in the literature, I thought that readers of the *Newsletter* might find these comments of interest.

✳ ✳ ✳

Marc A. Schuckit, "Chasing the Dragon," *Drug Abuse and Alcoholism Newsletter*, (3) XXII, (June 1993). Published by the Vista Hill Foundation, San Diego, California. Copyright © 1993 by the Vista Hill Foundation. All rights reserved. Reprinted by permission.

References

Griffiths, P., et al. Extent and nature of transitions of route among heroin addicts in treatment. *British Journal of Addiction* 87:485-491, 1992.

Gossop, M., et al. Chasing the dragon: characteristics of heroin chasers. *British Journal of Addiction* 83:1159-1162, 1988.

Oliver, R. Bronchospasm and heroin inhalation. *Lancet 1*:915, 1986.

Battersby, M., et al. Pharmaceutical heroin and chasing the dragon. *British Journal of Addiction* 85:151, 1990.

Gregg, J., et al. Inhaling heroin during pregnancy. *British Medical Journal 296*:754, 1988.

Madden, S. Chasing the dragon. *British Journal of Addiction 84*: 697-698 (letter), 1989.

Saxena, S. Chasing the dragon: Indian experience. *British Journal of Addiction 84*:699-700 (letter), 1989. ✦

18. Nonaddictive Opiate Use

Norman E. Zinberg

Most research and public opinion support the belief that people who try heroin either stop using it after the first "taste," or they continue using it to the point of addiction. Controlled heroin use, on the other hand, assumes that some people can use the drug frequently without becoming addicted. Little is known about this group of users, perhaps because they are less often found among treatment and jail populations.

Norman Zinberg reviews the literature on the topic and notes several references to nonaddictive opiate users. The sample upon which this article is based includes controlled users only, the majority of them women and many of them employed. The author argues that three factors determine whether individuals are able to control their use of heroin, the most important one being the social setting in which drug use occurs. Zinberg describes the rituals and sanctions embedded in the social settings that allow for controlled use of opiates.

Both the viewpoint and the data presented in this chapter are the outcome of my 4-year investigation of controlled opiate use, beginning with the pilot project sponsored by the Drug Abuse Council and continuing in the NIDA-sponsored projects. The first section of the chapter will consider the evidence presented by the literature for the existence of extensive nonaddictive opiate use. Second, the chapter will describe several broad patterns of opiate use that have come to light during project interviews with a variety of users. Third, it will discuss the importance of the social-setting variable; and fourth, it will briefly outline further areas of research that need to be undertaken, emphasizing the questions raised by my investigation. Finally, the fifth section will make some suggestions concerning public policy and education.

Evidence of Nonaddictive Opiate Use

The existence of occasional or controlled opiate use has long been recognized by experienced observers, in spite of the traditional view that chipping or chippying—that is, experimental or casual use—was a relatively brief way station leading either back to abstinence or quickly forward to habitual, chronic, heavy use, or regular abuse. The National Commission on Marijuana and Drug Abuse reported in 1973 that 90 percent of Americans disagreed with the statement, "You can use heroin occasionally without ever becoming addicted to it." The existence of hundreds of articles about heroin addiction, as opposed to only a few on any other pattern of use, attests to the research community's agreement with that view. For example, Chein's group, while noting the existence of "long-continued nonaddictive users," concluded that their numbers were insufficient to warrant investigation and that in all likelihood the large majority who continued use went on to addiction (Chein et al. 1964).

Lindesmith (1957) likewise had drawn a distinction between pleasure users of opiates, whom he called "joy poppers," and the prototypical addict. "A 'joy popper,'" he wrote, "is simply an individual who uses the drug intermittently and who has never been hooked." He too suspected that most continuing "joy poppers" went on to addiction. By 1972, Goode was stating the same traditional position somewhat more ambivalently: "The occasional (weekend) heroin user is probably a good deal more common than most of us realize, although an extraordinarily high percentage of those who 'chippy' (experiment) with heroin eventually become addicted."

Of greater importance, however, is a rigorous retrospective study by Robins and Murphy (1967) of a normal population of young Negro males in St. Louis. They found that 13 percent of the total sample had tried heroin and that all but 3 percent had become addicted. All those who had used heroin more than six times had gone on to become addicts.

Any literature search that attempts to determine the extent to which observers have recognized long-term, nonaddictive opiate use is hampered by the unwavering acceptance of this traditional view of chipping, which is reinforced by three factors: the concern that the mere recognition of such use might encourage experimentation by the unwary; the difficulty of arriving at any reasonable, quantitative estimates of such use; and the multiplicity and impreciseness of the terms employed to describe drug-using styles. This last point caused Chein et al. to note, as long ago as 1964, that the apparently specific term "heroin addict" had been used in so many different ways that "it is meaningless to identify an individual as an 'addict.'" In addition, and perhaps most important, the literature, because of the time lag both in the development and funding of studies of changing patterns of drug use and in publication, includes little up-to-date information on the swiftly changing patterns of drug use of the past 7 years.

Nevertheless, a careful literature review does indicate that patterns of long-term controlled opiate use have existed for some time. Although the literature does not provide quantitatively specific evidence, it does show that there is a considerably higher percentage of opiate users than had previously been supposed. This, however, has not been recognized by physicians and medical clinics, other than those concerned with heroin use alone.

In 1961, while working at the Cook County jail, Scher reported on a group of heroin users whom he described as having "what might be called a regulated or controlled habit." Later on, when considering the life cycle of addiction, Alksne et al. (1967) noted with some surprise that "although no research reports are available for this kind of user, our own observations indicate that some persons continue in occasional or limited use for an indefinite period of time without going on to more regular use." These observations almost exactly parallel those reported in 1974 by Newmeyer of the Haight-Ashbury Free Medical Clinic in San Francisco, concerning individuals who, he said, could "be characterized as persons who sample heroin without becoming addicted."

A perspective different from the medical profession's excessive fear of addiction is presented by medical personnel who screen applicants for methadone maintenance programs. Even the guidelines suggested by the American Medical Association (1972) state: "The mere use of a morphine-type drug, even if periodic or intermittent, and/or violation of drug laws cannot be equated with drug dependency. In each instance, a specific medical diagnosis is required." The same theme was brought up by Dobbs (1971), who warned that some people applying for methadone maintenance should be rejected, because they are only occasional users. It also led to a suggestion by Blachly (1973) that naloxone was useful in distinguishing between addicts and occasional users. Blachly noted that "a significant hazard exists in creating addicts to methadone hydrochloride, since a third of those applying to a methadone clinic without prior documentation of withdrawal in an institution showed no evidence of physical dependence." Glaser (1974), too, suggested that 45 percent of the applicants to a Philadelphia maintenance program were not addicts, although he gave no data on their frequency of use.

The interesting and paradoxical recognition that there are occasional users who, for reasons of their own, present themselves as addicts is not new. Zinberg and Lewis reported on such a group in 1964. In addition, Gay et al. (1974) have published case histories of occasional users who presented themselves as addicts, although urinalysis belied their claims. Such individuals were labeled "pseudo junkies" to indicate that they assumed the trappings of addiction without the necessary opiate use.

The reports mentioned so far have simply noted the existence of nonaddicted opiate users. Several other reports, however, have introduced an experimental or quantitative dimension.

Hughes et al. (1971), while studying addicts, used 15 occasional users as a comparison group. Eleven of that comparison group, they stated, became regular, frequent users without progressing to addiction.

In 1971–72, Levengood et al. (1973) conducted a study of single white male heroin users between the ages of 15 and 24 who lived in a Detroit suburb. Although their sample comprised multiple drug users, they examined three distinct subsamples classified by frequency of heroin use. Of the 60 subjects interviewed, 22 individuals (or 37 percent) used "regularly or on a daily basis"; 24 (40 percent) used occasionally, with quantity and frequency of use varying widely; and 14 (23 percent), who had used within the last year but not during the month prior to study, were considered "former users." Some who had recently been using on a daily basis were included in this last group, but none of them had received any form of treatment.

Graeven and Jones (1976), who examined adolescent heroin use in a suburban San Francisco high school between 1966 and 1974, reported that occasional use was almost as prevalent as addiction (49 percent as compared with 51 percent). Of the 143 "experimenters" identified, 33 percent had used between 3 and 30 times, 19 percent had used from 31 to 100 times, and 10 percent had used more than 100 times. Furthermore, by 1974, 24 percent of the addict group were using between once a month and twice a week, with only 47 percent using three or more times a week.

A study of Abt Associates Inc. (1975) on drug use in the state of Ohio showed that 1.39 percent of their respondents admitted having used heroin. If this figure were extrapolated to the general population of the state, the number of users would clearly be greater than any previous estimate of the number of actual addicts. Moreover, the survey indicated that among heroin users, occasional use predominated: 8.7 percent used "several times per week or more"; 17.4 percent "a few times per month"; 34.8 percent "a few times per year"; and 65.2 percent "less frequently." The Ohio results are not drastically different from data reported by Abelson and Fishburne (1976) from their 1975-76 nationwide study, which showed that 0.5 percent of youth under age 18 and 1.2 percent of all adults had had experience with heroin. Although generalizations made from such data are hazardous, these findings, together with the less comprehensive studies just described, suggest that many more nonaddicts use heroin than has been supposed.

Bourne et al. (1975) made an interesting survey of heroin use in Wyoming, where, to their surprise, they found heroin use greater than expected, as well as many different use patterns, including occasional use. Their work contains few counts of the numbers of such users, but it is of particular importance that they take issue with the conventional view that most users are known to the authorities. They uncovered significant numbers of users and addicts who were unknown to the police or to the community health facilities responsible for treatment of drug problems. Hunt, one of the participants in the Wyoming study, used these data, along with other data collected with Chambers (1976), to place the heroin-using population of the United States at 3 to 4 million, of whom they claimed that only 10 percent were addicted.

Probably, the most important study in this group is that which Robins made of Vietnam veterans 3 years after their return to the United States. Not only is it a more rigorously designed work than any described so far, but it specifically contradicts Robins' own previous work. She found in 1976 that 20 percent (114) of the 571 previously addicted veterans had used opiates occasionally after their return. Of these, only about 12 percent (14) had had any period of stateside addiction. In her study, she concludes that this ratio of addiction to occasional use was consistent with patterns noticed in the general U.S. population. Furthermore, she explains that the discrepancy between these conclusions and her ear-

lier St. Louis study (Robins and Murphy 1967) is due to the changing patterns of drug use. While the earlier study had shown that nonaddictive use among blacks was infrequent between the 1930s and the 1950s, such use had become widespread by 1976.

Perhaps the most convincing data showing widespread nonaddictive heroin use come from studies, reporting its appearance in other treatment modalities. Minkowski et al. (1972) found more than twice as many occasional heroin users as daily heroin users in a random sample of clients visiting the Los Angeles Health Department Youth Clinic. Excluding experimenters (those using fewer than 3 times), who constituted 12 percent of the 300 respondents, 4.6 percent used between more than once a week and less than once a month, while only 1.7 percent used once a day.

Health consequences usually associated with heroin addiction have been reported to affect occasional users. Kersh (1974) states that 70 percent of the narcotic overdose cases treated in a New York hospital emergency room were occasional users. Light and Dunham (1974) have reported on two cases of vertebral osteomyelitis due to septic intravenous administration of heroin in individuals who had not used heroin for at least 8 weeks preceding the onset of symptoms and who were "definitely not addicts." Lewis et al. (1972) reported that they encountered five occasional users in 1 year who had spinal chondro-osteomyelitis; they were not addicted, but all had used heroin intravenously within the week prior to their hospital admission. An independent medical biostatistician is currently studying all these medical figures more closely, and his initial response has supported the conclusions of Hunt and Chambers (1976).

Before my work began, only one study, that by Powell (1973), seems to have been made that was specifically oriented to the occasional heroin user. Of the dozen subjects he recruited through placing advertisements in a counter-culture newspaper, none reported previous addiction to heroin and each had used the drug for at least 3 consecutive years. Judging these scanty data by my standards, I would classify only a few of Powell's subjects as strictly controlled users and the others as having a more unstable or "marginal" use pattern.

Patterns of Use

As originally conceived, my DAC and NIDA studies were designed to deal only with individuals whose opiate use was carefully controlled. In selecting subjects, stringent criteria were used to define controlled use. Subjects were required to be over 18, and to have used opiates at least 10 times per year for more than 2 years and at least 2 times during the 6 months preceding the interview. They must not have had more than one "spree"—an instance of from 4 to 15 consecutive days of opiate use—in any of these years. With the exception of tobacco, they must have been using all drugs, licit and illicit, in a controlled way and must not have been in a drug-free or methadone-maintenance program, in jail, or in any other confining institution during their years of controlled use.

These conditions or standards were laid down to include regular weekend users who often use 3 days in a row, as well as spree users, who may use for a number of days in a row on a vacation but then demonstrate equally prolonged periods of abstinence. The limit of one spree per year excluded users who might be intermittently addicted.

Finding controlled users who were willing to participate in the research project was at first a time-consuming process. But as project workers grew more adept and also came across subjects who could help in finding other subjects by penetrating different social networks, it became clear that locating responsive interviewees was difficult not because they were so few in number, but because under present social conditions which condemn and punish any opiate use at all, they were terrified of being discovered. This secretive attitude and fear of discovery stand in sharp contrast to the attitude of the usual addict found in a drug-treatment program.

So far, the project has located and interviewed 90 opiate users who have been controlled for between 3 and 23 years. They have been found through advertising in newspapers (both regular and counter-cultural), through community agencies, by professional contacts, and by subject referral. All subjects have been interviewed for approximately 2 hours, 60 have been followed up between 6 months and 1 year later, and 25 of these have had still another interview 1 year after that. In addition, at least 1 friend of each of 45 of our subjects has been interviewed as a way of understanding these subjects' social interactions and as a check on the reliability of the data. The requirement that friends be interviewed has been added in the NIDA project only during the last 2 years; hence, the smaller number of subjects so treated. Interestingly enough, two of the

occasional users had participated in the study of controlled use made by Zinberg and Lewis 14 years ago (1964). That they have continued their patterns of control over such a long period of time indicates the high degree of consistency such patterns can attain.

The following descriptive data are based on my combined DAC and NIDA samples. Because the NIDA project is ongoing, these data are necessarily approximations.

Of the 90 controlled opiate users I have studied to date, some 30 percent are males and 70 percent are females. Their ages range from 17 to 50 years, with a mean of 27 years. Approximately 40 percent come from lower-class or lower-middle-class families, and the remainder are almost equally split between the middle-middle class and the upper-middle class. Of those subjects who are not currently in school, one-quarter did not complete 12 years of schooling, one-third did complete 12 years (high school), and the remainder completed more than 12 years. All those who are currently in school had previously finished high school.

As for my subjects' living situations and current activities, one-quarter are single and the remainder are divided almost equally between those who are married and those who are living with a mate. About 66 percent are working full- or part-time, approximately 15 percent are currently employed, and 10 percent are in school either full- or part-time. Nine of the 90 (10 percent) are engaged in crime or drug dealing, more than half of them on a part-time basis, and these 5 are members of the middle class, whose drug dealing is done to help out friends at little or no profit. Of those currently employed, 58 percent are blue-collar workers. The bulk of the white-collar workers hold either clerical or managerial positions. Only 10 percent of the employed are in professional positions, such as nursing. Concerns about confidentiality and about the consequences of disclosure of their opiate use seem to have discouraged the professional, well-educated, and upper-class users from entering my project.

Turning to the actual case of opiates by my subjects, heroin ranks first not only in current use, but also as the opiate used most intensively during the subjects' using careers. Well over 80 percent of the sample use heroin. The mean current period of controlled opiate use is 5 years. Most subjects use opiates infrequently. About 20 percent use less than monthly (one to three times a month); 40 percent use monthly; 20 percent use weekly (once or twice a week); and the remainder use in various patterns, combining sprees with more regulated periods of use. More than 25 percent of my subjects have either a history of addiction to opiates or a history of compulsive use of another drug, or both. Their periods of compulsive use, however, have been significantly (at the 0.05 level) shorter than their current period of controlled use, a fact that underscores the importance of controlled use as a comparatively stable using style.

Despite the careful attention paid to personality description and personality formulation in the initial interview, and the additional data supplied by the follow-up interview and interviews of friends, correlations have not been found between occasional opiate use and specific personality types. At the same time, the interviews have revealed important similarities which have served to indicate the problems users have in maintaining a stable chipping pattern. Surprisingly, with but three exceptions, my subjects have reported a greater fear of being forced into abstinence than of losing control and becoming addicted. The chief difficulty in maintaining a pattern of occasional use seems to be the user's need to determine, either alone or in conjunction with a peer group, how to integrate the drug high into his or her regular pattern of work and social relationships. All of my subjects first tried an opiate as part of a series of drug experimentations and found the experience particularly pleasing. They all recognized that they had no social or psychological preparation for opiate use. Their anxious attempts to learn all they could about the drug's actions and effects from peers indicate that they had not gone through the kind of social drug-education process that is available to alcohol users in our culture.

Although my sample of 90 controlled users is small, the interview material appears consistent. Taken along with the data obtained by Robins and other researchers, and with a growing body of confirming reports that I have received as personal communications, it reveals the existence of a category of people who have succeeded in setting up a stable pattern of controlled opiate use that does not necessarily lead to addiction. It is impossible to say what percentage of all opiate users this group represents. Some of the data mentioned in the literature review suggest that quite a high percentage of heroin users may not be addicts. But if this finding is correct, and I believe it is, it still does not mean that all of those who are not addicts fall into the category

of stable controlled users, nor does it indicate which of the potential experimenters may be reasonably expected to be able to exercise the stringent sanctions necessary for controlled use. As an unexpected byproduct, our research has uncovered several different patterns of use falling between the extremes of control and non-control.

In the course of recruiting controlled subjects, I unintentionally interviewed people who did not meet the stringent qualifications for controlled users. Rather than discarding these recorded interviews, I decided to analyze and use them as comparative cases. In this way, I not only found out that even physiologically addicted users showed some evidence of control and reacted to changes in their social setting, but I also recognized a number of diverse using patterns that, while falling short of my definition of control, did not fit the addict stereotype. Of the 90 primarily opiate-using subjects who were rejected as controlled users by my standards, 18 (approximately 20 percent) reported addiction within the previous 2 years but were not currently addicted, 15 (roughly 17 percent) reported current daily use of a single dose but also did not regard themselves as addicted, and 13 (or about 14 percent) had used occasionally for less than 2 years. Others used different drugs, used them less frequently than my standard required, or had "spreed" more frequently. Fourteen (about 16 percent) regarded themselves as currently addicted, and more than half of these addicts were not affiliated with a treatment program.

Thus, my investigation revealed greater differentiation among the various levels of control and non-control than I had expected. First, some subjects used heroin several times a day, were physiologically addicted, and showed the stereotypical pattern of using as much of the drug as was available. (Most heroin users, who at one time or another have been under treatment, probably fall into this category.) Second, some, though physiologically addicted, placed limits on their use. (Sometimes this type is also found in the treatment population.) Third, there were those whose physiological addiction did not disrupt their functioning. (Although users of this type are rarely found in the treatment population in this country, they are found in England.) Fourth, some subjects were not addicted, but their history of addiction was so recent that they could not be considered controlled users. Fifth, some used heroin only occasionally but were more or less compulsive users of other drugs. Sixth, some users could not be defined as either clearly controlled or clearly addicted. These I called "marginal users," thus adding a third category to the two basic types of opiate users (controlled and compulsive) that I had been aware of originally (Zinberg et al. 1977). Not only have many professionals in the field overlooked stable, controlled use as a basic category of nonaddictive opiate use, but they have also overlooked a complex and diverse group of "marginal users" who, while clearly at risk of addiction, must still be considered generally nonaddicted.

The Importance of the Social Setting Variable

Once it is recognized that responses to opiate use are far more complex and varied than has usually been assumed, the next essential is to consider those factors that determine the potential for controlled use. It is my contention that three variables determine the style and consequence and, therefore, the degree of control of drug use: drug (the pharmacological properties of the drug itself), set (the user's personality and his or her attitudes toward taking the drug), and setting (the characteristics of the physical and social setting in which use occurs). In theory, each of these three variables can be manipulated to prevent abuse or to improve treatment methods. In fact, however, it is not easy to manipulate the first two.

In the case of the drug variable, attempts to prevent abuse by reducing the supply of opiates have proved costly and only partially successful because of the high demand for the drug, the windfall nature of black-market profits, and the permeability of national borders. Even if the supply is reduced, opiate users tend to substitute alcohol, barbiturates, pharmaceutical opiates, or other drugs, instead of stopping compulsive use or going into treatment (Association of the Bar of the City of New York 1977; Newman 1974). Similarly, attempts to improve treatment methods solely through manipulating the drug variable, such as the use of methadone and other agents, have been only partially successful. Drug therapy programs appear to work well for only a portion of the client population, and those who enter such programs probably constitute only a small fraction of those who are genuinely addicted (Chambers and Inciardi 1972; Nightingale 1977).

Prevention and treatment strategies grounded in the relationship between drug use and the set variable are also inadequate. Although some opiate abuse undoubtedly is related to personality disorders or social deprivation (Chein et al. 1964; Khantzian 1974; Khantzian et al. 1974; Yorke 1970), it is difficult to see how those who are "addiction prone" by psychological makeup and social background can be identified and persuaded to remain abstinent. In addition, it is by no means clear how many opiate users are or have been deficient in these areas. When prospective work has been done with subjects who later turn out to be addicted, the personality aspects accounting for their addiction have not been clear (Zinberg 1975).

Because of the difficulty in manipulating the drug and set variables in order to prevent abuse or improve treatment, my research has emphasized the importance of the third variable—the physical and social setting. This work has shown that embedded in the setting in which use takes place are a number of social sanctions and social rituals that influence individuals' decisions to use a particular drug and also the way in which they use it. Social sanctions are the norms and beliefs concerning not only the ways in which a particular drug should be used, but also the ways in which its harmful physiological and psychological effects can be avoided. Rituals are stylized drug-using behaviors and practices, including the means by which the drug is obtained and administered, the physical setting chosen for use, the using circumstances and using companions selected, the user's activities when intoxicated, and any specific activities undertaken after intoxication that the user regards as part of the using process (Harding and Zinberg 1977). For example, a primary sanction of controlled opiate users is "Don't use enough to become addicted," which is reflected by the rituals and behaviors related to frequency and time of use, such as use on weekends only.

Nevertheless, rituals do not act to control use unless they are based on limiting sanctions. Although addicts follow some of the rituals adopted by controlled users, deciding who "gets off" first, sharing "works," "tying off" with belts, or "booting," these rituals do not operate as controls, because they are not grounded in sanctions. On the other hand, the controlled opiate users I have studied have internalized the social sanctions or precepts that tend to control drug use. They are even able to articulate these sanctions, sometimes explicitly and consciously, and sometimes in fragmented form, without conscious knowledge that they are following certain rules.

Thus, social sanctions, internalized by the user, are the predominant sources of control, and rituals buttress, reinforce, and symbolize these sanctions. Rituals and social sanctions seem to function in four distinct ways. The following list explains these functions by referring to my research subjects.

1. Sanctions define moderate use and condemn compulsive use. (Most of my subjects follow sanctions that limit use to frequencies well below those required for addiction. Many have special sanctions, such as "Don't use every day" or "Never use on more than two consecutive days.")

2. Sanctions limit use to physical and social settings that are conducive to a positive or "safe" drug experience. (Some subjects refuse to use in the company of addicts from whom they have bought the drug, and most avoid driving a car when high.)

3. Sanctions and rituals identify potentially untoward drug effects and prescribe precautions to be taken before and during use. (Some subjects minimize the risk of an overdose by using only a portion of their drug and waiting to gauge its effect before taking more. Others avoid mixing certain drugs, boil their works before injection, or refuse to share works.)

4. Sanctions and rituals operate to compartmentalize drug use and support the users' everyday obligations and relationships. (Some subjects avoid using opiates on Sunday night, so that they will not be too tired to go to work on Monday morning. Some carefully budget the amount of money they spend on drugs.)

The process by which controlling rituals and social sanctions are acquired varies from subject to subject. Most users come by them gradually during the course of their drug-using careers. But peer-using groups seem to be the most important source of practices and precepts for safer use. Most of my subjects appear to require the assistance of other controlled users to construct appropriate and effective rituals and sanctions out of the folklore and practices circulating in the various drug-using subcultures (Harding and Zinberg 1977; Zinberg et al. 1977).

Directions for Further Research

Because the samples studied in my DAC and NIDA projects were not random, and there is no assurance that they are representative, they do not provide generalizable data on five important topics: (1) the extent of opiate use; (2) the rapidity with which using patterns change; (3) the relationship of opiate use to other drug use and the stability of that relationship; (4) the connection between opiate use and demonstrable psychological difficulty; and (5) the leading demographic and social characteristics of users. The lack of such knowledge is serious (Heller 1972); it would be extremely helpful both in identifying the difficulties that lead to and result from opiate use and also in deciding public policy issues. It is unfortunately true that the criteria being used in 1978 to determine the extent of opiate use, such as arrest rates, overdose deaths, and applications to treatment programs, relate only to the stereotypical addict and ignore the broad range of users (Greene et al. 1975; Johnson 1977; Weissman and Edie 1976).

The best way to provide information on the first four topics would be to construct and survey a carefully designed random sample of opiate users. The sample would need special construction because, even including the one-time experimenters, opiate users make up only a tiny fraction of the population (Robins et al. 1977). But such survey data would provide little information on the fifth topic, the main characteristics of users: who can use, their degrees of control over use, and how they maintain control (Hunt and Chambers 1976). Only a qualitative and precise study of the concept of control itself could explain why some users do well at maintaining control, while others control their use only moderately well, poorly, or very poorly (Zinberg et al. 1977).

To indicate and understand some of the ways in which control functions, and to test the general applicability of concepts of control, as well as the variations within the range of opiate-using types, information should be gathered on the extent to which all types of users have been exposed, knowingly or unknowingly, to sanctions and rituals and to what degree they have followed them. Information is also needed on the extent to which style of use is affected by background and personality and by the individual's decision to center control outside himself or herself, perhaps by letting someone else keep the drug supply. Groups of addicts, both outside and within treatment programs, should also be investigated, both for the purpose of comparing them with controlled and marginal users and as a potential measure of the social evolution of the drug-using process. Interviews with addicts who have never been in treatment show that they feel greater concern about controlling their use than do those within treatment programs, who hardly believe that control is possible.

Long-term longitudinal studies are needed to investigate these subtle aspects of control. At the same time, such studies could provide information on two other important topics: patterns of drug use and the ability of users to predict their future use patterns.

Longitudinal studies would be useful in measuring the stability of the various drug-using styles and detecting changes in the three basic variables of drug, set, and setting. In such a study, the following kinds of life changes should be considered in relation to their impact on subjects' using patterns: death of mate, spouse, or other family member; change in health; change in job; geographic move; change in schooling; change in friends; change in drug supply; and change in using group or groups. A longitudinal approach which would allow subjects to be interviewed during these life changes or soon after they had occurred would elicit more reliable data than a strictly retrospective approach.

A longitudinal approach could also be used to test the subjects' own predictive abilities. It would indicate how correct subjects are in predicting what their future drug use will be and in projecting the effect of various changes on their use. Simultaneously, it would permit observation of the extent to which subjects' rules for use (social sanctions and rituals) become more internalized and often more conscious.

Public Policy and Education

The review of the existing literature, the research described here, and a spate of personal communications show that not all groups of opiate users become addicts. Until longer-term, more quantitative studies are completed, it is impossible to predict what percentage of experimenters will become addicted and what percentage will not. It is my impression that one of the most critical factors contributing to the development of controlled use, not only of the opiates but of any drug, is the attitudes and values of the larger social setting, which in turn are translated into social sanctions and rituals. In part, these attitudes and values are expressed in public policies and in the education about drug use that is offered by official bodies.

Until now, public policy has been essentially prohibitionist. Grounded in the conviction that all opiate use leads to addiction, and that addiction is the whole problem, it has dealt solely with the fraction

of dysfunctional addicts in the population and has failed to take account of the range of users who are not addicted but are capable of stable, controlled use. Moreover, public policy has been almost exclusively directed toward the drug variable. Policymakers have recommended reducing supplies, so that addicts cannot get their drugs and will be forced into treatment situations, an outcome that is expected to improve the set variable. So far, policy has made only negative use of the setting variable, which admittedly can have either a reinforcing or a restricting effect upon the individual's potential to exercise control. Policymakers, instead of considering the possibility that use can be controlled, have attempted to inhibit all use. While searching for methods of dealing with the heroin issue that would calm public fears, they have failed to realize that their own policy may be stimulating those fears.

If, as I contend, the use of opiates and other illicit drugs is indeed an evolving social process, the recognition that the social setting strongly influences the capacity for control offers an alternative to prohibition. Elements of potential control are active in all groups of opiate users, even among addicts. Many opiate users representing many different styles of use have precepts, however punitive, that dictate how they can use their drug without becoming addicted or suffering physical and psychological damage, or, at least, how they can use the drug in order to get what they desire from it. Is it not possible that using groups will gradually develop these ideas into social sanctions and rituals similar to those that govern acceptable alcohol use (Zinberg et al. 1975)? Although the sample studied in my NIDA project is small, the fact that many of those who fulfilled the project's stringent criteria for controlled use had formerly been addicted suggests the need to consider approaches other than abstinence. For example, assisting the maintenance of controlled use could be a practical means of preventing drug abuse with the least social cost; and experimenting with this alternative in a careful and gradual way would not obstruct the effort to discourage the use of the opiates generally.

If, as I contend, the use of opiates is a socially evolving process in which the social setting variable plays an important part, it is essential to reassess the current treatment programs for addicts. The bulk of these programs has grown out of the public policy decision implicit in the creation of the Special Action Office for Drug Abuse Prevention (SAODAP) in 1971. That policy decision to make drug treatment available to all who needed it may have been a forward step in 1971, but in 1978 it has very different implications.

Recently, Nightingale (1977) reported that, while there are approximately 150,000 to 170,000 persons in treatment and another 100,000 in jail for opiate addiction at any one time, there are "another 300,000 to 400,000 not in treatment, the majority of whom have never been in treatment." This strongly supports the following conclusion of Bourne et al. (1975), regarding opiate use in Wyoming: "Very little is known about the characteristics of undetected opiate users," particularly by official bodies, such as the Drug Enforcement Administration, and treatment programs.

Another even more recent study of treatment programs (Millman and Khuri 1977) also seems to suggest that the way in which opiate users view treatment has changed sufficiently to warrant a reassessment of treatment per se, as well as of the public policies determining its form. In sharp contrast to earlier studies by Vaillant (1966), who found few, if any, seriously emotionally disturbed clients in treatment programs, Millman and Khuri suggest that treatment programs are becoming wastebaskets for those addicts who have been remanded by the law enforcement system or who, because they are also in serious psychological difficulty, are incapable of functioning elsewhere.

If approaches to treatment were to be reassessed from the viewpoint of the social-setting variable, it would first of all be necessary to combat the belief that heroin is "the devil drug." True, heroin is a powerful, highly addictive substance whose potential for individual destruction in this country, as it is now used and as it is now viewed, is enormous. But, like many other drugs used medically, it is deadly only when used improperly. In other countries, such as England and some of the European states, heroin is regarded as medically useful.

At this time, heroin maintenance is not a viable treatment alternative in this country because of the public attitude toward the drug, the well-entrenched black market, the sheer numbers of addicts, and the difficulties of administration. But with a change in public policy, I can imagine a series of small, carefully designed experiments intended to determine whether the many addicts now avoiding treatment could be brought into treatment. Those experiments would try to determine and give to addicts what they want from the street-drug experience, such as getting their preferred drug on a weekend, in the morning, or at night, while maintaining them on oral methadone the rest of the time. It is a measure of our tremendous overconcern with heroin that, during the last 10 years of high levels of addiction, not one small experiment of this kind has been carried out.

The National Institute on Drug Abuse has responded to the slight change in public attitude by funding a study of the efficacy of heroin as an analgesic. If heroin indicates any advantage over other available analgesics for even a small percentage of patients in pain, its use should be permitted. Also, the drug is much favored in other countries as an anti-tussive. The increased medicinal use of heroin, along with its experimental use in drug-treatment programs, would not only add another substance that could be used humanely to alleviate suffering, but would also begin to provide some knowledge of the drug's advantages, disadvantages, and side effects, as well as of individual differences in toleration. Objective knowledge about a drug, whether it is alcohol, strychnine, cortisone, or heroin, enables individuals to decide about its use in a more realistic way than when they are influenced by users, who view it as a god, or by the general public, which views it as a devil. The hyper-emotional atmosphere surrounding the present use of heroin may actually be causing those to try it who can handle it least well.

The use of heroin in the ways just mentioned will only be possible, if the prevailing view about drug use (abstinence versus addiction) can be shaken. The medical profession, in particular, must reassess its position, because its cooperation will be critical in bringing about any change in heroin use and in the public understanding of that use.

My informal survey of medical teaching in this area in 1976 has shown why physicians feel insecure about the illicit drug issue. Every one of the medical lectures and courses I surveyed discussed the various addictions (opiates, barbiturates, alcohol), the noxious sequelae of use of certain drugs (psychedelics, cocaine, amphetamines), and the health hazards surrounding marijuana use. But none of them threw any light on the using patterns that lead to responsible use and even to beneficial relaxation.

Thus, medical education provides physicians with little of the information that they need when called upon to prescribe drugs now used illicitly. It prepares them inadequately for the frequent questions and requests for advice about the use of these drugs. The great majority of doctors seem to have accepted the abstinence-addiction alternative that has led to a prohibitionist public policy, and to be answering the public's questions from that position.

Such a response, in the face of the constantly increasing use of illicit drugs, has shaken public confidence in physicians. Their constant call for abstinence, except in the case of medical use, may even have led to a general weakening of their ability to promulgate social sanctions about drug use in general.

A good example would be the considerable misprescribing of amphetamines and barbiturates by physicians a few years ago. Physicians' overprescribing may well have occurred partly as a defense against patients seeking psychoactive drugs from other sources, or partly as an unconscious, exaggerated response to the lessened power of physicians' instructions, or both. Whatever the specific reasons for the difficulty, the problem not only left the profession generally looking incompetent but, more important, exposed the extent to which most doctors did not understand the management of psychoactive drugs. Broadening physicians' education in this area and enhancing their role as purveyors of moderation, rather than abstinence, may help restore their reputation for wisdom in this field.

A new awareness of the existence of nonaddictive opiate use, of its complexity, and of the need for a broad study of control factors may bring about small changes in public attitudes and may help the medical profession and policymakers to see that the time is ripe for change and experimentation. An investigation of the exercise of control, particularly in relation to social sanctions and rituals, could have far-reaching effects. Long-term studies of controlled use, though considering primarily the opiates and other illicit intoxicants, may also have important implications for alcohol use and many other habitual behaviors.

* * *

Norman E. Zinberg, "Nonaddictive Opiate Use," in Robert I. DuPont, Avram Goldstein, and John O'Donnel (eds.), Handbook on Drug Abuse (Rockville, MD: National Institute on Drug Abuse, 1979), pp. 303-313.

For Discussion

Most of the controlled opiate users were employed in Zinberg's study. How might nonaddictive opiate use be related to employment?

References

Abelson, H. I., and Fishburne, P. M. *Non-medical Use of Psychoactive Substances: 1975/1976 Nationwide Study Among Youth and Adults*. Princeton, NJ: Response Analysis Corporation, 1976.

Abt Associates, Inc. *Drug Use in the State of Ohio: A Study Based Upon the Ohio Drug Survey*. Cambridge, MA: Abt Associates, Inc., 1975.

Alksne, H., Lieberman, L., and Brill, L. A conceptual model of the life cycle of addiction. *Int J Addict, 2*:221-240, 1967.

American Medical Association, Council on Mental Health and Committee on Alcoholism and Drug Dependence. Oral methadone maintenance techniques in the management of morphine-type dependence. *JAMA, 219*:1618-1619, 1972.

Association of the Bar of the City of New York. *Drug Law Evaluation Project*. New York: The Association, 1977.

Blachly, P. H. Naloxone for diagnosis in methadone programs. *JAMA, 224*:334-335, 1973.

Bourne, P. G., Hunt, L. G., and Vogt, J. *A Study of Heroin Use in the State of Wyoming*. Report prepared for Department of Health and Social Services, Wyoming. Washington, DC: Foundation for International Resources, Inc., 1975.

Chambers, C. D., and Inciardi, J. A. An empirical assessment of the availability of illicit methadone. In National Association for the Prevention of Addiction to Narcotics. *Proceedings of the Fourth National Conference on Methadone Treatment*. New York: The Association, 1972.

Chein, I., Gerard, D. L., Lee, R. S., and Rosenfield, E. *The Road to H*. New York: Basic Books, 1964.

Dobbs, W. H. Methadone treatment of heroin addicts. *JAMA, 218*:1536-1541, 1971.

Gay, G. R., Senay, E. C., and Newmeyer, J. A. The pseudo junkie: evolution of the heroin lifestyle in the non-addicted individual. *Anesth Analg, 53*:241-247, 1974.

Glaser, F. B. Psychologic vs. pharmacologic heroin dependence. *N Engl J Med, 290*:231-233, 1974.

Goode, E. *Drugs in American Society*. New York: Knopf, 1972.

Graeven, D. B., and Jones, A. "Addicts and experimenters: dynamics of involvement in an adolescent heroin epidemic." Paper presented at National Drug Abuse Conference, San Francisco, CA, May 1976.

Greene, M., Nightingale, S., and DuPont, R. L. Evolving patterns of drug abuse. *Ann Int Med, 83*:402-411, 1975.

Harding, W. M., and Zinberg, N. E. The effectiveness of the subculture in developing rituals and social sanctions for controlled use. In du Toit, B. M., ed. *Drugs, Rituals, and Altered States of Consciousness*. Rotterdam, Netherlands: A. A. Balkema, pp. 111-133, 1977.

Heller, M. *The Sources of Drug Abuse*. Addiction Services Agency Report. New York: The Agency, 1972.

Hughes, P. H., Crawford, G. A., Barker, N. W., Schumann, S., and Jaffe, J. H. The social structure of a heroin-copping community. *Am J Psychiatry, 128*:43-50, 1971.

Hunt, L. G., and Chambers, C. D. *The Heroin Epidemics: A Study of Heroin Use in the United States, 1965-1975*. New York: Spectrum, 1976.

Johnson, B. D. "Once an addict, seldom an addict." Paper presented at National Drug Abuse Conference, San Francisco, CA, May 1977.

Kersh, E. Narcotic overdosage. *Hosp Med, 10*:3-6. 1974.

Khantzian, E. J. Opiate addiction: a critical assessment of theory and some implications for current treatment approaches. *Am J Psychother,* 28:59-70, 1974.

Khantzian, E. J., Mack, J. E., and Schatzberg, A. F. Heroin use as an attempt to cope: clinical observations. *Am J Psychiatry,* 131:160-164, 1974.

Levengood, R., Lowinger, P., and Schooff, K. Heroin addiction in the suburbs—an epidemiologic study. *Am J Pub Health,* 63:209-213, 1973.

Lewis, R., Gorbach, S., and Altner, P. Spinal pseudomonas, chondro-osteomyelitis in heroin users. *N Engl J Med,* 286:1303-1307, 1972.

Light, R. W., and Dunham, T. R. Vertebral osteomyelitis due to pseudomonas in the occasional heroin user. *JAMA, 228:* 1272-1275, 1974.

Lindesmith, A. R. *Opiate Addiction.* Evanston, IL: Principia, 1957.

Millman, R. B., and Khuri, E. T. "Therapeutic detoxification in an adolescent program." Paper presented at Conference on Recent Developments in Chemotherapy of Narcotic Addiction, sponsored by The New York Academy of Sciences, Washington, DC, November 1977.

Minkowski, W. L., Weiss, R. C., and Heidbreder, G. A. A view of the drug problem: a rational approach to youthful drug use and abuse. *Clin Pediatr, 11:*376-381, 1972.

National Commission on Marijuana and Drug Abuse. *Drug Use in America: Problem in Perspective.* Washington, DC: U.S. Government Printing Office, 1973.

Newman, R. G. Involuntary treatment of drug addiction. In Bourne, P. G., ed. *Addiction.* New York: Academic Press, pp. 174-205, 1974.

Newmeyer, J. Five years after: drug use and exposure to heroin among the Haight-Ashbury free medical clinic clientele. *J Psychedel Drugs,* 6:61-65, 1974.

Nightingale, S. Treatment for drug abusers in the United States. *Addict Dis, 3:*11-20, 1977.

Powell, D. H. Occasional heroin users: a pilot study. *Arch Gen Psychiatry,* 28:586-594, 1973.

Robins, L. N., Heizer, J. E., Hesselbrock, M., and Wish, E. Vietnam veterans three years after Vietnam: how our study changed our view of heroin. In Brill, L., and Winick, C., eds. *Yearbook of Substance Abuse.* New York: Human Sciences Press, in press.

Robins, L. N., and Murphy, G. E. Drug use in a normal population of young Negro men. *Am J Pub Health, 570:*1580-1596, 1967.

Scher, J. M. Group structure and narcotics addiction: notes for a natural history. *Int J Group Psychother, 11:*81-93, 1961.

Vaillant, G. E. A twelve-year follow-up of New York narcotic addicts. IV. Some characteristics and determinants of abstinence. *Am J Psychiatry, 123:*573-584, 1966.

Weissman, J. C., and Edie, C. A. Undetected opiate use in the Southwest: comparison of official opiate-user files and treatment program patient records. *Am J Drug Alcohol Abuse, 3:*235-242, 1976.

Yorke, C. A critical review of some psychoanalytic literature on drug addiction. *Br J Med Psychol, 43:*140-159, 1970.

Zinberg, N. E. Addiction and ego function. *Psychoanal Study Child, 30:*567-588, 1975.

Zinberg, N. E., Harding, W. M., Stelmack, S. M., and Marblestone, R. A. "Patterns of heroin use." Paper presented at Conference on Recent Developments in Chemotherapy of Narcotic Addiction, sponsored by the New York Academy of Sciences, Washington, DC, November 1977.

Zinberg, N. E., Harding, W M., and Winkeller, M. A study of social regulatory mechanisms in controlled illicit drug users. *J Drug Iss,* 7:117-133, 1977.

Zinberg, N. E., Jacobson, R. C., and Harding, W. M. Social sanctions and rituals as a basis for drug-abuse prevention. *Am Drug Alcohol Abuse, 2:*165-181, 1975.

Zinberg, N. E., and Lewis, D. C. Narcotic usage. I. A spectrum of a difficult medical problem. *N Engl J Med, 270:*989-993, 1964. ✦

Part V

Cocaine

Although chewing coca leaves for their mild stimulant effects had been a part of South America's Andean culture for perhaps a thousand years, for some obscure reason the practice had never become popular in either Europe or the United States. During the latter part of the nineteenth century, however, Angelo Mariani of Corsica brought the unobtrusive Peruvian shrub to the notice of the rest of the world. After importing tons of coca leaves to his native land, he produced an extract that he mixed with wine and called *Vin Coca Mariani*. The wine was an immediate success, publicized as a magical beverage that would free the body from fatigue, lift the spirits, and create a lasting sense of well-being. Vin Coca brought Mariani immediate wealth and fame, a situation that did not go unnoticed by John Styth Pemberton of Atlanta, Georgia. In 1885, Pemberton developed a product that he registered as *French Wine Coca—Ideal Nerve and Tonic Stimulant*. It was originally a medicinal preparation, but the following year, he added an additional ingredient, changed it into a soft drink, and renamed it *Coca-Cola*. And although the extracts of coca may have indeed made Pemberton's cola "the real thing," the actual cocaine content of the leaves was (and remains) quite low—one percent or less by weight.

The full potency of the coca leaf had remained unknown until 1859 when cocaine was first isolated in its pure form. Yet little use was made of the new alkaloid until 1883 when Dr. Theodor Aschenbrandt secured a supply of the drug and issued it to Bavarian soldiers during maneuvers. Aschenbrandt, a German military physician, noted the beneficial effects of cocaine, particularly its ability to suppress fatigue. Among those who read Aschenbrandt's account with fascination was a struggling young Viennese neurologist, Sigmund Freud. Suffering from chronic fatigue, depression, and various neurotic symptoms, Freud obtained a measure of cocaine and tried it himself. Finding the initial results to be quite favorable, Freud decided that cocaine was a "magical drug."

In July 1884, less than three months after Freud's initial experiences with cocaine, his first essay on the drug was published. Freud then pressed the drug onto his friends and colleagues, urging that they use it both for themselves and their patients; he gave it to his sisters and his fiancée, and continued to use it himself. By the close of the 1880s, however, Freud and the others who had praised cocaine as an all-purpose wonder drug began to withdraw their support for it in light of an increasing number of reports of compulsive use and undesirable side effects. Yet by 1890, the patent-medicine industry in the United States had also discovered the benefits of the unregulated use of cocaine. The industry quickly added the drug to its reservoir of home remedies, touting it as helpful not only for everything from alcoholism to venereal disease, but also as a cure for addiction to other patent medicines. Since the new tonics contained substantial amounts of cocaine, they did indeed make users feel better, at least initially, thus spiriting the patent-medicine industry into its golden age of popularity.

By the early years of the twentieth century, however, the steady progress of medical science had provided physicians with an even better understanding of the abuse liability of cocaine. In 1906, furthermore, the Pure Food and Drug Act was passed, bringing about a significant decline in the use of cocaine. The use of the drug did not entirely disappear during the early years of the new century. Rather, the drug moved underground, to the netherworlds of crime, the bizarre, and the avant garde, where it remained for some forty years. There, its major devotees included prostitutes, poets, artists, writers, jazz musicians, fortune tellers, and criminals. By the 1950s, cocaine use had spread to such other exotic groups as the "beatniks" of New York's Greenwich Village and San Francisco's North Beach, the movie colony of Hollywood, and to such an extent with the urban "smart set" that coke became known as "the rich man's drug." During the late 1960s and early 1970s, cocaine use began to move from the underground to mainstream society.

At this time, most users viewed cocaine as a relatively "safe" drug. They inhaled it in relatively small quantities, and use typically occurred within a social-recreational context. But as the availability of cocaine increased during the late '60s, so too did the number of users and the mechanisms for ingesting it. Some users began to sprinkle street cocaine on tobacco or marijuana and smoke it as a cigarette or in a pipe, but this method did not produce effects distinctly different from inhalation or "snorting." But a new alternative soon became available, *freebasing*, the smoking of "freebase cocaine."

Freebase cocaine is actually a different chemical product than cocaine itself. In the process of freebasing, street cocaine—which is usually in the form of a hydrochloride salt—is treated with a liquid base (such as ammonia or baking soda) to remove the hydrochloric acid. The free cocaine, or cocaine base (and hence the name "freebase"), is then dissolved in a solvent, such as ether, from which the purified cocaine is crystallized. These crystals are then crushed and used in a special glass pipe. Smoking freebase cocaine provides a more potent rush and a more powerful high than regular cocaine. By 1977, it was estimated that there were some 4,000,000 users of cocaine, with as many as 10 percent of these freebasing the drug exclusively. Yet few outside of the drug-using and drug research and treatment communities were even aware of the existence of the freebase culture. Further, an even lesser number had an understanding of the new complications that freebasing had introduced to the cocaine scene.

The complications are several. First, cocaine in any of its forms is highly seductive. With freebasing, the euphoria is more intense than when the drug is inhaled. Moreover, this intense euphoria subsides into irritable craving after only a few minutes, thus influencing many users to continue freebasing for days at a time—until either they, or their drug supplies, are fully exhausted. Second, the practice of freebasing is expensive. When snorting cocaine, a

single gram can last the social user an entire weekend or longer. With street cocaine ranging in price anywhere from $50 to $200 a gram, depending on availability and purity, even this method of ingestion can be a costly recreational pursuit. Yet with freebasing, the cost factor can undergo a geometric increase. Habitual users have been known to freebase continuously for three or four days without sleep, using up to 150 grams of cocaine in a 72 hour period. Third, one special danger of freebasing is the proximity of highly flammable ether (or rum when it is used instead of water as a coolant in the pipe) to an open flame. This problem is enhanced since the user is generally suffering from a loss of coordination produced by the cocaine or a combination of cocaine and alcohol. As such, there have been many freebasing situations where the volatile concoction has exploded in the face of the user.

Freebasing is but one variety of cocaine smoking. Common in the drug-using communities of Colombia, Bolivia, Venezuela, Ecuador, Peru, and Brazil is the use of coca paste, known to most South Americans as "basuco," "susuko," "pasta basica de cocaina," or just simply "pasta." Coca paste is an intermediate product in the processing of the coca leaf into cocaine. In the initial stages of coca processing, the leaves are pulverized, soaked in alcohol mixed with benzol (a petroleum derivative used in the manufacture of motor fuels, detergents, and insecticides), and shaken. The alcohol/benzol mixture is then drained, sulfuric acid is added, and the solution is shaken again. Next, a precipitate is formed when sodium carbonate is added to the solution. When this is washed with kerosene and chilled, crystals of crude cocaine, or coca paste, are left behind. While the cocaine content of leaves is relatively low—1/2 to 1 percent by weight—paste has a cocaine concentration ranging up to 90 percent, but more commonly about 40 percent. Coca paste is typically smoked straight, or in cigarettes mixed with either tobacco or marijuana.

The smoking of coca paste became popular in South America, beginning in the early 1970s. It was readily available, inexpensive, had a high cocaine content, and was absorbed quickly when smoked. As the phenomenon was studied, however, it was quickly realized that paste smoking was far more serious than any other form of cocaine use. In addition to cocaine, paste contains traces of all the chemicals used to initially process the coca leaves—kerosene, sulfuric acid, methanol, benzoic acid, and the oxidized products of these solvents, plus any number of other alkaloids that are present in the coca leaf. One analysis undertaken in Colombia in 1986 found, in addition to all of these chemicals, traces of brick dust, leaded gasoline, ether, and various talcs.

Beyond coca, cocaine, freebase, basuco, there is also *crack-cocaine*. Contrary to popular belief, crack is not a product of the 1980s. Rather, it was first reported in the literature during the early 1970s. At that time, however, knowledge of crack, known then as "garbage freebase," seemed to be restricted to segments of cocaine's freebasing subculture. Crack is processed from cocaine hydrochloride by using ammonia or baking soda and water, and heating it to remove the hydrochloride. The result is a pebble-sized crystalline form of cocaine base.

Contrary to another popular belief, crack is neither "freebase cocaine" nor "purified cocaine." Part of the confusion about what crack actually is comes from the different ways that the word "freebase" is used in the drug community. "Freebase" (the noun) is a drug, a cocaine product converted to the base state from cocaine hydrochloride *after* adulterants have been chemically removed. Crack is converted to the base state without removing the adulterants. "Freebasing" (the act) means to inhale vapors of cocaine base, of which crack is but one form. Finally, crack is not purified cocaine, since when it is processed the baking soda remains as a salt and reduces the overall purity of the product. And, interestingly, crack gets its name from the fact that the residue of baking soda often causes a crackling sound when heated.

The rediscovery of crack during the early 1980s seemed to occur simultaneously on the East and West Coasts. As a result of the Colombian government's attempts to reduce the amount of illicit cocaine production within its borders, it apparently, at least for a time, successfully restricted the amount of ether available for transforming coca paste into cocaine hydrochloride. The result was the diversion of coca paste from Colombia, through Central America and the Caribbean, into South Florida for conversion into cocaine. Spillage from shipments through the Caribbean Corridor acquainted local island populations with coca paste smoking, which developed the forerunner of crack-cocaine in 1980. Known as "baking-soda base," "base-rock," "gravel," and "roxanne," the prototype was a smokable product composed of coca paste, baking soda, water, and rum. Immigrants from Jamaica, Trinidad, and locations along the Leeward and Windward Islands chain introduced the crack prototype to Caribbean inner-city populations in Miami and New York, where it was ultimately produced from cocaine hydrochloride rather than from coca paste.

Apparently at about the same time, a Los Angeles basement chemist rediscovered the rock variety of baking-soda cocaine, and it was initially referred to as "cocaine rock." It was an immediate success, as was the East Coast type, for a variety of reasons. First, it could be smoked rather than snorted. When cocaine is smoked, it is more rapidly absorbed and reportedly crosses the blood-brain barrier within a few seconds. Hence, an almost instantaneous high. Second, it was cheap. While a gram of cocaine for snorting may cost $50 or more depending on its purity, the same gram can be transformed into any number of "rocks," depending on their size. For the user, this meant that individual "rocks" could be purchased for as little as $2, $5, $10, or $20. For the seller, $50 worth of cocaine hydrochloride (purchased wholesale for $30) could generate as much as $150 when sold as rocks. Third, it was easily hidden and transportable, and when hawked in small glass vials, it could be readily scrutinized by potential buyers.

By the close of 1985, crack had come to the attention of the media and was predicted to be the "wave of the future" among substance abusers. By mid-1986, national headlines were calling crack a glorified version of cocaine and the major street drug of abuse in the United States. There was also the belief that crack was responsible for rising rates of street crime. As a cover story in *USA Today* put it:

> Addicts spend thousands of dollars on binges, smoking the contents of vial after vial in crack or "base" houses—modern-day opium dens—for days at a time without food or sleep. They will do anything to repeat the high, including robbing their families and friends, selling their possessions and bodies.

As the media blitzed the American people with lurid stories depicting the hazards of crack, Congress and the White House began drawing plans for a more concerted war on crack and other drugs. At the same time, crack use was reported in Canada, England, Finland, Hong Kong, Spain, South Africa, Egypt, India, Mexico, Belize, and Brazil.

The following essays and articles examine the history of cocaine, the effects of cocaine use, and patterns of behavior associated with the use of both *powder*-cocaine and *crack*-cocaine. ◆

19. Cocaine: Recreational Use and Intoxication

RONALD K. SIEGEL

Ronald K. Siegel offers a brief history of cocaine use, with early reports suggesting that it was used initially for sustenance. Contemporary research demonstrates that the effects of cocaine are both intoxicating and exhilarating, and that chronic use produces many negative effects. Siegel explores the effects of cocaine in his study of mostly male users with a history of multiple-drug use. He describes drug usage in terms of dosage, and set and setting. Five categories of use are discussed: experimental, social-recreational, circumstantial-situational, intensified, and compulsive. Siegel compares his findings for user groups with the previous literature on cocaine effects.

Cocaine is one of several alkaloids obtained from coca leaves (*Erythroxylon Coca* Lam.). The function of alkaloids in plants is generally unknown, as is the reason plants produce them. Alkaloids taste bitter, often produce numbing sensations, and are physiologically active with psychologic, teratogenic, and toxic effects. They act as extremely effective feeding deterrents; it has been argued that naturally occurring plant drugs, such as cocaine, are justified evolutionarily by their potentially maladaptive effects on herbivores (Bever 1970; Eisner and Halpern 1971). The major questions concerning the use of cocaine alkaloid by humans are: (1) why did man bypass these deterrent effects and initiate use of cocaine; (2) why is use of cocaine maintained; and (3) what are the consequences of such continued use? These questions are addressed in this chapter. It will presently be seen that the psychological intoxication resulting from cocaine use is a primary reason for its continued use. The nature and extent of this intoxication in a group of contemporary users will also be explored. These users reflect social-recreational patterns of intranasal use, and they differ substantially from more compulsive intravenous users.

Discovery and Initial Use

Folklore and mythology are replete with examples of man's discovery of plant alkaloids through observation and modeling of animal behavior (cf., Siegel 1973). The legendary discovery of coffee, purportedly around 900 A.D., was made by an Abyssinian tending his herd of goats. The herder noticed that his animals became abnormally "frisky" after eating the bright red fruit of a tree that was later isolated and identified as coffee (Taylor 1965). In Yemen, another herder discovered that his goats exhibited signs of extraordinary stimulation after eating certain leaves. The shepherd tried the leaves himself and found them quite stimulating, even after a day's work. Since that time, the use of those leaves (qat leaves which contain the alkaloids cathine, cathedine, and cathenine) has spread through the entire country (Abdo Abbasy 1957).

Similarly, several stories are told of coca's discovery based on modeling of animal behaviors. One story—told by an informant from Huanuco, Peru—claims that coca was first used by pack animals traveling in the mountains and deprived of their normal forage. The coca leaves sustained the animals, and humans quickly copied the coca-eating behavior. Indeed, Mortimer (1901; reprinted 1974) notes that coca was used by man, and perhaps by beast, when traveling in the mountains, where ingestion was probably induced by irregular eating, improper diet, and lack of oxygen at higher altitudes. Such use is similar to that of peyote used in small doses by Huichol Indians traveling in the Sierra Madre mountains of Mexico (Lumholtz 1902). Recent nutritional analysis has revealed that, since 100 grams of coca leaves contains 305 calories, 18.9 grams of protein, and 46.2 grams of carbohydrates, and satisfies the Recommended Dietary Allowance for calcium, iron, phosphorus, vitamins A, B_{12}, and E (Duke et al. 1975), the coca leaves could, indeed, have sustained Peruvian travelers. However, the full complement of nutrients present in coca leaf may not be fully absorbed in the normal chewing-sucking extraction employed by man.

Another story, told by informants from Cuzco and Lima, Peru, claims that a number of birds and insects are fond of coca seeds and leaves and the speed with which they devour the plant suggested the stimulant properties to early man. Mortimer (1901; reprinted 1974) indicated that ants and other insects avidly devoured the leaves, but there was no indication of psychoactive effects from this ingestion. However, he did note that "the birds are great lovers of coca seeds, and when these are lightly sown on the surface of the nursery, it is necessary to cover the beds at night with cloths to guard against 'picking and stealing'. . . ." One may speculate that early man modeled his coca use after such observations, much like the Greeks who adopted the habit of eating hempseeds—and, later, other parts of the cannabis plant—after watching finches do so (Schultes 1970).

Man's inevitable ecological encounters with coca would have brought him into contact with the highly reinforcing properties of the cocaine alkaloid. Independent of the nutritional value, the psychoactive effects are considerably more direct and immediate. Animal studies are rich with examples of cocaine's powerful psychoactive and reinforcing effects (cf., Preclinical Behavior, Chapter 4). Lewin (1931) reports a case of an animal modeling human use:

> The case is, however, on record of a monkey which became a cocaine-eater through imitation. . . . The animal searched the pockets and the cupboards of its mistress for cocaine, which it voraciously consumed. The consequences were the same as in man.

Maintenance of Use

These consequences or effects are undoubtedly responsible for maintaining cocaine use. The effects can be interpreted as a state of intoxication with high reinforcement potential. Indeed, animals, such as rats and monkeys, having once experienced unlimited access to cocaine, will self-administer the drug until they die, often ignoring food and water. While many non-pharmacologic factors (e.g., individual and environmental variables) may affect man's use of a drug, such as cocaine, psychological intoxication appears to be the primary reinforcing effect.

Freud described the intoxication in *Uber Coca*, his famous 1884 monograph on coca:

> The psychic effect [of cocaine] consists of exhilaration and lasting euphoria, which does not differ in any way from the normal euphoria of a healthy person. . . . One senses an increase of self-control and feels more vigorous and more capable of work; on the other hand, if one works, one misses the heightening of the mental powers which alcohol, tea, or coffee induce. One is simply normal, and soon finds it difficult to believe that one is under the influence of any drug at all. . . . Long-lasting, intensive mental or physical work can be performed without fatigue; it is as though the need for food and sleep, which otherwise makes itself felt peremptorialy (sic) at

certain times of the day, were completely banished. (Byck 1974)

Aleister Crowley (1917) offers a more romantic description of cocaine intoxication:

> The melancholy vanishes, the eyes shine, the wan mouth smiles. Almost manly vigor returns, or seems to return. At least faith, hope and love throng very eagerly to the dance; all that was lost is found. . . . To awe the drug may bring liveliness, to another languor, to another creative force, to another tireless energy, to another glamour, and to yet another lust. But each in his way is happy. Think of it!—so simple and so transcendental! The man is happy!

Throughout the 19th and 20th centuries, the literature on coca and cocaine contained many references to the reinforcing nature of this intoxication. Even current patterns of recreational use appear to be initiated and maintained by the psychoactive effects (Phillips 1975). A number of recent studies of cocaine users have confirmed the experience of positive drug effects which appear to maintain continued use. Ashley (1975) interviewed and observed 81 cocaine users and found that they experienced euphoria, sexual stimulation, increased energy, and a reduction in fatigue and appetite. In another study of 17 cocaine users, Grinspoon and Bakalar (1976) reported additional phenomenological data on the intoxication, and these authors emphasized their agreement with reports from literary sources and other studies.

In yet another interview study with 32 intranasal cocaine users, the subjective effects reported included a subtle exhilaration, increased energy and sociability, and a pleasant feeling of well-being and mastery (Waldorf, pers. comm. 1976).

Consequences of Continued Use

Despite the obvious appeal and romantic attraction of this state of intoxication, the consequences of continued use have been the subject of over a century of research and debate. Most researchers agree that the pleasurable effects diminish with continued use and are replaced by an increasing number of adverse effects which can only be alleviated through its cessation. Crowley (1917, reprinted 1973) describes this state in a highly stylized account:

> But to one who abuses cocaine for his pleasure, nature soon speaks and is not heard. The nerves weary

of the constant stimulation; they need rest and food. There is a point at which the jaded horse no longer answers whip and spur. He stumbles, falls a quivering heap, gasps out his life. . . . So perishes the slave of cocaine. With every nerve clamoring, all he can do is to renew the lash of the poison. The pharmaceutical effect is over; the toxic effect accumulates. The nerves become insane. The victim begins to have hallucinations. . . . And alas! The power of the drug diminishes with fearful pace. The doses wax; the pleasures wane. Side-issues, invisible at first, arise; they are like devils with flaming pitchforks in their hands. (Crowley 1917)

Unfortunately, the language of this passage and others like it, with its connotations of cocaine addiction and psychosis, have influenced many of the medical and scientific opinions to date. With a similar "data base" of self-experimentation, Freud described the state as one of agitation characterized by persecution and hallucinations, but he used less emotional language for his observations (Freud, 1887). Others call the condition one of "delirium" (e.g., Mantegazza 1859) or "extreme alarm due to false impressions" (Lewin 1931). Still others write about mania and psychoses (cf., Grinspoon and Bakalar 1976). But for most, the critical diagnostic features of this state are the hallucinations, and the presence of tactile hallucinations are the most conspicuous.

One of the more consistent findings is that continued use is associated with tactile hallucinations of animals moving in the skin, or bugs or insects moving under the skin. This phenomenon was described by Magnan and Saury (1889) and has since been known as "Magnan's sign" or "cocaine bugs." Magnan and Saury noted that these symptoms are the first hallucinatory phenomena to develop with chronic use while hallucinations of sight, hearing, and smell come later. Although Magnan's sign and allied symptoms are usually associated with chronic use, a number of hallucinatory experiences have been reported with large acute doses of cocaine (e.g., Mortimer 1901; reprinted 1974; Eggleston and Hatcher 1919). According to Magnan and Saury, the hallucinations subsequently lead to difficulties in thinking and orientation.

Indeed, the diagnosis of psychosis often emerges from the presence of these tactile sensations, independent of other changes. But psychosis involves more than hallucinations and usually implies dysfunction in an individual's mental processes, emo-

tional responses, memory, communication skills, sense of reality, and behavior. Furthermore, psychosis is often characterized by regressive behavior, inappropriate mood, diminished impulse control and delusional thinking (cf., American Psychiatric Association 1969). The presence of such a wide range of phenomena in cocaine intoxication is less clear than the presence of hallucinations. Indeed, descriptions of cocaine hallucinations often include references to clear mental ability (e.g., Mantegazza 1859).

Variables Affecting Use and Intoxication

The precise description of this state of cocaine intoxication requires information about concomitant variations between the characteristics of the behavior and of the drug. Information about the behaviors should be specific with respect to individual variability, type of behavior, and behavioral history. Information about the drug should be specific with respect to dose, adulterants, routes of administration, dose-response, and time-response relations, among others. Such variables can be further modified by environmental variables, such as set and setting. While a full understanding of these interactions is presently restricted by the limited knowledge about cocaine, the presence of such a myriad of interacting variables should temper a desire to simplify use and intoxication with succinct labels, such as "euphoria," "mania," or "psychosis." The study described below was undertaken in an attempt to elucidate some of these variables in relation to the psychological intoxication.

The Sample

A large population of recreational drug users, recruited through advertisements in several Los Angeles-area newspapers, was initially screened by a telephone interview and a subsequent drug-history questionnaire. A total of 85 social-recreational cocaine users were eventually selected for the study. All subjects in the sample met the initial requirement of having used a minimum of 1 gram of cocaine per month for 12 months (range = 1-4 grams). All subjects were male, 21-38 years old, and were examined and tested in the Neuropsychiatric Institute at UCLA. Examination procedures included a personal-history questionnaire, drug-history questionnaire, mental-status examination, Minnesota Multiphasic Personality Inventory (MMPI), Experiential World Inventory (EWI) (El-Meligi and Osmond 1970), in-depth interview, physical examination (for most subjects), and visual imagery and perception tests. Two additional groups of subjects were recruited for interview and questionnaire study only. One group consisted of 14 female social-recreational users, who all satisfied the 1-gram-per-month minimum requirement. The second group consisted of both male and female experimental users (n=19), who had only used cocaine 10 times or fewer with a total intake of no more than 1 gram.

Unless otherwise specified, the data discussed below are from the group of 85 male social-recreational users.

Preparations and Purity

All subjects used the hydrochloride salt of cocaine available through illicit markets. The LAC-USC Medical Center street-drug analysis laboratory has found that the average purity of street cocaine in the Los Angeles area is 63 percent (Montgomery, personal communication 1976). Another street-drug assay laboratory in Northern California (Pharm Chem, Palo Alto) found that the average street cocaine was 53 percent for samples received in that area. The most common adulterants in these samples are sugars (lactose, mannitol, and inositol); local anesthetics (procaine, lidocaine, benzocaine, and tetracaine); and, albeit rarely, other drugs (amphetamine, caffeine, phencyclidine, acetaminophen, salicylamide, pemoline, and heroin). Several other non-drug adulterants may be present, such as flour and talc, but analysis for these is rarely done (Perry 1974). Of the 85 subjects, 4 had used the free base of cocaine (primarily for smoking, as discussed below), while 6 had occasionally chewed coca leaves, primarily during travels in South America.

Multiple Drug Use

All subjects had histories of multiple drug use. Concomitant with their use of cocaine, 85 percent were using alcohol; 66 percent, cannabis preparations; 57 percent, caffeine (coffee, tea, chocolate, and cola beverages); 8 percent, amphetamines; and 5 percent, hallucinogens other than cannabis. Surprisingly, the figure for caffeine is considerably below national averages, which are estimated to be as high as 90 percent for adults (Gilbert 1976). It is possible that this represents a substitution of cocaine for caffeine as a stimulant of choice. Further-

more, caffeine interacts with drugs that affect neural transmission, and this interaction with cocaine may have undesirable or non-preferred effects on users.

Prior to their cocaine use, subjects reported experiences with amphetamines and related stimulants (27 percent), barbiturates (20 percent), hallucinogens other than cannabis (10 percent), and opiates (2 percent). All subjects had tried cannabis in the past.

During the 12-month period of the survey, all 85 subjects reported that cocaine was their recreational drug of choice, and 73 subjects identified themselves as regular cocaine users and only casual users of other drugs. The average frequency of drug use per week was: caffeine, 5x; cocaine, 3x; alcohol, 2x; and marijuana or other cannabis preparations, 0.25x (1/4x).

Routes of Administration

All subjects employed the intranasal route of self-administration, while a few (n=12) had also experimented with smoking cocaine on tobacco or marijuana cigarettes and chewing coca leaves (n=6). One subject had several experiences with intravenous, intramuscular, and subcutaneous injections of cocaine. Four subjects had experimented with topical applications of cocaine to the genitalia.

Dosages

When cocaine was used intranasally, subjects self-administered one "cokespoonful" per nostril or one "line" per nostril. The amount of pure pharmaceutical cocaine hydrochloride (crushed, flaky crystals) in commercially available "cokespoons" has been determined to range from 5-10 mg for a level cokespoon. Assuming an average street purity of roughly 58 percent, this amounts to an average intranasal dose of 8.7 mg (total for both nostrils) per administration. The average "line" of cocaine is about 1/8 inch wide by 1 inch long (Gottlieb 1976) and amounts to approximately 25 mg of cocaine, if pure, or 14.5 mg of cocaine, if street cocaine. When cocaine hydrochloride was used for smoking, small amounts were placed on the burning end of a marijuana or tobacco cigarette or sprinkled throughout the cigarette. When cocaine base was used with tobacco or marijuana for smoking, users distributed approximately 1/3 gram of base throughout a cigarette for each person smoking (cf. Siegel et al. 1976). Cocaine base is an intermediate compound in the manufacture of the hydrochloride salt and is less susceptible to decomposition upon heating. It can be re-obtained from street cocaine via simple chemical procedures.

Dose Regimes

While subjects in this sample used 1-4 grams of cocaine per month, doses were not evenly distributed across time. Generally, subjects purchased cocaine in gram quantities, sometimes referred to as "bindles" or "spoons," although a spoon could vary from 0.5 to 2.0 grams (Lee 1976). This amount was generally consumed in less than one week (49 percent); some subjects used it within two days (34 percent). When cocaine was used intranasally, most subjects repeated the self-administration an average of 3 times per night, usually at 15 or 30 minute intervals (range = 10 minutes to 2 hours). When cocaine base was used for smoking, a cigarette containing approximately 1 gram of cocaine base was smoked by two or three persons over an average period of four hours.

Patterns of Use

The dose regimes, together with the set and setting, define the pattern of drug use. Five patterns of drug use have been designated by The National Commission on Marijuana and Drug Abuse (1973) and will be used for discussion here.

Experimental Use

The group of 19 subjects, classified as experimental users, engaged in short-term, non-patterned trials of cocaine with varying intensity and a maximum frequency of 10 times (or a total intake of less than 1 gram). These users were primarily motivated by curiosity about cocaine and a desire to experience the anticipated drug effects of euphoria, stimulation, and enhanced sexual motivation. Their use was generally social and among close friends. Only four of these individuals purchased their own cocaine, and these, together with two subjects given gifts of cocaine, were the only ones who engaged in individual (non-social) trials. Most (68 percent) expressed a desire to use cocaine more often but were restricted by economic and supply considerations. The remainder (32 percent) experienced little or no drug effect and felt no desire to continue use. Interestingly, most of the experimental users endorsed the street myth that cocaine is a subtle drug (cf.,

Phillips 1975), but only those individuals who expressed a desire to continue cocaine use also believed that cocaine gives a "kick" or "rush." This latter finding suggests the importance of psychological set in determining drug reactions.

Social-Recreational Use

All 85 subjects in the formal study were classified as social-recreational users who engaged in more regular use than experimenters. Use generally occurred in social settings among friends or acquaintances who wished to share an experience perceived by them as acceptable and pleasurable. These users were primarily motivated by social factors, and their use was always voluntary. It did not tend to escalate to more individually oriented patterns of uncontrollable use. Many of these subjects started as experimental users and many (71 percent) engaged in episodes of more frequent use (see below), although their primary pattern was social-recreational. Most (75 percent) purchased their own cocaine, while the remainder shared use with others in social settings. All 85 subjects experienced drug effects and varying degrees of intoxication (described below).

When asked to rank all drugs in terms of recreational drugs of choice, all users ranked cocaine first. However, when asked to rank all drugs used in terms of potency in producing euphoria and ecstasy, 69 percent of the males and 95 percent of the females ranked cocaine first. Other drugs ranked above cocaine in this category included LSD, marijuana, and methamphetamine. Nonetheless, cocaine retained popularity as a recreational drug of choice for these reasons:

1. Cocaine was viewed by users as a social drug which facilitated social behavior. Conversely, LSD and marijuana were generally viewed as individually-oriented and asocial drugs.

2. Cocaine was viewed by users as the "ideal" drug, in terms of convenience of use, minimal bulk, rapid onset of effects, minimal duration of action with few side effects, a high degree of safety, and no after effects.

3. Cocaine was viewed by users as an exotic drug which had appeal because of its rarity, high price, and historical-contemporary associations with popular and often high-status folk heroes.

In connection with this latter attitude, users spent an average of $30 on cocaine paraphernalia during the period surveyed, compared to only $4 on marijuana paraphernalia. While cokespoons, vials, mirrors, and other cocaine paraphernalia are more expensive than marijuana rolling papers or pipes, users consistently claimed that the cocaine paraphernalia was not essential to their drug use, but represented a desire to share in the illicit status associated with such devices.

Undoubtedly, these attitudes contributed to stable patterns of social-recreational use which did not escalate to individually oriented patterns of uncontrollable use. In addition, most users felt that the high cost and inconsistent quality of street cocaine, together with the short duration of action, were rate-limiting determinants of cocaine use. They also felt that cocaine was not addictive, except perhaps with intravenous use, and thus, social-recreational intranasal use would not result in escalating patterns of use. A number of these subjects were re-interviewed at various times during the months following this study, and none of them manifested any signs of increased usage.

Circumstantial-Situational Use

Approximately 53 percent of the males engaged periodically in circumstantial-situational use, defined as a task-specific, self-limited use, which was variably patterned, differing in frequency, intensity, and duration. This use was motivated by a perceived need or desire to achieve a known and anticipated drug effect deemed desirable to cope with a specific condition or situation. The motivations cited by male users, in order of decreasing frequency, were: to increase performance at work (89 percent); to enhance mood during periods of situational depression (69 percent); and to enhance performance at play (e.g., sports, hiking, sex) (42 percent). Approximately 68 percent of the females engaged in situational use, and they cited the following motivations: to enhance mood (90 percent); to increase performance at work (particularly housework) (90 percent); to suppress appetite (60 percent); and to enhance sexual performance (20 percent).

Intensified Drug Use

Fifteen males (18 percent) and two females (14 percent) engaged in intensified use characterized by long-term patterned use of at least once a day. Such use was motivated chiefly by a perceived need to achieve relief from a persistent problem or stressful situation or a desire to maintain a certain self-prescribed level of performance. Nonetheless, users here still referred to their intensified use as "runs" or "binges"—terms normally used for periods of repeated dosing found in all groups of cocaine users. Only this group of intensified users reported hallucinations (discussed below) and tolerance to behavioral effects. Tolerance was chiefly reported as a lessening in perceived stimulation and anti-fatigue effects, with no loss in euphoric effects. While behavioral tolerance to cocaine has been demonstrated in three animal species (Matsuzaki et al. 1976; Moerschbaecher 1976; Whyte 1976; Thompson, in press), reports of tolerance in man are still purely anecdotal at this time (cf., Grinspoon and Bakalar 1976).

Compulsive Drug Use

None of the subjects studied engaged in compulsive use, which is characterized by high-frequency and high-intensity levels of relatively long duration, producing some degree of psychological dependence.

Phenomonology and Incidence of Intoxication Effects

The acute physiological and psychoactive effects reported by social-recreational users did not differ substantially from those described in the historical literature or elsewhere in this volume (cf., Byck and Van Dyke, Chapter 5). Briefly, subjects repeatedly sought and experienced euphoria (100 percent), stimulation (82 percent), reduced fatigue (70 percent), diminished appetite (67 percent), garrulousness (59 percent), sexual stimulation (13 percent), increased mental ability (12 percent), alertness (7 percent), and increased sociability (6 percent). A number of untoward effects were also reported by users: restlessness (70 percent), anxiety (34 percent), hyperexcitability (28 percent), irritability (16 percent), and paranoia (5 percent). Taken together, individuals reported experiencing some positive effects in all intoxications and negative or untoward effects in only 3 percent of the intoxications.

The chronic effects reported by these social-recreational users were also similar to those reported elsewhere (Grinspoon and Bakalar 1976). In addition to acute intoxication phenomena, users experienced both desired and undesired effects. The desired effects included: a generalized feeling of increased energy (65 percent), increased sensitivity to acute effects of cocaine (60 percent), and weight loss (21 percent). The undesired effects included: nervousness and irritability (44 percent), perceptual disturbances (44 percent), nasal problems (28 percent), fatigue or lassitude when effects wore off (26 percent), and situational sexual impotency (4 percent). Overall, chronic positive or desired effects were experienced in all intoxications, while negative effects were experienced in approximately 5 percent of the intoxications.

Perceptual Changes

Of the phenomena reported above, the perceptual changes are perhaps the least understood but also among the most important in understanding the precise nature and form of cocaine intoxication. Indeed, Post (1975) has suggested that cocaine users may manifest an orderly progression of clinical syndromes, including euphoria, dysphoria and paranoid psychosis. Furthermore, the presence of perceptual changes, including hallucinations, are key diagnostic criteria in the determination of the psychotic phase. Therefore, these perceptual changes were the subject of concentrated examination and testing in the study.

A total of 37 subjects (44 percent) experienced some perceptual phenomena, consisting chiefly of increased sensitivity to light, halos around bright lights, and difficulty in focusing the eyes. Some of these subjects were experiencing chronic mydriasis, caused by cocaine-induced enhancement of norepinephrine, tonically released from sympathetic fibers that innervate the radial muscle of the iris (Woods and Downs 1973). The mydriasis may have contributed to these perceptual effects. Several users also experienced exophthalmos (protrusion of the eyeball) and cycloplegia (paralysis of the ciliary muscle of the eye), which may have further contributed to these effects.

All 37 subjects of this subsample experienced some lapses of attention, but only 16 of these reported any difficulty in thinking associated with such changes. Such experiences included difficulty in maintaining attention during complicated tasks; difficulty in maintaining thoughts during conversation; and general preoccupation with personal problems. These effects are similar to what Post (1975) has described as "inability to concentrate," a component of cocaine dysphoria.

A total of 15 subjects (18 percent) reported hallucinatory experiences in several modalities, including vision, touch, smell, hearing, and taste. These phenomena were first noticed after approximately six months of recreational use, and subjects usually became aware of them only during episodes of intensified use. Subjects described these events as pseudohallucinations, lacking the concomitant delusion that such events really existed. Pseudohallucinations are characteristic of many drug intoxications (e.g., marijuana) and differ from psychotic or true hallucinations which are accompanied by delusions or beliefs that the perceptions are real (Siegel and Jarvik 1975).

Visual

Thirteen subjects (15 percent) reported visual hallucinations associated with the use of cocaine. Effects were reported both with the eyes open and closed. In the eyes-open condition, subjects reported the sensation of object movement in their peripheral visual fields. For example, subjects stated, "Something just went by the corner of my eye," "Something just flew by," "I feel like something or someone just moved over there," etc. In dim illumination or with eyes closed, these sensations of movement were extremely weak and often appeared only as flashes or spots of light (cf., Wilson 1973). Indeed, several subjects coined the phrase "snow lights" to indicate the origin and nature of these events. Snow lights were described as similar to, but less intense than, the twinkling of sunlight as it is reflected from frozen snow crystals. They were also described as similar to the sparkling of cocaine (i.e., "snow") crystals.

During later stages of use, subjects reported seeing geometric patterns in their peripheral visual field, usually only with open eyes. These patterns were usually black and white and were composed of straight lines, points, and curves. Patterns reported by subjects included stars, stripes, zigzags, herringbones, checkerboards, and lattices. Such patterns are virtually identical to those patterns seen as normal entopic phenomena, as well as those experienced in states of migraine. Subjects did not report "complex" hallucinations of fully formed or recognizable objects, although such reports are found in the literature (Woods and Downs 1973).

Four subjects reported occasional polyopia. For example, one subject saw a duplication of a painting hanging on the wall, another subject claimed that a telephone dial appeared to have hundreds of holes, etc. Three subjects experienced the rare phenomenon of dysmegalopsia, including micropsia and macropsia, in which objects and people appeared distorted in size. Only the subjects who smoked cocaine base or injected cocaine had any dysmorphopsia. The single subject who injected cocaine reported seeing an ashtray change into a frying pan and then into a chicken! The phenomena of polyopia, dysmegalopsia, and dysmorphopsia are described by Kluver (1942) as appearing in incipient toxic psychoses, as well as in cocaine intoxication. Such phenomena are also common in other states of central nervous system excitation where zoopsia—or hallucination of animals—are conspicuous (Wolf and Curran 1935; Feldman and Sender 1970; Ey 1973).

Tactile

Eleven subjects reported tactile hallucinations after several days of intensified use. These hallucinations included, in order of occurrence: itching of the skin, primarily of the hands but also including legs and back; the sensation of "moving itches" or foreign particles moving under the skin; the sensation of small insects moving under or on the skin, primarily confined to the face and hands but including all parts of the body; and the sensation of objects or people brushing against the body. None of the subjects reported any concomitant visual hallucinations; nor did they believe that insects or objects were actually present, although they often scratched or rubbed the skin. Thus, the phenomena seen here appear to be simple pseudohallucination. Interestingly, one subject who had experience with smoking opium and the consequent itching associated with opium-induced histamine release found the cocaine experience identical. S.A.K. Wilson (1955) describes this paresthesia of pricking, "working" or "crawling" under the skin, as eventually developing into hallucinations of sight and hearing. However, none of the survey subjects experienced this development. Subjects always described the tactile sensations in terms of the similes "like," "as if," or "it is as though," and they insisted that they never suffered from the delusion that insects were, in fact, really present.

Olfactory

Six subjects reported olfactory hallucinations. In most instances, subjects interpreted the perception of smell and odors which were not consensually validated as simply an increased awareness or sensitivity to smells actually present. Smells reported included smoke, gasoline, natural gas, feces, urine, and garbage. At the time of examination, three of these subjects had noticeable rhinitis (inflamed nasal mucous membranes), while a fourth had several sores and scars on the interior nares. Such damage to the nasal mucosa may also have caused degenerative changes in olfactory receptors, leading to abnormal firings (input) to the olfactory bulb. The presence of "bad" or "foul" odors is strikingly similar to those odors which precede uncinate fits which are also linked to olfactory receptors as well as abnormal brain activity.

Auditory

Three subjects reported auditory hallucinations. One of these experienced recurrent perceptions of a voice calling his name when he was alone in the house. Another subject occasionally heard a noise "like" whispering which appeared to come from fans and ventilation ducts. The third subject heard whispering while lying in bed alone at night. These whisperings, while unintelligible, often kept the subject awake. Interestingly, he interpreted the noises as "the sound of coke."

Gustatory

Three subjects reported strong gustatory (taste) hallucinations occurring during acute intoxications. In every case, these were negative hallucinations—the subjects failed to detect strong tastes in foods and drinks, tastes which others could readily perceive. Such negative hallucinations may be associated with olfactory changes, as well as with attentional dysfunction.

Hallucinosis or Psychosis?

Taken together, the results of this study of perceptual changes in users suggest an orderly progression of hallucinations from simple "snow lights" through geometric forms to tactile sensations. The subjects frequently described the "snow lights" and geometric patterns as being "like" insects, especially in their darting and fleeting movements. Unlike previous accounts of "cocaine bugs," subjects did not see insects but did feel itches and other sensations which were "like" insects crawling on the skin. Nevertheless, none of the subjects, while manifesting these behaviors, showed any abnormal profiles on either the MMPI or the EWI. Indeed, the EWI scales indicated some elevation of sensory perception scales with no concomitant elevation of time perception, body perception, self-perception, perception of others, ideation, dysphoria, or impulse regulation (El-Meligi and Osmond 1970). This latter configuration would seem to indicate that the reported phenomenology may be simply an acute psychopharmacologic effect of cocaine and not a symptom of incipient psychosis. Since the dysphoria generally seen in the development of cocaine clinical syndromes (Post 1975) was not present here, it is also possible that the recreational doses and patterns of use reflected in this population of subjects were insufficient to produce psychosis. Thus, the perceptual changes suggest only the presence of an hallucinosis, events which users found to be transient and which disappeared when they went from periods of intensified use back to more moderate social-recreational use.

Overview

The initial use of cocaine by humans appears to have been the result of accidental self-administration of coca, perhaps modeled from animal use of the coca plant. Early coca use was initially maintained by nutritional and psychoactive effects, which were instrumental in sustaining work activity. Use of cocaine itself in the 19th and 20th centuries was primarily maintained by the reinforcement value of the intoxication state itself. This state is characterized by euphoria and stimulation. Contemporary experimental use appears to be initiated by a curiosity about the drug and a desire to experience the effects of euphoria and stimulation. Use among social-recreational users is maintained by the social sharing of this highly pleasurable experience. Some negative effects are also reported among this group, and these include irritability, perceptual disturbance, nasal problems, and fatigue. When use is intensified, negative effects, particularly perceptual changes, are more noticeable. Such perceptual changes, which include "snow lights" and geometric patterns in the visual modality, are pseudohallucinations which users can accurately judge as unreal. Magnan's sign, or "cocaine bugs," appear to be little more than tactile sensations of itching. Among social-recreational users, these pseudohallucinatory events appear to be more acute psychopharmacologic effects than signs of incipient psychosis. Psychometric instruments failed to detect the pres-

ence of dysphoria or psychosis in this population. Adverse effects, including perceptual disturbances, seem to disappear when use is shifted from intensified patterns back to more moderate recreational regimes. In this sense, users are capable of titrating their doses, so as to circumvent adverse reactions. An important caveat is that these effects are neither uniformly negative nor uniformly predictable. The number of variables affecting their production is presently unknown.

* * *

Ronald K. Siegel, "Cocaine: Recreational Use and Intoxication," in Robert C. Petersen and Richard C. Stillman (eds.), *Cocaine: 1977* (Rockville, MD: National Institute on Drug Abuse, 1977), pp. 119-136.

For Discussion

How might the set and setting have different effects for male and female cocaine users?

References

Abdo Abbasy, M. The habitual use of "qat." *Internationales Journal fur Prophylaktische Medizin und Sozialhygiene, 1*:20-22 (1957).

American Psychiatric Association. *American Psychiatric Glossary*. Washington, DC: American Psychiatric Association, 1969.

Ashley, R. *Cocaine. Its History, Uses, and Effects*. New York: St. Martin's Press, 1975.

Bever, O. Why do plants produce drugs? Which is their function in the plants? *Quarterly Journal of Crude Drug Research, 10*:1541-1549 (1970).

Crowley, A. *Cocaine*. San Francisco, CA: Level Press, 1973.

Duke, J. A., Aulik, D., and Plowman, T. Nutritional value of coca. *Botanical Museum Leaflets*, Harvard University, *24*(6):113-119 (1975).

Eggleston, C. and Hatcher, R. A. A further contribution to the pharmacology of the local anesthetics. *Journal of Pharmacology and Experimental Therapeutics, 13*:433-487 (1919).

Eisner, T., and Halpern, B. P. Taste distortion and plant palatability. *Science, 172*:1362 (1971).

El-Meligi, L. M., and Osmond, H. *Manual for the Clinical Use of the Experiential World Inventory*. New York: Mens Sana Publishing, 1970.

Ey, H. *Traite des hallucinations*. Volume 1. Paris, France: Masson et Cie, 1973.

Feldman, M., and Bender, M. B. Visual illusions and hallucinations in parieto-occipital lesions of the brain. In Keup, W. (ed.), *Origin and Mechanisms of Hallucinations*. New York: Plenum Press, 1970, pp. 23-35.

Freud, S. *Uber Coca*. In Byck, R. (ed.), *Cocaine Papers: Sigmund Freud*. New York: Stonehill Publishing Co., 1974, pp. 49-73.

Freud, S. Contributions about the applications of cocaine. *Second Series*. I. Remarks on craving for and fear of cocaine, with reference to a lecture by W. L. Hammond. In Byck, R. (ed.), *Cocaine Papers: Sigmund Freud*. New York: Stonehill Publishing Co., 1974, pp. 171-176.

Gilbert, R. M. Caffeine as a drug of abuse. In Gibbins, R. J., Israel, Y., Kalant, H., Popham, R. E., Schmidt, W., and Smart, R. G. (eds.), *Research Advances in Alcohol and Drug Problems*. Volume III. New York: John Wiley and Sons, 1976, pp. 49-176.

Gottlieb, A. *The Pleasures of Cocaine*. San Francisco, CA: Golden State Publishing Company, 1976.

Grinspoon, L., and Bakalar, J. B. *Cocaine: A Drug and its Social Evolution*. New York: Basic Books, 1976.

Kluver, H. Mechanisms of hallucinations. In McNemar, Q., and Merrill, M. A. (eds.), *Studies in Personality*. New York: McGraw Hill, 1942, pp. 175-207.

Lee, D. *Cocaine Consumer's Handbook*. San Francisco, CA: And/Or Press, 1976.

Lewin, L. *Phantastica. Narcotic and Stimulating Drugs*. London, England: Kegan Paul, Trench, Trubner and Co., 1931.

Lusholtz, C. *Unknown Mexico*. Volume 1. New York: Scribner, 1902.

Magnan et Saury. Trois cas de cocainisme chronique. *Comptes Rendus des Seances de la Societe de Biologie, 1*(4):60-63 (1889).

Mantegazza, P. On the hygienic and medicinal virtues of coca. In Andrews, G., and Solomon, D. (eds.), *The Coca Leaf and Cocaine Papers*. New York: Harcourt Brace Jovanovich, 1975, pp. 38-42.

Matsuzaki, M., Spingler, P. J., Misra, A. L., and Mule, S. J. Cocaine: Tolerance to its convulsant and cardiorespiratory stimulating effects in the monkey. *Life Sciences, 19*:193-204 (1976).

Moerschbaecher, J. M. Repeated acquisition and performance of conditional discriminations as a behavioral baseline for studying drug effects. (Doctoral dissertation, American University, 1976). *Dissertation Abstracts International, 37*:1009B (1976). (University Microfilms No. 76-18, 865).

Mortimer, W. G. *History of Coca The Divine Plant of the Incas*. 1901, reprinted, San Francisco, CA: And/Or Press, 1974.

National Commission on Marijuana and Drug Abuse. *Drug Use in America: Problem in Perspective. Second Report*. Washington, DC: U.S. Government Printing Office, 1973.

Perry, D. C. Heroin and cocaine adulteration. *Clinical Toxicology, 8*(2):239-243 (1975).

Phillips, J. L. *Cocaine: The Facts and Myths*. Washington, DC: Wynne Associates, 1975.

Post, R. M. Cocaine psychoses: a continuum model. *American Journal of Psychiatry, 132*:225-231 (1975).

Schultes, R. E. Random thoughts and queries on the botany of Cannabis. In Joyce, C. R. B., and Curry, S. (eds.), *The Botany and Chemistry of Cannabis*. London, England: J and A Churchill, 1970, pp. 11-38.

Siegel, R. K. An ethnologic search for self-administration of hallucinogens. *International Journal of the Addictions, 8*:373-393 (1973).

Siegel, R. K. Cocaine hallucinations. Manuscript in preparation.

Siegel, R. K., and Jarvik, M. E. Drug-induced hallucinations in animals and man. In Siegel, R. K., and West, L. J. (eds.), *Hallucinations: Behavior, Experience, and Theory*. New York: John Wiley and Sons, 1975, pp. 81-161.

Siegel, R. K., Johnson, C. A., Brewster, J. M., and Jarvik, M. E. Cocaine self-administration in monkeys by chewing and smoking. *Pharmacology, Biochemistry, and Behavior, 4*:461-467 (1976).

Taylor, N. *Plant Drugs that Changed the World*. New York: Dodd, Mead, 1965.

Thompson, D. M. Stimulus control and drug effects. In Blackman, D., and Sanger, D. (eds.), *Contemporary Research in Behavioral Pharmacology*. New York: Plenum Press, in press.

Whyte, A. A. Acute and chronic administration of cocaine and damphetamine in rats on a multiple schedule. Unpublished doctoral dissertation, American University, 1976.

Wilson, R. A. *Sex and Drugs*. Chicago, IL: Playboy Press, 1973.

Wilson, S. A. K. Cocainism. In Bruce, L. N. (ed.), *Neurology*. Baltimore, MD: Williams and Wilkins, 1955, pp. 832-834.

Wolf, H. G., and Curran, D. Nature of delirium and allied states. *Archives of Neurology and Psychiatry, 33*:1175-1215 (1935).

Woods, J. H., and Downs, D. L. The psychopharmacology of cocaine. In *Drug Use in America: Problem in Perspective. Appendix Volume 1: Patterns and Consequences of Drug Use*. Washington, DC: U.S. Government Printing Office, 1973, pp. 116-139. ✦

20. Survival Sex: Inner-City Women and Crack-Cocaine

H. Virginia McCoy,
Christine Miles,
  and
James A. Inciardi

Media reports and anecdotal evidence from the early 1980s suggested that prostitutes were often a source of HIV transmission and that this group posed great risk for the heterosexual population. More recent research, however, suggests that most prostitutes are not infected with HIV and that HIV prevalence among prostitutes is due largely to the needle sharing that is associated with their injection drug use.

The emergence of crack-cocaine has led many women users to engage in sex-for-drugs exchanges to support addiction. This issue is the focus of the following article. The authors' sample targeted women who were not enrolled in drug treatment at the time of study but were recruited by street outreach workers in Miami as part of a larger study of injection drug users and their sex partners. The authors found a number of differences between women who use crack-cocaine and women who do not. Crack users report significantly more sex partners and have a higher prevalence of HIV infection and other sexually transmitted diseases. Finally, the authors provide a brief discussion of the effects of crack-cocaine on sexual functioning as well as the risk for HIV infection among heterosexuals.

Crack-cocaine poses a threat to inner-city communities in general, and to many of the women in those communities in particular. The drug's ready availability and low price (as little as $2 per vial in some locales) fueled its flow into numerous low-income neighborhoods during the mid- and late-1980s. In at least a few cases, shrewd mass-marketing procedures may have been involved. An Oklahoma City detective was told by one informant, for example, that his crew had test-marketed the area in a matter not unlike that in his previous work selling vacuum cleaners door-to-door (Witkin, 1991).

There are diverse reasons for the popularity of crack. Most notably, when crack is heated and its vapors are inhaled, the drug crosses the blood-brain barrier in only a few seconds, providing a virtually instantaneous "high" and intense gratification, often described as a "sexual euphoria," or orgasm. Or, as a Miami crack user commented in late 1990:

> Man, when you load and light the devil's dick [crack pipe] and *draw a hard one* [inhale deeply], it's like, like one big mind and body fuck, an' both at the same time. You know, I mean it's like, it's like the greatest sex, like your whole body is gonna come. It starts in your head and your tail, and then moves up and down and around, and out, and to the tips of your fingers. All of a sudden, you are electrified all over, and, for a few minutes, you're on top of the whole world.

Cocaine in general, and crack in particular, has a high abuse potential precisely because it is such a powerful reinforcer. But for the user, the mood elevation is as temporary as it is extreme, and is quickly followed by a depression or "crash" characterized by acute malaise and intense craving. This cycle of euphoria and craving typically promotes patterns of compulsive use (Inciardi 1992; Wallace 1991).

Users typically smoke crack for as long as they have supplies of the drug or the resources to obtain more. For many women, a common way to finance a chronic crack habit is "sex." For example, the program manager of an AIDS-prevention center in Belle Glade, Florida, during her discussion of the high rates of HIV infection among local heterosexuals, explained that a "survival instinct" was responsible for much of the sexual activity:

> A woman who needs Pampers and food for her baby gets a boyfriend. When she needs money for rent, she gets another boyfriend. She might have three or four boyfriends, but what she's doing isn't considered to be prostitution. It's *survival*. (Rozsa 1991)

In early 1991, a 17-year-old Miami crack user put it even more directly:

> When you needs the cracks, and you needs money for other things 'cause your rent money *went on the boards* [was used to buy crack], you got to survive, and *you* know, to do that, the pussy works!

The apparent association between crack use and sexual behaviors has been discussed at length in the literature. In one recent study, for example, sex-for-drugs exchanges were found to be far more common among contemporary female crack addicts than they ever were among female narcotics users, even at the height of the 1967-1974 heroin epidemics (Inciardi, Lockwood, and Pottieger 1991). Moreover, it appears that crack has generated a subculture that both endorses and promotes sexual activities, while also exploiting many of the women involved. Women in the San Francisco area who exchange sex for crack, for example, are referred to as "tossups,"—literally, something to be used and then thrown away (Fullilove et al. 1990). In other locales, they are called "skeezers," "gut buckets," "rock monsters," "base whores," "freaks," and other highly pejorative appellations (Inciardi 1991). Moreover, some women become "house girls," kept in crack houses for providing sex for clients, in exchange for drugs, wine, junk food, and a place to sleep (Inciardi 1991). The disinhibiting effects of crack seem to make these exchanges and conditions more psychologically tolerable to women. Furthermore, crack reportedly enables both male and female users to engage in sexual acts that they might not otherwise consider (Inciardi 1991; Wallace 1991).

It has been suggested that women may be especially vulnerable to the lure of crack-cocaine. Depression, low self-esteem, and learned helplessness are problems that typically affect women more often then men. It has been suggested that cocaine, in any of its forms, can provide these women with a temporary sense of accomplishment, self-worth, and potency. Some women have reported that they felt worthwhile for the first time in their lives, while high on crack (Mondanaro 1989). Others value cocaine's appetite suppressant and energizing effects. An additional attraction is the avoidance of the stigma associated with needle use. The intersection of these factors has caused crack to be viewed as the perfect trap for women.

Within this context, this analysis targets selected effects of crack use on women. Specifically, the connections between crack use, increased sexual activity, and the spread of sexually transmitted diseases (including HIV) are examined, including factors related to the spread of sexually transmitted diseases (STDs) in general, such as condom use and number of sex partners.

Methods

Data for this analysis were taken from the Miami Community Outreach Study, a National AIDS Demonstration Research project funded by the National Institute on Drug Abuse, in which intravenous and other injection drug users (IDUs) and their primary female sex partners were randomized into alternative types of HIV/AIDS prevention/intervention initiatives. Subjects who had *not* been in a drug-treatment program during the prior six months were recruited from inner-city street settings by indigenous outreach workers. After an explanation of the study at the project's local assessment center, informed consent was elicited, pre-HIV test counseling was provided, and a voluntary blood sample was drawn. A nationally standardized questionnaire—the AIDS Initial Assessment—was then administered to each subject, focusing on basic demographic characteristics, current and past drug use, and sexual behaviors, including number of sex partners and condom use. Interviews were conducted under conditions where privacy could be maintained, and subjects were assured that all information would be kept strictly confidential. In addition to a small cash stipend for coming to the assessment center, all participants received intervention counseling, literature on AIDS-prevention measures and the effect of AIDS on the immune system, and drug-treatment and social-service referral information.

Study subjects were re-interviewed at six-month intervals, at which time a follow-up questionnaire was administered in order to determine the effectiveness of the intervention in modifying risky behaviors. Follow-up data were elicited for drug use, needle use, and sexual activities during each six-month time period.

Out of the total Miami Community Outreach population of 1,359 male and female IDUs and sex partners, there were 929 crack users and 430 non-crack users. For this analysis, all men, as well as women who were drug injectors, were eliminated from the data set in order to more clearly identify HIV risks associated with crack-cocaine use. Of the remaining 235 women, 40.9 percent used crack and 59.1 percent were non-users of crack. Chi-square statistics were calculated to assess statistical significance of differences between users and non-users.

Table 1
Female Users & Non-Users of Crack Cocaine
(N = 235)

RACE**	Crack Users N = 289	Non-Crack Users N = 203
Black	84.4	96.4
Hispanic	4.2	2.9
White	10.4	0.7
Native American	1.0	0
AGE		
18-29	50.0	56.1
30-39	41.7	33.8
40-49	7.3	7.9
50+	1.0	2.2
EMPLOYMENT		
Unemployed	75.0	79.9
INCOME*		
Job	14.6	18.6
Welfare	28.0	44.2
Spouse/Partner	17.1	17.7
Illegal	18.0	0.9
Other	22.0	18.6
EDUCATION		
1-8	8.6	8.4
9-11	51.1	49.5
HS Graduae	32.4	23.2
Some College	7.2	14.7
College Grad.	0.7	4.2

** p <.01
*** p <.001

Table 2
Exchange of Sex for Money or Drugs
Female Users and Non-Users of Crack Cocaine

	Crack Users	Non-Crack Users
Sex for Money***	64.5	18.4
Sex for Drugs**	24.2	2.7

*** p <.001
** p <.01

Results

As indicated in Table 1, the study sample as a whole was predominantly black (84.4 percent of the crack users and 96.4 percent of the non-crack users), approximately half of each group were in the 18-29-year age range, and most had either a high-school diploma or at least some high school. Three-fourths of both groups were unemployed, and a legal job was the major source of income for only 14.6 percent of the crack users and 18.6 percent of the non-users. An interesting demographic difference is that 18.0 percent of the crack users, as opposed to only 0.9 percent of the non-crack users, reported illegal activities as their primary source of income.

The significance of crack use in the intensification of behavioral risks is illustrated by the exchange of sex for either drugs or money. The exchange of sex for *money* was reported by 64.5 percent of crack users and 18.4 percent of non-crack users. The difference is even more pronounced when exchanges of sex for *drugs* are considered— reported by 24.2 percent of the crack users but only 2.7 percent of non-crack users (Table 2).

Both groups in this study had a high degree of HIV risk associated with having sex partners who were injection drug users. As indicated in Table 3, almost 90 percent of the non-crack users and 96 percent of the crack users reported having one or more IDU sex partners—an expected finding since the Miami Community Outreach Study targeted IDUs and their sex partners from the outset. And interestingly, of those who reported *no* sexual risk, 3.1 percent were crack users and 8.6 percent were non-crack users.

Table 3
Sexual Risk Related to IDU Partners
Female Users and Non-Users of Crack Cocaine***

	Crack Users	Non-Crack Users
No Sexual Risk	3.1	8.6
No IDU Partners	1.0	1.4
1 IDU Partner	66.7	82.7
2 or More IDU Patners	29.2	7.2

Since the amount of HIV/STD risk associated with almost all sexual activities can depend on whether or not barrier protection is used, subjects were questioned about their use of condoms. Crack users reported higher rates of condom use, perhaps reflecting higher frequencies of bartered sex (sex for drugs/money). However, at baseline interviewing, both users and non-users of crack reported that they used condoms less than half the time (Table 4). Such infrequent use of condoms clearly increases the risk for HIV.

Table 4
Mean Condom Use Frequency by Condom Use@

	Crack Users	Non-Crack Users
Baseline	1.2	0.7
6 Month AFA	2.3	1.9
12 Month AFA	2.3	2.5
18 Month AFA	2.4	1.9

@ Explanation of codes: 0 = Never, 1 = Less than half the time, 2 = About half the time, 3 = More than half the time, 4 = Always.

Since condom use was not high, it was important to probe the reasons for their non-use. Interestingly, there was very little difference between the two groups. The most important reasons were "not liking them," reported by 36.4 percent of the crack users and 36.5 percent of the non-users, and "partner not liking them," reported by 38.8 percent and 34.0 percent, respectively. Additionally, a small percentage (7.8 percent of crack users and 3.8 percent of non-users) reported that discussing condom use made them "uneasy" (Table 5).

Table 5
Reasons for not Always Using Condoms
Female Users and Non-Users of Crack Cocaine

	Crack Users	Non-Crack Users
Not Like	36.4	36.5
Uneasy	7.8	3.8
Partner Not Like	38.8	34.0

Just as the opportunity for acquiring the more common sexually transmitted diseases increases with the number of a person's sex partners, it is logically assumed that the degree of sex-related HIV risk also increases with the number of partners. Interestingly, the number of partners reported by the study subjects was radically different for users and non-users of crack-cocaine. At baseline, crack users reported a mean of 13.6 sex partners, while non-crack users reported 1.6 (Table 6). These means decreased for both groups over the course of the 18-month follow-up period. There was less difference in the number of *IDU sex partners* at baseline, with crack users reporting a mean of 2.1 and non-crack users reporting 1.2. Over the 18-month period, these figures decreased as well.

Table 6
Mean Number of Sexual Partners and IDU SPs
Female USers and Non-Users of Crack Cocaine

	Crack Users		Non-Crack Users	
	SPs	IDU SPs	SPs	IDU SPs
Baseline	13.6	2.1	1.6	1.3
6 Months AFA	18.1	0.6	1.8	0.8
12 Months AFA	6.9	1.1	1.6	1.0
18 Months AFA	10.1	0.7	1.2	0.5

Heterosexual contact is the primary mechanism of HIV transmission in several parts of the world, and is becoming increasingly prominent in the United States. For this reason, it is important to note that the baseline seropositivity for HIV was 19.8 percent among women crack users and 10.8 percent for non-crack users (Table 7). As such, it would appear that crack puts women at risk for contracting HIV infection, and that the source of the risk lies in the apparently special relationship between crack use and sexual behavior. Some confirmation for this hypothesis can be found in crack users' higher rates of other sexually transmitted diseases. The STD found most common among study subjects was gonorrhea, reported by 42.7 percent of the crack users, compared to 23.7 percent of the non-users. Similarly, syphilis was reported by 30.2 percent of the crack users, compared to 13.8 percent of the non-users, and genital sores were reported by 17.7 percent and 6 percent, respectively (Table 8).

Table 7
Serostatus
Female Users and Non-Users of Crack Cocaine

	Crack Users	Non-Crack Users
Positive*	19.8	10.8
Negative**	80.2	89.2

* $p < .05$

Table 8
History of Sexually Transmitted Disease
Female Users and Non-Users of Crack Cocaine

	Crack Users	Non-Crack Users
Genital Herpes	1.0	0.7
Gonorrhea**	42.7	23.7
Syphilis**	30.2	13.8
Genital Sores***	17.7	3.6

** $p < .01$
*** $p < .001$

Discussion

In this sample of women drawn from inner-city areas of Miami, Florida, the use of crack would appear to be closely associated with a variety of HIV-risk behaviors—unprotected sex with multiple partners, including injection drug users. Much of the multiple-sex-partner activity is the product of increased sexual activity through the numerous sex-for-drugs (or money) exchanges associated with crack dependence.

It would appear that there are both psychopharmacological and economic explanations for the sex/crack association. All forms of cocaine, including crack, engender a release of inhibitions on behavior, and especially sexual behavior (Smith, Wesson, and Apter-Marsh 1984; Gawin 1991; Siegel 1982). Not only is the loss of inhibitions rapid, but among novice users, there is *increased* sexual functioning, in the form of more intense orgasms. Combined with the profound elation engendered by the drug, there is the tendency to desire more frequent sexual activities. Among long-term cocaine and crack addicts, however, sexual capabilities are se-

verely diminished—among men, the inability to achieve and/or maintain an erection, and among both sexes, the inability to reach a climax. Among males in crack houses, nevertheless, there remains the desire to have vaginal, and particularly oral, sex while smoking crack. Moreover, in some locales the crack house has become the new "brothel," where the potential cheap sex with many partners reportedly abounds. Thus, many male non-users seek out female crack addicts in crack houses.

Going further, the crack/sex association involves the need by female users to pay for their drugs. Crack's rapid onset and short duration of effect engender compulsive use, and a willingness to obtain the drug through any means. Compulsive use results in a staggering financial burden, and historically, prostitution has been the most lucrative, reliable, and readily available way for many women to finance drug use (Goldstein 1979).

As such, the relationships among crack use, unsafe sex, and injection drug use suggest that the use of crack-cocaine will increase heterosexual transmission of HIV among crack users, drug injectors, and their sex partners, and outward from crack-using and drug-injecting networks to other populations.

* * *

H. Virginia McCoy, Christine Miles, and James A. Inciardi, "Survival Sex: Inner-City Women and Crack-Cocaine." Copyright © 1995 by Roxbury Publishing. All rights reserved.

For Discussion

What types of policy initiatives might be effective in curbing sex-for-crack exchanges among inner-city women?

References

Bollinger, A. V., and R. Pierson (1990). "Children of the Damned: Crack Binge Dooms Her Unborn Child." *New York Post*, May 10, pp. 4, 33.

Fullilove, R. E., M. T. Fullilove, B. Bowser, and S. Gross (1990). "Crack Users: The New AIDS Risk Group?" *Cancer Detection and Prevention*, 14 (3), pp. 363-335.

Gawin, F. H. (1991). "Cocaine Addiction: Psychology and Neurophysiology." *Science*, 251, pp. 1580-1586.

Goldstein, P. J. (1979). *Prostitution and Drugs* (Lexington, MA: Lexington Books).

Inciardi, J. A. (1991). "King Rats, Chicken Heads, Slow Necks, Freaks, and Blood Suckers: A Glimpse at the Miami Sex-for-Crack Market." Paper Presented at the Annual Meeting of the Society for Applied Anthropology, Charleston, March 13-17.

Inciardi, J. A. (1992). *The War on Drugs II: the Continuing Epic of Heroin, Cocaine, Crack, Crime, AIDS, and Public Policy* (Mountain View, CA: Mayfield).

Inciardi, J. A., D. Lockwood, and A.E. Pottieger (1991). "Crack-Dependent Women and Sexuality: Implications for STD Acquisition and Transmission." *Addiction and Recovery*, July/August, pp. 25-28.

Mondanaro, J. (1989). *Chemically Dependent Women: Assessment and Treatment* (Lexington, MA: Lexington Books).

Rozsa, L. (1991). "Town's AIDS Figures 'Horrible,' Panel Says." *Miami Herald*, February 6.

Siegel, R. K. (1982). "Cocaine and Sexual Dysfunction: The Curse of Mama Coca." *Journal of Psychoactive Drugs*, 14, pp. 71-74.

Smith, D. E., D. R. Wesson, and M. Apter-Marsh (1984). "Cocaine and Alcohol Induced Sexual Dysfunction in Patients with Addictive Disease." *Journal of Psychoactive Drugs*, 16, pp. 359-361.

Wallace, B. C. (1991). *Crack Cocaine: A Practical Treatment Approach for the Chemically Dependent* (New York: Brunner/Mazel).

Witkin, G. (1991). "The Men Who Created Crack." *U.S. News and World Report*, August 19, pp. 44-53. ✦

21. How Women and Men Get Cocaine: Sex-Role Stereotypes and Acquisition Patterns

PATRICIA J. MORNINGSTAR

AND

DALE D. CHITWOOD

Stereotypes are often false representations of a particular group. In the following article, Patricia J. Morningstar and Dale D. Chitwood explore the sex-role stereotypes among 170 cocaine users in Miami, Florida. The cocaine subculture is characterized by two sex-role stereotypes: the "Cocaine Cowboy," a stereotypical male cocaine user who exhibits characteristics of toughness and machismo; and the "Coke Whore," a stereotypical female cocaine user who obtains cocaine through sexual manipulation.

The authors note that most of the cocaine users in their study were familiar with these representations; however, few fit the stereotypical profile. While significantly more women than men reported having traded sex for cocaine on at least one occasion, many women had also obtained cocaine through other methods. The authors also comment on a gender-based hierarchy in drug dealing; for example, more males than females acquired cocaine for personal use through dealing, and females reported that males often controlled cocaine use among women.

Anyone who has had extensive experience with cocaine knows that the use of the drug transforms relationships, including relationships between men and women. This transformation is epitomized and exaggerated by two complementary sex-role stereotypes of the cocaine-using subculture: the cocaine cowboy and the coke whore. It will be demonstrated in this article that, while these images reveal a considerable amount of information regarding the way people think about behavior, they provide a distorted picture of observable behavior patterns.

Since Walter Lippmann coined the term "stereotype" in 1922, the relationship between cultural images and actual behavior patterns has been a sub-

ject of ongoing investigation. Early research developed the notion that stereotypes contain a kernel of truth. While some findings support the kernel-of-truth hypothesis (Schuman 1966), studies demonstrating the inaccuracy of stereotypes are more common. O'Leary (1977), in her review of sex-role stereotyping, noted that "whatever the weight of the grain of truth at the basis of every stereotype, it appears that the extent of the misperception far outweighs the actual divergence between the sexes."

Recent research on stereotypes takes a different approach. Stereotypes are seen as a single example of the cognitive distortion and remolding of reality inherent in any type of classification or information processing. This orientation shifts the focus of interest: distortion is taken for granted. The researcher focuses on the forces that shape the stereotype.

These forces appear to have their roots in the framework of cultural knowledge, beliefs, and standards that provides the context for stereotyping. Thus, the interpretation of stereotypes depends on understanding social dynamics. For example, Barth (1969) viewed ethnic identity as a product of boundary maintenance between competitive or interacting groups. He regarded the content of social differentiations to be less significant than their role in the maintenance of a social ecology. Following the same theme, Campbell (1967) developed a series of propositions concerning in-group and out-group interactions. Some of these propositions suggested that the social context of interaction guides the formation of stereotypes. Three of these propositions are relevant to the present discussion: (1) mutual stereotypes are likely to include traits that are dimensions of real contrast; the more real contrast there is, the more likely it is to appear in the stereotype; (2) trait differences directly involved in intergroup interaction will be most strongly represented; and, (3) given trait differences of equal contrast, those that are most relevant to the desires and needs of the groups are most apt to be included in stereotypes.

The stereotypes discussed in the present article reflect a complementary relationship between male cocaine users, who tend to control the supply of the drug, and female cocaine users, who often depend on men for access to the drug. This relationship is dramatized in the role of the cocaine cowboy, the dangerously macho egomaniac who deals cocaine, and the coke whore, the degraded slave of cocaine who will trade sex for the drug. While the images do not accurately represent majority behavior among men and women, they do depict dimensions of real contrast, because—as will be seen—more men are involved in dealing activity and more women receive cocaine in the form of gifts. Also, these stereotypes focus on aspects of the subculture that govern male-female interactions and highlight the particular needs of the two groups.

These stereotypes were identified during a general study of patterns of cocaine use in Miami, Florida, conducted between 1979 and 1981 for NIDA. The study employed both survey and ethnographic techniques to investigate a wide range of behaviors related to drug use among 170 users whose primary drug of choice was cocaine. The sample included users who employed a variety of routes of administration, including shooting, snorting, and freebasing. Participants were selected to represent Hispanics (primarily Cubans), non-Hispanic blacks, and non-Hispanic whites. Those sampled were predominantly lower- or middle-class. The sample included 91 men and 79 women. The primary objective of the study was to examine various types of drug-using behaviors as they related to sociocultural factors. Men and women in the study did not differ in overall use patterns (as measured by an additive scale that combined measures of quantity, frequency, and route of administration). However, there were variations in acquisition patterns. Such variations are focal areas of contrast depicted in the stereotypes and are discussed below. However, it is important to keep in mind that these stereotypes do not represent typical behaviors. A discussion of behavior patterns measured in this survey will follow the descriptions of the stereotypes.

The Stereotypes

Each of the two stereotypes includes descriptive and prescriptive information woven together into a Gestalt impression. In addition, each contains an inner logic that makes sense in the context of the requirements of subcultural behavior. The following are descriptions of the cocaine cowboy and the coke whore as they emerged from unstructured interviews.

The Cocaine Cowboy

The cocaine cowboy stereotype is that of a male, usually Hispanic and relatively high up in the cocaine-distribution structure, who is aggressive,

tough, and macho. This image had so permeated the popular press at the time of the study that Miami had acquired the nickname of Dodge City.

While there are women dealers, the cocaine-distribution system is, as one user put it, "a male market," especially at the higher-quantity levels. One woman who was interviewed was the wife of a dealer who was involved in considerable "weight" or quantity. Her description of the scene and her bitter feelings about it provide some idea of behavior at this level of distribution:

> All the men I knew were very sort of manly; had a lot of women. The women kissed their ass . . . you never really heard them talk. They would wait in the cars for them to come back out. See, where the conflict with me and my husband was always that I wanted to be there, that was my coke, that was my money. Basically all of his friends would end up saying, keep the bitch off in the back room. There are many times that I've walked in, and they would be dealing. They'd tell me that my house was off limits. . . . Basically, I'll tell you, the only time I saw them give us coke was right before going to bed, was like after the party was over, the male party, sitting there and telling war stories and blah, blah, blah . . . when that ended, it was time to give the girls some coke. . . . The lines would be longer and higher for the males. The females didn't need as much, that was basically their rationalization for the smaller lines for the women. We were mainly made to stay in cars; a lot of men told their wives to stay home, and that was that.

The above description is an extreme example. The man mentioned in the story eventually died from a cocaine overdose that his wife suspected was an intentional homicide. She herself explained that the more people are involved in this lifestyle and the upper levels of distribution, the more the network is dominated by males and an ethic of aggressive sex discrimination.

Sex segregation and extreme aggressive behavior affects interaction in all areas of this lifestyle. This is illustrated by the same woman's description of an incident involving her son:

> I've seen a lot of guns, too. I remember one day a bunch of people were sitting on black suitcases, guns in their pockets, three-piece suits, and my son comes walking out with a gun. He's just a little kid, and he holds it at these three people, and no sooner did he do that they all pulled their guns out and held

them at him. So, it was like the old standoff . . . who was going to shoot who. . . . Like, all of us froze. We're watching these men sitting there and my son pointing a gun at them, going "hee, hee, hee." I know they would've killed him like that. You got to think that all that they probably've been seeing, since they've been in the business, is guns, and fear and paranoia, and basically a feeling that anybody is going to hurt them, don't trust anybody . . . including a five year old, with a gun.

Even less aggressive men who deal find themselves involved in situations in which confrontation and escalating aggression is a real possibility. A respondent described the role of guns in negotiating a deal:

Respondent: You just get into details.

Interviewer: What sort of details?

Respondent: Just make sure that the merchandise is good. That nobody's got guns. Everybody had them anyway, but . . . those were things like you would lay out. Like your friends might have them, but when you go in there . . . you and him . . . he ain't got a gun and you ain't got a gun.

Interviewer: What happens if the coke isn't good? Respondent: Then you end up getting shot or killed. Anything could happen.

Interviewer: And if you found out that it wasn't good. What would you do?

Respondent: I'll probably pull out a gun for trying to make a fool or a sucker out of me. Maybe it'd be like $5,000, and that was all my money that I'd worked for, and I'd earned it and saved it. So I have to show that . . . I've got respect for myself. That I ain't gonna let somebody steal money from me.

The young man who made these statements did not fit the cocaine-cowboy stereotype. He was an 18 year old who had to maintain his reputation in a situation of potential confrontation. This issue is woven into the very fabric of the cocaine-distribution system. The process of buying any quantity of cocaine has an inner logic that makes aggressive or defensive behavior comprehensible. The following is a typical rationale for this type of behavior: cocaine-dealing involves a lot of money; transactions are conducted outside legal protection; enough money is involved to warrant confrontation in order to obtain or protect it; therefore, it is necessary to

be suspicious and to protect oneself. As one respondent stated,

In some respects you do have to . . . if you're going to deal, you have to protect not your honor, but your name. If you get ripped off, then other people think that you're an easy rip-off target. So I've had that happen to me, to the point where I had to either . . . myself get nasty or have other people do it for me.

In addition to this situational component, users often mention an affective component that they claim is present when any quantity of cocaine is distributed. The theme of suspiciousness, paranoia, and violence recurs again and again. One commonly held theory among users is that the effect of cocaine itself, producing paranoia and agitation, combined with the dangerous circumstances, produces behaviors that are commonly labeled as "macho." Another respondent said that

when you get people who are doing quantities, who do coke every day, and who're a bit crazy to begin with . . . they start playing like they're Jessie James or something . . . and they start thinking that they can outfox everybody and they can do anything they want to, and they can have anybody they want to. And that's crazy! There is so much trouble right now with the cocaine cowboys. They get burned on a deal and . . . they don't like the quantity or something, so they just blow somebody away.

From the descriptions above, it should be apparent that the cocaine-cowboy stereotype addresses a character trait that is of primary concern in the distribution process and the social ecology of the cocaine trade. Despite the apparent justifications for so-called macho behavior, aggressiveness in dealing interactions is generally regarded as "uncool." On the other hand, the right balance is regarded as appropriate. When asked why he admired the cocaine cowboy, one Hispanic interviewee stated:

Well, he's the type of guy that won't let anyone play dirty on him. He's a man that will face anything.

The Coke Whore

The coke whore is another stereotype that reflects a situational tension in the cocaine subculture. On the one hand, there is the mythology that cocaine can be used to arouse women sexually. On the other hand, there is the real possibility that a woman will pretend to be interested in order to obtain cocaine. For example, one respondent remarked:

> I know a lot of people who think that coke makes women horny. I don't really think that's true. I was saying these coke whores . . . they just want the coke and they'll put out if they have to for it.

The behavior of the coke whore is generally regarded as a nuisance, much like other mooching behavior, although the term may also carry a denigrating connotation:

> Unfortunately, now you find so many . . . what I call coke whores . . . it's like, if you don't have cocaine, you ain't worth shit. Right after 'What's your sign?' comes 'Do you have any coke?' . . . I know the type all too well.

Some of this behavior is a straightforward exchange of sexual favors for cocaine in a situation of prostitution, because

> you can buy anything with coke; you can even buy a woman with coke.

One black male dealer explained:

> Sex is regarded as a salable item to dealers. And I got my kicks off that night, 'cause a lot of people came by with things to sell. A lot of girls would come by, you know, offer their bodies for bags.

Several black street users who were interviewed expressed the opinion that the cocaine dealer was replacing the pimp as the man of status on the streets of Miami. One of them said:

> It used to be that cocaine was for the big-style hustler . . . who had the ladies, and maybe he was a pimp or something like that. A man can hardly make a woman do anything now. A woman is for herself . . . you know, and just makes love for cocaine with dudes that have coke.

One woman's explanation of cocaine dealers who snort the drug makes it clear that this street image is the direct descendant of the pimp image, and the coke whore is a role that is played opposite the role of the cocaine dealer:

> They like to ride around and show folks, and put on airs, especially for the pretty girls, you know. Bring out their little plastic bags and give it to the chicks . . . a lot of the so-called big-timing chicks, they think that's super . . . see a dude with his own personal

stash, you know, of cocaine, just giving it away. That's how a lot of them bull the girls.

However, actual prostitution is not what is meant by the image of the coke whore. The coke whore is a woman who knowingly and consciously takes a man's cocaine and then goes to bed with him, or simply goes out with a man because he has cocaine. These women do not view their activity to be the same as prostitution. While both behaviors may have similar forms, there are some important differences. The trading of sexual favors that cocaine whores engage in is often quite ambiguous compared to actual prostitution. First, the rate of exchange is not made explicit in the coke whore's interaction with her provider. Second, there is considerable variation in the degree to which the provider is aware of the exact nature of the interaction with the coke whore. She may attempt to manipulate the situation, such that the man believes that he is seducing her with the drug.

Some men believe that they can seduce women with cocaine, just as in the dominant society where they might seduce women with money. Examples of this belief abound in the interviews, especially among younger men in the sample. As one of them said,

> Men use cocaine as bait. The majority of women who are periqueras [cocaine users], they go easier . . . if they want to go and have a nice time . . . they know that you have perico [cocaine] . . . they'll go with you wherever you want. They will . . . be easier to make a sexual pass at once they know, well, 'If he gives me some cocaine, I might give him some ass.' Something along those lines. It's like holding the golden rod. Anything you want . . . to kind of get your wishes.

A Hispanic woman explained the potential shallowness of this sort of relationship, as well as explaining how such men might be vulnerable to the coke-whore gambit:

> It was because they had coke around, they were fun to be with. They'd go out and party and they'd go out and eat, just do coke all the time. They were caught up in this syndrome of . . . their dealings and coppings, and that was their excitement. But there was some kind of charisma about them . . . it was only because of their coke. . . . I always categorized them as "cocaine cowboys." Take their coke away, and they were nothing to me. Because everything that I was attracted to them about was surrounded

around their coke and their dealings of coke, their monetary status, the places they went to, you know. Without coke, to me they were really boring people. They gave you coke, because they thought you'd be easier to go to bed with that. And a bunch of times that was the case, sure, you'd go to bed with them, yeah. If they didn't have the coke, you probably would've said, "Forget it." And that definitely made them more attractive.

For some women, this blended exchange of cocaine and sexuality is even less like a business or quasi-business exchange:

> Men use coke to lure women away. I've been lured away many times. I keep doing coke and I get horny, so that makes it easier even. And it breaks down a lot of barriers, you can talk to people, you get interested in talking to them. It's fun to make love with coke, so sometimes I've found, even when I'm with somebody I don't want to go to bed with, I end up going to bed with [that person] because we've been sitting there talking and becoming friends. We talk for hours and hours, you know, and find out you think a lot of the same things . . . have a lot of the same experiences in life, and become friends.

In society in general, women deal with an ambiguous expectation that, if a man takes a woman out, the woman should respond with affections. This same issue is extended to the cocaine culture:

> We used to snort a lot of coke together, and we'd go to bed sometimes, and sometimes we'd be up all night. But he won't snort any with me or sell me any 'cause I won't go to bed with him now.

The coke whore per se is the woman who uses a man for cocaine, who has sex with him, not in appreciation of him, but for the cocaine he has. In a sense, she turns her would-be suitor into a trick (for a complete discussion, see Milner and Milner 1972). Women who are in the habit of doing this may or may not feel that what they are doing is appropriate; but just as some men purposely tried to seduce women with coke, some women purposely tried to find men who would give them coke:

> I still felt that I was choosy, but I was choosy, because I was only sleeping with the people that could support my habit, because I got to the point where a gram was not enough, and two grams wasn't enough.

However, not all women appreciated men using cocaine as a seduction device:

> I knew that this guy had cocaine, because sometimes he used to see me and he used to say, "You want to get high?" . . . and I said, "No" . . . you know, 'cause I knew he wanted to lay up and I didn't want to lay up just to get no dope . . . at least not with him. Any man can pick you up, and he's got coke. It used to be so neat when a guy told me he had coke. Now, when I'm in a bar, the second line he says is "I have coke."

Here, an ironic full circle may be seen, in which both men and women are vulnerable to these stereotypes.

Table I
Person Who Provided Cocaine for
First Occasion of Use by Sex of User*

Person Who Provided Cocaine	Sex	
	Male (N = 91) (%)	Female (N = 79) (%)
Male friend	68	43
Spouse or intimate other of the opposite sex	1	34
Other male relative	10	5
Other female relative	11	9
Female friend	3	1
Other (dealer, coworker)**	7	8
Total	100	100

* $\chi^2 = 35.09$, df = 5, a<.01
** The sex of those providers listed under this category is unknown.

The Behavior Pattern

The stereotypes of the cocaine cowboy and the coke whore appear to reflect a variety of issues that are significant in mainstream society and other drug-using environments, as well as the cocaine scene. For example, research on heroin addicts has demonstrated a general pattern of women's dependence on men for access to drug experiences. Female addicts commonly begin use through male associates (Rosenbaum 1981) and resort to prostitution as one of several means of support (James 1976). Distribution and access to drugs are generally controlled by males (Hildred and Washington 1976). According to the Women's Drug Research Coordinating Project (Finnegan 1979), social factors affect women addicts, including that women often derive their status from men, are more stigmatized than men for deviant behavior, and have fewer, as well as less, lucrative vocational options than men.

The cocaine-using arena is also dominated by a degree of male control. One indication of this is the tendency for men to be the gatekeepers of the subculture or scene. Table I summarizes survey findings on the sex of the person who provided cocaine to the respondent on the first occasion of use. Men accounted for a significant percentage of providers for both male (78 percent) and female (82 percent) users.

Another aspect of women's essentially dependent position is the economic condition of women cocaine users. One black woman user characterized this dependence by generalizing that all the women she used cocaine with

> . . . are either prostitutes or have husbands. The money that their husbands give them, they use for drugs, right. And a lot of them have to sell their bodies to get it. It's different, because they be able to buy more cocaine than the ones that have husbands.

The survey data demonstrate that this characterization is an exaggeration. To establish each respondent's primary source of income, everyone was asked to select from a list of possible sources the one source from which they obtained most, if not all, of their income (see Table II). A plurality of both the men and women obtained their income from legitimate employment or investments. Of the remainder, women were more likely to receive income from other people or social welfare agencies, while men were more likely to engage in illegal activities.

Any difficulties a woman might have acquiring drugs are exacerbated in the cocaine-using arena. In addition, any drama that might be involved in dealing among men is intensified. This is because of the expense of cocaine. Although the price appears to have fallen somewhat since the time when these data were collected, the generalization that cocaine is an expensive drug and one of extravagant luxury

probably still holds in most drug-using circles. More than any other drug, cocaine has been associated with money. A report in the popular press (Unsigned 1981) compared the price of cocaine with gold, noting that at $2,200 an ounce, it is five times more expensive than gold, and stated that, if the cocaine trade were to be listed in the Fortune 500, it would rank seventh.

Table II
Major Source of Income by Sex*

	Sex	
	Male (N=91)	**Female (N=79)**
Income Source	(%)	(%)
Job/Investments	48	43
Spouse/Family/Friend	9	25
Welfare/Unemployment/VA/ADC	3	18
Illegal sources	40	14
Total	100	100

$*\chi^2 = 26.13$, df=3' $\alpha < .001$

The high cost of the drug is reflected in the fact that, on the average, the study respondents had spent $912/month on cocaine in the three months prior to the interviews. Among users interviewed, it is called the "connoisseur's drug," the "millionaire's drug" and the "rich man's high." A common response to the question of what type of people are suited to cocaine use was "rich people," "people who have money," or "you have to be rich." Expense and reputation appear to contribute greatly to cocaine's desirability as a commodity. Cocaine's association with money designates it as a status marker in a culture in which financial and material achievement are highly valued. The use of cocaine is one way, albeit a peculiar one, of raising social status, and hence, self-esteem.

The expense of cocaine is a condition that brings issues of exchange and acquisition into focus. The effect of purchasing cocaine on the overall financial condition of the user is striking. Sixty percent of the survey sample reported that cocaine had caused them money problems. Of those with families or

intimate relationships, 67 percent reported that cocaine use had "harmed the family budget."

Acquisition interactions are an elaborate, infor-
mation-rich domain of the cocaine subculture. Interviewees had many stories about acquiring cocaine, including concerns about risk and rules for
proper conduct. Eighteen general types of acquisition were discussed in open-ended interviews, ranging from a valet receiving cocaine as a tip for park-
ing cars to customary cutting or adulteration of the
drug and taking a quantity off the top for resale.

In the context of a subculture in which acquisition strategies play a major role, it is not surprising
that sex roles should be interpreted in these terms.
The patterns of acquisition measured in the survey
demonstrate that women and men have somewhat
different approaches, but again the plurality of men
and women have common patterns (see Table III).
While 43 percent of the men and 42 percent of the
women almost always acquired cocaine through
trade or purchase, men were twice as likely as
women to depend on dealing as their primary
source for the drug. Conversely, women were twice
as likely as men to receive cocaine from someone
else who shares with them or gives them a gift of
cocaine. The difference between men and women is
made more clear by the findings of whether or not
they had ever traded sexual favors for cocaine.
Twenty-eight percent of the men and 47 percent of
the women answered affirmatively ($X^2 = 5.25$, .05).

Table III
*Percent Reporting That All or Almost All (80%-100%) of
Their Cocaine Comes from One Specific Source**

	Sex	
	Male (N=91)**	Female (N=79)***
Source	(%)	(%)
Given to respondent as a gift or shared with respondent	18	35
Traded for goods and services or bought not for resale	43	42
Taken off the top of cocaine for sale	21	11
Total	82	88

* $\chi^{2=6.80,\ df=2,}$ $\alpha < .05$
** 18 percent of the men reported no single or usual source.
***12 percent of the women reported no single or usual source.

This difference between men and women in acquisition patterns forms the kernel of truth, to
which a variety of cognitive associations attach
themselves in completing the stereotype. That these
associations are part of a more general belief system
is illustrated in the following comments by one
user, who viewed the subculture as a part and intensification of mainstream society:

> Respondent: Men are more aggressive than women
> in my observations. . . . The women that I've known
> that have been involved use their own techniques
> to manipulate.

> Interviewer: Like, what would be an example of a
> woman's technique to get some coke?

> Respondent: Obviously sex . . . just any other way
> that a woman might want to manipulate a man, say,
> in a given situation no matter what it is . . . if it's
> her husband and she wants a new dress . . . she
> might stroke him in the right ways, you know, use
> her sex.

Conclusion

The data presented in this article make it clear
that the complementary sex-role stereotypes of cocaine cowboy and coke whore are not representative
of the majority of men and women's acquisition
patterns. Rather, they appear to be an exaggeration
and intensification of observable but unrepresenta-
tive differences. In order to interpret these cultural
images, one may refer back to Campbell's propositions (1967).

First, the cowboy and whore represent a dimension of real contrast in a situation in which the majority of men and women do not differ. In other
words, where there is a difference, it is reflected in
the stereotype.

Second, interaction between the two groups occurs along dimensions of acquisition and sex. Thus,
one would expect these two elements to be emphasized in the stereotype. In the case of the female
stereotype, the two elements are combined in a
characterization of a woman who offers sex in order
to acquire cocaine. In the male case, masculine
traits are grossly exaggerated in acquisition transac-

tions. In general, the position of male dominance is maintained in the complementary stereotypes.

Third, one learns something of the desires and needs of cocaine users through the two stereotypes. For the male stereotype, cocaine emerges as both a power in itself and as a tool of power, sexual and otherwise. This desire and need for cocaine by men is set in sharp relief by the female stereotype.

Finally, the above analysis suggests that in the cocaine-using subculture, as in other drug and criminal subcultures, women have less power than men and tend to function as the out-group or minority, while men maintain control of access to the drug.

* * *

Patricia J. Morningstar and Dale D. Chitwood, "How Women and Men Get Cocaine: Sex-Role Stereotypes and Acquisition Patterns." This article appeared in the *Journal of Psychoactive Drugs*, Volume 19(2), April-June 1987 and is reprinted with permission. Copyright © 1987 by Haight-Ashbury Publications.

For Discussion

What are some possible reasons for excluding women from cocaine sales transactions?

References

Barth, F. (ed.). 1969. *Ethnic Groups and Boundaries: The Social Organization of Cultural Difference*. Boston: Little, Brown.

Campbell, D. T. 1967. Stereotypes and the perception of group differences. *American Psychologist* 22:817-829.

Finnegan, L. P. 1979. Women in treatment. In DuPont, R. L., Goldstein, A., and O'Donnell, J. (eds.), *Handbook on Drug Abuse*. Rockville, MD: NIDA.

Hamilton, D. (ed.). 1981. *Cognitive Processes in Stereotyping and Intergroup Behavior*. Hillsdale, NJ: Lawrence Erlbaum.

Hildred, C. A., and Washington, M. N. 1976. Interpersonal relationships in heroin use by men and women and their role in treatment outcome. *International Journal of the Addictions* 11(1):117-130.

James, J. 1976. Prostitution and addiction: An interdisciplinary approach. *Addictive Disease* 2(4):601-618.

LaPiere, R. 1936. Type-rationalizations of group antipathy. *Social Forces* 15:232-237.

Lippmann, W. 1922. *Public Opinion*. New York: Harcourt Brace.

Milner, R., and Milner, M. 1972. *Black Players*. Boston: Little, Brown.

O'Leary, V. 1977. *Toward Understanding Women*. Monterey, CA: Brooks/Cole.

Rosenbaum, M. 1981. Sex roles among deviants: The woman addict. *International Journal of the Addictions* 16(5):859-877.

Schuman, H. 1966. Social change and the validity of regional stereotypes in East Pakistan. *Sociometry* 29:428-440.

Tajfel, H. 1969. Cognitive aspects of prejudice. *Journal of Social Issues* 25:79-97.

Taylor, S. 1981. A categorization approach to stereotyping. In Hamilton, D. (ed.), *Cognitive Processes in Stereotyping and Intergroup Behavior*. Hillsdale, NJ: Lawrence Erlbaum.

Unsigned. 1981. Cocaine. *Time*, July 6. ✦

Part VI

Hallucinogenic Drugs

During the 1960s, the use of drugs seemed to have leapt from the more marginal zones of society to the very mainstream of community life. No longer were drugs limited to the inner cities, the half-worlds of the jazz scene, and the underground bohemian protocultures. Rather, their use had become suddenly and dramatically apparent among members of the adolescent and young-adult populations of rural and urban middle-class America. By the close of the decade, commentators on the era were maintaining that ours was "the addicted society," that through drugs millions had become "seekers" of "instant enlightenment," and that drug-taking and drug-seeking would persist as continuing facts of American social life.

In retrospect, what were then considered the logical causes of the new drug phenomenon now seem less clear. A variety of changes in the fabric of American life had occurred during those years which undoubtedly had profound implications for social consciousness and behavior. Notably, the revolution in the technology and handling of drugs that had begun during the 1950s was of sufficient magnitude to justify the designation of the 1960s as "a new chemical age." Recently compounded psychotropic agents were enthusiastically introduced and effectively promoted, with the consequence of exposing the national consciousness to an impressive catalog of chemical temptations—sedatives, tranquilizers, stimulants, antidepressants, analgesics, and hallucinogens—which could offer fresh inspiration, as well as simple and immediate relief from fear, anxiety, tension, frustration, and boredom.

Concomitant with this emergence of a new chemical age, a new youth ethos had become manifest, one characterized by a widely celebrated generational disaffection, a prejudicial dependence on the self and the peer group for value orientation, a

critical view of how the world was being run, and a mistrust of an "establishment" drug policy, the "facts" and "warnings" of which ran counter to reported peer experiences.

Whatever the ultimate causes of the drug revolution of the sixties might have been, America's younger generations, or at least noticeable segments of them, had embraced drugs. The drug scene had become the arena of "happening" America; "turning on" to drugs to relax and to share friendship and love seemed to have become commonplace. And the prophet—the "high priest" as he called himself—of the new chemical age was a psychology instructor at Harvard University's Center for Research in Human Personality, Dr. Timothy Leary.

The saga of Timothy Leary had its roots not at Harvard in the 1960s, but in Basel, Switzerland, just before the beginning of World War II. It was there, in 1938, that Dr. Albert Hoffman of Sandoz Research Laboratories first isolated a new chemical compound which he called D-lysergic acid diethylamide. Known now as LSD, it was cast aside in his laboratory where, for five years, it remained unappreciated, its properties awaiting discovery. On April 16, 1943, after absorbing some LSD through the skin of his fingers, Hoffman began to hallucinate. In his diary, he explained the effect:

> With closed eyes, multihued, metamorphizing, fantastic images overwhelmed me. . . . Sounds were transposed into visual sensations, so that from each tone or noise a comparable colored picture was evoked, changing in form and color kaleidoscopically.

Hoffman had experienced the first LSD "trip."

Dr. Humphrey Osmond of the New Jersey Neuropsychiatric Institute coined a new name for LSD. He called it "psychedelic," meaning mind-expanding. But outside of the scientific community, LSD was generally unknown—even at the start of the 1960s. This was quickly changed by Leary and his colleague at Harvard, Dr. Richard Alpert. They began experimenting with the drug—on themselves and with colleagues, students, artists, writers, clergymen, and volunteer prisoners. Although their adventures with LSD had earned them dismissals from Harvard by 1963, their message had been heard, and LSD had achieved its reputation. The messages had been numerous and shocking to the political establishment and to hundreds of thousand of mothers and fathers across the nation.

In *The Realist*, a radical periodical of the 1960s, Leary commented:

> I predict that psychedelic drugs will be used in all schools in the near future as educational devices— not only marijuana and LSD to teach kids how to use their sense organs and other cellular equipment effectively—but new and more powerful psychochemicals. . . .

And then, perhaps most frightening of all to the older generation, were Leary's comments to some 15,000 cheering San Francisco youths on the afternoon of March 26, 1967. As a modern-day Pied Piper, Leary told his audience:

> *Turn on* to the scene, *tune in* to what's happening, and *drop out*—of high school, college, grad school . . . follow me, the hard way.

The hysteria over Leary, LSD, and other psychedelic substances had been threefold. First, the drug scene was especially frightening to mainstream society because it reflected a willful rejection of rationality, order, and predictability. Second, there was the stigmatized association of drug use with anti-war protests and anti-establishment, long-haired, unwashed, radical "hippie" LSD users. And third, there were the drug's psychic effects, the reported "bad trips" that seemed to border on mental illness. Particularly in the case of LSD, the rumors of how it could "blow one's mind" became legion. One story told of a youth, high on the drug, who took a swan dive in front of a truck moving at 70 mph. Another spoke of two "tripping" teenagers who stared directly into the sun until they were permanently blinded. A third described how LSD's effects on the chromosomes resulted in fetal abnormalities. The stories were never documented and were probably untrue. What *were* true, however, were the reports of LSD "flashbacks." Occurring with only a small percentage of the users, individuals would re-experience the LSD-induced state days, weeks, and sometimes months after the original "trip," without having taken the drug again.

Despite the lurid reports, as it turned out, LSD was not in fact widely used on a regular basis beyond a few social groups that were fully dedicated to drug experiences. In fact, the psychedelic substances had quickly earned reputations as being dangerous and unpredictable, and most people avoided them. By the close of the 1960s, all hallucinogenic drugs had been placed under strict legal control, and the number of users was minimal.

In the years since, interest in LSD and other hallucinogens periodically re-emerge for short periods of time. Every few years, a new "psychedelic" is introduced to the American drug scene. Without question, however, LSD has remained the best known, and perhaps the most mysterious. ✦

22. Ethnographic Notes on Ecstasy Use Among Professionals

Marsha Rosenbaum,
Patricia Morgan,
and
Jerome E. Beck

Because much of the research on the American drug scene concentrates on dysfunctional users in inner-city urban areas, there is the erroneous perception among many observers that drug use occurs primarily among low-income persons. In fact, however, drug use occurs in all socio-economic groups. Nevertheless, little is known about patterns of use in middle- and upper-income groups. Marsha Rosenbaum, Patricia Morgan, and Jerome E. Beck report findings from their study of MDMA (Ecstasy) use among working professionals. The users in their sample were college-educated and employed in such professions as law, academia, and medicine.

The informants in this study reported that an important reason for their use of Ecstasy was to escape, at least temporarily, from their stressful and structured lifestyles. Daily schedules and responsibilities do not permit spontaneous use of the drug; therefore, "trips" were planned carefully and users were well-prepared for the drug's effects. Not unlike users of other drugs, the social setting was important for these Ecstasy users. However, the setting was planned to ensure that "trips" were rewarding. On the basis of their findings, the authors conclude that all drug use is not necessarily abhorrent behavior.

Current "war on drug" rhetoric informs us that any use of illegal drugs is by definition harmful, if not dangerous. Users are seen as out-of-control abusers whose lives are either on the road to destruction or already chaotic. Indeed, most ethnographic drug research has focused on "deviants" whose lives are shaped by their drug use. These individuals are otherwise known as "drug addicts" and have been targeted for research because their use, primarily of opiates, has been seen as a major social problem; and as sub-jects with little to lose, they have been accessible to researchers. A result of this research (some of which has been our own) is the creation of a "model" of the drug user as an addict whose life is consumed with drugs.

Recently, we have had the opportunity to undertake an ethnographic-type study of a group of the drug users whose lives are much more focused around career than any drugs: professionals who use MDMA, or "Ecstasy."[1] This group, we discovered, has been able to integrate drug use into their busy lives, scheduling it in much like any other appointment or activity. It is, in the words of one respondent, "controlled hedonism," or the ability to choose selectively where, when, and how one experiences a rare moment of "time out" behavior with drug-induced altered states of consciousness.

The research upon which this paper is based is part of an ongoing study of the world of MDMA users.[2] It is an exploratory project involving historical/comparative, ethnographic, and in-depth interviews of users of Ecstasy. The research includes one hundred in-depth interviews as well as ethnography. The snowball method was used to procure subjects. The purpose of this study is to begin mapping the types of users, their motives for using the drug, and their patterns of use.

Professionals' Use of Ecstasy

About a third of the way through the study, we began to notice a particular type of drug user. We found that several middle/upper-middle class professionals were using Ecstasy on a regular basis[3] and had integrated its use into very busy and complicated lives. In many ways, these professionals seemed to think of Ecstasy as "their" drug. It's not a "street" drug and is not very well known in the usual drug-using culture. As one professional man told us:

> . . . they [users] would be professional people, like real estate brokers, nurses, doctors, lawyers, entrepreneurs in businesses; there is this group. . . . There is another group which is not professional. They're people who have been doing drugs and everything else on and off, and they try everything that comes their way. But they're not the majority [of Ecstasy users]. Basically the professional, young professional working class that I know are using it.

As part of our study, we followed up on these professionals to examine (1) how they organized their lives around this illegal activity; and (2) the implications of using an illegal psychedelic substance.

Using the "Chicago tradition" in sociology, we observed groups of these professionals as they planned and executed their Ecstasy trips. This paper describes professionals' use of MDMA. We begin with motivations for use; planning the trip; the trip itself; and the aftermath of the trip.

Motivations for Use

Ecstasy presents an opportunity to be open and relaxed within the context of a professional lifestyle that is stressful and very regulated. It provides a chance for individuals to be hedonistic under controlled circumstances and time frames. One 38-year-old woman described Ecstasy as "time-out behavior":

> To me, this is time-out behavior. My life is very full, and I have lots of responsibility, I've got a lot of work that I need to do, I have a lot of deadlines. So to me, it's like time out . . . it's like taking a vacation in Mexico for a week, only I'm going to do it in a day, because that's all I've got.

It is also a part of the "good life" that these professionals have come to enjoy:

> It's like you haven't been to a ball game for three or four months, or you haven't gone out to a real fancy dinner in three or four months, or you haven't gone to a good movie in three or four months. This is part of those things outside of my workaday world that I look forward to. . . . I look forward to being around the people that I'm with when I'm on it, and it's like going to summer camp.

Another motivation for use is time-related and bears directly on the busy schedules and lives lead by these professionals. These individuals complained that they did not seem to have time anymore to let friendships or relationships develop slowly and naturally. As a 30-year-old civil engineer put it, Ecstasy tends to depress time and accelerates interpersonal processes:

> In addition to making you open, it seems to depress time and the ability to cover a lot of ground in this flurry of experience that you might take quite a long time to get to or may not get to without it. I think the world we live in right now seems too busy with our lives.

For those who are therapeutically oriented, MDMA has the potential to allow the individual to "work through" a lot of material in a short time. As this 46-year-old Ph.D. told us:

> I'm not a drug person. I don't use drugs regularly and I don't particularly like getting "high." But the thing I like about Ecstasy is that it allows you to do two years of therapy in one afternoon.

Finally, these professionals see themselves as creative or adventuresome. They are "evolving." As one 38-year-old psychotherapist said:

> I think . . . that was part of the context of the group that was using it on a regular basis, that it was an evolving type drug. Not that the drug itself evolved, but it was an evolutionarily pushing drug. We were evolving.

Planning the 'Trip'

Ecstasy trips are well-planned, often months in advance. Although younger, career-oriented Ecstasy users tended to be more spontaneous in general, spontaneity was something our professionals had long ago forsaken. Like middle-class professionals everywhere, they tend to schedule everything. Most tend to use Ecstasy very sparingly—every three to four months. This spacing is a result of a combination of concerns about the physiological effects of the drug and, equally as important, time constraints. Thus, as this 40-year-old Ph.D. commented:

> . . . if you want to do it, it's gotta be a full-day trip. We always do it with this couple. There's a lot of preparation and also some concern about what are the effects of a lot of use.

Users' age (which is not unrelated to professional status) seems to be an important overriding variable, as 35-year-old-plus bodies do not recover from drugs as quickly as those which are more youthful. According to one middle-aged respondent, these professionals also tend to be more discriminating. In this 51-year-old airline pilot's life, more is not necessarily better:

> . . . the spacing out, I don't know, it's as if you need that period in between to get the effect that I'm looking for.

Thus, busy professionals do not have the time necessary to do more than three or four trips per year. They are too busy, too discriminating, and a bit too old.

Professionals cannot afford to lose sleep. Thus, although it is understood that a "trip" technically lasts four hours, with boosters of more MDMA or marijuana, it can be extended to eight to ten hours. Thus, people very often take Ecstasy early in the day, often between noon and 4:00 p.m., and rarely later than 6:00 or 7:00 p.m. This requires scheduling a whole day and night, rather than just an evening. Given that many of these people, aside from having demanding jobs, also have children, finding a mutually acceptable day and night can be quite a task. They report that usually five or six appointment books have to be consulted in order to find a date that works. And then numerous arrangements have to be made, clearing of calendars, procurement of babysitters, hotel accommodations, if the group is going away for the trip. As one Ph.D. notes:

> . . . just to schedule it is a major problem, like scheduling anything else, like scheduling a dinner. Say you were to schedule a weekend trip with another couple; that's the kind of thinking and work that needs to go into it. Because it is . . . it's like a two-day experience. There's the day of the drug and then the day after.

When a professional is planning his or her first trip, much research on the drug and its effects is done. These individuals have a healthy respect for the power of drugs, and want to know exactly what to expect. They tend not to like surprises and do not want to lose control. Consequently, they attempt to learn as much as possible about the drug before taking it.[4] Generally, one friend will use the drug and tell another about it, describing the effects in particular and the experience in general. S/he may talk about its bonding power, euphoria, spirituality, oneness with nature, etc. Once interested, the friend may decide to do Ecstasy and want to procure the drug. Now the friend becomes the middle-person in procurement, as well as the quasi-guide. S/he buys the drug and sells it to the friend at the same price, making no money.[5] Once the friend has the drug and is getting ready for the trip, s/he is informed about the logistics of taking Ecstasy— what to do to ensure a "good trip," proper dosage (often the first time, the experienced friend will measure out the dose), time of day, emptiness of stomach, setting. Printed "flight instructions" have circulated among some circles of users, describing ways to maximize the trip's benefits and minimize

the possible dangers. Professionals tend to take these instructions quite seriously and often literally. In fact, most of the professionals we interviewed and observed were initiated through friends and relied upon these friends to provide them with the blueprint.

Once the trip has been planned by first-time or subsequent users, there is a waiting period between the plan and the execution. During this period, while professionals are immersed in their work and social worlds, there might be light use of other drugs, particularly alcohol and sometimes marijuana or perhaps some cocaine, although the latter is somewhat out of fashion. However, most of the professionals we talked with indicated that their drug use had lessened considerably since their college days, when many had experimented with psychedelics, cocaine, and other illegal substances.

Some users begin to look forward to the trip weeks before. If the professional is planning an Ecstasy trip for specific goals, such as personal growth, awareness, or building or patching up a relationship/friendship/marriage, often lists are made of items to address. Many professional couples, for example, use this opportunity to explore issues and/or problems in their relationship. As the day of the trip approaches, excitement begins to mount. On the eve of the trip, some professionals make a special effort to preserve their stamina. They have a quiet evening, do not use other drugs, and get a good night's sleep. Often, trips are planned in three-day increments, so that the first day can be spent "resting," the second for the actual trip, and the third for recovery and gearing up for the following week's work. Again the airline pilot comments:

> I'll try and plan . . . ideally to have three days, a day before to come down, in other words, to sort of slow down, so you don't just rush into it, a day before it actually happens, and a day to sort of relax and see what happens if there's any secondary effects. So three days to me is ideal.

The Trip

Finally, the day of the trip arrives. There is excitement in the morning. Many eat a "good breakfast," and often about noon, when the stomach has emptied, the group is ready to "drop" (a word borrowed from old psychedelic lore). Leaving little to chance, they will proceed to the designated spot and set up. A trip to the beach, for example, includes comfortable chairs, plenty of water to counter dehydration, blankets (the body feels colder as the sun sets), and often music. The idea of a retreat, whether indoor or outdoor, is a crucial part of the package. Professionals make these elaborate plans, so that they can "trip" uninterrupted and unencumbered by controllable factors, such as physical comfort. They also choose out-of-the-way locations so they will not have to deal with intrusions and responsibilities, especially children. As one 41-year-old woman, a physician, told us:

> . . . to me it just fits into my realm of playing, really playing, playing and not having the responsibility of taking care of my children.

All settled in, the group takes the MDMA in tablet or capsule form. It can take as long as one hour to "come on," as the users wait in anticipation. They talk, listen to music, get comfortable. Whereas the logistics of planning an Ecstasy trip may be unique to professionals due to their responsibilities and tight schedules, the actual trip and the experience of the drug is similar to others who use it. As each begins to feel the effects, usually at different times (depending on individual weight and dosage), comments such as "I think I'm coming on" and then "It's definitely here" are common. Individuals report that the MDMA come on in waves, beginning with sweaty palms, and then an almost nauseous feeling in the stomach-chest area. Finally, the user fully experiences the effect, and there is no doubt that s/he is "loaded." Almost everyone we've observed and/or interviewed has reported feeling euphoric: all is well with the world, one is part of nature, things are seen clearly, "I'm okay, you're okay—even if we can't live together."

Depending on their motivation, Ecstasy users in general may (1) shut off outside stimuli and interaction in an effort to go inward; (2) sit for hours in a beautiful setting, listening to music, talking with friends; (3) become intimate with another person, sometimes sexually; (4) party, often dancing for hours; (5) do some physical activity, such as skiing. Professionals tend to fall into the first three categories, primarily due to the time of day that they take Ecstasy (daytime) and because they tend not to want to be out in public, dealing with normal interaction. They are much more quiet and private about their drug use than other types of users and have too much to lose if it is publicly exposed.

The hours pass quickly. Some enjoy a "booster" at the beginning of the trip (if they want to get higher initially) or in the middle (if they want to prolong the experience). Others use alcohol to quench thirst and "take the edge off" if the MDMA is creating physiological tension, such as jaw-grinding. Many smoke marijuana at the end of the trip to bring them back up and to prolong the "high."

During the trip, there is much warm, affectionate conversation, a feeling of bonding and closeness with friends. Generally, the spirit is positive and euphoric. There is much affirmation—of life, of relationships.

Afterwards

Finally, the trip is winding down. Some users feel ravenous after a trip; others continue to feel the methamphetamine effects for days after and cannot eat. Some take sleeping pills in order to sleep. Others have no trouble sleeping ten hours after "dropping." Most feel very tired.

As noted, professionals often set aside not one but two or three days for the entire experience. The day after is spent quietly. Some claim they are able to feel the euphoric effects, in a subdued way. Others argue that the best interactive "work" can be done on the day after, when the individual is not so "high" but continues to be clear and forgiving.

Finally it is over, and the professional who uses MDMA occasionally is back to work and the numerous responsibilities which characterize his/her life. There is rarely a "crash," and the benefits seem to far outweigh the costs, which few could elaborate upon.

Implications and Conclusions

"Stress" is commonplace in 1989 America, where keeping up has replaced getting ahead. We are technologically more advanced, and there is more to do, more that can be done, more that has to be done. Technology has helped to create, and is used to sustain, a hurried world. Microwave ovens which speed the cooking process are standard kitchen items. The "black box" accelerates the meditation process and produces the same effect. Computers which speed the writing process are necessities in the office, and those which "save" material in seconds are seen as vastly superior to those which take a few moments. There is more to do, less time to do it, and many, especially those in "high-stress" occupations, wonder how to "kick back" and relax. Many no longer know how, although they are told that "stress reduction" is crucial to good health.

Some professionals, particularly those whose ideas about drugs were formulated during the 1960s, quietly view psychoactive substances as one of many ways to relax, to relate, to "kick back." It is within this context, coupled with the need to relax fast and relate quickly, that Ecstasy is used.

As described in this paper, the professionals studied are able to use this psychoactive substance (and others, such as marijuana) in a rational, controlled, highly organized way. These patterns are in sharp contrast to the multitudinous "war on drugs" messages being forced upon this society, which make claims about the inherent dangers—both social and physiological—of drugs.

The notion of drug use by persons in positions of public health and safety is seen as abhorrent; thus, the institution and proliferation of widespread drug testing. Yet, we have found, upon interviewing and observing professionals in just such positions (e.g., airline pilots, physicians), that their drug use is anything but irresponsible. They use Ecstasy as a way to take time from very busy, stressful lives filled with responsibilities. Their "trips" are well-planned so as not to interfere with these responsibilities. Ironically, their ability to have a "picnic with no food" for a day every few months may have beneficial effects on their performance.

Unfortunately, the irrational rhetoric of the war on drugs has created a hysteria in which it has become impossible to have an open dialogue about drugs. In this McCarthyesque era, dissenting voices are labelled "soft on drugs" and discounted. Perhaps the last item on the agenda should be a better understanding of drugs and how they are used.

One importance of this study is that an examination of professionals' use of Ecstasy illustrates not only the possibility of using drugs in a controlled and responsible way, but the necessity in a hurried world for condensed "time-out" behavior.

*   *   *

Marsha Rosenbaum, Patricia Morgan, and Jerome E. Beck, "Ethnographic Notes on Ecstasy Use Among Professionals," *The International Journal on Drug Policy, 1* (September/October 1989), pp. 16-19.

For Discussion

Why would the working professionals in this study be less likely than other drug users to be arrested, prosecuted, and convicted for drug offenses?

Notes

1. Ecstasy is a mild psychedelic drug with some properties common to methamphetamine. Although first synthesized in 1914 in Germany, Ecstasy enjoyed a resurgence in the mid-to-late 1970s among psychotherapists and "New Age Seekers" for its therapeutic qualities. After a brief spurt of nationwide publicity stemming from more recreational use of the drug among gays and party-goers in Texas, the drug was made illegal (Schedule I) in July, 1985. The user experiences a euphoria lasting four to five hours and reports feeling more communicative and closer to the people s/he happens to be with.

2. NIDA Grant #R01 DA 0440801, "Exploring Ecstasy: A Descriptive Study of MDMA Users," Marsha Rosenbaum, Principal Investigator; Pat Morgan, Co-Principal Investigator; Jerome Beck, Project Director.

3. For the purposes of this study, we have identified "professionals" as those whom we have interviewed and observed who have at least eighteen years of education, and are currently fully engaged in a professional career, such as academia, medicine, law, etc. Most of our professional respondents in the interview portion of the study are married and report making over $35,000 per year, with several reporting an annual income of over $75,000.

4. A major rationale for using Ecstasy, rather than one of the other psychedelics, is that it is shorter-acting and does not render the user confused and out of control.

5. There is an entire middle-class distribution system operating here, in which by definition friends are doing favors for each other, while protecting the money-making distributor. ✦

23. Misuse and Legend in the 'Toad Licking' Phenomenon

Thomas Lyttle

The parotoid glands of the bufo toad contain various substances, and, according to some accounts, "toad licking" produces hallucinogenic reactions among users. In the following article, author Thomas Lyttle describes the media reports of this phenomenon. He claims, however, that these reports were exaggerated, yet embedded in various cultural legends. Initial media coverage led to a wave of "toad licking" accounts by law-enforcement officials and drug-treatment experts. Lyttle concludes by suggesting that the "toad licking" phenomenon is not based on factual evidence.

Introduction

"Toad licking" is a contemporary colloquial euphemism given to the oral ingestion of the glandular secretions of the bufo toad. The genus Bufo includes *Bufo marinus* (the common marine toad.) and related species (e.g., the European *Bufo vulgaris*, the Amazonian *Bufo aqua*, and the North American *Bufo alvarius*).

All have paratoid glands located on their backs. These glands produce a wide variety of biologically active compounds including dopamine, epinephrine, norepinephrine, and serotonin (Boys 1959; Marki et al. 1961).

These compounds are all neurotransmitters found in animal tissue. Other compounds secreted by the bufo toads include the extremely cardioactive steroids bufogenin and bufotoxin (Gessner et al. 1961; Erspamer et al. 1967; Turner and Merlis 1959). The genus *bufo* also produces the possibly hallucinogenic compound bufotenine (5-hydroxy-dimethyltryptamine) See Table 1.

I say "possibly," because there exists a plethora of confusing and contradictory studies, news reports, and anecdotal accounts surrounding various uses of bufotenine and toad secretions generally. See Table 2.

These many studies include the purely pharmacological, the anthropological, the religious, and most recently report on unusual illicit uses or misuses by the general public to get "high," etc. The latter is reportedly done by "licking" the parotoid glands of live bufo toads.

Table 1
Major Categories of Constituents of Toad Venoms

I. Toxic Venoms

A. Bufogenins—Generally known as bufagins. This class of organic molecules represents the major cardioactive principle biosynthesized from cholesterol, containing 24 carbon atoms in their structure. These may be distinguished from the 23 carbon steroids of digitalis and strophanthus. These do not contain nitrogen and are generally labeled with alphabetic letters.

B. Bufotoxins—These molecules contain nitrogen and are conjugates of the steroidal bufogenins with suberic acid/arginine (suberylarginine).

  1. Vulgarobufotoxin—First isolated from the European Toad, *Bufo bufo bufo* in 1922.

  2. Cinobufotoxin—first isolated by Chen and Chen from Chinese medicinal preparation ch'an su, (Japanese senso) from 1929-1931. Identified by K. K. Chen (1931-1933) as coming from skin preparation of Asian toad, *B. gargarizans*.

  3. Gamabufotoxim—First isolated from Asian toad, *B. formosus* in 1930. Its steroid residue is called gamabufotalin.

  4. Marinobufotoxin—First given the name of bufagin by Abel and Macht in 1911. Isolated from *B. marinus* in 1930.

  5. Alvarobufotoxin—First isolated in a very small amount as an amorphous form by Chen and Chen in 1933; recently isolated from *B. alvarius*, along with cholesterol.

An unconjugated cardiotonic steroid molecule was extracted from *B. marinus* in 1988 and named bufalin. The bufotoxins are generally distinguished by the number and location of hydroxyl radicals.

Table 1–Continued

II. The Phenethylamine Bases—The Catecholamines

	Isolated from *Bufo marinus*, *B. aqua*: the American tropical toad	Isolated from ch'an su; *B. gargarizans*
A. Dopamine	X	
B. N-Methyl-dopamine (epinine)	X	
C. (-)Noradrenaline; (-)norepinephrine	X	X
D. (-)Adrenaline; (-)epinephrine;	X	X
E. Corresponding enzymes:		
1. Catechol-*O*-methyl transferase	X	
2. Phenylethanolamine-*N*-methyl transferase	X	
3. Nonspecific *N*-methyl transferase	X	
4. Imidazole-*N*-methyl transferase	X	

III. The Tryptamine Bases

	A[a]	B[b]	C[c]	D[d]
1.[e] Serotonin, enteramine, 5-hydroxytryptamine, 5-IIT	X	X	X	X
2.[e] N-Methyl-serotonin, N-methyl-5-HT	X	X	X	X
3.[f] Bufotenine, *N*-dimethyl-5-HT	X	X	X	X
4. Bufotenidine, *N*-trimethyl-5-HT	X		X	X
5.[g] *N*-Methyl-5-methoxy-tryptamine		X		
6.[g] *O*-Methyl-bufotenin, *N*, *N*-dimethyl-5-methoxy-tryptamine		X		
7[h] Dehydrobufotenine	X		X	X
8.[i] Bufothionine				X
9.[j] Bufoviridine		X		

---

[a]*Bufo marinus*—American tropical toad.

[b]*B. alvarius*—Colorado River toad.

[c]*B. bufo bufo*—European toad.

[d]*B. gargarizans*—Asian toad; probable source of ch'an su.

[e]Vasoconstrictive agents, producing autonomic and cardiovascular distress.

[f]Paradoxical hallucinogenic agent with pressor effects.

[g]Hallucinogenic.

[h]Convulsant agent with a novel tricyclic structure.

[i]Sulfate ester of dehydrobufotenine.

[j]Sulfate ester of bufotenine.

Table 2
Pharmacological Profiles of Bufotenine/Bufotenin

A. Bufotenin isolated from paratoid glands of *Bufo bufo bufo B. vulgaris*, the European toad, and *B. aqua*, *B. marinus*, the giant tropical toad:

1. Phisalix, C.; Bertrand, G. (1893). *C. R. Soc. Biol. 45*:477; *C. R. Acad. Sci. 116*:1080.
2. *Idem*. (1902). C. R. Soc. Biol. 54:932; *C. R. Acad. Sci. 135*:46.
3. Handovsky, H. (1920). *Arch. Exp. Pathol. Pharmakol. 86*:138.
4. Wieland, H.; Hess, G.; Mittasch, H. (1931). *Bericht 64B*(2):2099.
5. Jensen, H.; Chen, K. K. (1932). *Bericht 63*:1310-1314.
6. Wieland, H.; Konz, W.; Mittasch, H. (1934). *Annalen 513*:1-25.
7. Jensen, H.; Chen, K. K. (1936). *Jour. Biol. Chem. 116*:87.
8. Erspamer, V. (1954). *Pharmacol. Rev. 6*:425.
9. *Idem*. (1959). *Biochem. Pharmacol. 2*:270.

B. Bufotenin isolated from fungi:

1. Wieland, T.; Motzel, W.; Merz, H. (1953). *Annalen 581*: 10-16; extracted bufotenin from *Amanita mappa A. muscaria* and *A. pantherina*.

C. Bufotenin containing fungi associated with shamanistic and social pharmacologic rites:

1. Bourke, John Gregory; Captain, U.S. Army (1891, 1934). *Scatologic Rites of All Nations*; Washington, DC.
2. Heizer, Robert F. (February 1944). Mixtum Compositum. The use of narcotic mushrooms by primitive peoples; *Ciba Symposia 5*(11): 1713-1716.
3. Fabing, Howard D. (1956). On going berserk: a neurochemical inquiry; *Scientific Monthly 83*:232-237.

D. Bufotenin isolated from *Piptadenia perigrina*; cohoba snuff:

1. Stromberg, Verner L. (1954). *J. Am. Chem. Soc. 76*:1707; Bufotenine constitutes 1 percent of the weight of seeds of *P. perigrina*.
2. Fish, M. S.; Johnson, N. M.; Lawrence, E. P.; Horning, E. C. (1955). *Biochim. Biophys. Acta 18*:564; isolated from *P. Perigrina* seeds: DMT, DMT-oxide; 5-OH-DMT (bufotenine); 5-OH-DMT-oxide; and a fifth unidentified indole.
3. Fish, M. S.; Johnson, N. M.; Horning, E. C. (1955). *Jour. Amer. Chem. Soc. 77*:5892-5895.
4. Fish, M. S.; Horning, E. C. (1956). *Jour. Nerv. Ment. Dis. 124*:33-37.
5. Fish, M. S.; Johnson, N. M.; Horning, E. C. (1956). *Jour. Amer. Chem. Soc. 78*:3668-3671.
6. Stowe, B. (1959). Occurrence and metabolism of simple indoles in plants; *Forschr. Chem. Org. Naturst. 17*:248-297.
7. Iacobucci, G. A.; Ruveda, E. A. (1964). *Phyrochemistry 3*:465.

E. Bufotenine effects in animals:

1. Evarts, E. (1954). *Jour. Med. Chem. 4*:145. Intravenous injections of bufotenin in the monkey produce a splaying out of hind legs in a pseudoparaplegic manner, and the animal becomes indifferent to noxious stimuli.
2. *Idem*. (1955). *Am. J. Physiol. 182*:594-598. Bufotenine causes a delay in *trans*-synaptic transmission in the optic tract of the cat.
3. *Idem*. (1956). *Arch. Neurol. Psychiat. 75*:49-53. Comparative behavioral effects of LSD and bufotenin; both result in similar behavioral response in the monkey.

F. Bufotenin and related tryptamines urinary excretion associated with states of mental illness:

1. Haddox, C. H.; Saslaw, M. S. (1963). *Journ. Clin. Investiga. 42*:435. 5-MeO-Tryptamine was found in the urine of patients with rheumatic fever—30-210 micrograms/24 hours.
2. *Idem*. (1963). *Jour. Neuropsychiatry 5*:14. Bufotenine is reported in urine of mentally defective patients.

Table 2—Continued

3. *Idem.* (1967). *International Jour. Neuropsychiat. 3*:226. Bufotenine is reported in the urine of chronic schizophrenics; and, by innuendo, it is alleged to be associated with the genesis of this disease.

4. *Idem.* (1967). *Nature 216*:490. Bufotenin is reported in the urine of mentally defective patients.

5. *Idem.* (1967). *Nature 216*:1110. In chronic schizophrenics, excretion of bufotenine and N-methyl-tryptamine should be less than 10 micrograms, if they occur.

6. Fischer, E.; Spatz, H. (1970). Studies on urinary elimination of bufotenine-like substances in schizophrenia; *Biol. Psychiat. 2*:235-240.

7. Heller, B.; Narasimhachari, N.; Saide, J.; Haskovec, L.; Himwich, H. E. (1970). *N*-Dimethylated indoleamines in blood of acute schizophrenics. *Experientia 25*:503.

8. Cottrell, A. C.; McLeod, M. F.; McLeod, W. R. (1977). A bufotenine-like substance in the urine of schizophrenics. *American Jour. Psychiat. 134*:322-323.

9. Raisanen, M.; et al. (1984). Increased urinary excretion of bufotenin by violent offenders with paranoid symptoms and family violence. *Lancet 2*:700-701.

G. Bufotenin—psychotomimetic effects in humans:

1. Fabing, H. D.; Kropa, E. L.; Hawkins, J. R. (March 1956). Bufotenine effects in humans. *Federation Proceedings 15*:421.

2. Fabing, H. D.; Hawkins, J. R. (May 18, 1956). Intravenous bufotenine injection in the human being. *Science 123*:886-887.

3. Fabing, H. D. (May 1957). Toads, mushrooms, and schizophrenia. *Harper's Magazine*, pp. 50-55.

4. Naranjo, Plutarco (July/September 1958). *Archivos de Cnminologia, Neuropsiquiatria y Disciplinas Conexas*, 2nd epoca, *VI*(no. 23):358-379. Psychotomimetic effects of DMT and bufotenin.

5. Costa, E.; Himwich, W. A.; Himwich, H. E. (1959). *Neuropsychopharmacology*, pp. 299-303. Psychotomimetic effects of injected bufotenin.

6. Gessner, P. K.; McIsaac, W. M.; Page, I. H. (1960). *Jour. Pharm. Elp. Ther. 130*:126-133. ". . . it has been known for some time . . . that bufotenine . . . is somewhat psychotomimetic."

7. *Idem.* (1961). Pharmacological actions of some methoxyindolealkylamines. *Nature 190*:179-180. Including serotonin, bufotenine, and 5-MeO-DMT.

8. Anonymous (November 11, 1967). Hallucinogens and psychosis. *Nature 216*:538. Reference is made to psychotomimetic properties of bufotenine.

9. Anonymous (1968). The chemistry of the brain. *Nature 219*:838. Bufotenin is referred to as a well-known hallucinogen.

10. Ahlborg, U.; Holmstedt, B.; Lindgren, J. (1968). Fate and metabolism of some hallucinogenic indolealkylamines. *Advances in Pharmacology 6B*:213-229. Including DMT, 5-OH-DMT (bufotenin), and 5-MeO-DMT.

11. *Encyclopedia Britannica*, 15th ed. (1975). *Micropedia 11*:349-350. Bufotenin identified as a mild hallucinogen.

12. McLeod, W. R.; Sitaram, B. R. (1985). Bufotenine reconsidered. *Acta Psychiatr. Scandin. 72*:447-450. Intravenous bufotenin at 2 mg and 4 mg show no hallucinogenic effects. 8 mg i.v. results in profound emotional and perceptual changes, extreme anxiety, a sense of imminent death, visual disturbance associated with color reversal and distortion, severe flushing of cheeks and forehead. Suggests bufotenin is a psychotomimetic under some circumstances (high dose, i.v.).

13. Kysilka, R.; Wurst, M. (March 3, 1989). High-performance liquid chromatographic determination of some psychotropic indole derivatives. *Jour. Chromatog. 464*(2):434-437. Including bufotenin, psilocybine, and psilocin.

H. Bufotenin—nonpsychotomimetic effects in humans:

1. Turner, W. J.; Merlis, S. (January 1959). *Arch. Neurol. Psychiat. 81*:121-129. Tried Cohoba snuff; reported no hallucinogenic activity due to bufotenin.

2. Hofmann, A. (1963). Psychotomimetic substances. *Indian Journal of Pharmacy 25*:245-256. Bufotenine is not psychotomimetic.

Table 2—Continued

3. Fischer, Roland (1968). Chemistry of the brain. *Nature 220*:411-412. Bufotenin is not a true psychotomimetic compound in the sense that LSD, mescaline, and psilocybin are.

4. Schultes, R. E.; Hofmann, A. (1973). *The Botany and Chemistry of Hallucinogens*, p. 90. It seems probable that 5-OH-DMT (bufotenin) does not contribute to the psychotomimetic activity of cohoba or virola snuffs.

5. Stafford, Peter (1978, 1983, 1992). *Psychedelic Encyclopedia*. Bufotenin is uninteresting and not psychedelic.

6. Grinspoon, L.; Bakalar, J. B. (1979). *Psychedelic Drugs Reconsidered*. Bufotenin is not psychedelic.

7. Shulgin, A. T. (October/December 1981). Bufotenine. *Jour. Psychoactive Drugs 13*(4):389. Bufotenin is not orally active; at high dose i.v. (16 mg), there is face purpling, difficulty in focusing, physical tension, anxiety and dopiness.

Shulgin, A. T. (1988). The controlled substances act; p. 317. 32 Federal Register (FR) 10308 (July 13, 1967): The initial proposal for placing bufotenine, diethyltryptamine (DET), and ibogaine into Schedule 1 as controlled drugs. 32 FR 13407 (September 23, 1967): Final action on proposal. 32 FR 15340 (November 3, 1967): Official final word on the listing of bufotenine, DET, and ibogaine.

The first wave of news reports regarding "toad licking" or the oral ingestion of bufotenine occurred in the mid-1980s in the popular press, where it was highly sensationalized, and it has continued to the present (Anonymous 1986, 1991). The story is developing still, and it holds implications of interest to serious drug researchers and sociologists.

The "toad licking" stories themselves are usually reported in areas (South or Central America, Canada, the United States, and Australia) where the bufo toad is either indigenous or is easily transported from an indigenous environment. Reports have also appeared where the bufo has been artificially introduced into an ecosystem for reasons of pest control, as in Australia (Lewis 1989; Anonymous 1990a; Ebert 1988).

The practice of "toad licking" seems to have developed out of legendary and mythological uses of toads through history. Reports of bufo uses as a poison, as well as a magical tool, go back as far as Roman times (Davis 1985). The poet Robert Graves (1948) cites Gwion regarding "the toad" and its uses in sorcery. He states:

> . . . Gwion implies that a single gem can enlarge itself under the influence of "the toad" or "the serpent" into a whole treasury of jewels. His claim to be as learned in math and to know myriads of secrets may also belong to the toad/serpent sequence. . . .

Boetius de Boot, in his *Parfait Joallier* (1644), describes "the toad stone" alleged to ". . . exist in the toad's head . . . another sure talisman for obtaining perfect Earthly happiness. . . ." (de Givry 1963). Johannes de Cuba, in his *Hortus Sanitatus*

(1498), ". . . has indicated a method, at once both practical and elegant, of extracting this stone, which I especially recommend to my readers. . . ." (de Givry 1963).

The bufo toad was reintroduced to Western Europe by Christopher Columbus on a return voyage from America (Davis 1985). "The toad" remained a legendary ingredient in witches "philtres" or "brews," supposedly used at Sabbaths for magical purposes (Fabing 1956; Wilson 1973; Chilton et al. 1979; Lee and Schlain 1986). This was probably as an admixture.

In 1986, both the *New England Journal of Medicine* and *Discover* magazines reported that "classic German violinists used to handle toads before their performances because the toxins reduced the sweat on their palms. . . ." (Anonymous 1986).

"Toad licking" also seems to have developed out of Central and South American religious uses. It also has precedents in Southeast and Southwest North American Indian tradition.

The Choco Indians of West Colombia learned to "milk" these bufo toads to obtain the glandular secretions. In *The Serpent and the Rainbow* by Wade Davis (1985) is this description:

> . . . the Choco Indians learned to milk these toads by placing them in bamboo suspended over flames. The heat caused them to extrude a yellow liquid which dripped into ceramic vessels. . . .

The venom was then used for a variety of purposes, divinatory, hunting, etc.

The bufo toad also seems to have played important roles in Central American religions. Virtually *all* the amphibian remains at the post-classic Maya sites at Cozumel (Mexico) are bufo. There is even conjecture that this toad played some "narcotic-like" role in ancient Olmec traditions (Chilton et al. 1979; Davis 1985). There is, however, no conclusive evidence so far as to the true meaning(s) of the bufo toads in these cultures.

North American Indian tribes of the Southeast and Southwest have also implemented bufo into their cultures. In 1981, several reports surfaced regarding the discoveries of anthropologist Dr. Jean Rundquist who discovered ". . . over 10,000 toads" in an Indian burial site in South Carolina, United States. In *Omni* magazine (August 1981) Maurer reported that

> . . . excavating a Cherokee Indian burial site in South Carolina, Dr. Jean Rundquist found something she did not expect . . . the skeletal remains of 10,000 toads. She discovered that the Indians in New Mexico and the Caribbean . . . snorted a chemical in the dried toad skins . . . that they used the chemicals in ceremonies. . . .

In 1984, author and researcher Albert Most revealed his The Church of The Toad of Light with his publication of his book *Bufo alvarius: Psychedelic Toad of the Sonoran Desert* (Venom Press 1984). This small book detailed how to use the bufo toad for ritual and pleasure. Shown was how to catch the toad, extract or "milk" the glandular secretions, dry them, and then "enjoy" the smoked vapors. His book claims that 5-MeO-DMT (5-methoxy-N, N-dimethyltryptamine) is the active hallucinogen, not bufotenine. 5-MeO-DMT is the O-methyl ether of bufotenine (Gessner et al. 1961; Marki et al. 1962).

The subject of clandestine or cult uses of bufo presents an interesting dilemma for researchers. The very nature of such illicit activity makes open, usually easy data-gathering troublesome. Anecdotal or "word-of-mouth" descriptions often prove invaluable, so far as providing a profile of the activity itself.

A private letter to the author talks about the introduction of hallucinatory toad venom to well-known American (Indian) artist Christobal. This letter details Christobal's "yarn art" (an innovative stylized art form) based on his bufo exposures. Letter-writer Jacaeber Kastor (1989) states:

> . . . the colors are very subdued in the Polaroid . . . they are vibrant and fluorescent in the yarn painting, etc. This piece has to do with Leo (Mercado) turning Christobal on to the toad secretions and Christobal incorporating the desert toad into his technology/iconography, etc. . . . A very interesting mixology. . . .

In another note to researcher B. J. Ridge, Kastor states that "the toad is in their (Huichol) cosmology, but I don't think that any of the older Huichols ever tried smoking it. . . ." (Kastor 1989).

Christobal's (1989b) actual description of his bufo toad visions are as follows:

> The symbol of brother toad and the mushroom which are Gods to give wisdom of the shamanism and to study how to be able to communicate and be able to receive direction and encounter the sacred places that exist. Because not all [places] serve for that which one wants to know. For the Gods say in which place one can ask for that which one in reality wants to know, to be able to learn here is when the shaman are in the sacred places with their candles praying to wait for the hour when the Gods arrive to be able to communicate for their power and ask luck for their shamanism. . . . And when the hour arrives, they see that the candles surge . . . the life force appears, as if it explodes, and from the sparks the force which comes out is seen, and that is the way it is where the transformation occurs. . . . It is power which the brother toad and the mushroom have . . . because in this way . . . the Gods speak. . . .

Another more recent anecdotal account showing bufo venom use comes from *The Village Voice* (July 10, 1990). Author G. Trebay describes art critic Carlo McCormick's sojourn with the hallucinogenic toad: "the group drank tincture of peyote, chewed dried peyote buttons, and smoked the dried secretions of a desert toad, whose toxins produce . . . 'an effect,' etc." (Trebay 1990). The non-oral, psychoactive uses of bufo toads (smoking, enema,

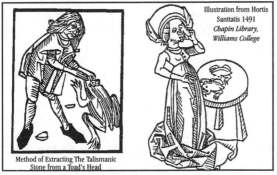

Illustration from Hortis Santtatis 1491
Chapin Library, Williams College

Method of Extracting The Talismanic Stone from a Toad's Head

Figure 1

snuffs, etc.) are well-documented. What are the implications of these non-oral uses of bufo in relation to supposed "toad licking," etc?

A number of reports show bufotenine itself to be totally inactive orally (McKim 1986; Root 1990; Horgan 1990). Toxic reactions have been reported in humans and animals after oral ingestion, however (Anonymous 1986, 1988; Uzelac 1990).

If this is true, then where did the whole "toad-licking" scenario emerge from? What are the implications, so far as drug reporting and research, legal studies, placebo theory, and urban legends, etc.?

The Contemporary Situation

In 1967, the Food and Drug Administration and the Drug Enforcement Administration placed bufotenine (the supposed main psychoactive in the bufo toad) on its Controlled Substances List. It was assigned to Schedule One, making it highly illegal to possess.

In the mid-1980s, the newspaper *USA Today* reported that Australian "hippies" were forsaking traditional drugs for "cane toads," which they "boil for a slimy, potentially lethal cocktail" (Anonymous 1988). A later corresponding report described "the Drug Squad in Brisbane (Australia) as having . . . a Heinz Baby Food jar which carried the label Venom Cane Toad: Hallucinogenic; Bufotenine" (Lewis 1989).

A few months later, a Dr. Inaga gave a lecture in Baltimore, Maryland, in which he "comically" mentioned the "phenomenon" (Horgan 1990). Almost simultaneously, Dr. Alex Stalcup, of the Haight Ashbury Free Medical Clinic, gave this statement to reporters: ". . . it is amazing the lengths that people will go to, to get high. . . ." He was referring to the recent "toad licking stories" that were starting to circulate in the media (Seligman 1989).

This media interest became the topic of discussion at a 1989 conference on crack cocaine in San Francisco (Seligman 1989; Presley 1989). Berkeley police chief R. Nelson was there and commented that "[toad licking] . . . is a problem that comes up from time to time," legitimizing the rumors. Pressed at a news conference, Robert Sager, head of the DEA's Western Regional Laboratory, said "[bufo toad venom] . . . is in the same legal category as heroin or LSD," further confusing the issue through incomplete comparisons (Seligman 1989). While all three are in the same legal category, only LSD and heroin are widely used drugs.

A New York City DEA spokesman also stated to the press "that we have heard of it . . . but have yet to make an arrest" (Carillo 1990), implying that there was some sort of active problem.

The rumors now circled back to the Haight Ashbury Clinic. In response to the press releases, the Clinic stated that "ironically . . . the DEA's actions have inspired a few people to try licking live toads" (Carillo 1990).

Reporters now pressed any expert they could find to investigate the apparently "legitimate" stories. Back in Australia, Glen Ingram, a herpetologist at Queensland Museum, stated to the press that "it [toad venom] gives them a kick like alcohol. . . ." This and other wire service stories led some Australians to react with "panic," according to *Scientific American*. Alarmed at the newest "drug craze," some people in Australia formed "toad-eradication leagues" (Horgan 1990).

Back in California, a probation officer stated to the media, "We hear of youngsters who do this frequently [lick toads]. . . . It is not as strong as LSD, but it's free" (Montgomery 1990).

At this point, little in the way of names, precise locations, fatalities, or witnesses had appeared in the legitimate press. The press had, presumably with the help of so-called "experts" in related drug-misuse fields, fueled partial rumors and misinformation. As well, most of the press reports lacked the solid primary sources needed to trace back for facts.

Later in 1990, this started to change when reports naming P. Cherrie and G. Murphy appeared in *The Albany Times Union*. The story reported that "Gary Murphy and Paul Cherrie saw a TV show about 'toad licking' and decided to experiment." They scraped some toad secretions from the backs of the cane toads in Cherrie's pet collection and spread it on a cracker (Anonymous 1990c). Murphy, 21, said that after an hour of "deep hallucinations" he awoke "bam!" in the hospital. Both men suffered severe vomiting (Anonymous 1990c). The story was amended a few days later in the tabloids, which reported that Murphy had killed himself, after being prematurely released from the hospital (Alexander 1990).

Stanton Geer was next named, awaiting trial in Colombia after being arrested on "toad licking" charges. He faced a sentence of "two years and a $10,000 fine," if convicted, for "drug abuse" (Street 1990). Other names also started appearing.

During all this, Dr. Stalcup from the Haight-Ashbury Clinic in San Francisco complained that "we were getting calls from all over the world—Germany, England, South America, etc. from reporters wondering about this new high" (Dorgan 1990).

Then, once again, the rumors started to circle. According to Dr. Sager of the DEA, Australian journalists were now studying the United States situation to see "if there was a cane toad problem in California" (Dorgan 1990).

The main problem with substantiating the original and later reports was "that they are all based on other reports . . . and that there is no evidence to support them," said writer Michael Dorgan (Dorgan 1990). Writer Eileen Uzelac said this was a case of "media feeding on media" (Dorgan 1990). Words like "urban legend" were now being used, along with other explanations.

In all this confusion, a number of legislators were convinced that where there was smoke, there might be fire. Not to be beat to the punch for solutions to the newest drug "epidemic," Representative Beverly Langford (D, Calhoun, Georgia) introduced legislation to the State General Assembly regarding "toad licking" (Secrest 1990):

> In a resolution introduced Monday, apparently with a straight face, Rep. J. Beverly Langford (D, Calhoun) called on the General Assembly to look into "the extreme danger of toad licking becoming the designer drug of choice in today's sophisticated society. . . . [The Assembly] has been very diligent in finding and proposing a legitimate solution to every conceivable type of drug problem. . . .

The next legislative attempt to curb this new drug menace appeared in Vancouver, British Columbia (Canada). The report states (Anonymous 1991):

> . . . Vancouver police today said that they want the Canadian government to ban imports of the potentially lethal giant toad blamed on the deaths of several Australian drug users. . . .

> . . . Cpl. John Dragoni said the city police force is applying to Ottawa to prohibit ownership of . . . the toads . . . by outlawing them under The Federal Narcotics Control Act, etc.

Trying to lend some credibility to what was becoming an embarrassing flurry of misinformation, George Root, a former administrator at SP Labs in Miami, Florida, stated (Root 1990):

> . . . there has been speculation in the anthropological literature regarding the possible hallucinogenic use of bufo, but this debate is largely based upon the fact that bufo is a common representation in the art of some Meso-American peoples . . . and the fact that bufo skeletal remains have been found at archaeological sites.

> Speculations aside, there is a very good reason why licking toads will not get you high. The toxic compounds are likely to kill you before you could possibly consume enough bufotenine to have a hallucinogenic effect (if there is a hallucinogenic effect).

Conclusion

Within the space of four years, an informational epidemic based in "toad licking" lore and legendry played minor havoc among supposedly "professional" drug experts and journalists. This led to incidents of public concern and actually stirred legislative debate among lawmakers in the United States and Canada. An examination of the media frenzy, and the willingness of our culture to support such unfounded conclusions, points to weaknesses in our public policies and attitudes about illicit drug use/misuse. We cannot fathom existing drug use/misuse problems if we base our understanding on false or confused premises. "Toad licking" is an example of this.

Future Research Needs

Scholars in the future must diligently pursue primary sources for facts, not hearsay. In the case of the ongoing "toad-licking" phenomenon, this led to outlandish and distorted stories which may or may not have had a basis in fact. Future reporting and information-gathering should be weighed against this profile.

This article should be seen as a preliminary profile of an ongoing cultural phenomenon involving drug use/misuse. Future surveys of this particular topic must include a solid bibliography showing primary, secondary, as well as "hearsay" accounts, police and medical statistics, and in-depth interviews with key participants. Future research must also study this phenomenon in relation to other aspects of cultural life.

Understanding drug use/misuse issues—both legitimate as well as clandestine—is a complicated undertaking. Let us hope that future scholars will gain a better understanding through our current diligence.

Acknowledgments

The assistance of researchers David Goldstein, Roger Knights, Charles Andrew, and B. J. Ridge in obtaining newspaper accounts, bibliographic material, and some anecdotal accounts is appreciated.

✳ ✳ ✳

For Discussion

How might the media contribute to the creation of a drug problem?

References

Abel, J., and Macht, D. (1911). The poisons of the tropical toad: *Bufo aqua. J. Am. Med. Assoc. 56*:1531.

Alexander, J. (1990). Toad-licker kills himself. *The Weekly World News*, October 2, p. 21.

Anonymous (1981). Toad away. *Drug Survival News* (October).

Anonymous (1986). It could have been an extremely grim fairy tale. *Discover 12*.

Anonymous (1988). Terror toads. *The New York Times*, June 28, p. A24.

Anonymous (1989a). Drug experts warn of new high—Toad licking. *San Francisco Examiner*, June 1, p. H10.

Anonymous (1989b). Colorado River toad licking. *The National Enquirer*, August 8, p. 6.

Anonymous (1990a). Australia's investments in cane toads. *The Chicago Tribune*, April 9, p. 14A.

Anonymous (1990b). Toad-lickers gamble with death. *Sea Frontiers*, June, p. 36.

Anonymous (1990c) Minds go loose from toad juice. *The Albany Times Union*, no date, p. A2.

Anonymous (1991). Toad addicts licking giant toads to get high. *The Palm Beach Post*, July 31, p.9A.

Boys, F. (1959). *Poisonous Amphibians and Reptiles*. Springfield, IL: Thomas.

Carillo, C. (1990). Toads take a licking from desperate druggies. *The New York Post*, January 31, p. 4.

Chen, K., and Jensen, H. (1929). A pharmacognostic study of Ch'an Su, the dried venom of the Chinese toad. *J. Am. Pharm. Assoc. 23*:244-251.

Chilton, W., Bigwood, J., and Jensen R. (1979). Psilocin, bufotenine, and serotonin: Historical and biosynthetic observations. *J. Psychedelic Drugs 11*(1-2):61-69.

Christobal (1989a). Photo of stylized yarn art featuring bufo visions (from the collection of Thomas Lyttle).

Christobal (1989b). One-page handwritten note describing bufo visions (from the collection of Thomas Lyttle).

Davis, W. (1985). *The Serpent and the Rainbow*. New York: Simon and Schuster.

Davis, W. (1988). *Passage of Darkness: The Ethnobiology of the Haitian Zombie*. Chapel Hill: The University of North Carolina Press.

deGivry (1963). *Picture Museum of Sorcery, Magic, and Alchemy*. New York: New York University Press.

Dorgan, M. (1990). Nobody, but nobody licks toads in California. *The Sunday Albany Times Union*, February 18, p. A24.

Ebert, R. (1988). Hungry toads raising cane. *The New York Post*, October 1, p. 2.

Erspamer, V., Vitali, T., Rosenghini, M., and Cei, J. (1965). 5-Methoxy- and 5-Hydroxyindolealkylamines in the skin of *Bufo alvarius. Experientia 21*:504.

Erspamer, V., Vitali, T., Rosenghini, M., and Cei, J. (1967). 5-Methoxy- and 5-hydroxyindoles in the skin of *Bufo alvarius. Biochem. Pharmacol. 16*:1149-1164.

Fabing, H. (1956). Intravenous bufotenine injection in the human being. *Science 123*:886-887.

Fabing, H. (1967). Toads, mushrooms, and schizophrenia. *Harper's 214*:51-55.

Furst, P. (1976). The virola tree as a source for hallucinogenic snuffs. In *Hallucinogens and Culture*. Novato, CA: Chandler and Sharp.

Gessner, P., McIsaac, W., and Page, I. (1961). Pharmacological actions of some methoxyindolealkylamines. *Nature 190*:179-180.

Goldstein, D. (1992). *The PHD (papers from the history of drugs) Catalog*. New York: privately published.

Graves, R. (1948). *The White Goddess*. New York: Farrar, Straus, and Giroux.

Hofmann, A. (1963). Psychotomimetic substances. *Indian J. Pharm. 25*:245-256.

Horgan, J. (1990). Bufo abuse: A toxic toad gets licked, boiled, tee'd up, and tanned. *Sci. Am. 263*(2):26-27.

Kanus, L. (1989). Review of *Cane Toads: An Unnatural History. Libr. J. 114*:122.

Kastor, J. (1989). Private correspondence to Thomas Lyttle.

Kennedy, A. (1982). Ecce bufo: The toad in nature and Olmec iconography. *Curr. Anthropol. 23*(3):273-290.

Lee, M., and Schlain, B. (1986). *Acid Dreams*. New York: Grove Press.

Lewis, S. (1989). *Cane Toads: An Unnatural History*. New York: Dolphin Press.

Lyttle, T. (1989a). Private correspondence.

Lyttle, T. (1989b). Drug-based religions and contemporary drug taking. *J. Drug Issues 18*(2):271-284.

Lyttle, T., and Montagne, M. (1992). Drugs, music, and ideology: A social pharmacological interpretation of the acid house movement. *Int. J. Addict. 27*(10):1159-1177.

Marki, F., Axelrod, J., and Witkop, B. (1961). Dehydrobufotenine: A novel type of trycyclic serotonin metabolite from *Bufo marinus. J. Am. Chem. Soc. 83*:3341.

Marki, F., Axelrod, J., and Witkop, B. (1962). Catecholamines and methyltransferases in the South American toad (*Bufo marinus*). *Biochim. Biophys. Acta 58*:367-369.

Maurer, A. (1981). Ancient pyschedelics. *Omni*, August, p. 38.

McKim, W. (1986). *Drugs and Behavior: An Introduction to Behavioral Pharmacology*. Englewood Cliffs, NJ: Prentice-Hall.

Montgomery, C. (1990). Druggies find new way to get high: They lick toads. *Weekly World News*, October 28, p. 6.

Most, A. (1984). *Bufo alvarius: Psychedelic Toad of the Sonoran Desert*. New Mexico: Venom Press.

Most, A. (1985). Advertisement for *The Church of the Toad of Light* T-shirts (from the collection of Thomas Lyttle).

Mugger (1989). Colorado River toad licking. *The New York Press*, August 11.

O'Shea, B. (1990). A year of political pageantry and toad licking. *Atlanta Journal and Constitution*, March 11, p. C5A.

Presley, D. (1989). Toad licking poses threat to youth of America. *The Weekly World News*, July 11.

Root, G. (1990). First the bad news, toad licking will not get you high. *New Times* (letter).

Schultes, R., and Hofmann, A. (1980). *The Botany and Chemistry of the Hallucinogens*. Springfield, IL: Thomas.

Secrest, D. (1990). Bill gets hopping mad on way to lick toad problems. *Atlanta Journal and Constitution*, February 13, p. D1F.

Seligman, K. (1989). The latest high—Warts and all: Thrill seekers risk death to lick toads. *The San Francisco Examiner*, May 29, p. A10.

Shulgin, A. (1988). *The CSA (Controlled Substances Act) Manual*. LaFayette, CA: privately printed.

Street, M. (1990). Toad lickers get busted. *The Weekly World News*, March 13, p. 12.

Trebay, G. (1990). Mexican standoff: Carlo McCormick's bad trip. *The Village Voice*, July 10, p. 19.

Turner, W., and Merlis, S. (1959). Effects of some indolealkylamines on man. *Arch. Neurolog. Psychiatry 81*:121-129.

Uzelac, E. (1990). A desperation high: Crack, coke, croak? *The Baltimore Sun*, January 30, p. 5.

Wilson, R. A. (1973). *Sex and Drugs: A Journey Beyond Limits*. Chicago: Playboy Press. ✦

24. The Dusting of America: The Image of Phencyclidine (PCP) in the Popular Media

JOHN P. MORGAN

AND

DOREEN KAGAN

P*CP, or more formally* phencyclidine, *is a central nervous-system excitant agent having anesthetic, analgesic, and hallucinogenic properties. Originally, PCP was used as an anesthetic agent in surgical procedures. Although it was found to be generally effective, the drug often produced a number of unpleasant side effects—extreme excitement, visual disturbances, and delirium. As a result, in 1967 the use of phencyclidine was restricted to "veterinary use only," as an animal tranquilizer. The initial street use of PCP (also known as rocket fuel, horse tranquilizer, animal trank, aurora borealis, DOA, elephant, elephant juice, dust, goon, green snow, mist, sheets, angel dust, fairy dust, dummy dust, monkey dust, devil's dust, devil stick, hog, THC, tic, tic tac, supergrass, flakes, and buzz), appeared in the Haight-Ashbury underground community of San Francisco and other West and East Coast cities during 1967. It was first marketed as the* PeaCe *Pill; hence, the name PCP quickly became popular. In the following essay, authors John P. Morgan and Doreen Kagan review the history of PCP in the American drug scene, focusing on its image as a "devil drug."*

"The Devil Drug of All Time," "Violence Increases Due to Angel Dust," "Person High on PCP Gouges Out His Own Eyes."

These recent headlines were easily selected from a panoply of similar frightening stories about phencyclidine, America's newest important drug of abuse. PCP, 1-(1-phencyclohexyl)piperidine, was first synthesized in 1958 (Domino 1964). It was widely tested in humans between 1959 and 1962 because it suppressed perception of painful (and other) stimuli and made possible surgery in patients who were not suppressed to the point of full stupor, as is usually required in surgery. Its clinical use was curtailed because patients often emerged from surgery or other treatments with excitation, fearful delusions, or complete psychosis (Luby et al. 1959). The drug's originators, Parke-Davis, ceased clinical testing in 1962 but for years the drug was available to veterinarians who used it to anaesthetize large animals, particularly primates. It was sold to this market as Sernylan®. PCP emerged as a street drug in San Francisco in 1967 (Meyers, Rose and Smith 1967-1968). After that first use, it surfaced periodically; it was often deceptively sold as THC, the active ingredient of cannabis products. In the last years of the 1970s, however, its use became very widespread in America and to many it became our most important drug problem (Luisada 1978).

Our purpose here is not to describe the pharmacology or patterns of use of PCP but to describe how America learned about the drug and how it earned its status as the "devil drug." Early medical reports concerned with street use and abuse of PCP used the customary medical-scientific-journalistic style, a non-emotive style. By the mid-1970s, however, a few reports published for medical readers began to cite a number of horror stories. In 1976 an article appeared in *Emergency Medicine* entitled "High on PCP" (Unsigned 1976). This presentation featured an interview with R. Stanley Burns who with other workers had published the first extensive clinical article on PCP in *Western Medicine* the preceding year (Burns et al. 1975). The 1975 article did not detail stories of crimes, rapes, and murders, but the *Emergency Medicine* article did present a number of PCP horror tales told by Burns. While discussing a group of chronic users he referred to patients who died.

> . . . all three died because of behavioral toxicity. Two drowned in swimming pools while under the influence and the other burned to death in a fire.

Burns also referred to several homicides and suicides resultant from the use of the drug.

The emergence of this style of material in the medical literature regarding drug abuse was not without precedent, but this was the first signal of a now predominant theme regarding PCP that emerged in newspapers, magazines, and TV shows. We decided to survey *popular* media sources of PCP stories to identify both this pattern of emergence and the predominant themes presented to the larger public.

Methodology

We surveyed published newspaper reports for the period of 1957-1979. We then expanded the survey to popular periodicals, television news, and dramatic shows and finally included popular music.

Newspapers

The most extensive survey was carried out on newspaper articles. The "underground press" would have constituted an interesting source but existing indexes are far from comprehensive and we reluctantly confined this search to the established press. Indexes are maintained by a number of major newspapers and we searched the following ones:

- *Atlanta Constitution*
- *Chicago Tribune* Index
- *Detroit News*
- *Houston Post*
- *Los Angeles Times*
- *New Orleans Times-Picayune*
- *New York Times*
- *San Francisco Chronicle*
- *Washington Post*

We found one extremely valuable source, Newsbank. This microfiche collection catalogs articles from more than 250 major and minor national newspapers. A search of the "health" category revealed valuable indexing of drug and drug-addiction articles.

We obtained two large clipping files from Dr. Richard E. Garey of Tulane University and from "The Bridge," a drug-information service of the Town of North Hempstead, Manhasset, New York. The New York office of the Associated Press (AP) supplied us photocopies of their wire stories on PCP. Each news article was obtained and analyzed. We recorded the city of origin (national wire service or local) and the thematic treatment.

Most of the cited indexes were first organized in 1972 except the *New York Times Index* (1851) and *Newsbank* (1970). Therefore most pre-1970 data come from the *New York Times*. The geographic distribution of the major indexes is uneven and our data focus prominently on large cities. The study does not encompass every PCP article printed but any errors from omission are probably negligible.

Popular Periodicals

Indexing services were also important in locating articles published by magazines. Some sources used were:

- *Access*
- Catholic Periodical Literature Index
- Humanities Index
- Index to Little Magazines
- Magazine Index
- New Periodicals Index
- Popular Periodical Index
- Reader's Guide to Periodical Literature
- Social Science Index

The Magazine Index provided the most comprehensive compilation of popular journals and supplied most of our citations. It indexes on microfilm approximately 370 periodicals.

Television News and Entertainment

Comprehensive indexing tools for this important area of American media do not exist. We obtained some information from:

- Television News Index and Abstracts
- Vanderbilt Television News Archives
- Radner Corporation (publisher of TV Guide)
- Program information units of ABC, NBC, and CBS
- Television Information Office, NYC
- Museum of Broadcasting, NYC

The Vanderbilt service catalogs evening network news broadcasts. The Television Information Office (TIO), whose files were incomplete, retains some information on network television shows. Most other sources were, like TIO, parochial, incomplete, or both. We probably located more television shows that focused on PCP from friends who paid attention to the TV listings in newspapers than from any other source.

Results

We read 323 newspaper articles that focused on PCP between 1958 and 1979.[1] Twenty-seven states plus the District of Columbia were represented by newspaper articles. Table I indicates the total number of articles found in the established press for the period 1958-1979. An obvious explosion of coverage occurred in 1978 and the subsequent reporting has begun to diminish. Most notable was the fact that the presentation and representation of horror stories became a most important theme. These narrative accounts dealt with acts of violence by users on others or themselves. Often such stories were shocking and even repugnant and loathsome. We were able to identify 59 different stories involving violent or shocking themes during this time. One narrative horror tale occurred in 25 percent of all newspaper articles and some articles recounted as many as 15. Even when the news report did not utilize a narrative horror tale, the articles often focused on violence secondary to the drug. Table II presents the dates and locations of horror tales and Table III identifies those stories recounted five or more times.

Table I
National News Articles About PCP: 1958-1979

Year	Number of Articles	Percentage of Total
1958	1	–
1970	1	–
1973	5	2%
1974	2	1%
1975	4	1%
1976	3	1%
1977	18	6%
1978	247	76%
1979	42	13%
Totals	323	100%

The most repeated tale was that of self-removal of eyes which was cited 17 times during a three-year period. Different versions gave specific origins and identification. The victim was said to be a Baltimore college student (Brown 1978), the son of a Massachusetts Congressman (Charcot 1978), a man in a midwestern city (Oswald 1978), or a man from San Jose (Green 1978).

Table II
Locations* and Dates of Newspaper Horror Tales

State	1977	1978	1979
Alabama		1	
California	3	14	4
Florida		1	
Georgia		1	
Illinois	1	4	
Indiana		1	1
Kentucky		1	
Louisiana		11	
Maryland		1	
Massachusetts		1	
Michigan		3	1
Minnesota			1
Missouri		2	
New Hampshire		1	
New York		5	3
Pennsylvania		1	
South Carolina		1	
Texas		8	
Utah		1	
Washington, D.C	2	.2	

* In only seven instances did the story appear in a wire service (AP or UPI) report. However, this does not mean that the stories were given a local setting. The writer of the local story merely recounted the tale sometimes giving a locale—sometimes not.

Magazines

We located 23 magazine articles in the 1977-1979 period: seven in 1977, 13 in 1978, and three in 1979. Table IV lists these sources. Horror stories appeared in 10 of these 23. The "gouged eye" theme was again most popular and appeared in seven stories. Two new versions appeared: *Sepia* (Gay 1978) stated that the incident occurred in 1971 when a young woman, following arrest for assault, gouged out her eyes in jail; and *New Times* (Koper 1978) identified a young man by name who, following arrest for indecent exposure, gouged out his eyes in jail.

Table III
Popular Horror Tales of PCP Users

Horror Tales	Number of News Accounts
1. Person gouges out own eyes	17
2. Nude, unarmed man refuses to halt on police command. Dies after varying number of police bullets are fired.	13
3. Person drowns in shower stall with four inches of water	12
4. Young man shoots and kills own father, mother, and grandfather	9
5. Person sits engulfed in flames, unable to perceive danger.	9
6. Person amputates a bodily part: nose, breast, or penis.	9
7. Man crosses eight-lane freeway, enters a house, randomly stabs pregnant woman and toddler. Toddler and fetus die; mother survives.	8
8. Pulls out own teeth with pliers.	7
9. Small 14-year-old girl requires many police to subdue her.	6
10. Seventeen-year-old runs naked through streets in deep snow.	6
11. Motorcyclist points vehicle head-on into Trailways bus (or tree).	6
12. Person pops handcuff restraints.	5
13. Mother puts baby in cauldron of steaming water.	5
14. Person wanders onto freeway and does push-ups	5

quently told horror stories and, in fact, focused on them as part of the dramatic setting and urgency that accompanies TV news. Nine horror stories were presented by Walter Cronkite on *The CBS Evening News* in 1978.

Table IV
Popular Journals

1977	
7/18/77	*Time*
8/8/77	*U.S. News & World Report*
8/77	Human Behavior
12/12/77	Village Voice
12/19/77	*Time*
12/77	*Current Health*
1978	
3/13/78	*Newsweek*
3/20/78	*New Times*
4/78	*Conservative Digest*
6/14/78	*Woman's Day*
6/78	Human Behavior
7/13/78	*Rolling Stone*
8/78	*Sepia*
9/4/78	*People*
9/11/78	*New West*
9/78	*Playboy*
9/78	Reader's Digest
1979	
1/79	*Chemistry*
4/79	*Reader's Digest*
10/79	Reader's Digest

Television

Table V lists television news programs that featured PCP stories. Most listed were national news programs such as Today, *Tomorrow*, and *60 Minutes*, or network national evening shows. We were able to find, because of our location, a number of local NYC features as well. In most instances we were able to view these presentations. There were certainly many other local telecasts about PCP throughout the nation. Those shows we saw fre-

The *60 Minutes* show of October 23, 1977, devoted one-third of its time to PCP. It featured reputed live filming of a drug seller's arrest in San Jose, California. Mike Wallace interviewed two men accused of murder who were supposedly under the influence of PCP at the time of their crimes. Wallace also interviewed R. Stanley Burns and his associate Steven Lerner. Both men were co-authors of the *Western Medicine* article in 1975 and they, with associate Ronald Linder, had formed a private corporation to carry out training, educational, and treatment services related to PCP. Lerner told two of the horror stories we have mentioned, perhaps promoting their retelling. The gouged eye story was told by a Hayward, California, drug worker. The show featured a lengthy interview with Barry Braeske, a young man who had murdered his mother, father and, grandfather while under the influence of PCP. This horror story, made more compelling by Braeske's quiet recitation, was retold nine times in our newspaper survey. As Table V indicates, Lerner made frequent appearances on national television where he essentially always illustrated the PCP story by the telling of violent tales. He even achieved an unusual notoriety for a scientist by being featured in *People* magazine in September, 1978 wherein more horror stories were featured.

Table V
TV News

1977		
Geraldo Rivera	10/12/77- 10/14/77	ABC
Mike Wallace (*60 Minutes*) with Steven Lerner* and Stanley Burns*	10/23/77	CBS
Tom Brokaw (*Today*) with M. Rosenthal* and R. DuPont*	11/10/77	NBC
1978		
Don Harris	2/16/78	NBC
Don Harris (*Today*)with Steven Lerner* and Gerald DeAngelis*	2/21/78	NBC
Eye On	3/78	CBS
Walter Cronkite	3/10/78	CBS
Ed Bradley	4/19/78	CBS
Tom Snyder (*Tomorrow*) with two users and Steven Lerner* and T. Ogelsby*	5/24/78	NBC
Tom Snyder (*Tomorrow*) with Steven Lerner*	6/5/78	NBC
Walter Cronkite	6/21/78	CBS
Barry Serafin	8/8/78	CBS
Susan Spencer	8/25/78	CBS

*All these men are experts in the field of drug abuse. Most have lectured and written about PCP and some have served as witnesses in trials regarding the drug. Lerner and Ogelsby have (with others) served as consultants for some of the TV dramas listed in Table VI.

Table VI
TV Dramas and Documentaries

1979	
February	*Quincy*
March	*Chips*
May	"Narc" (*Police Story*)
October	*Angel Death*
October	*The Wack Attack*
1980	
February	*The White Shadow*

TV Dramatic Presentations

By early 1979 PCP had become a thematic concern in fictionalized television drama (see Table VI). Sometimes it was central to the theme, at other times, peripheral. The compelling effects of the drug and its ability to induce mindless violence and self-destructive acts were widely exploited in most. *The Man Undercover* show opened with a young man taking two or three hits of a joint of "angel dust" and becoming psychotic and raging.[2] *The Wack Attack*, a made-for-television movie, featured a preposterous scene inside a "PCP treatment ward" where a group of young people enact a gathering of chronic psychotics *a la Snakepit*. *The White Shadow* episode featured two reifications of horror stories. In one a young woman tried to fly off the roof of her high school and in another a young man removed (most of) his clothing and ran about overwhelming and evading his pursuers. The *Quincy* show focused on the strength and invincibility of the user. Two popular horror stories were dramatized: an oncoming dope-crazed fiend required multiple police bullets to halt his advance; and handcuffs and leg restraints were broken by users crazed and fortified by the drug. A special case of "documentary entertainment" was provided by the David Begelman documentary *Angel Death* narrated by Joanne Woodward and Paul Newman. This documentary was not fictionalized but was a telling of the PCP story. Many of the horror stories were retold and some footage purported to show a naked young man under the influence of "dust" whose superhuman strength made him difficult to subdue. We were also shown the actual handcuffs that an enraged person had broken while under PCP's influence.

Miscellaneous Media

Three not easily categorized 1979 items were found. The National Institute on Drug Abuse (NIDA) funded a short television public service announcement in which Robert Blake, very much in his role as Baretta, warns people away from angel dust ("It's a rattlesnake and it'll kill you"). Also during 1979 some New York City radio stations played another public service announcement by musician Gil Scott-Heron warning about the "dangerous powder." Scott-Heron's song "Angel Dust" was played behind the spot. The recording achieved, on its own, fairly wide play and was listed on the *Billboard* Soul Charts as a hit record.[3] Scott-Heron was also an in-studio commentator following the first New York City showing of Begelman's documentary in October of 1979.

Discussion

The abuse of phencyclidine emerged as a national problem in the 1970s. The volume of newsprint devoted was large and the story has moved steadily through all forms of media. In this video age the attention paid by television news and drama has been important and probably validated for many people the importance of the drug and its story. The style of presentation in all media has encompassed a dramatization of the dangers of the drug by focusing on individual, supposedly true, stories of violent, even loathsome behavior carried out by individuals intoxicated by the drug. It is erroneous to think of this approach as unprecedented.

The Case of Cocaine

In 1908 the *New York Times* printed an article that described "Jew peddlers" selling cocaine to drug-crazed Southern Negroes (Stickgold 1977). Another *New York Times* account in 1914 attributed to the "drug-crazed [cocaine] fiend": superhuman strength, cunning, sexual rapaciousness, and a temporary immunity to shock so as to withstand .32 caliber bullets. The murders of 17 Southern Whites were blamed on Negro cocaine-sniffing parties (Williams 1914). Musto believes that White fears of released Black aggression secondary to cocaine use strongly contributed to state and national anti-cocaine legislation (Musto 1973).

The Case of Marijuana

Anti-marijuana slogans and posters signaled the governmental campaign against marijuana prior to the 1937 Marijuana Tax Act. One famous poster portraying a marijuana cigarette read:

> Beware! Young and Old—People in All Walks of Life. This may be handed you by the friendly stranger. It contains the killer drug marijuana—a powerful narcotic in which lurks Murder! Insanity! Death!
>
> —Fort 1978

Federal Agents kept an up-to-date gore file listing accounts of vicious crimes committed by users of marijuana. The most famous case described Victor Licata, 21, who with his axe killed his father, mother, sister, and two brothers while they slept. Another tale described a user who smashed a man's face and head to a pulp. Not satisfied with murder, he then extracted the tongue and the eyes from the victim (Sloman 1979).

The Case of LSD

The PCP story of the 1970s was probably matched in volume by the media attention to LSD in the 1960s. Multiple stories of murders committed by LSD-influenced people were reported. Few of these cases were ever documented by the measurement of LSD in the bloodstream of the killer, although this finding would scarcely prove that LSD caused the killing.

LSD often was stated to have caused individuals to remove their eyes. Grinspoon and Bakalar (1979) in fact tried to document the self-enucleation stories and found only three cases about which any information existed. All three events involved hospitalized individuals who may have used LSD previously, but at the time of the incident there was no evidence that they were intoxicated. All three were ruminating on sexual guilt and two cited the Biblical edict "If thy right eye offend thee, pluck it out."

The Case of Other Drugs

Siegel (1980) cites the following:

> A powerful vineyard worker fought wildly against an imaginary tiger, smashing chairs against the wall. A normally quiet garage worker thought he was a circus performer and walked along the cable of a suspension bridge.... A man yelled, "Look at me! I'm an airplane and I can fly!" and jumped from a win-

dow to the ground below and then ran 50 meters on two broken legs while unaware of any pain. . . . The attacks were fluctuating while the intoxicated broke out of their bonds and restraints, attacking firemen and police who were forced to use manual restraint by gangs of men in order to control those with "superhuman strength." At least two people ripped out of their straitjackets with bare hands.

These familiar episodes grew out of ergotism, the consumption of fungus-contaminated rye in Pont-Saint-Esprit, France, in 1951.

Every new drug experience in America is handled in a stereotyped fashion by the media. Emphasis is placed on individual tales of dangerous, criminal, or self-destructive behavior by the drug-crazed. The myth is newly erected and slightly embellished with each new drug, and the stories come to resemble the myths, ballads, and folk-tales previously generated and transformed by oral transmission. Indeed, the best model seems to be the Frankenstein monster who advances impervious to pain, bullets, and this time to fire, in order to murder, dismember, or bugger men, women, children, and the household pets. The myths are compelling because they touch an emotional core that has meaning in the individual and in the culture, and they exploit our fascination with horror. The user commits wanton rape and murder, the murders often encompass fratricide, matricide, or infanticide. The monster must die bizarrely: drowning in inches of water, attempting to fly from a building, or trying to halt a speeding two-ton vehicle with its bare hands or body. If it lives it should commit the most sexually meaningful self-mutilations—removal of the eyes or castration. These tales are the archetypal expressions of human inner terrors and exist in the preserved ballads and epic tales of most languages. Jung would have loved to analyze the "facts" about PCP presented by American media.

Are some of these stories true? Probably so; myth feeds on fact nearly as well as it feeds on fancy. But if they were not true we would make them up—as we have in the past. The multiple sources of the gouged-eyes does not mean that the event did not happen, merely that it is so meaningful that facts cannot constrain it. The story moves from anecdote to apocrypha.

Charles Innes, a Baltimore student, did blind himself in jail in 1971 and his story served as a model for some retellings of this legend (Smith

1980; Green 1971). A 1977 AP wire story quoted Dr. Regine Aronow:

> She said a Baltimore college student who took an overdose [of PCP] tore his eyes out of their sockets. (Carter 1977)

The photocopy of the AP story we obtained has the following notation above the text:

> Editor: Material in the tenth graf (sic) may be objectionable to some readers.

The warning about the gouged-eye tale might also have predicted that the retelling would be extremely popular.

Charles Innes had dropped out of college by 1971 but he did live in Baltimore and was the son of a Massachusetts state legislator. He swallowed a film canister of drug during a police raid on his home. Some of the material removed by gastric suction was analyzed chemically as LSD. No tests for PCP were carried out because the drug had attained little publicity in the East in 1971. Four days after the ingestion Innes was incarcerated after a nude appearance in public and blinded himself while in jail; he did not remove his eyes from their sockets. He denied that the drug was PCP and claimed that it was PCPA (parachlorphenylalanine). This agent, which increases copulatory behavior in rats and is unrelated to PCP, was claimed to be available on the street in the late 1960s and early 1970s but there is no proof that it was ever available. As late as 1978, during his interview for Koper's article in *New Times*, Innes apparently denied that PCP caused his behavior and indeed the case was initially listed in the LSD horror tales. Green, the journalist who described the events in 1971, was correct in listing PCP as a potential cause. He had learned that the drug at times caused severe disruption of behavior and that it was sometimes misrepresented as other street drugs. Despite this careful speculation by Green, there is no proof that Innes ever ingested PCP. Seven years after the fact, the case was exhumed, polished, and transformed into part of the horrific PCP mythology.

We found one other important example of mythic transformation. During the *60 Minutes* portrayal of PCP, Mike Wallace interviewed Barry Braeske who confessed on national television that he had murdered his mother, father, and grandfather. Wallace then interviewed Steven Lerner who stated that Braeske had been using PCP (it had been found in his urine) and that he had been under its influence when these crimes were committed. The Braeske story was then repeated multiple times in newspaper stories essentially as Wallace and Lerner (and the *60 Minutes* editors) told it. In reality, there was much more to the story. Far from an unpremeditated act, Braeske planned the murders with an accomplice who assisted in the killings. The motive was to collect Braeske's inheritance. The two killers then ransacked the house to create the appearance of a burglary, removed some items from the house, and hid these "stolen" goods with the rifle used for the murders. They then went to the movies to establish an alibi and returned to the house. Braeske phoned the police stating that he had just come home and "discovered" the bodies (People vs. Braeske 1979). I do not wish to imply that Braeske could not have been influenced by the PCP. However, the testimony of the behavior above may have influenced the jury to discount Lerner's expert testimony at the trial and convict Braeske of the murder.[4] The portrayal on *60 Minutes* was deceptive because of the exclusion of this material, but it is doubtful that the deception occurred because Wallace or Lerner wished to lie. They wished to participate in the telling of a myth too meaningful to be altered by a few inconvenient facts.

Martin Phillips, the producer of the PCP segment for *60 Minutes*, states that he knew of these characteristics of Braeske's crime. He denied that the withholding of them was in any way deceptive. Phillips believes that "everyone" associated with the case knew that Braeske committed the crime because of PCP. Not only Lerner and the defense attorney but the prosecution and even the jury believed that Braeske was under the drug's influence. Because of this unanimity of opinion that he perceived, Phillips did not feel leaving out the associated facts we've cited was deceptive.[5]

This event signals another difficulty in television portrayals of fact. Television, like any visual medium, best makes any statement by focusing on the particular rather than explaining the general. One picture is indeed worth better than a thousand words and infinitely more deceptive. The visual artist attempts in this focus on the particular or the individual instance to illuminate an issue on which the historian or social scientist may expend many thousands of words. Additionally, of course, the display of the individual provokes in us an identification with the character that exceeds anything presentable by the writer constrained by fact. The young woman falling off the building in *The White*

Shadow and the young musician killed in *The Wack Attack* are immediately more recallable than documented facts about PCP, just as Garbo's *Camille* is more recallable than documented facts about tuberculosis. The danger is that putative documentary fact as presented by Mike Wallace on *60 Minutes* may be reshaped to accomplish "artistic goals" while we believe that the material is straight truth from something akin to the *International Journal of the Addictions*.

There are two other points to be made about the terrifying presentation we have described. Even those caught up in drug lies may justify their behavior by claiming that if the tale scared one individual away from using the drug then the distortion of fact was entirely justified. A scientist active in the black community of Los Angeles told me that *The Wack Attack*, which is so distorted and laughable that it will become the *Reefer Madness* of the "angel dust" generation, scared some users away from the drug. The oft-stated problem is that scare factors do not seem to work. One motivation for the street-drug user is the thrill of danger, and scare stories may actually offer a challenge to some (Franklin 1978; Unsigned 1978). The scare approach works on those who have some prior agreement with the message; in others resistance to the message develops. Potential users know that there are people who have used the drug without these disastrous events and resist the message. The story is discounted and the source discredited. Furthermore, there are data that strongly emotional presentations regarding pain and disfigurement provoke tension in the recipient sufficient to generate psychological resistance to the communication's messages (Janis and Terwilliger 1962).

The horror tale has another apparent utility. Young quotes Dr. Gerald DeAngelis:

> [There are] irresponsible people in my profession who want publicity to attract dollars to their programs. . . . Spoonfeeding sensational stories to the media to keep themselves in grant money. . . . If I go to you with a list of 80 kids that killed their mothers because of PCP and tell you all I need is money to solve the problem, my chances of getting it are good. . . . (Young 1978)

DeAngelis' words are nearly a horror story, and they may apply to some situations. Someone has to perceive a problem to get money to solve the problem. Since its inception, the problem of drug abuse has been exploited and sensationalized for some of the reasons we have stated in this article and for some pecuniary goals.

Although we have not focused on the reality of danger with PCP (and we believe the reality of danger has little to do with media handling) some comments on that danger are appropriate in this conclusion. We believe that PCP is probably the most dangerous drug, other than alcohol, that has been widely utilized by the recreational drug culture. Our criticism of media exaggeration and exploitation does not alter that assessment. However, there is reason to believe that morbidity secondary to the drug has been overestimated and is declining. Those who worked in hospital emergency rooms in the late sixties will recall that numerous young people were seen with "bad trips" secondary to LSD. Such a clinical event is now rare because, in part, the culture has learned to use the drug and has learned to anticipate its effects and to deal with them. There is evidence that a similar pattern is now operating in the PCP culture. During late 1978 and early 1979 the Harlem Hospital Emergency room saw approximately 60 cases per month of apparent PCP intoxication. The late 1979 admission rate is closer to 10 cases per month (Sixsmith 1979). Additionally, the publicity of the problem may well have led to overdiagnosis. The psychosis that may occur with PCP is distinguished only with difficulty from nondrug psychosis. Few clinical centers confirmed a clinical diagnosis of PCP with detection of the drug in bodily fluids.

Finally, as in other "drug epidemics," professionals in the drug field decide that the entire population of drug users resemble those whose self-selection brings them to where we work. For instance Wesson (1979) has described his experience in a private psychiatric hospital where his PCP patients have been chiefly auto workers whose insurance enables them to be treated at his hospital. Many workers, according to him, came to the attention of supervisors because of erratic work performance or accidents. They often had used the drug for periods of time without trouble and described friends and fellow employees who had not had particular difficulty. There may well be many such "functional" users who have never presented to emergency departments or murdered their mothers. This again does not mean to imply that such users are safe from long-term hazard with use of the drug.

Conclusion

The media presentation of PCP has been conditioned by mythic perceptions of the drug users and should have been predictable in light of previous drug-abuse stories. Malcolm Muggeridge once described journalists feverishly looking at previous newsclips to give them perspective on a story, comparing the recycling journalist to the parched desert traveler consuming his own urine (Muggeridge 1979). The particular character of the randomly violent PCP user has also attracted much attention in television drama. In fact, PCP is the ideal American television dramatic drug because it fits so many violent stereotypes. PCP *may* be the drug that the American media hoped LSD would be.

* * *

John P. Morgan and Doreen Kagan, "The Dusting of America: The Image of Phencyclidine (PCP) in the Popular Media." This article appeared in the *Journal of Psychoactive Drugs*, Volume 12(3-4), July-December 1980 and is reprinted with permission. Copyright © 1980 by Haight-Ashbury Publications.

Notes

1. The first article in the *New York Times* described the hope of Sernyl® as a new anesthetic development (March 27, 1958).
2. It later evolved that he faked this attack because he was an undercover narc who carried out the charade to escape the consequences of having blown his cover.
3. Scott-Heron has previously composed anti-heroin and anti-alcohol songs.
4. The conviction was later overturned on appeal because of the irregularity by officers in informing Braeske of his rights. He awaits trial.
5. Phillips made these statements in a phone conversation with J.P.M. on Thursday, May 8, 1980.

References

Brown, M. 1978. Angel dust abusers winging way to a harp. *Evansville (Indiana) Courier and Press* March 19.

Burns, R.S.; Lerner, S.E.; Corrado, R.; James, S.H. and Schnoll, S.H. 1975. Phencyclidine—states of acute intoxication and fatalities. *Western Journal of Medicine* Vol. 123(5): 345-349.

Carter, M.N. 1977. Its name is heavenly but angel dust can be a deadly high. *AP Wire Story* November 10.

Chargot, P. 1978. The cheap street drug PCP: A little bit of this angel dust can bring on a whole lot of hell. *Detroit Free Press* January 15.

Domino, E.F. 1964. Neurobiology of phencyclidine (Sernyl), a drug with an unusual spectrum of pharmacological activity. *International Review of Neurobiology* Vol. 6: 303-347.

Fort, J. 1978. Pot: A rational approach. *Playboy* Vol. 25: 131+.

Franklin, S. 1978. USA panics: Angel Dust burns out teenagers. *Philadelphia Evening Bulletin* January 1.

Gay, B. 1978. The evils of angel dust and other "street drugs." *Sepia* Vol. 27: 17-19.

Green, B. 1978. Angel dust: A teenage drug epidemic. *San Francisco Chronicle* June 1.

Green, D.S.A. 1971. Charlie's awful "trip": He blinded himself in a Baltimore jail. *National Observer* November 6.

Grinspoon, L. and Bakalar, J.B. 1979. *Psychedelic Drugs Reconsidered*. New York: Basic Books, Inc.

Janis, I.L. and Terwilliger, R.F. 1962. An experimental study of psychological resistances to fear-arousing communications. *Journal of Abnormal and Social Psychology* Vol. 65: 403-410.

Koper, P. 1978. Angel death. *New Times* March 20.

Luby, E.D.; Cohen, B.D.; Rosenbaum, G.; Gottlieb, J.S. and Kelley, R. 1959. Study of a new schizophrenic drug—Sernyl. *Archives of Neurology and Psychiatry* Vol 81: 363-369.

Luisada, P.V. 1978. The phencyclidine psychosis: Phenomenology and treatment. In: Petersen, R.C. and Stillman, R.C. (Eds.). *Phencyclidine (PCP) Abuse: An Appraisal*. NIDA Research Monograph 21. Rockville, Maryland: NIDA.

Meyers, F.H.; Rose, A.J. and Smith, D.E. 1967. Incidents involving the Haight-Ashbury population and some uncommonly used drugs. *Journal of Psychedelic Drugs* Vol. 1: 139-146.

Muggeridge, M. 1979. *Things Past*. New York: William Morrow and Company.

Musto, D.G. 1973. *The American Disease*. New Haven, Connecticut: Yale University Press.

Oswald, J. 1978. Use of unheavenly dust is on the rise here. *St. Louis Globe-Democrat* March 17.

People vs. Braeske. 1979. App., 154 Cal. Rstr. 619.

Siegel, R.K. 1980. PCP and violent crime: The people vs. peace. *Journal of Psychedelic Drugs* Vol. 12(3-4).

Sixsmith, D. 1979. Personal Communication.

Sloman, L. 1979. *The History of Marijuana in America: Reefer Madness*. Indianapolis, Indiana: Bobbs-Merrill, Inc.

Smith, D.E. 1980. Personal communication.

Stickgold, A. 1977. Dope scoreboard: Coke comes of age. *Los Angeles Free Press* June 10-16.

Unsigned. 1978. If the drug is angel dust, heaven may not wait. *Kansas City (Missouri) Star* October 5.

Unsigned. 1977. PCP treatment. *AP Wire Story* January 8.

Unsigned. 1976. High on PCP. *Emergency Medicine* Pp. 265-279.

Wesson, D.R. 1979. PCP Abuse: A Skeptic's Appraisal. Unpublished manuscript.

Williams, E.H. 1914. Negro cocaine fiends are a new Southern menace. *New York Times* February 8.

Young, D. 1978. PCP horror stories a plug for money? *Seattle Post Intelligencer* April 8. ✦

25. 'More Than Medical Significance': LSD and American Psychiatry 1953-1966

JOHN R. NEILL

In *"More Than Medical Significance,"* author *John R. Neill traces the history of LSD as it related to psychiatric patients and clinicians. Early reports suggested numerous benefits of LSD use; in subsequent writings, however, researchers modified the preliminary views of the drug. Nonmedical use in the 1960s dramatically altered the beliefs of the therapeutic effects of LSD, and new reports resulted in government regulation. A major focus of this article is Neill's presentation of the reasons that led to the changing views of LSD among psychiatrists.*

Lysergic acid diethylamide (LSD) was synthesized in 1938 by Albert Hofmann for Sandoz, a Swiss pharmaceutical company. In 1943, Hofmann accidentally absorbed or inhaled a small amount (in the microgram range) of the substance and soon after experienced perceptual distortions. He even left an account of this, the world's first LSD trip (Hofmann 1959). From the beginning, psychiatry was interested in LSD. The first clinical paper was published in Switzerland. Stoll (1947), the investigator, gave LSD to various psychotic patients and produced what he thought was a non-specific toxic delirium. Sandoz marketed the drug in tablets and in injectable form under the name of Delysid® (Hollister 1968), and it became available by prescription in Europe. In North America, work with LSD lasted more than 10 years, from 1953 through 1966. During this period, several thousand research communications were published regarding the substance. Yet after 1966, when it was banned by federal law in the United States as an illicit substance, research virtually ceased.

LSD sparked some of the most acrimonious debate seen within the young specialty of psychiatry. That LSD proved to be a drug of "more than medical significance," in Humphry Osmond's phrase (1957), casts a revelatory light on psychiatry's rela-

tion to medicine, its patients, and the government. Within the profession, LSD brought into question the difference between *therapist* and *patient*, the distinction between the *crazy* and the *sane*, and in the end tested the boundaries of the profession quite profoundly. *Scientific* methodology used by psychiatry would be found wanting, and the myth of a profession operating scientifically, untrammeled by the government, would be found to be false.

In this article, the history of LSD in American psychiatry will be briefly documented, concentrating on attitudes and responses by members of the profession expressed in the mainstream professional literature. Next, it will look at what was revealed about the profession in its encounter with LSD, especially points bearing on its relation to clients, the rest of medicine, and the government. The literature dealing with the acid culture of the 1960s is not directly relevant to the purposes of this article and has been excluded.

When LSD first came to the U.S., it was given to normal volunteers, including Mennonite conscientious objectors, at the National Institute of Mental Health (NIMH) (Meyer 1969) and, rather indiscriminately, to "volunteer patients" at St. Elizabeth's Hospital (Katzenelbogen and Fran 1953). The development of the neuroleptic antipsychotic chlorpromazine (Thorazine®) at about this time had renewed interest in psychosis, especially schizophrenia. Researchers sought substances that would produce a *model psychosis* against which these antipsychotic drugs could be tested.

Although mescaline and other substances were known to produce perceptual distortions, LSD—now classed as "psychotomimetic" or "hallucinogen"—seemed the best candidate (Hollister 1968). Given to animals, schizophrenics, and normal volunteers as a psychotomimetic, the drug produced symptoms but not the clinical syndrome of schizophrenia. Hollister, an early and persistent worker in the area, wrote that interest in the use of LSD to reveal the biochemical basis of psychosis was on the wane by the mid-1950s. LSD thus entered psychiatry as an investigational agent, a status it has never entirely lost.

It is to LSD's ill-fated career as an investigational drug in psychotherapy that this article now turns. As early as 1953, there were published reports of psychotherapeutic success with LSD in Europe and North America. In 1955, it was a discussion topic on the program of the American Psychiatric Association Meeting held in Atlantic City, New Jersey. Two symposiums followed in the early 1960s on LSD and psychotherapy: the Göttingen Symposium in West Germany in 1960 and the Royal Medical Psychological Conference in England in 1961.

The symposiums were conducted mainly by and for clinicians who spoke about their work. These clinicians used LSD as an adjuvant to existing therapies, principally Freudian and Jungian psychoanalysis. Therapists felt the drug could facilitate regression to obtain early-childhood memories, shorten therapy, and, in particular, open up heretofore difficult patients, such as obsessive-compulsives and alcoholics. As LSD passed into the hands of therapists, who were not laboratory researchers, it came to be called a psycholytic, a term adopted at the 1960 Göttingen Symposium (Crockett, Sandison, and Walk 1963).

Psycholytic therapy was being conducted in ways that made some uneasy. Martin Roth (1963) of the University of Newcastle reported, "My first introduction to the treatment of alcoholics was a certain university in North America [probably University of Saskatchewan's project, run by Abram Hoffer and Humphry Osmond], where I was assured by one of the therapists that it was essential for the therapist to take the drug himself—otherwise, he was totally incapable of empathizing with the patient." Other therapists reported using other approaches, such as conversation between therapist and patient, a supportive group, and a permissive environment (Crockett, Sandison, and Walk 1963). They found that they had to discard the analytic stance of free-floating attention, the cornerstone of psychoanalytic technique. To skeptics and critics alike, the experienced LSD therapist answered as the early psychoanalysts had: "If you haven't used LSD [been analyzed], you can't really understand." Sandison (1963) attempted to be understanding:

Finally, religious and ethical considerations may lead to uncertainties through arousing emotional and biased attitudes in others, or particularly those whose experience of psycholytic drugs has only been from the outside or experimental situation. We would do well to clear our minds of any unduly mystical or ritualistic approach to this treatment. To do so at once leads to comparisons of other systems of thought and belief [Was he referring to psychoanalysis?] which confuses the proposition that LSD, as used by the psychiatrist, is intended to lay bare the origins of neurosis and, thus assisted by the natural healing powers of the unconscious thus revealed,

cures the patient. If one might conclude, by meeting a challenge sometimes offered by theologians, that work and suffering are essential ingredients for salvation, I would suggest that successful psycholytic therapy involves a great deal of work on the part of the patient, sometimes accompanied by suffering. But the will to work is derived from the same source as that of healing, from the unconscious.

It seemed that scientific psychiatry was treading on dangerous ground. An embarrassing number of patients were having religious or conversion experiences in therapy with LSD, the erstwhile psychotomimetic. How were these to be understood when the framework of Freudian theory left no room for accommodation to religious or aesthetic discourse? Too many patients were having unitive experiences, too few were having recollections of the primal scene. At this point in the late 1950s, LSD was about to escape the sole purview of psychiatry. It was to become a drug of "more than medical significance."

Humphry Osmond (1957) provided the final transformation of LSD in an article in the *Annals of the New York Academy of Sciences*. Osmond had begun early in LSD work. He worked with Abram Hoffer, a former physical chemist, and had conducted the first group treatments with LSD outside of Europe. Osmond argued that LSD and related substances were not *psychotomimetic*, for they did not produce the model psychosis schizophrenia researchers had sought. Nor was it properly a hallucinogen, for hallucinations were not generally an effect of LSD. Nor, finally, was LSD merely a substance that lysed repressive bonds to bring Freudian material into consciousness. Osmond wrote:

If mimicking mental illness were the main characteristic of these agents, "psychotomimetics" would indeed be a suitable term. Why are we always preoccupied with the pathological and the negative? Is health only the lack of sickness? Is good merely the absence of evil? Is pathology the only yardstick? Must we ape Freud's gloomier moods that persuaded him that a happy man is a self-deceiver, evading the heartache for which there is no anodyne? . . . I have tried to find an appropriate name for these agents under discussion: a concept that will include the concepts of enriching the mind and enlarging the vision. . . . My choice, because it is clear, euphonius, and uncontaminated by other associations, is psychedelic, mind-manifesting.

Osmond went on to state that "these agents have a part to play in our survival as a species." In apocalyptic voice, he described the coming perils to humanity's existence, and how the greater awareness of what humans can truly be will be aided in its birth by these drugs of greater than medical significance.

The Josiah Macy, Jr., Symposium, sponsored in part by the CIA (Marks 1979), was published as a book titled *The Use of LSD in Psychotherapy* (Abramson 1960). The conference, which consisted of several days of informal discussion, began with each participant, at the chairman's request, telling how s/he became involved in LSD work. Many admittedly came in by the back door, from other areas of psychiatry or other disciplines. The clinical perspective was well-represented here, but not dominant, and the group was preoccupied with the role of LSD in psychotherapy and psychiatry.

So, within the psychiatric profession over a period of 10 years, LSD had gone through three transformations. As a psychotomimetic, LSD was for, if anyone, mental patients, especially the more severely disturbed ones. Perhaps a substance like LSD caused their disease, or perhaps they had chemical psychotogens already in their blood. As a psycholytic, it was of use to psychiatric patients and their therapists, for therapy and training, respectively. In either case, it was a medical therapeutic tool, part of a technique, and professional property. When LSD became a psychedelic, it moved beyond the bounds of control of the professional elite and its clientele, as well as psychiatry and psychology.

For the federal government and the psychiatrists who were its employees, LSD had become a public health problem. Reacting to what they thought was epidemic use that was sustaining a counterculture that was opposed to its policies, they sought to ban the use of LSD and related drugs. In 1965, the 89th Congress passed the Drug Abuse Control Amendment (Public Law 89-74), which went into effect in May 1966. It banned the use and sale of peyote, mescaline, and several other similar drugs by the public.

Reacting to what they considered to be unwarranted and inaccurate publicity by the lay press (e.g., Dahlberg, Mechanek, and Feldstein 1968) and hasty policymaking on the part of the federal government, legitimate researchers became bitter. They felt that legitimate research was endangered, as was clearly evidenced by its precipitous decline. Unger (1969a), a researcher, wrote that "qualified,

recognized researchers who would be or are authorized to do the work, apparently, do not seem to want to risk the possible notoriety of, or taint of, or embroilment in the controversy and mass-media confrontations that surround the psychedelic use of LSD. I cannot say I blame them; often it's a great emotional strain." Times had changed. In regard to his first LSD trip at NIMH, Unger (1969b) stated that "it seems necessary, unfortunately, in 1968, to say at the time, 1962, [that trying LSD] seemed not only logical or desirable, but even a respectable course of action." He reported that, after trying LSD, his section chief at NIMH and the director of clinical investigation quickly followed in succession.

By the mid-1960s, non-medical use of LSD, especially by young people, seemed nearly epidemic, although this was later shown not to be so (Freedman 1968). Mass-circulation magazines (e.g., Ungerleider 1966) ran articles, documenting its use apart from the image of the medical establishment. For many during this time, LSD developed a sinister connotation, whether based on myth or fact. Now, of more than medical significance, LSD was experiencing difficulty within the profession of psychiatry.

Also, by the mid-1960s, experienced workers could agree that there were no specific reactions to LSD based on personality or disease classifications. Its therapeutic property (Grinspoon and Bakalar 1979; Abramson 1960) was the ability to "facilitate an altered state of consciousness." Federally funded research continued, however, in the face of mounting criticism within and without the profession. A symposium held in 1967, a book published in 1968, and a review article that appeared in 1968 reflected the growing tensions.

The 1967 Hahnemann Conference Proceedings, which bore the enigmatic subtitle "The Look Before the Leap," showed the new extramedical interest in LSD. Fully one half of the published proceedings (Hicks and Fink 1969) was devoted to side effects, illicit use, and legal matters. One finds a clergyman speaking out against "psychedelic religion," an anthropologist who believes LSD can be used as a path for spiritual growth, an educator who deplores its destruction of critical thinking, and a psychologist who believes that it fosters "antinomianism," mysticism and psychosis due to a withdrawal from the "real" world. The drug's clinical use is limited in this volume to only 44 of 243 pages.

The book published that year was by Leo Hollister (1968), perhaps the only experienced clinical psychopharmacologist to work with LSD in America.

He found that research was uniformly of poor quality, due to the lack of specialized training of investigators. No adequate clinical trials had yet been performed. Yet, LSD would seem, in its idiographic and unpredictable effects, as suitable to group clinical trial as a movie or a novel.

Hollister cautioned that ". . . the more things change, the more they remain the same"; and "the interplay between drugs which produced chemical psychosis and religion persists even until the present, as evidenced by the current interest in LSD." He concluded that, therapeutically, for producing insight, "candy is dandy but liquor is quicker," might be pertinent to the facilitation of psychotherapy by LSD. He believed existing drugs could duplicate each of LSD's alleged therapeutic effects. In addition, he rejected the notion that mystical religious experiences might help in the therapeutic endeavor for these cures; but like Lourdes, they do not last. He felt that those who are looking for a psychedelic experience were looking for "an easy way to change the personality." Hollister's concluding chapter, "Drugs in Our Culture," is alarmist in tone, warning of a sort of cultural regression, the loss of rational thought, especially lamentable and unexpected when "we are truly entering a scientific age."

In a long review article, "On the Use and Abuse of LSD," Freedman (1968), a politically influential LSD laboratory researcher, sought to dissociate psychiatry from the LSD controversy. Only one page out of 15 dealt with LSD in psychiatry: "In the late 1950s some physicians thought they had discovered a new reality of the mind and were not only struck by the drug induced phenomena, but apparently addled by them. Perhaps they were simply jealous of the subject when they insisted on taking the drug concurrently with him."

Freedman wanted the drug to be federally regulated (as it then was). He thought that in proper hands it could be a "tool" to study the mind. The present problem was that "the real danger of LSD is that the wrong people seem to be taking it at the wrong time for the wrong reason." Furthermore, he wrote, "We must ask whether a stable person is really under sufficient control of his motives and shifting circumstances, let alone the dosage, to take these drugs as a civil right for whatever personal reason he wishes."

According to Freedman, the popular acid culture was steering young people, in particular, the wrong way when it took the use of these drugs out of professional hands: "We seem to have forgotten that there are trained persons who, in fact, have more experience than the self-appointed gurus in coping with adolescent turmoil and the more serious dysfunctions. There are scholars in disciplines knowledgeable about man's attempts to understand subjective experience and its manifold aesthetic, literary, and expression. Finally, he warned, "We should not forget to assess the cost of sustained euphoria or of pleasure states. We can seriously wonder if man is built to endure more than a brief, chemically induced glimpse of paradise."

When, in 1967, evidence came to light of the mutagenic effect of LSD on human chromosomes (Cohen and Marmillo 1967), the federal government seized on these findings as part of its antidrug campaign. Despite cautionary pleadings by psychiatrists that the government would lose its credibility and that the propaganda was not based on confirmed evidence, the public was warned of genetic damage as a payment for its pleasure. Later shown to be neither a mutagen, teratogen, or carcinogen in humans (Dishotsky et al. 1971), the idea that, as one editorial (Ungerleider 1967) in the *New England Journal of Medicine* put it, "a decision today [to use LSD] may very well be reflected by the biologic fitness of the next generation," was probably most effective in curbing casual use of LSD.

With its ostracism from psychiatry, its banishment from use under penalty of law, and reports of genetic damage, use of LSD within and outside of the psychiatric profession ceased to be of significance. In the 15 years since that time, there has been little added to document its usefulness or danger. Yet, by examining the psychiatric encounter with LSD, one can learn something about American psychiatric modes and morals.

First, there is what the author of the present article calls the scientific problem. In the study of a new drug, clinical researchers attempt to emulate, in their setting, the technique of the laboratory. Groups of patients, rather than individuals, are studied in the clinic, much as groups of small animals are studied in the laboratory. Changes measured must have statistical significance (i.e., be molar) in order to study a drug whose effect was so protean or, in pharmacological parlance, "nonspecific." That the drug's effects were unpredictable, even within the individual across time, rendered it suspect as a candidate for study.

A particularly maddening problem was the experiential, rather than the behavioral, nature of the drug effect. Reports of behavioral changes pale in significance before those of subjective experience. Nonpharmacologic researchers—by definition unequipped to conduct drug research—felt early on that they needed a whole new methodology to study the effects of LSD. Things could not be put into the right words or were completely ineffable (Abramson 1960).

At Spring Grove State Hospital in Baltimore, where the greatest amount of systematic work was done with LSD over a 10-year period, researchers under the direction of Albert A. Kurland tried to develop such a method. Kurland's group gave LSD to alcoholics, neurotics, and later to drug addicts (Savage and McCabe 1973; Savage et al. 1973; Kurland et al. 1971). Kurland's group (1967) found context, not LSD, to be critical (viz., LSD had no inherent therapeutic effect):

> In conclusion, it should be emphasized that LSD is *not* conceived to have any inherent beneficial effects, i.e., its use is different from that of other drugs or chemotherapeutic agents. LSD affects the brain of man in widespread and unusual ways, many of which are irrelevant to its therapeutic use (the production of so-called hallucinations, etc.). The history of experimental work with this compound has abundantly indicated that beneficial results do occur from its mere administration—in fact, indication is quite clear that without therapeutic intent, preparation, and management, administration of the drug to human subjects is definitely dangerous. The therapeutic potential of LSD depends primarily on its ability to activate in the patient a period of intense emotionality, while still allowing for control, direction, and guidance by the therapist. It is the sequence of psychological experience upon which the therapeutic intent and structuring is focused. The analogy that we have sometimes used to try to convey the role of LSD in therapy is that of a scalpel in surgical intervention: the scalpel is helpful, but without the skilled surgeon, it is merely a dangerous instrument.

Another psychiatrist, working as a laboratory psychopharmacologist, described the Spring Grove program in a rather skeptical tone (Freedman 1968): "In the so-called psychedelic therapies as they are now being tested, there is an awareness of an immense amount of preparation, of salesmanship with an evangelical tone, in which the patient is confronted with hope and positive displays of it before he has his one great experience with a very high dose of drug. The drug's experience is structured by music and by confident good feelings."

A third element in the scientific problem was that it was not always clear what LSD was supposed to do. Was it itself, or as an adjunct, curative, facilitator, augmenter? Experienced therapists who were not trained as pharmacologists felt that context or ritual were important for the drug to work, but ran afoul of the charge of being unscientific. In standard laboratory methodology transposed to the clinic, one tries to match drug effects to symptoms (target symptoms) or diagnoses. Contextual effects are supposed to be constant or ignored. If there are contextual changes, they are incorporated into the placebo effect, which is considered to have no direct bearing on the actions of the drug itself.

Psychiatry's psychedelic experience points to the limitations imposed by tending to bring laboratory methods into the clinic, by using molar methods and ignoring contexts. Certainly applicable in some situations, these methods proved to be of little use to the LSD researchers. Perhaps more noteworthy is the fact that over a 10- to 15-year period, when these drugs were under active investigation, although there was an awareness of a need for a method, none was forthcoming that was acceptable.

The second question that LSD raised for the profession of psychiatry was what the author of the present article calls the problem of boundaries. LSD blurred the boundaries of the profession between doctor and patient, and the sick and the well. Osmond began the controversy in his 1957 article, insisting that the golden rule for psychedelic therapists was to "start with yourself" (Unger 1969b). One can see from the list of Macy Conference participants and infer from other presentations that this, indeed, was common practice. Some therapists took LSD before seeing their patients (Kafka and Garder 1964). Certainly, LSD was used by some researchers recreationally. In public, this was denied, if mentioned at all. Unger (1969b) wrote that "Jonathan Cole [a government psychopharmacologist], at one point, noted with a certain vague sense of misgiving that psychedelic LSD investigators tended to communicate 'an implicit or explicit attitude . . . that these drugs may be of value or benefit to individuals who do not ordinarily consider themselves to be psychiatrically ill.'" It is probably safe to assume that Unger spoke the feelings and experiences of many of his more reticent colleagues.

In effect, LSD created a subgroup within the psychiatric profession which had had a rather special experience that set them apart from their colleagues and moved them closer to their patients. They were enthusiastic about their experience, but in public tempered their enthusiasm, striving to maintain the image of sober scientific investigators.

The reaction to LSD within the profession was much like that of the reaction within the profession to psychoanalysis 40 years before. Psychoanalysts had insisted on the special experience of being analyzed before treating patients. This special experience departs from the realm of rational, objective, impersonal operations, the grounding of a truly scientific psychiatry, a psychiatry that separates the sick from the well and the patient from the doctor. In moving too close, the boundaries blur, one has to fight the attempt to "go native."

Another element of the problem with boundaries is the image of the therapist invoked by the use of LSD. With his/her special experience, the therapist emerges as a healer—an actual taker of potions, the master of a ritual. This harks back to the pre-scientific era and could only seem dangerously atavistic to the majority in a profession struggling for recognition as a science.

Although many would allow that psychiatry is more art than science, few would admit its kinship to that bugbear of the Enlightenment, religion. Yet, patients and therapists were often brought back to the domain of the religious by their experiences, another blurring of the boundaries. Rebirth, union, transcendence, conversion, and unity are all words used by patients and therapists to describe the LSD experience, and they are in the domain of religious and not scientific discourse. Some outside of the psychiatric profession, such as Timothy Leary, did indeed see LSD as the basis for a new religion, and it was against "the religious cultist" that psychiatrists directed their strongest invective (Freedman 1968; Ungerleider 1968).

The problem of the boundaries lingered on through the entire period of LSD's residence with psychiatry. Like the scientific problem, it was handled with a conspicuous lack of creativity, in the presence of fear and rigidity, and was never solved. The integration of persuasion, suggestion, and ritual, the use of aesthetic devices, such as music, and the penetration by religious discourse were all successfully resisted by psychiatry.

The final problem is labeled the political problem. The susceptibility of the LSD researchers, indeed, the entire professions to political pressures was quite evident. Part of it may be ascribed to the atmosphere of a nation at war and being faced with a fractious internal protest movement. Perhaps if times were more peaceful, the federal government's handling of LSD might have been more gentle. However, having come to symbolize rebellion and obstruction of its policy, the substance was doomed to extinction.

It may be that the relationship between organized psychiatry and the federal government was particularly close during this time, for millions of dollars were being poured into community mental health centers that were being run by psychiatrists. This move, initiated by the Mental Health Act of 1963 (the culmination of years of lobbying), put psychiatry on the map, so to speak, with thousands of community mental health centers. Perhaps the most accurate thing to say is that psychiatry's closeness to the federal government and researchers' susceptibility to political pressures were much greater than was commonly thought.

LSD raised problems for psychiatry, among them the scientific, boundary, and political problems that have been described. Yet, one must say that LSD was given a good chance to prove itself within the profession, and that many leaders—perhaps not the most vocal—were all continuing study, despite controversy. Perhaps, if controversy had been kept within the bounds of the profession, a different resolution would have been reached in a scientific manner. Perhaps it would have taken longer, on the order of decades, for LSD research and its conclusions to gain legitimacy. It could be argued that the acceptance of psychoanalytic thinking by the profession took 20 to 30 years. Instead, the use of LSD as a drug of more than medical significance occurred. It occurred at the most inopportune time for the profession which could be accused of bringing LSD into the world. For now, that same profession was to be charged by the state with controlling its use and with eradicating its effect as a public health problem. Psychiatry was somewhat in the position of the tobacco industry when it was called on to do research on the effects of smoking.

It has been suggested recently that LSD should again be studied. Psychedelic drug therapy still goes on unofficially. People would not still continue to practice it under difficult conditions unless they believed that they were accomplishing something. Many regard it as an experience worth having, some as a first step toward change, and a few as a turning point in their lives (Grinspoon and Bakalar 1981). Indeed, the battle against the LSD culture is long over. That psychiatry has much to learn both clinically and in basic research from the psychedelics seems likely. Whether or not psychedelic research will be revived from where it fell by the wayside almost two decades ago remains to be seen.

* * *

John R. Neill, "'More Than Medical Significance': LSD and American Psychiatry 1953 to 1966." This article appeared in the *Journal of Psychoactive Drugs,* 19(1), January-March 1987, and is reprinted with permission. Copyright © 1987 by Haight-Ashbury Publications.

References

Abramson, H. A. (ed.). 1960. *The Use of LSD in Psychotherapy*. New York: Josiah Macy Jr. Foundation.

Cohen, M. M., and Marmillo, M. J. 1967. Chromosomal damage and human leukocytes induced by lysergic acid diethylamide. *Science 155*(3768):1417-1419.

Crockett, R., Sandison, R. A., and Walk, A. (eds.). 1963. *Hallucinogenic Drugs and Their Psychotherapeutic Use*. London: H. K. Lewis.

Dahlberg. C. C., Mechanek, R., and Feldstein, S. 1968. LSD research: The impact or lay publicity. *American Journal of Psychiatry 125*(11):685-689.

Dishotsky, N. I., Loughman, W. D., Mogar, R. E., and Lipscomb, W. R. 1971. LSD, and genetic damage. *Science 172*(3982):431-440.

Freedman, D. X. 1969. In Meyer, R. E. (ed.), *Adverse Reactions to Hallucinogenic Drugs*. Washington, DC: U.S. GPO.

Freedman, D. X. 1968. On the use and abuse of LSD. *Archives of General Psychiatry 18*(3):330-347.

Grinspoon, L., and Bakalar, J. B. 1981. The psychedelic therapies. *Current Psychiatric Therapies 21*:275-283.

Grinspoon, L., and Bakalar, J. B. 1979. *Psychedelic Drugs Reconsidered*. New York: Basic Books.

Hicks, R. E., and Fink, P. J. (eds.) 1969. *Psychedelic Drugs*. New York: Grune and Stratton.

Hofmann, A. 1959. Psychotomimetic drugs, chemical and pharmacological aspect. *Acta Physiologica Pharmacologica Neerlandica 8*:240-258.

Hollister, L. E. 1968. *Chemical Psychosis*. Springfield, IL: Charles C. Thomas.

Kafka, J., and Garder, K. R. 1964. Some effects of the therapist's LSD experience in his therapeutic work. *American Journal of Psychotherapy 18*(2):236-243.

Katzenelbogen, S., and Fran, A. D. 1953. Narcosynthesis effects of sodium amytal, methedrine, and LSD-25. *Diseases of the Nervous System 14*(1):85-90.

Kurland, A. A. 1967. The therapeutic potential of LSD in medicine. In De Bold, R. C., and Leaf, R. C. (eds.), *LSD, Man, and Society*. Middletown, CT: Wesleyan University Press.

Kurland, A. A., Savage, C., Pahnke, W., Grof, S., and Olsson, J. 1971. LSD in the treatment of alcoholics. *Pharmakopsychiatrie Neuropsychopharmakologie 4*:83-94.

Mark, J. 1979. *The Search for the Manchurian Candidate*. New York: Times Books.

Meyer, R. E. (ed.). 1969. *Adverse Reactions to Hallucinogenic Drugs*. Washington, DC: U.S. GPO.

Osmond, H. 1957. A review of the clinical effects of psychotomimetic agent. *Annals of the New York Academy of Sciences 66*(3):418-434.

Roth, M. 1963. In Crockett, R., Sandison, R. A., and Walk, A. (eds.), *Hallucinogenic Drugs and Their Psychotherapeutic Use*. London: H. K. Lewis.

Sandison, R. A. 1963. Certainty and uncertainty in the LSD treatment of psychoneurosis. In Crockett, R., Sandison, R. A., and Walk, A. (eds.), *Hallucinogenic Drugs and Their Psychotherapeutic Use*. London: H. K. Lewis.

Savage, C., and McCabe, O. L. 1973. Residential psychedelic (LSD) therapy for the narcotic addict: A controlled study. *Archives of General Psychiatry 28*(6):808-814.

Savage, C., McCabe, O. L., Kurland, A. A., and Hanlon, T. 1973. LSD-assisted psychotherapy in the treatment of severe chronic neurosis. *Journal of Altered States of Consciousness 1*(1):31-47.

Stoll, W. A. 1947. Lysergsäure-diäthylamid, ein phantastikum aus der mutterkorngruppe. *Schweizer Archiv für Neurologie und Psychiatrie 60*:279-323.

Unger, S. 1969a. Panel discussion. In Hicks, R. E., and Fink, P. J. (eds.), *Psychedelic Drugs*. New York: Grune and Stratton.

Unger, S. 1969b. The psychedelic use of LSD: Reflections and observations. In Hicks, R. E., and Fink, P. J. (eds.), *Psychedelic Drugs*. New York: Grune and Stratton.

Ungerleider, J. T. (ed.). 1968. *The Problems and Prospects of LSD*. Springfield, IL: Charles C. Thomas.

Ungerleider, J. T. 1967. Radiomimetic properties of LSD. *New England Journal of Medicine 277*(20):1090-1091.

Ungerleider, J. T. 1966. A remarkable mind drug suddenly spells danger: LSD. *Life 25*(3). ✦

Part VII

Drugs and Crime

For generations, while commentators on the American drug scene were sensationalizing the crimes committed by users of heroin, cocaine, and other drugs, researchers and clinicians argued a related series of issues in question. Is criminal behavior antecedent to addiction; or, does criminality emerge subsequent to addiction? More specifically, is crime the result of, or a response to, a special set of life circumstances brought about by the addiction to narcotic drugs? Or conversely, is addiction per se a deviant tendency characteristic of individuals already prone to offensive behavior? Moreover, and assuming that criminality may indeed be a pre-addiction phenomenon, does the onset of chronic narcotics use bring about a change in the nature, intensity, and frequency of deviant and criminal acts? Does criminal involvement tend to increase or decrease subsequent to addiction? Furthermore, what kinds of criminal offenses do addicts engage in? Do they tend toward violent acts of aggression? Or are their crimes strictly profit oriented and geared toward the violation of the sanctity of private property? Or is it both?

As early as the 1920s, researchers had been conducting studies seeking to unravel these very questions. Particularly, Edouard Sandoz at the Municipal Court of Boston and Lawrence Kolb at the U.S. Public Health Service examined the backgrounds of hundreds of heroin users, focusing on the drugs-crime relationship. What they found within criminal-justice and treatment populations were several different types of cases. Some drug users were habitual criminals, and likely always had been; others were simply violators of the Harrison Act, having been arrested for no more than the illegal possession of narcotics. Moreover, among both types a record of violent crimes was absent.

The analyses provided by Sandoz, Kolb, and others established the parameters of several points of view:

- Addicts ought to be the object of vigorous law-enforcement activity, since the majority are members of a criminal element, and drug addiction is simply one of the later phases of their deviant careers.

- Addicts prey upon legitimate society, and the effects of their drugs do indeed predispose them to serious criminal transgressions.

- Addicts are essentially law-abiding citizens who are forced to steal to adequately support their drug habits.

- Addicts are not necessarily criminals but are forced to associate with an underworld element that tends to maintain control over the distribution of illicit drugs.

The notion that addicts ought to be the objects of vigorous police activity, a posture that might be called the *criminal model of drug abuse*, was actively and relentlessly pursued by the Federal Bureau of Narcotics and other law-enforcement groups. Their argument was fixed on the notion of criminality: on the basis of their own observations, the vast majority of heroin users encountered were members of criminal groups. To support this view, the Bureau of Narcotics pointed to several studies that demonstrated that most addicts were already criminals before they began using heroin. Addicts, the Bureau emphasized, represent a destructive force confronting the people of America. Whatever the sources of their addiction might be, they are members of a highly subversive and antisocial group. For the Bureau, this position did indeed have some basis in reality. Having been charged with the enforcement of a law that prohibited the possession, sale, and distribution of narcotics, what bureau agents were confronted with were *criminal* addicts, often under the most dangerous of circumstances. It was not uncommon for agents to be wounded or even killed in arrest situations, and analyses of the careers of many addicts demonstrated that their criminal records were lengthy. But the Bureau was incorrect in its belief that all drug users were from the same mold. Studies of drug-using populations have referenced the existence of numerous and alternative patterns of narcotic addiction.

During the years between 1900 and 1960, for example, there was a pattern of addiction characteristic of a core of *middle-aged white southerners*. Identified through patient records at federal drug-treatment facilities, they were usually addicted to morphine or paregoric, and their drugs had been obtained from physicians through legal or quasi-legal means. As "patients" under treatment for some illness, these addicts were not members of any deviant subcultures and did not have contacts with other addicts.

There were also groups of *hidden addicts* who, because of sufficient income and/or access to a legitimate source of drugs, had no need to make contacts with visibly criminal cultures to obtain drugs. Among these were musicians, physicians, and members of other segments of the health professions.

Finally, there was the stereotyped *heroin street addict*—the narcotics user of the American ghetto of whom the mass media spoke. Heroin street addicts were typically from the socially and economically deprived segments of the urban population. They began their careers with drug experimentation as adolescents for the sake of excitement or thrills, to conform with peer-group activities and expectations, and/or to strike back at the authority structures which they opposed. The use of alcohol, marijuana, codeine, or pills generally initiated them into substance abuse, and later drug intake focused primarily on heroin. Their status of addiction was often said to have emerged as a result of an addiction-prone personality, and they supported their habits through illegal means. Also among this group were *poly-drug users*—those who concurrently abused a variety of drugs.

By mid-century, most law-enforcement agencies focused their attention and commentary on those who manifested the pattern of heroin street addiction. Their judgments and assertions were often a response to the clinicians and social scientists of the time, who had put forth the notion of what might be called a *medical model of addiction*, as opposed to the *criminal* view by law enforcement. The medical model, which physicians first proposed in the late nineteenth century, held that addiction was a chronic and relapsing disease. The addict, it was argued, should be dealt with as any patient suffering from some physiological or medical disorder. At the same time, numerous proponents of the view sought to mitigate addict criminality by putting forth the "enslavement theory of addiction." The idea here was that the monopolistic controls over the heroin black market forced "sick" and otherwise law-abiding drug users into lives of crime to support their habits.

In retrospect, from the 1920s through the close of the 1970s, hundreds of studies of the relationship between crime and addiction had been conducted. Invariably, when one analysis supported the medical model of addiction, the next would affirm the criminal model. Given these repeated contradictions, something had to be wrong—and, indeed, there was. The theories, hypotheses, conclusions, and other findings generated by almost the entire spectrum of research were actually of little value, for there were awesome biases and deficiencies in the very nature of their designs. Data-gathering enterprises on criminal activity had usually restricted themselves to drug-users' arrest histories, and there can be little argument about the inadequacy of official criminal statistics as measures of the incidence and prevalence of offense behavior. Those studies that did manage to go beyond arrest figures to probe self-reported criminal activity were invariably limited to either incarcerated heroin users or addicts in treatment settings. The few efforts that did manage to locate active heroin users in the street community typically examined the samples' drug-taking behaviors to the exclusion of their drug-seeking behaviors. Given the many methodological difficulties, it was impossible to draw many reliable conclusions about the nature of drug-related crime—about its magnitude, shape, scope, or direction. Moreover, and perhaps most importantly, the conclusions being drawn from the generations of studies were not taking a number of important features of the drug scene into account: that there were many different kinds of drugs and drug users; that the nature and patterns of drug use were constantly shifting and changing; that the purity, potency, and availability of drugs were dynamic, rather than static; and that both drug-related crime and drug-using criminals were undergoing continuous metamorphosis. It was not until the 1970s that research began to reliably address these issues to generate a better understanding of the drugs/crime connection in the American drug scene. In the essays that follow, aspects of this research are presented. ✦

26. The Drugs-Crime Connection

DAVID N. NURCO,
TIMOTHY W. KINLOCK,
AND
THOMAS E. HANLON

The nature of the drug-crime relationship is not altogether clear. Is addiction another expression of a criminal lifestyle? Or do addicts commit crime to support their addictions? In the opening essay of this section, David N. Nurco and his colleagues address these important questions, while discussing a number of problems associated with previous studies. Addicts, they argue, should not be classified as a homogeneous group. Some drug users do not commit crime except for drug possession and sale. For others, criminal activity occurs before the onset of addiction, while some commit crimes to support their addictions. The authors conclude with suggestions for improving our knowledge of the drug-crime connection.

The first recorded speculation regarding a link between narcotic drugs and crime appeared more than a hundred years ago.[1]

Since that time, there has been a long and continuing controversy in the United States about the relationship between narcotic addiction and crime. On one side were those advocating the "criminal model of addiction,"[2] who regarded addicts as confirmed criminals who endanger society by their anti-social behavior. This viewpoint was epitomized by the late Harry J. Anslinger, the first head of the Federal Bureau of Narcotics, who served in this capacity from 1930 to 1962. Similar viewpoints were publicly expressed as early as 1924.

As David Musto noted in his comprehensive historical account, *The American Disease*, it was stated in testimony before Congress that heroin was a stimulus to the commission of crime.[3] In this testimony, Dr. Alexander Lambert, the head of the Mayor's Committee on Drug Addiction for New York City, expressed the view that heroin tended to destroy the sense of responsibility to the herd. The commissioner of health of Chicago,

Dr. Herman Bundesen, went even further, stating that "the root of the social evil is essentially in our dope, our habit-forming drugs [the] main cause of prostitution and crime."[4] Although there were differences in emphasis and interpretation among those who held that heroin use promoted crime, it was generally agreed that heroin was destructive and criminogenic.

The other side in this historical controversy took the position that narcotic addicts were not criminals, but deprived or mentally ill individuals who were "forced" into the commission of petty theft in order to support their habit. This viewpoint was emphatically presented by Harry Barnes and Negley Teeters of Temple University in their 1945 textbook, *New Horizons in Criminology*:

> It is now definitely demonstrated that most serious cases of drug addiction are the result of neurotic conditions, namely, mental and nervous disorders growing out of deep-seated mental conflicts in the individual. . . . It is not likely, however, that a normal person will become an addict. . . . Alarmist literature and the propaganda of the crusaders against drug addiction have created a grotesquely exaggerated impression of the danger to society from the drug addict.[5]

This notion has been frequently referred to as the "enslavement theory of addiction."[6] It was based on a medical model, and the proponents of this view advocated the treatment of narcotic addiction by psychiatrists or other physicians. Those who supported this idea included many clinicians and social scientists of the 1950s and 1960s.

Regardless of which side one took in this controversy, it was often assumed that all narcotic addicts were alike. This concept of uniformity was tacitly assumed by most researchers of the drugs-crime connection before the 1970s.

As researchers from the National Institute of Justice summarized in a comprehensive literature review published in 1980, the majority of studies concentrated on how certain factors affect most addicts, largely ignoring the fact that "these factors all affect addicts differently" and that addicts "should not be viewed as a homogeneous group that follow the same career paths."[7] This appears to be one of the major flaws inherent in earlier research.

Research on the Drugs-Crime Connection

Literature reviews have documented that hundreds of studies of the relationship between addiction and crime were performed from the 1920s to the late 1970s.[8] Several reviewers have commented that these studies contained numerous flaws. As James A. Inciardi has summarized elsewhere,[9] the theories, hypotheses, conclusions, and other findings generated by these studies were of little value, since there were considerable biases and deficiencies in their designs. Given the many methodological difficulties, it was impossible to draw reliable conclusions about the magnitude, shape, scope, or direction of drug-related crime.

In their 1987 review article, "Characterizing Criminal Careers," Alfred Blumstein and Jacqueline Cohen maintained that "even though the subjects of crime and crime control have been major issues of public debate, and despite their regular appearance as one of the nation's most serious problems, significant advances in empirical research related to these issues are relatively recent. . . ." They also emphasized that "more effectively disentangling the apparent drug-crime nexus is of particular concern."[10]

Not until the 1970s and 1980s were more sophisticated studies of the relationship between drug use and crime finally undertaken. In their book, *Taking Care of Business*,[11] published in 1985, Bruce D. Johnson and his associates at the New York State Division of Substance Abuse Services noted that earlier literature reviews had concluded that little was known about the crime rates of heroin abusers and emphasized the need for improved information about the criminal behavior of drug users. They cited the 1967 report of the President's Commission on Law Enforcement and the Administration of Justice: "Only minimal comprehensive data are available relative to the issue of the drugs/crime relationship";[12] and the 1976 Panel on Drug Use and Criminal Behavior: "Convincing empirical data on drug abuse and crime . . . are generally unavailable—the principal reason being the lack of a long-term, research program in the area."[13]

While there were some notable exceptions, the results of studies revealing differential characteristics among narcotic addicts were usually ignored by policy makers. Examples of these exceptions were the works of Edward Sendoz at the Municipal Court of Boston and Lawrence Holt from the U.S. Public Health Service.[14] Both series of studies suggested that there were different types of addicts. Some were habitual criminals and were so before becoming addicted. On the other hand, others were simply violators of the Harrison Act, having been arrested for illegal possession of narcotics. Unfortunately, the notion of heterogeneity of addicts did not become evident until much later.

Methodological Deficiencies of Early Studies

Evidence of criminal activity among narcotic users is longstanding and abundant; however, it is apparent that relationships among the important variables involved are much more complex than were initially believed. As mentioned, literature reviews of studies conducted on the relationship between narcotic addiction and crime found that these investigations contained several important methodological deficiencies. Among the most commonly mentioned problems were the following:

1. The employment of seriously deficient measures of criminality.

2. The preoccupation with the single-cause issue or the "chicken-egg" question of which came first, crime or drugs.

3. The use of "captive" samples of narcotic addicts.

4. The failure to apply measures of criminal activity over time.

5. The failure to correctly identify the empirical precursors, correlates, possible determinants, and patterns of criminality, and the ignoring of the co-variation of such factors within an addict population.

Measurement of Crime Among Narcotic Addicts

Probably the most serious methodological problem contained in early studies of the relationship between drug use and crime has been the use of official arrest records, or "rap sheets," as indicators of criminal activity. In a review of sixty-five studies to determine the methods of measuring individual criminal behavior, James J. Collins and his coworkers concluded that "arrest data are a seriously deficient indicator of criminal involvement—in fact, it is more accurate to view arrest data as an indicator of criminal justice *system* involvement."[15] In other words, arrest data more properly measure how often one *gets caught* for committing crime, and there is far from a one-to-one relationship between how often someone is caught and how much crime he or she commits.[16]

Several studies employing confidential self-report interview methods have shown that the use of arrest data as an indicator of the amounts and types of crimes actually committed results in gross underestimates.[17] These investigations have found that less than 1 percent of all offenses reported by addicts resulted in arrest. Typical of findings emphasizing the inadequacy of official statistics as measures of the incidence and prevalence of criminal behavior are those of Inciardi.[18] In one of his studies, Inciardi noted that his sample of 573 Miami narcotic abusers had engaged in criminal activity for an average of two years before their first arrest. Also, he indicated that subsequent arrest rates were extremely low. Of 215,105 offenses reported by the respondents over a one-year period, only 609, or one arrest for every 353 crimes committed (0.3 percent), resulted in arrest.[19]

A common finding of the research of Jan M. Chaiken and Marcia R. Chaiken has been that number of arrests is a poor predictor of who the most dangerous criminals are. Analyzing arrest data and self-reported crime in a Rand Corporation study of over two thousand offenders in three states, these investigators concluded that it was impossible to identify serious and frequent offenders from official records, since "the vast majority of those who do commit all of these crimes (robbery, assault, and drug sales) have not been convicted of them."[20] Although all respondents had been arrested, it was found that arrests were so infrequent and the official records so inadequate that it was impossible to distinguish the serious and persistent offenders from the less serious ones. Chaiken and Chaiken found that only about 10 percent of self-reported violent predators could be so identified by arrest records.[21]

In our studies of narcotic addicts in Baltimore, we have obtained similar results.[22] In one of these studies, we analyzed the self-reports and arrest data of a sample of 243 addicts. While these addicts had a total of 2,869 arrests over an eleven-year period, they also had accumulated 473,738 days of crime, resulting in a ratio of arrests to crime days of .006. Not only were arrests an extreme underestimate of

how much crime was committed, but also the arrests were biased with regard to both the type of offense committed and the frequency of offenses. Violent crimes were more likely than other crimes to result in arrest, and the probability of arrest decreased for addicts with high crime rates.[23]

The Validity of Self-Reported Crime

Any study relying primarily on informant self-disclosure must eventually come to grips with the issue of the accuracy, or veridicality, of such information.[24] In this context, the self-reports of drug addicts are particularly suspect because of the deviant and illegal nature of their lifestyles. In addition to possible distortions introduced in order to conceal unsavory aspects of their lives, genuine errors in recalling information about events that occurred years earlier can further affect the accuracy of the information obtained. However, evidence in the literature indicates that addicts, as a group, tend to be surprisingly truthful and accurate in their replies to a wide range of questions when interviewed under non-threatening conditions.[25] Validation studies that have been conducted have used the following methods: comparing self-reports of arrests with official records, comparing information on drug use with urinalysis results, and using repeat-interview procedures.

It is, of course, clear that the social context and the conditions under which interviews are conducted may affect the addicts' motivation to be candid, equivocal, or deceitful. Thus, even though interview information is obtained in the context of research, it would be just as unwarranted to maintain that addicts' responses are invariably valid as it would be to assume that they are invalid. Research procedures that appear to be particularly important to the securing of valid interview data include the following: the addict's recognition of the availability of an official record (that allows corroboration of self-report information); the interviewer's thorough knowledge of the addict subculture, as well as his or her competence, experience, and training in interviewing procedures; the absence of an authoritarian or retribution function in the interview; the assurance of confidentiality; and the use of a structured instrument that enables internal consistency checks and the offering of meaningful time-reference points to assist in the recall of information. (The "addict career" interview, which will be discussed in more detail later, is especially useful in this respect.)

The Crime-Days per Year-at-Risk Concept

Several investigators of the drugs-crime connection have been striving to develop a meaningful application of what has been termed "lambda"—the rate of offending per unit of time (usually a year) for a given population at risk. Our own calculations involving a variation of this index have used self-reported information from narcotic addicts, covering varying periods, while addicted and not addicted to narcotics over a lifetime of narcotic drug use. Because narcotic addicts may engage in hundreds of offenses per year, it has proved useful to express the magnitude of their criminal behavior in terms of the number of crime-days per year-at-risk (while at large in the community), rather than in terms of the total number of offenses committed per year. A *crime-day* is conceptually defined as a twenty-four-hour period, during which one or more crimes are committed by a given individual. Thus, crime-days per year-at-risk is a rate of occurrence that varies from 0 to 365.

Our use of the crime-days per year-at-risk measure has served to document the continuity of high crime rates among narcotic addicts over extended periods. Although there are differences in the types of crimes that individual addicts engage in, their overall high rates of criminality characteristically persist throughout their periods of addiction. The continuity of these high crime rates is remarkable. An analysis of crime-days per year-at-risk for 354 addicts interviewed between 1973 and 1978 revealed that the crime-day means for the first seven addiction periods were 255, 244, 259, 257, 254, 336, and 236, respectively. Thus, the high rate of criminality reported not only was persistent on a day-to-day basis, but also tended to continue over an extended number of years and periods of addiction.[26]

Use of the crime-days per year-at-risk approach has also enabled us to document a reduction in crime when individuals are not actively addicted. Inasmuch as the life course of narcotic addiction or "addict career," while in the community, is characterized by numerous periods of addiction and nonaddiction, it is feasible to compare the amounts of crime committed by individuals when they are addicted and when they are not.[27] When crime rates were compared in this manner, it was found that the number of crime-days per year-at-risk averaged 255 during periods of active addiction and only 65 during periods of nonaddiction.[28] There was, then, a 75-percent decrease in criminality from addiction to nonaddiction. Further analysis showed that there was a decline in annualized crime rates during successive nonaddiction periods as well. Conversely, crime rates during successive addiction periods remained high.

A subsequent study of 250 addicts in Baltimore and New York whom our staff interviewed between 1983 and 1984 provided similar results. It was found that the number of overall crime-days per year-at-risk during periods of addiction averaged 259, while the rate for periods of nonaddiction was 108.[29]

Narcotic Addict Types

There has long been a nagging concern about the order of first occurrence of drug abuse and crime, and about the directional nature of the relationship between the two. Many early studies of the drugs-crime connection were preoccupied with this question. The inquiry was typically stated as an either-or, mutually exclusive one. Addicts either committed crimes to support their habits or were criminals to begin with, addiction merely being one more manifestation of a deviant lifestyle. As mentioned, regardless of whatever side one took, there was general consensus that addicts basically comprised a homogeneous group. Only recently (since the 1970s) have researchers begun to systematically evaluate the differential characteristics of narcotic addicts. A major outgrowth of research, based on an assumption of heterogeneity, has been the derivation of narcotic addict types. Such information is just beginning to be available for consideration by policy makers.

Our own work in this area of research has determined that addicts vary along a host of dimensions, including the degree to which they engage in crime.[30] Some individuals are extremely criminal before they become addicted, while others turn to criminal behavior only as a result of their addiction. There are addicts who do not commit any crime, except for possession of illegal drugs, while others commit several crimes per day and carry weapons while doing so. Certain addicts may maintain rather stable levels of crime, while the criminal behavior of others may trend upward or downward, as addiction careers extend over time. Also, many addicts undergo treatment for their addictions, while others remain addicted for long periods of time, with no intention of being treated for their drug problems. Only by carefully examining the various kinds of narcotic addicts will more effective use be made of treatment facilities and correctional resources.

In one of our studies of addicts, we classified a sample of 460 individuals, according to criminality, employment, and adequacy of income to meet needs.[31] Two of the types generated by this classification were so different from one another that they suggested two distinct ways of dealing with drug activities. The first type, the "successful criminal," is accustomed to having more than enough money from illicit sources to meet his needs. The second type, the "working addict," is employed at least eight hours a day and is only involved minimally in criminal activities. The successful criminal would appear to be a poor candidate for treatment that counsels him to seek a legitimate job, paying far less than his illegal income. For such a strategy to succeed, this type of addict would have to be monitored closely to ascertain whether or not he was returning to drug abuse and crime. Should reinvolvement occur, he should be promptly referred back to the court for disposition. In contrast, the working addict attempts to live in two worlds, the "straight world" and the drug subculture; his struggle to maintain this precarious balance makes him a prime candidate for receiving help in planning for a more legitimate lifestyle. It is believed that such meaningful, pragmatic typologies will ultimately serve to increase the effectiveness of prevention, rehabilitation, and correctional efforts with respect to the individual at risk.

Use of 'Captive' Samples

Several literature reviews have reported that most investigations of the criminal behavior of narcotic addicts have ignored the problem of population representativeness.[32] Many researchers have studied only "captive" addicts (those in jail or in treatment) who may possess characteristics quite different from those of addicts at large in the community. This fact obviously compromises the generalizability of results.

While a truly random sample of narcotic addicts is apparently impossible to achieve, since the activity is illegal and therefore often unseen, making the population incapable of complete enumeration, in the 1970s, attempts were begun to minimize these difficulties. One example was our own study, which employed a "community-wide" population, consisting of all individuals identified as narcotic addicts by the Baltimore City Police over a twenty-year period.[33] Another approach to the representativeness problem has been the use of samples of narcotic abusers "on the street." In this type of research, ethnographic methods have been used. Often researchers employ ex-addicts or become familiar themselves with the addict subculture in various ways. An example of the latter, the setting up of "storefronts," is exemplified by the work in New York City of Edward A. Preble and John J. Casey[34] in the 1960s and of Bruce Johnson, Paul Goldstein, and others in the 1970s and 1980s.[35]

Ethnographic research may provide a means of obtaining valuable insights into the procurement of information regarding the drugs-crime connection that has not been possible through traditional research. As Goldstein summarized in 1982:

> Careful and probing research is needed to explicate the dynamics underlying both drugs and crime, and the multi-faceted relationship between the two phenomena. Ethnographic techniques may well hold the most promise in this regard. Interviewing subjects in institutional settings, or perusing official statistics, is a poor substitute for being with subjects on a daily basis.[36]

Measures of Criminal Activity Over Time

Career patterns of criminal behavior and drug use were typically ignored in earlier research,[37] most studies having dealt with single-event, pre- and post-intervention comparisons of criminal behavior.[38] Systematically measuring criminal activity over time is a relatively new development. As William H. McGlothlin[39] and other reviewers have noted, however, unless suitable adjustments are made, the age of the addict may become a confounding variable. Since research has shown that many individuals tend to "mature out" of both crime and addiction over time, the decreased prevalence of illicit behavior among older (more experienced) addicts may be a phenomenon associated with age. One way of dealing with this methodologically, as Blumstein and Cohen have suggested, is by "tracking carefully the patterns of offending by individual criminals in order to collect reliable data," which "involves the characterization of the longitudinal pattern of crime events for offenders and assessment of factors that affect that pattern."[40]

A way of applying this method to the joint study of crime and addiction over time has centered around the notion of "addict careers." As mentioned earlier, the addict career, or the time from the first regular narcotic use to the present, is divided into periods of addiction and nonaddiction. Using this longitudinal method, crime rates can be compared between different addiction status periods, as well as over successive periods of addiction and nonaddiction.[41] This form of interview schedule has also been successfully used by McGlothlin, and later by Douglas Anglin, at UCLA in their follow-up studies of addicts.[42]

Types and Extent of Drug-Related Crime

Many researchers have concluded that the prevalence and diversity of criminal involvement by narcotic addicts are high, and that this involvement is primarily for the purpose of supporting the use of drugs. Further, it has been a consistent finding that initiation into both substance abuse and criminal activity occurs at an early age. In particular, several investigators have found that, among samples of drug-using offenders, those who reported the most crime as adults, including the most violent crime, were characteristically precocious in their drug use and illegal activity.[43]

It has also been a uniform finding that frequency of narcotic use is generally associated with higher crime rates. Johnson and his associates[44] found that the heaviest heroin users were more likely to be classified as serious offenders. In their research, such individuals were found to be disproportionately represented in the highest categories of criminal involvement and had the highest incomes from major crime. Examining a broader range of drug abusers, the Research Triangle Institute group[45] reported that "expensive" drug use was at least a partial explanation for income-generating crime. These investigators found that more-than-once-a-day heroin and cocaine use predicted comparatively high levels of illegal income. Further examination of the drug-use-frequency/income-from-crime relationship suggested that, whereas low-use levels are supportable without resort to illegal activity, frequent daily use rarely is. And Chaiken and Chaiken,[46] classifying prison and jail inmates as addicted heroin users, nonaddicted heroin users, nonheroin drug users, and nondrug users, found that addicted

heroin users had markedly higher levels of criminal activity than did nonheroin drug users.

In explanation of the above results, one might argue that those individuals prone to be heavy drug users are also innately prone to become involved in criminal activity. Evidence of a more direct relationship between narcotic drug-use frequency and crime requires longitudinal, intra-subject information on narcotic-abusing individuals over periods varying with respect to frequency of narcotic drug use. In our own studies of addict careers, the consistently high rates of criminality associated with addiction periods and the markedly lower rates found in the nonaddiction periods provide substantial support for a causal component in the relationship of drug use to crime. The most parsimonious explanation of these within-group changes in crime rates with varying amounts of narcotic use is that narcotic addiction contributes to an increase in crime. Without engaging in a discussion of causal analysis, it seems evident from the totality of the data that heroin addiction is criminogenic in the same sense that cigarette smoking or air pollutants are carcinogenic—they can, and often do, lead to increased incidence, although they are not the only causal agents.

Although individual addicts vary with respect to the crime they engage in, narcotic addicts as a group engage in many different types of criminal activity. Examining a sample of male and female narcotic users in Miami between 1978 and 1981, Inciardi found that over a preceding twelve-month period, the 573 individuals in this sample were responsible for over 82,000 drug sales, nearly 6,000 robberies and assaults, 6,700 burglaries, and 900 car thefts, as well as for more than 25,000 instances of shoplifting and 46,000 other types of larceny and fraud. Overall, they were responsible for a total of 215,105 criminal offenses of all types during the twelve-month reporting period, or an average of 375 offenses per narcotic user.[47]

Drug-Distribution Crimes

Drug-distribution crimes (e.g., dealing, copping, tasting) appear to account for a sizable proportion of all crimes performed by narcotic abusers. For Inciardi's sample, drug sales was by far the most frequent crime, accounting for 38 percent of all offenses. The respondents averaged 144 drug sales per year.[48] A sample of 201 heroin abusers studied by Johnson reported committing, on the average, 828 crimes per year per user. The most frequent crime was drug sales, or dealing, which accounted for 34 percent of all crimes. The second most frequent crime was copping (buying for others), which constituted 28 percent of all crimes. Taken together, these and other drug-distribution offenses accounted for 65 percent of all crimes reported.[49]

Our recent studies of addicts interviewed in Baltimore and New York, during 1983 and 1984, also documented the dominance of drug-distribution crimes. This sample of 250 male addicts reported performing drug-distribution crimes on nearly 48,000 days while addicted, the average time spent addicted being nearly eight years. On average, the addicts were involved in drug-distribution crimes 191 days per year. For the entire sample, drug-distribution crimes accounted for 48.3 percent of all crime-days. Comparisons of crime-days frequencies with those reported by an earlier sample of addicts interviewed, during 1973-1978, revealed a higher proportion of drug-distribution crimes and a lower proportion of theft crimes in the more recent sample. In the earlier sample, drug-distribution crimes accounted for only 27 percent of the crime-days, while theft crimes made up 38 percent of the crime-days.[50]

The 100 subjects interviewed in Baltimore were also examined in a separate series of analyses, comparing crime-days results with those for an earlier sample of Baltimore addicts.[51] It was found that, for both black and white addicts, crime increased overall, with the greatest area of increase in drug-distribution crimes. This was true of crimes committed during both addiction periods and nonaddiction periods. Minor differences in study procedures, however, render these findings tentative rather than conclusive.

Violent Crimes

Obviously, because of their severe consequences to victims, policy makers and the media have emphasized violent drug-related crimes. While investigations by us and others have reported that violent crimes make up a small proportion of all crimes committed by addicts, the actual number of such offenses is still large, since addicts commit so many crimes. For example, in Inciardi's sample of 573 narcotic users, the proportion of violent crimes committed in the year before the interview constituted only 2.8 percent of all offenses, but this amounted to nearly six thousand offenses, since a total of 215,105 crimes were committed.[52]

Paul Goldstein[53] has recorded many ethnographic accounts of violent drug-related acts from both perpetrators and victims in New York City. Resulting from this research is his theory that violent crime and drugs can be related in three different ways. The psychopharmacological model of violence implies that individuals act violently because of the short- or long-term effects of the ingestion of certain substances. Crimes resulting from withdrawal effects of heroin or directly related to barbiturate or PCP use are examples of this. The economically compulsive model suggests that violent crime is committed to obtain money to purchase drugs. This applies primarily to expensive drugs, such as heroin and cocaine. The systemic model purports that violence results from the traditionally aggressive patterns of interaction within the drug-distribution system. Killing or assaulting someone for distributing "bad" drugs is an example of this.

A study of 578 homicides in Manhattan in 1981 found that 38 percent of the male victims and 14 percent of the female victims were murdered as result of drug-related activity.[54] This report, published in 1986, stated that the observed proportion of homicides related to drug and other criminal activities was higher than had been reported previously in the United States. The authors concluded that rather than being related to pharmacological actions producing aggressive and homicidal behavior, the effects of drugs were probably indirect and related to drug-seeking activities. They concluded that "the fact that over one-third of male homicide victims in Manhattan in 1981 died in drug-related homicides attests to the magnitude and the impact of the drug problem, particularly with narcotics."[55]

Non-Narcotic Drug Use and Crime

While it has been acknowledged that a substantial relationship exists between narcotic addiction and crime, the situation has been somewhat less clear with regard to non-narcotic drugs. In a comprehensive review of the literature published in 1980, Robert P. Gandossy and his associates found the evidence connecting the use of various non-narcotic drugs to crime to be inconclusive.[56] A further problem concerning this issue is that narcotic and non-narcotic drugs are often used in combination. Thus, disentangling their joint relationship to criminal behavior, let alone resolving the issue of cause and effect, is problematical. Research endeavors in the past decade, however, have made several advances in addressing these difficulties.

One method of approaching the issue has been to study the crime rates of individuals, during a particular period in which they were strictly non-narcotic users and had never become addicted to narcotics. Inciardi interviewed a sample of 429 such individuals in the years 1978-1981.[57] Reporting both a high prevalence and a diversity of crimes, these individuals admitted to committing a total of 137,076 offenses, for an average of 320 crimes per user, over a one-year period. This rate was slightly lower and the diversity of crimes somewhat less than those found for a sample of narcotic users interviewed during the same period. Of the crimes committed by the non-narcotic users, drug sales accounted for 28 percent, prostitution for 18 percent, and shoplifting for 16 percent.[58]

Another way of studying the non-narcotic, drug-crime relationship has been to correlate rates of various types of crime with the use of non-narcotic drugs during periods of addiction and nonaddiction to narcotics. Our own findings from this type of approach have consistently indicated that the use of certain non-narcotic drugs by narcotic addicts is associated with the commission of certain types of crime, although this varied somewhat by ethnic group and narcotic addiction status.[59] Cocaine use was found to have a particularly high association with several different types of crime, including theft, violent crimes, drug dealing, and confidence games. This association appeared to be stronger in black and Hispanic addicts than in white addicts.[60]

Treatment and Rehabilitation

Most of the addicts we have studied in over twenty years of research have been arrested a number of times and have spent considerable time in prison. Many addicts have also had at least one treatment experience for narcotic drug abuse. However, these arrests, periods of incarceration, and treatment experiences appear to have had little deterrent effect on subsequent criminal behavior in the community for a good many addicts. As we have indicated elsewhere,[61] the finding of continuity and persistence of criminal behavior among narcotic addicts stands out as a major conclusion of our research.

Some encouraging findings concerning rehabilitation efforts have involved the use of legal pressures accompanied by a monitoring or surveillance component. Studies of the California Civil Addict Program by McGlothlin and Anglin[62] found that court-ordered, drug-free outpatient treatment accompanied by supervision, including urine testing and weekly visits to a parole officer, was associated with reduced criminal activity. Other studies, conducted by investigators at the Research Triangle Institute (RTI) in North Carolina, found that legal pressure was positively related to retention in treatment programs, and that time in treatment was a significant factor in the reduction of criminal behavior following treatment.[63] And, encouraged by their findings in a recently reported study of legal pressure and methadone-maintenance outcome, Anglin and his colleagues[64] argue for greater utilization of community drug treatment by pretrial, probation, and parole agencies.

By far the most ambitious series of studies of the influence of treatment on the behavior of the narcotic addict has been that conducted by the Institute of Behavioral Research at Texas Christian University in Ft. Worth.[65] Based on a client reporting system for community-based drug abuse programs, titled Drug Abuse Reporting Program (DARP), this treatment-outcome evaluation research involved a comparison of the effectiveness of methadone-maintenance programs, therapeutic communities, outpatient drug-free treatments, outpatient detoxification clinics, and intake only (i.e., no treatment). Major criteria of effectiveness included illicit drug use and criminality, along with alcohol use, employment, and need for further treatment. Post-treatment results over a three-year follow-up period were available for four to five thousand clients, with many individuals being followed for as long as six years after treatment admission.

Findings of the DARP revealed a clear-cut superiority of methadone maintenance, therapeutic community, and outpatient drug-free treatment over outpatient detoxification and no treatment. No further differentiation was made among the three effective treatment approaches, all of which produced a marked reduction in self-reported narcotic drug use and criminal behavior. Regardless of treatment type, outcomes associated with treatments of less than ninety days tended to be poor. Persons with less criminal involvement before treatment and persons employed before treatment were more likely to demonstrate favorable outcomes. As apparent in our own research, criminal activity during follow-up was related to daily drug use. And, consistent with the results of other studies, there was no obvious interaction between client and treatment types in terms of outcome.[66]

For DARP clients, during-treatment performance, including longer program involvement and completion of the program, was also positively related to outcome. As in the RTI studies, the marked improvement that tended to occur after the first few months of treatment, particularly with methadone maintenance, suggested a compliance factor associated with coercive entry and program surveillance. After this marked change, there was continued improvement over time in treatment, which suggested a therapeutic effect, due to the development of motivation that was also instrumental in the clients' remaining in treatment.[67]

Policy Implications

Although narcotic addicts as a group extensively engage in crime, the amounts and types of crimes committed vary considerably across individuals. The criminal activity of most addicts is strongly influenced by current addiction status. Narcotic addicts commit millions of crimes per year in the United States, and many of these offenses are of a serious nature. In a very real sense, it can be said that illicit narcotic drugs "drive" crime. Therefore, there is a pressing need to address the problem by continuing to inform the public and its leaders concerning the magnitude and perseverance of criminal behavior among heroin addicts.

As several recent writers have suggested,[68] one approach to a solution involves the early identification of those individuals prone to commit large numbers of serious crimes. Our studies, as well as those by Chaiken and Chaiken, have indicated that, among offenders, those who are precocious in crime and poly-drug use will most likely become the most dangerous, long-term criminals.[69] In addition, we are currently studying the etiology of drug abuse, with the goal of determining the distinguishing characteristics of those individuals who later become addicts, as opposed to their peers who do not. Such information will eventually be useful in planning prevention and intervention strategies.

Another policy with regard to drug abuse and crime centers on the targeted reduction of the amounts of illicit drugs, especially heroin and cocaine, consumed by daily users. Implementation of this policy would involve identifying criminally active, daily heroin and cocaine users and ensuring

that they are treated and closely monitored in order to alter their drug-abuse patterns. Our studies suggest that this particular strategy may work best with addicts minimally involved in crime before becoming addicted and during periods of nonaddiction (i.e., those whose criminal activity is more exclusively related to supporting a habit).[70]

In determining an appropriate disposition of a narcotic drug abuser after arrest, it should again be emphasized that there is not a one-to-one relationship between official arrest records and extent of criminal activity. For a more accurate estimate of the latter, it is important that frequency of narcotic abuse also be determined. From our experiences and those of Johnson and his associates, it appears that the more criminally prone, heaviest narcotic abusers are "slipping through the cracks of the criminal justice system."[71] These individuals are committing more crimes per arrest and are managing to avoid involvement in drug-abuse treatment efforts.

Identifying the "heavy" drug abuser is, however, problematic. While individuals tend to be truthful in reporting drug use in research situations, where confidentiality and immunity from prosecution are ordinarily guaranteed, there is evidence that, on arrest, they are likely to conceal their recent drug use.[72] As a result of this finding, urine testing of arrestees has been recommended as an additional means of identifying those who are habitual drug users. Urine testing has, therefore, been utilized in many jurisdictions as an additional means of identifying arrestees who are drug users. It has recently been estimated that approximately 70 percent of those arrested for serious crimes in major U.S. cities test positive for at least one illicit drug.[73] However, while a single positive urinalysis result is a valid indicator of recent drug use, it is not sufficient to identify an individual as a frequent and persistent drug user. As several researchers have indicated, a series of positive results over a long period of time tends to be a more accurate indicator.[74]

At the very least, it would be advisable for criminal justice authorities to give more concerted attention to evidence concerning the drug activity of individuals who are arrested. One useful approach to this task would be to develop a triage/liaison service within the criminal justice system that would deal exclusively with the disposition of drug-abusing offenders. This service would provide a much-needed link between the criminal justice system and a variety of drug-abuse treatment programs available for rehabilitation. Major functions of the service would include participation in decisions regarding sentencing, parole, and probation, as well as in implementation of procedures for the appropriate placement, monitoring, and evaluation of outcome for all narcotic addict arrestees. Thus, this service would be an important resource to clinicians who treat drug abusers, as well as to judges and other criminal justice system officials who are involved in the disposition of individual cases.

It is important to reiterate that all narcotic addicts are not alike. What works with one type of addict may not work with another. Some addicts commit a considerable amount of crime, regardless of whether they are addicted, and they may engage in crime several years before becoming addicted to narcotics. On the other hand, other addicts may not commit much crime and may only commit crimes directly related to their use of drugs; during periods of nonaddiction, their criminal activities may drop to trivial levels. As we have emphasized, there are clearly different types of addicts and different pathways to addiction. Effective strategies for dealing with the drugs-crime problem will depend, to a significant extent, on recognizing this diversity among addicts and on tailoring counter-measures, both therapeutic and judicial, to individual requirements.

Legalizing Drug Use

Some policy makers have proposed that drug-related crime be curtailed by legalizing the use of illicit drugs, making them openly available at little or no cost. This is offered as an admittedly simplistic solution that requires the development of strategies aimed at preserving the smooth functioning of society and mitigating damage to addiction-prone individuals. Outlandish as it may seem, this is an intriguing notion, the ramifications of which bear consideration, in view of the lack of effectiveness of current methods of controlling drug use that largely involve attempts at cutting off the sources of drug supply.

A look at history is particularly helpful in conceptualizing the polarity of this issue. During the era of prohibition of alcohol use in this country, emphasis was placed on eliminating sources of supply. As a consequence, alcoholism became less of a national problem, but organized crime flourished in its nearly exclusive role as distributor of alcoholic products. The subsequent repeal of the prohibition, while dealing a significant blow to the underworld,

undeniably increased the number of alcoholics and problematic drinkers in our society.[75]

We are now faced with an analogous situation. Unless innovative strategies are developed, the alternative to the high level of drug-related crime associated with strict drug control appears to be an inevitable rise in the number of drug-dependent individuals in society. Ignoring ethical and moral issues for the moment, from a purely pragmatic standpoint, there is the question of how many drug-dependent individuals society can tolerate.

Basic unresolved questions make any position taken, with regard to the impact of the legalization of drugs, a matter of educated opinion, at best. No one knows for certain the extent to which legalization of drugs in this country would increase the number of addicts, nor whether such a strategy would eventually undermine the integrity of our society. Few would deny, however, that the greater availability of, and easier access to, drugs would increase drug use (and addiction) beyond current levels. Whether this nation can be adequately prepared to deal with the consequences of this increase is, again, a matter of conjecture that is beyond the scope of this chapter. More pertinent is this question: What would be the impact of open drug availability on drug-related crime?

To a large extent, the amount of drug-related crime committed is proportional to the costs of drugs, and the latter depend to a large extent on supply and demand. On the supply side, there are two important considerations with regard to legalization, both of which have to do with the effects of a vigorously enforced policy of interdiction. When it is most effective, a policy of interdiction reduces the supply of drugs and, as a consequence, raises the prices people have to pay for them. It also increases the risks associated with drug production and distribution and thus increases the compensation demanded by drug suppliers for their services. Again, the end result is higher drug prices. Assuming that interdiction will never entirely eliminate the supply of drugs, the ironic conclusion is that vigorously enforced interdiction may very well be instrumental in increasing drug-related crime.

In view of the above, some would argue that legalizing drugs would lead to substantial reductions in drug costs and a corresponding reduction in drug-related crime. Such an argument, however, assumes exclusive, trouble-free governmental regulation of the drug supply. Such an assumption would appear to be untenable. The possibility of providing a more desirable drug price and/or purity, unrestricted quantity, personal anonymity, lack of restrictions with regard to age, and other similar inducements could readily lead to black-market competition in drug sales and thus continue the involvement of illegitimate sources of drug supply. Also, the argument ignores the impulsivity and lack of control associated with the use of certain drugs and the crime-linked effects of such drugs as PCP (which produces both self-destructive and assaultive behavior) and cocaine (the excessive use of which has been associated with violence stemming from affective disturbance and paranoid ideation).

This leads us to a consideration of the demand side of the equation, relating supply and demand to drug cost and attendant crime. In view of the above, and the fact that greater demand is associated with increased cost, adoption of intervention strategies aimed at diminishing demand for illicit drugs appears to be the most suitable approach to dealing with the issue of drugs and crime. Consequently, an appropriate policy recommendation would be that concerted attempts be made to dissuade individuals from becoming involved with drugs, along with persistent efforts to wean them off drugs when and if they do become involved. Drug-prevention and treatment programs employing both novel and already proven approaches should, therefore, be targeted for increased support on a national level by both governmental agencies and private funding sources. To the extent that it is drug-related, criminal activity in this country should show discernible signs of abatement with any subsequent decrease in drug demand that can thus be effected.

* * *

David N. Nurco, Timothy W. Kinlok, and Thomas E. Hanlon, "The Drugs-Crime Connection," in James A. Inciardi (ed.), *Handbook of Drug Control in the United States* pp. 71-90, Greenwood Press, an imprint of Greenwood Publishing Group, Inc., Westport, CT. Copyright © 1991 by Greenwood Publishing Group. All rights reserved. Reprinted with permission.

Notes

1. James A. Inciardi, ed., *The Drugs-Crime Connection* (Beverly Hills, CA: Sage, 1981), 7.

2. James A. Inciardi, *The War on Drugs: Heroin, Cocaine, and Public Policy* (Palo Alto, CA: Mayfield, 1986), 106.

3. David F. Musto, *The American Disease: Origins of Narcotic Control* (New Haven, CT: Yale University Press, 1973).

4. *Ibid.*, 326.

5. Harry E. Barnes and Negley K. Teeters, *New Horizons in Criminology* (New York: Prentice-Hall, 1945), 877.

6. Inciardi, *The War on Drugs*, 148.

7. Robert P. Gandossy, Jay R. Williams, Jo Cohen, and Henrick J. Harwood, *Drugs and Crime: A Survey and Analysis of the Literature* (Washington, DC: U.S. Department of Justice, National Institute of Justice, 1980), 67.

8. See Harold Finestone, "Narcotics and Criminality," *Law and Contemporary Problems 22* (Winter 1957):72-85; Gregory A. Austin and Dan J. Lettieri, *Drugs and Crime: The Relationship of Drug Use and Concomitant Criminal Behavior* (Rockville, MD: National Institute on Drug Abuse, 1976); Inciardi, *The Drugs-Crime Connection*; David N. Nurco, John C. Ball, John W. Shaffer, and Thomas E. Hanlon, "The Criminality of Narcotic Addicts," *Journal of Nervous and Mental Disease 173* (1985):94-102; Inciardi, *The War on Drugs*.

9. Inciardi, *The War on Drugs*.

10. Alfred Blumstein and Jacqueline Cohen, "Characterizing Criminal Careers," *Science 237* (1987):985-91.

11. Bruce D. Johnson, Paul J. Goldstein, Edward Preble, James Schmeidler, Douglas S. Lipton, Barry Spunt, and Thomas Miller, *Taking Care of Business: The Economics of Crime by Heroin Abusers* (Lexington, MA: Lexington, 1985).

12. President's Commission on Law Enforcement and the Administration of Justice, *The Challenge of Crime in a Free Society* (Washington, DC: U.S. Government Printing Office, 1967), 229.

13. Robert Shellow, ed., *Drug Use and Crime: Report of the Panel on Drug Use and Criminal Behavior* (Washington, DC: National Technical Information Service, 1976), 5.

14. Inciardi, *The War on Drugs*.

15. James J. Collins, J. Valley Rachal, Robert L. Hubbard, Elizabeth R. Cavanaugh, S. Gail Craddock, and Patricia L. Kristiansen, *Criminality in a Drug Treatment Sample: Measurement Issues and Initial Findings* (Research Triangle Park, NC: Research Triangle Institute, 1982), 27.

16. Jan M. Chaiken and Marcia R. Chaiken, *Who Gets Caught Doing Crime?* (Los Angeles: Hamilton, Rabinovitz, Szanton, and Alschuler, Inc., 1985).

17. See James A. Inciardi and Carl D. Chambers, "Unreported Criminal Involvement of Narcotic Addicts," *Journal of Drug Issues 2* (1972):57-64; William H. McGlothlin, M. Douglas Anglin, and Bruce D. Wilson, "Narcotic Addiction and Crime," *Criminology 16* (1978):293-316; John C. Ball, Lawrence Rosen, John A. Flueck, and David N. Nurco, "Lifetime Criminality of Heroin Addicts in the United States," *Journal of Drug Issues 12* (1982):225-39.

18. Inciardi, *The War on Drugs*.

19. *Ibid.*, 127.

20. Jan M. Chaiken and Marcia R. Chaiken, *Varieties of Criminal Behavior: Summary and Policy Implications* (Santa Monica, CA: Rand, 1982), 18.

21. Chaiken and Chaiken, *Who Gets Caught Doing Crime?*

22. Ball, Rosen, Flueck, and Nurco, "Lifetime Criminality of Heroin Addicts."

23. *Ibid.*

24. Richard C. Stephens, "The Truthfulness of Addict Respondents in Research Projects," *International Journal of the Addictions* 7 (1972):549-58.

25. See John C. Ball, "The Reliability and Validity of Interview Data Obtained from Narcotic Drug Addicts," *American Journal of Sociology* 72 (1972):549-58; Stephens, "The Truthfulness"; Arthur J. Bonito, David N. Nurco, and John W. Shaffer, "The Veridicality of Addicts' Self-Reports in Social Research," *International Journal of the Addictions* 11 (1976):719-24.

26. John C. Ball, John W. Shaffer, and David N. Nurco, "The Day-to-Day Criminality of Heroin Addicts in Baltimore—A Study in the Continuity of Offense Rates," *Drug and Alcohol Dependence* 12 (1983):119-42.

27. See Ball, Rosen, Flueck, and Nurco, "Lifetime Criminality of Heroin Addicts"; Hall, Shaffer, and Nurco, "The Day-to-Day Criminality"; John W. Shaffer, David N. Nurco, and Timothy W. Kinlock, "A New Classification of Narcotic Addicts," *Comprehensive Psychiatry* 25 (1984):315-28; David N. Nurco, John W. Shaffer, John C. Ball, Timothy W. Kinlock, and John Langrod, "A Comparison by Ethnic Group and City of the Criminal Activities of Narcotic Addicts," *Journal of Nervous and Mental Disease* 174 (1986):112-16.

28. Ball, Shaffer, and Nurco, "The Day-to-Day Criminality," 123.

29. *Ibid.*

30. See David N. Nurco, Ira H. Cisin, and Mitchell B. Balter, "Addict Careers II: The First Ten Years," *International Journal of the Addictions* 8 (1981):1305-25; "Addict Careers II: The First Ten Years," *International Journal of the Addictions* 8 (1981):1327-56; "Addict Careers III: Trends Across Time," *International Journal of the Addictions* 8 (1981):1357-72; David N. Nurco and John W. Shaffer, "Types and Characteristics of Addicts in the Community," *Drug and Alcohol Dependence* 9 (1982):43-78; Shaffer, Nurco, and Kinlock, "A New Classification"; David N. Nurco, Thomas E. Hanlon, Mitchell B. Balter, Timothy W. Kinlock, and Evelyn Slaght, "A Classification of Narcotic Addicts Based on Type, Amount, and Severity of Crime," *Journal of Drug Issues* (in press).

31. Nurco and Shaffer, "Types and Characteristics."

32. See Gandossy, Williams, Cohen, and Harwood, *Drugs and Crime*; Anne E. Pottieger, "Sample Bias in Drugs/Crime Research: An Empirical Study," in *The Drugs-Crime Connection*, ed. James A. Inciardi (Beverly Hills, CA: Sage, 1981), 207-38; George Speckart and M. Douglas Anglin, "Narcotics and Crime: An Analysis of Existing Evidence for a Causal Relationship," *Behavioral Sciences and the Law* 3 (1985):259-82.

33. David N. Nurco and Robert L. DuPont. "A Preliminary Report on Crime and Addiction Within a Community-Wide Population of Narcotic Addicts," *Drug and Alcohol Dependence* 2 (1977):109-21.

34. Edward A. Preble and John J. Casey, Jr., "Taking Care of Business: The Heroin User's Life on the Street," *International Journal of the Addictions* 4 (1969):1-24.

35. See Paul J. Goldstein, "Getting Over: Economic Alternatives to Predating Crime Among Street Drug Users," in *The Drugs-Crime Connection*, ed. James A. Inciardi (Beverly Hills, CA: Sage, 1981), 67-84; Johnson et al., *Taking Care of Business*.

36. Goldstein, "Getting Over," 82-83.

37. Gandossy, Williams, Cohen, and Harwood, *Drugs and Crime*, 67.

38. See William H. McGlothlin, "Drugs and Crime," in *Handbook on Drug Abuse*, ed. Robert L. DuPont, Avram Goldstein, and John O'Donnell (Washington, DC: National Institute on Drug Abuse and Office of Drug Policy, 1979), 357-64; Gandossy, Williams, Cohen, and Harwood, *Drugs and Crime*, 110.

39. McGlothlin, "Drugs and Crime."

40. Blumstein and Cohen, "Characterizing Criminal Careers," 985.

41. See David N. Nurco, "A Discussion of Validity," in *Self-Reporting Methods in Estimating Drug Abuse*, ed. Beatrice A. Rouse, Nicholas J. Kozel, and Louise G. Richards (Rockville, MD: National Institute on Drug Abuse, 1985), 4-11.

42. See McGlothlin, Anglin, and Wilson, "Narcotic Addiction and Crime"; M. Douglas Anglin and George Speckart, "Narcotics Use, Property Crime, and Dealing: Structural Dynamics Across the Addiction Career," *Journal of Quantitative Criminology* 2 (1986):355-75.

43. See Chaiken and Chaiken, *Varieties of Criminal Behavior*; Shaffer, Nurco, and Kinlock, "A New Classification."

44. Johnson et al., *Taking Care of Business*.

45. James J. Collins, Robert L. Hubbard, and J. Valley Rachal, *Heroin and Cocaine Use and Illegal Income* (Research Triangle Park, NC: Research Triangle Institute, 1984).

46. Chaiken and Chaiken, *Varieties of Criminal Behavior*.

47. *Ibid.*

48. *Ibid.*

49. Johnson et al., *Taking Care of Business*, 77.

50. Nurco, Shaffer, Ball, Kinlock, and Langrod, "A Comparison by Ethnic Group and City."

51. *Ibid.*

52. Chaiken and Chaiken, *Varieties of Criminal Behavior*.

53. Paul J. Goldstein, "Drugs and Violent Behavior" (Paper presented at the annual meeting of the Academy of Criminal Justice Sciences, Louisville, KY, 28 April 1982).

54. Kenneth Tardiff, Elliot M. Gross, and Steven F. Messner, "A Study of Homicide in Manhattan, 1981," *American Journal of Public Health* 76 (1986):139-43.

55. *Ibid.*, 143.

56. Gandossy, Williams, Cohen, and Harwood, *Drugs and Crime*.

57. Inciardi, *The War on Drugs*, 128-30.

58. *Ibid.*

59. See John W. Shaffer, David N. Nurco, John C. Ball, and Timothy W. Kinlock, "The Frequency of Nonnarcotic Drug Use and Its Relationship to Criminal Activity Among Narcotic Addicts," *Comprehensive Psychiatry* 26 (1985):558-66; David N. Nurco, Timothy W. Kinlock, Thomas E. Hanlon, and John C. Ball, "Nonnarcotic Drug Use Over an Addiction Career—A Study of Heroin Addicts in Baltimore and New York City," *Comprehensive Psychiatry* 29 (1988):450-59.

60. *Ibid.*

61. Nurco, Ball, Shaffer, and Hanlon, "The Criminality of Narcotic Addicts."

62. See William H. McGlothlin. M. Douglas Anglin, and Bruce D. Wilson, *An Evaluation of the California Civil Addict Program* (Washington, DC: U.S. Government Printing Office, 1977); M. Douglas Anglin and William H. McGlothlin, "Outcome of Narcotic Addict Treatment in California," in *Drug Abuse Treatment Evaluation: Strategies, Progress, and Prospects*, ed. Frank Tims and Jacqueline P. Ludford (Washington, DC: U.S. Government Printing Office, 1984), 106-28.

63. See James J. Collins and Margaret Allison, "Legal Coercion and Retention in Drug Abuse Treatment," *Hospital and Community Psychiatry 34* (1983):1145-49; Robert L. Hubbard, J. Valley Rachal, S. Gail Craddock, and Elizabeth R. Cavanaugh, "Treatment Outcome Prospective Study (TOPS): Client Characteristics and Behaviors Before, During, and After Treatment," in *Drug Abuse Treatment Evaluation: Strategies, Progress, and Prospects*, ed. Frank Tims and Jacqueline P. Ludford (Washington, DC: U.S. Government Printing Office, 1984), 42-68.

64. M. Douglas Anglin, Mary-Lynn Brecht, and Ebrahim Maddahian, "Pretreatment Characteristics and Treatment Performance of Legally Coerced Versus Voluntary Methadone-Maintenance Admissions," *Criminology 27* (1989):537-57.

65. D. Dwayne Simpson and Saul B. Sells, *Highlights of the DARP Follow-Up Research on the Evaluation of Drug Abuse Treatment Effectiveness* (Ft. Worth: Institute of Behavioral Research, Texas Christian University, 1981).

66. Shaffer, Nurco, Ball, and Kinlock, "The Frequency of Nonnarcotic Drug Use and Its Relationship to Criminal Activity Among Narcotics Addicts."

67. Simpson and Sells, *Highlights of the DARP*.

68. See Chaiken and Chaiken, *Varieties of Criminal Behavior*; Peter W. Greenwood, Selective Incapacitation (Santa Monica, CA: Rand, 1982); Nurco, Ball, Shaffer, and Hanlon, "The Criminality of Narcotic Addicts."

69. *Ibid.*

70. See David N. Nurco, Thomas E. Hanlon, Timothy W. Kinlock, and Karen R. Duszynski, "Differential Patterns of Criminal Activity Over an Addiction Career," *Criminology* (in press).

71. Bruce D. Johnson, Paul Goldstein, Edward Preble, James Schneidler, Douglas S. Lipton, Barry Spunt, Nina Duchaine, Reuben Norman, Thomas Miller, Nancy Meggett, Andrea Kale, and Deborah Hand, *Economic Behavior of Street Opiate Users: Final Report* (New York: Narcotic and Drug Research, Inc., 1983), 232.

72. Eric Wish, "Drug-Use Forecasting: New York 1984 to 1986," *National Institute of Justice Research in Action*, February 1987.

73. James R. Stewart (director, National Institute of Justice), *NIJ Reports*, no. 213 (Washington: U.S. Department of Justice, March-April 1989), 1-3.

74. See Chaiken and Chaiken, *Varieties of Criminal Behavior*; Eric D. Wish, Mary A. Toborg, and John P. Bellasai, *Identifying Drug Users and Monitoring Them During Conditional Release* (Washington, DC: U.S. Department of Justice, 1987); Marcia R. Chaiken and Bruce D. Johnson, *Characteristics of Different Types of Drug-Involved Offenders* (Washington: U.S. Department of Justice, 1988).

75. Mark Moore and Dean Gerston, eds., *Alcohol and Public Policy: Beyond the Shadow of Prohibition* (Washington, DC: National Academy Press, 1981). ✦

27. Heroin Use and Street Crime

James A. Inciardi

Drugs-crime research often relies on official criminal statistics (e.g., arrest or criminal history data). Yet these data are generally biased in that many crimes do not result in arrest. Further, many studies draw from treatment samples or samples of individuals who are incarcerated in jail or prison. The degree to which we can generalize from these findings to the larger population of drug users is unknown. In this study, James A. Inciardi conducted personal interviews with male and female heroin users in Miami, Florida. His research subjects were identified through social networks of users. Inciardi describes patterns of drug-use onset, and the nature and extent of criminal activity among targeted heroin users. His findings document how criminally involved some heroin users are, and how effective they are in avoiding arrest. In fact, the heroin users in this study were arrested for less than 1 percent of the crimes they committed.

The relationship between heroin use and street crime represents an issue that has long been studied, argued, and reexamined—yet few definitive conclusions are apparent today. For more than six decades, researchers and opinion makers have addressed the subject, asking such questions as, do heroin use and addiction cause crime? If so, what ought to be done to manage the problem? Much of the research on this has attempted to determine the sequence of heroin use and criminal activity. Does addiction per se lead the user into a life of crime, or do the demands of the addict's lifestyle force him into criminal behavior? Or, alternatively, is heroin use simply an additional pattern of deviant activity manifested by an already criminal population? The catalog of research has been impressive, at least in terms of sheer quantity.[1]

The findings that have emerged, however, have led to a series of peculiar and contradictory perspectives. Some researchers have found that the criminal histories of their sample cases considerably preceded any evidence of drug use; thus, their conclusion has been that the heroin user is indeed a criminal, and should be treated as such. Others have found in their data that the sequence is in the reverse direction, and have offered us an "enslavement theory" of addiction. Within this perspective, it is suggested that the monopolistic controls over the heroin black market have forced the otherwise law-abiding user into a life of crime in order to support his habit. The answer to the "problem" is simple: legalize heroin, and the need for crime is removed. And still a third group finds conflicting data: some members of the samples were drug users first, other members were criminals first, and still others embraced both drug use and crime simultaneously. The conclusion here is that heroin use and crime may not be related at all, but instead result from some third, unknown variable, or some complex set of factors that pervade the user's operating social milieu and greater environment.

Yet, any conclusions, hypotheses, and theories from these efforts become meaningless when one considers the awesome biases and deficiencies in the information that has been generated. Data-gathering enterprises on criminal activity have usually restricted themselves to the heroin users' arrest histories, and there can be little argument as to the inadequacy of official statistics as measures of the incidence and prevalence of criminal behavior. Those studies that have gone beyond arrest figures to probe self-reported criminal activity invariably have been limited to small samples of either incarcerated heroin users or users placed in treatment programs. And the few efforts that have been made to locate active heroin users have generally examined their samples' drug-taking behaviors to the exclusion of their drug-seeking behaviors.

Method

In an effort to generate a preliminary and more realistic data-base descriptive of the criminal activities of active heroin users, the present study focused, during a twelve-month period ending in 1978, on the street community as an information source, using active cases in Miami, Florida.[2]

The peculiar lifestyle, illegal drug-taking and drug-seeking activities, and mobility characteristics of active drug users preclude any examination of this group through standard survey methodology. A sample based on a restricted quota draw was rejected in favor of one derived through the use of a sociometrically oriented model.

Table 1
Selected Characteristics of
356 Active Heroin Users

Characteristics	Males (n=239)	Females (n-117)
Age		
17 and under	.8%	3.4%
18-24	19.2%	34.2%
25-34	64.0%	51.3%
35 -49	14.2%	9.4%
50 and over	.8%	1.7%
Median	27.9 years	26.9 years
Ethnic background		
White	52.3%	55.6%
Black	33.5%	24.8%
Hispanic	14.2%	16.2%
Other	–	3.4%
Years of school (median)	11.8 years	11.7 years
Employment status		
Currently employed	49.3%	41.9%
Unemployed	48.5%	53.8%
Not in labor force	2.2%	4.3%
Marital status		
Never married	45.6%	46.2%
Married	25.9%	13.7%
Divorced/separated	26.4%	36.8%
Widowed	1.7%	2.6%
No data	.4%	.9%

Drug Use Patterns

The heroin users sampled in this study had long histories of multiple-drug involvement, following clear sequential patterns of onset and progression. Both males and females began the use of drugs with alcohol. Their first experiences with alcohol intoxication occurred at median ages of 13.3 and 13.9 years, respectively, with 39.3 percent of the males and 21.4 percent of the females having such an experience before age 12. Furthermore, as indicated in Table 2, progression into the other major drugs followed identical sequential patterns for both sexes. For example, based on median ages of onset, alcohol use was followed by initial drug abuse experimentation at 15.2 years of age, followed by marijuana use, barbiturate use, heroin use, and cocaine use:

Median Onset Age

Substance	Males	Females
Alcohol use	12.8	13.8
Alcohol intoxication	13.3	13.9
First drug abuse	15.2	15.2
Marijuana use	15.5	15.4
Barbiturate use	17.5	17.0
Heroin use	18.7	18.2
Cocaine use	19.7	18.7

In the field site, the author had established extensive contacts within the subcultural drug scene. These represented "starting points" for interviewing. During or after each interview, at a time when the rapport between interviewer and respondent was deemed to be at its highest level, each respondent was requested to identify other current users with whom he or she was acquainted. These persons, in turn, were located and interviewed, and the process was repeated, until the social network surrounding each respondent was exhausted. This method, as described, restricted the pool of users interviewed to those who were currently active in the given subcultural knit in the street community and who were "at risk." In addition, it eliminated former users, as well as those who were only peripheral to the mainstream of the subcultural half-world.

This selection plan does not guarantee a totally unbiased sample. However, the use of several starting points within the same locale eliminated the difficulty of drawing all respondents from one social network. Confidentiality was guaranteed to the respondents, interviewing was done in an anonymous fashion, and each respondent was paid a fee for participating.

This sampling technique resulted in an initial study population of 356 heroin users (see Table 1) who were active in the free community at the time of the interview. Not unlike other populations of drug users, most of the sample cases were males (67 percent), and the majority of both the males and females were unemployed whites, clustered in the eighteen- to thirty-four-year-old age group (see Table 1). Males and females did, however, evidence many pronounced differences in their criminal career patterns.

Table 2
Drug Use Histories

Drug Use Characteristics	Males (n=238)	Females (n=117)
Age of first alcohol use (median)	12.8	13.8
Age of first alcohol high (median)	13.3	13.9
Ever used alcohol	95.8%	98.3%
Age of first drug (excluding alcohol) use (median)	15.2	15.2
Age of first marijuana use (median)	15.5	15.4
Ever used marijuana	99.2%	99.1%
Age of first barbiturate use (median)	17.5	17.0
Ever used barbiturates	84.9%	88.0%
Age of first heroin use (median)	18.7	18.2
Age of first cocaine use (median)	19.7	18.7
Ever used cocaine	92.9%	92.3%
Median number of drugs ever used*	10.3	10.5
Median number of drugs "currently" being used**	5.0	5.6
Ever treated for drug use	56.9%	56.4%
Currently in treatment	.4%	.9%

* Includes alcohol, heroin, other narcotics, sedatives, stimulants, antidepressants, hallucinogens, analgesics, and solvents/inhalants.

** Current use refers to any intake during the ninety days before the interview.

Curiously, while the females began their careers of substance use one year later than the males, their progression was more rapid and the extent of their drug involvement seemed to be greater. A median of 5.9 years separated the males' initial alcohol experimentation from their first use of heroin at age 18.7. With the females, the onset of heroin use was at age 18.2, only 4.4 years after the first use of alcohol. Furthermore, as is shown in Table 2, the females were using a slightly wider variety of drugs than were the males.

Criminal Histories

Early involvement in criminal activity was characteristic of the great majority of the sampled heroin users. As shown in Table 3, 99.6 percent of the males and 98.3 percent of the females reported having ever committed a crime, with the median age of the first criminal act preceding the sixteenth year. The first crimes committed were generally crimes against property, although the specific kind of property crime varied between males and females.

As shown in Table 3, burglary was cited most often by males as the first crime (25.1 percent), followed by shoplifting (20.1 percent), other larcenies (11.7 percent), and drug sales (10.0 percent). In contrast, 38.5 percent of the females reported shoplifting as their first offense, followed by prostitution (18.8 percent) and drug sales (12.8 percent). It might also be noted here that the proportion reporting vehicle theft as the first crime was ten times higher among males than among females; the percentage of violent crime (robbery and assault) was also higher among the male group. For example, while 15.4 percent of the males specified robbery or assault as the first criminal offense, only 6.0 percent of the females indicated one or the other as the first offense.

Most of the heroin users studied here had arrest histories, but these typically began more than two years after the initiation of criminal activity (Table 3). Some 93.7 percent of the males reported having been arrested at least once, with the first arrest occurring at a median age of 17.2 years. Slightly fewer females (83.8 percent) had arrest histories, with the initiation into criminal justice processing beginning at a median age of 18.3 years. The data also indicate that the males had more frequent contacts with the criminal justice system (Table 3). The median number of arrests for the males was 3.5, with 81.2 percent having histories of incarceration. In contrast, the females reported a median of 2.6 arrests, with 62.4 percent having been incarcerated. Such differences might be explained by the younger age at which the males initiated their criminal activity and arrest histories, or by the slightly younger age of the female group. However, the expanded arrest figures below, reflecting the nature of the various arrests, may suggest the somewhat more serious, and hence more visible, nature of the males' criminal involvement. For example:

	Median Number of Arrests	
Nature of Arrest	*Males*	*Females*
Crimes against property	1.6	.5
Crimes against persons	.3	.2
Drug law violations	1.4	.8
Public order crimes	.2	1.1

Table 3
Criminal Histories

Criminal Characteristics	*Males* (n=239)	*Females* (n=117)
Ever committed offense	99.6%	98.3%
Age of first crime (median)	15.1	15.9
First crime committed		
Robbery	7.9%	3.4%
Assault	7.5%	2.6%
Burglary	25.1%	5.1%
Vehicle theft	9.2%	.9%
Shoplifting	20.1%	38.5%
Other theft/larceny	11.7%	6.9%
Prostitution	–	18.8%
Drug sales	10.0%	12.8%
Other/no data	8.1%	9.3%
Have arrest history	93.7%	83.8%
Age at first arrest (median)	17.2	18.3
Total arrests (median)	3.5	2.6
Ever incarcerated	81.2%	62.4%

While the male arrest data reflect a greater involvement in crimes against the person, property, or drug laws, the females were more often arrested for the less serious crimes against the public order, primarily prostitution. This would account for the higher rate of incarceration among the male group.

As indicated below, the heroin users reported a wide variety of sources of support for both their general economic needs and their drug use. For example:

Sources of Income	*Males*	*Females*
Family, friends	12.5%	31.6%
Legal employment	4 9.4	43.6
Public assistance	20.0	18.8
Criminal activity	97.4	94.9

While more than 90 percent of both groups relied upon criminal activity as a means of income, most had a second source of funds. However, some 98.7 percent of the males and 96.6 percent of the females reported some form of illegal activity during the twelve months before the interview, and more than 80 percent of this criminality was for drug-use support (80.5 percent for males, 87.7 percent for females).

Current Criminal Activity

The data on current criminal activity clearly demonstrate not only that most of the heroin users were committing crimes, but also that they were doing so extensively and for the purpose of drug-use support. Initially, some 98.7 percent of the males reported committing crimes during the twelve-month period prior to interviewer contact, with a median of 80.5 percent of such criminality undertaken for the purpose of supporting a drug habit.

As indicated in Table 4, the 239 male heroin users reported committing 80,644 criminal acts, averaging some 337 offenses per user. While this might be viewed as an astronomical sum, one must consider the relative proportions for each crime category. The violent crimes of robbery and assault, although reaching the considerable figure of almost 3,500, nevertheless represent only 4.3 percent of the total. Similarly, property crimes, while including some 17,846 thefts of various types, account for less than 25 percent of the total figure. On the other hand, a clear majority of the crimes by male heroin users were crimes without victims: almost 60 percent of the criminal behavior reported here was drug sales, prostitution, gambling, and alcohol offenses, with an additional 8.1 percent of criminal activity involving the buying, selling, or receiving of stolen goods—a secondary level of criminality, re sulting, in most instances, from the users' initial involvement in property crimes.

These comments are not intended to minimize the amount of serious crime among heroin users. Rather, they emphasize that such criminality is more often victimless crime than predatory crime. On the other hand, these data also indicate that male heroin users have diverse criminal careers. Almost all (91.6 percent) were involved in the sale of drugs; almost half (46.9 percent) also engaged in robberies; 59.4 percent also engaged in shoplifting; and more than two-thirds (69.0 percent) were also burglars. It might also be added here that 42.7 percent of these subjects used weapons during the commission of all or some of their crimes, the usual weapon being a handgun.

Strikingly, the incidence of arrest among these 239 male heroin users was extremely low. Of the 80,644 reported crimes, only .2 percent (n=189) resulted in arrest. More specifically, consider the following ratios of crimes committed to ensuing arrests:

Crimes against persons	293:1
Crimes against property	273:1
Drug sales	440:1
Forgery/counterfeiting	285:1

Table 4
Criminal Activity During Past Twelve Months, 239 Active Male Heroin Users

Crime	Total Offenses	Percentage of Total Offenses	Percentage of of Sample Involved	Percentage Offenses Resulting in Arrest
Robbery	3,328	4.1	46.9	.3 (n=11)
Assault	170	<.2	20.9	.6 (n=1)
Burglary	4,093	5.1	69.0	.7 (n=30)
Vehicle theft	398	.5	22.6	.5 (n=2)
Theft from vehicle	877	1.1	29.3	.7 (n=6)
Shoplifting	9,685	12.0	59.4	.2 (n=15)
Pickpocketing	11	<.1	.8	—
Prostitute theft	62	<.1	1.3	1.6 (n=1)
Other theft	1,009	1.3	35.1	.5 (n=5)
Forgery/counterfeiting	1,711	2.1	40.2	.4 (n=6)
Con games	1,267	1.6	30.1	—
Stolen goods	6,527	8.1	59.4	<.1 (n=3)
Prostitution	2	.1	.4	—
Procuring	2,819	3.5	30.5	<.1 (n=1)
Drug sales	40,897	51.0	91.6	<.2 (n=93)
Arson	65	<.1	2.9	—
Vandalism	58	<.1	8.8	1.7 (n=1)
Fraud	185	.2	12.1	1.1 (n=2)
Gambling	6,306	7.8	38.5	<.1 (n=3)
Extortion	648	.8	10.0	—
Loan sharking	463	.5	13.0	—
Alcohol offenses	58	<.1	6.3	10.3 (n=6)
All other	5	<.1	2.1	60.0 (n=3)
TOTAL	80,644	100.0	100.0	.2 (n=189)
Mean number of offenses per subject	337			

Table 5
Criminal Activity During Past Twelve Months, 117 Active Female Heroin Users

Crime	Total Offenses	Percentage of Total Offenses	Percentage of Sample Involved	Percentage of Offenses Resulting in Arrest
Robbery	573	1.5	17.1	.5 (n=3)
Assault	26	<.1	7.7	11.5 (n=3)
Burglary	185	.5	20.5	1.1 (n=2)
Vehicle theft	5	<.1	1.7	—
Theft from vehicle	182	.5	18.8	.5 (n=1)
Shoplifting	5,171	13.8	70.1	.3 (n=13)
Pickpocketing	162	.4	4.3	—
Prostitute theft	1,345	3.6	51.3	—
Other theft	182	.5	20.5	.5 (n=1)
Forgery/counterfeiting	888	2.4	29.9	.3 (n=3)
Con games	251	.7	17.1	—
Stolen goods	1,006	2.7	36.8	<.1 (n=4)
Prostitution	14,307	38.2	72.6	.3 (n=37)
Procuring	1,153	3.1	23.1	—
Drug sales	11,289	30.1	81.2	.2 (n=23)
Arson	88	.2	3.4	—
Vandalism	3	<.1	1.7	—
Fraud	34	<.1	6.0	—
Gambling	574	1.5	22.2	—
Extortion	41	.1	4.3	—
Loan sharking	1	<.1	.9	—
Alcohol offenses	22	<.1	6.8	22.7 (n=5)
All other	2	<.1	1.7	100.0 (n=2)
TOTAL	37,490	100.0	100.0	.3 (n=97)
Mean number of offenses per subject	320			

The level of criminal involvement among the female heroin users was also high, but with a different pattern (see Table 5). Some 96.6 percent of the females reported the commission of crimes during the twelve months preceding the interview, with a median of 87.7 percent of the criminal activity engaged in to support a drug habit. The 117 female heroin users admitted responsibility for 37,490 crimes, with prostitution and drug sales accounting for more than two-thirds (68.3 percent) of the total. Like the males, the female group manifested considerable diversity in their offense behavior, with 81.2 percent admitting drug sales, 72.6 percent engaging in prostitution, 70.1 percent reporting shoplifting, and 51.3 percent indicating prostitute theft. Fewer females participated in crimes of violence, and, while many engaged in burglaries and other types of theft, such larceny was notably less frequent than among males. Females, however, tended to be arrested more frequently than males during this twelve-month study period, with a ratio of 1 arrest for every 387 crimes committed. The highest rates of arrest involved assaults and alcohol; most arrests were for prostitution and drug sales; no arrests resulted from 1,345 cases of prostitution theft; and the ratio of shoplifting crimes to arrests was 398:1 for the more than 5,000 cases.

In sum, considering all crime categories, one arrest occurred for every 427 crimes committed, with the highest proportion of arrests following alcohol offenses, fraud, vandalism, and prostitutes' theft from clients; the lowest levels of arrest were in cases of extortion, loan sharking, prostitution and procuring, pickpocketing, con games, arson, and dealing in stolen goods. Finally, fewer females used weapons during all or part of their offenses (18.8 percent), with the most common weapon being a knife rather than a gun.

Discussion

These data suggest a number of considerations and implications relevant to the relationship between heroin use and crime, while at the same time indicating several areas for further research.

First, the data document a high incidence and diversity of criminal involvement among both male and female heroin users. The 356 persons studied here reported involvement in a total of 118,134 criminal offenses during a twelve-month period, most of these offenses committed for the purpose of supporting the economic needs of a drug-using career. Furthermore, while most of the criminal offenses were what are often referred to as victimless crimes, the 356 respondents were nevertheless responsible for some 27,464 instances of what the Federal Bureau of Investigation designates as index, or serious, crimes.[3] Numerous differences are apparent between males and females in this regard, with the males manifesting a greater involvement in predatory crime, especially violent predatory crime; however, the data also demonstrate that heroin users of both sexes manifest considerable participation in many different levels of criminal activity.

Second, it is evident in these data that arrest rates among heroin users are low. The 118,134 criminal events reported here resulted in a total of only 286 arrests, or a ratio of 1 arrest for every 413 crimes committed; with respect to the more serious index crimes, there was a ratio of 1 arrest for every 292 crimes. This low level of arrest is also apparent in the overall arrest histories of the subjects studied. Among the males, whose careers in crime spanned a median of 12.8 years, the median number of arrests was 3.5. Similarly, the median career in crime among the female heroin users was 11.0 years, and the median number of arrests was only 2.6.

Third, the data described here provide some information pertinent to the question about drug use and crime; namely, is crime a pre- or post-drug-use phenomenon? What the data suggest is that the question phrased in these terms is an oversimplification of a very complex phenomenon. By examining the median ages of initiation into various stages of substance abuse and criminal careers, the complexity becomes evident. For example:

	Males	Females
First alcohol use	12.8	13.8
First alcohol intoxication	13.3	13.9
First criminal activity	15.1	15.9
First drug abuse	15.2	15.2
First marijuana use	15.5	15.4
First arrest	17.2	18.2
First barbiturate use	17.5	17.0
First heroin use	18.7	18.2
First continuous heroin use	19.2	18.4

Among the males, there seems to be a clear progression from alcohol to crime, to drug abuse, to arrest, and then to heroin use. But upon closer inspection, the pattern is not altogether clear. At one level, for example, criminal activity can be viewed as predating one's drug-using career, since the median point of the first crime is slightly below that of first drug abuse, and is considerably before the onset of heroin use. But, at the same time, if alcohol intoxication at a median age of 13.3 years were to be considered substance abuse, then crime is clearly a phenomenon that succeeds substance abuse. Among the females, the description is even more complex. In the population of female heroin users, criminal activity occurred after both alcohol and drug abuse and after marijuana use, but before involvement with the more debilitating barbiturates and heroin.

In summary, these preliminary data suggest that an alternative perspective for research on the link between drugs and crime may be in order. Although the findings here are descriptive of only one popula-

between drugs and crime may be in order. Although the findings here are descriptive of only one population, which could be unique, they suggest that the pursuit of some simple cause-and-effect relationship may be futile. It is clear that heroin users are involved extensively in crime, and that their involvement is largely for the purpose of supporting the desired level of drug intake. It is also clear that users' initiation into substance abuse and criminal activity occurs at a relatively early age. But there are several things that are not clear. Do substance abusers, for example, alter the nature, extent, and diversity of their criminal behaviors at the onset of marijuana use, at the onset of heroin use, or after their initial criminal justice processing? Do adolescent predatory criminals alter the nature and extent of their criminal involvement at various stages of drug abuse? Does drug abuse involve a shifting from primarily predatory crime to victimless crime? Does drug-taking result in an increase or decrease in criminal activity? And finally, does a drug-taking career fix the criminal careers of adolescents who might otherwise shift into more law-abiding pursuits as they approach young adulthood? These questions can be answered only by turning away from existing notions about the drugs/crime nexus, generating a more comprehensive data base, pinpointing the locations where drug use and crime are highest, and circumscribing total criminal involvement at all stages of drug-using and non-drug-using adolescent careers.

* * *

James A. Inciardi, "Heroin Use and Street Crime," *Crime and Delinquency* (July 1979), pp. 335-346. Copyright © 1979 by James A. Inciardi.

For Discussion

1. How might the results of this study differ from results of a similar study in which heroin users were drawn from treatment programs?

2. Much of the research on drugs and crime shows disproportionate numbers of low income African-Americans are involved in drugs and crime. Is it possible that white middle and upper income users are just as prevalent among drug users but that individuals in these groups are less likely to come to the attention of criminal justice authorities?

Notes

1. For annotated bibliographies and analyses of these studies, see Research Triangle Institute, *Drug Use and Crime* (Springfield, VA: National Technical Information Service, 1976); Gregory A. Austin and Daniel J. Lettieri, *Drugs and Crime: The Relationship of Drug Use and Concomitant Criminal Behavior* (Rockville, MD: National Institute on Drug Abuse, 1976); S. W. Greenberg and Freda Adler, "Crime and Addiction: An Empirical Analysis of the Literature, 1920-1973," *Contemporary Drug Problems*, vol. 3 (1974), pp. 221-270; and James A. Inciardi, "The Villification of Euphoria: Some Perspectives on an Illusive Issue," *Addictive Diseases*, vol. 1 (1974), pp. 241-267.

2. These data were generated by DHEW grant #1-R01-DA-0-1827-02, from the Division of Research National Institute on Drug Abuse.

3. The FBI index crimes include homicide, forcible rape, aggravated assault, robbery, burglary, larceny-theft, and motor vehicle theft. ✦

28. Kids, Crack, and Crime

JAMES A. INCIARDI

AND

ANNE E. POTTIEGER

Media reports during the 1980s suggested that crack-cocaine was a root cause of crime and violence in urban areas, and that the drug was initially popular among inner-city youth. The following article by James A. Inciardi and Anne E. Pottieger focuses on a study of "serious delinquents" in Miami. Most of those interviewed reported extensive use of crack-cocaine. The authors report on the degree of involvement in crack distribution and relate this involvement to criminality. In general, the more involved the youths were in crack sales and distribution, the more crack and other drugs they used, and the more criminally involved they were.

Crack-cocaine is the newest substance included in discussions of the relationship between drug use and crime. Since it made its first appearance on the streets of urban America during the mid-1980s, media attention has focused on how the high addiction liability of the drug instigates users to commit crimes to support their habits, and how rivalries in crack-distribution networks have turned some inner-city communities into urban "dead zones," where homicide rates are so high that police have written them off as anarchic badlands.[1]

Of special emphasis in press reports on crack has been the involvement of inner-city youths in the crack business. As *Time* magazine explained in its 9 May 1988 cover story:

> With the unemployment rate for black teenagers at 37 percent, little work is available to unskilled, poorly educated youths. The handful of jobs that are open—flipping burgers, packing groceries— pay only minimum wages or "chump change," in the street vernacular. So these youngsters turn to the most lucrative option they can find. In rapidly growing numbers, they are becoming the new criminal recruits of the inner city, the children who deal crack. (p. 20)

Other stories have targeted the "peewees" and "wannabees" (want-to-be's), the street gang acolytes in grade school and junior-high who patrol the streets with walkie-talkies in the vicinity of crack houses, serving in networks of look-outs, spotters, and steerers, and aspiring to be "rollers" (short for high-rollers) in the drug-distribution business (*Newsweek*, 28 March 1988). Yet, with all the media attention on youths in the crack scene, only minimal empirical information has been collected on their use of the drug, their complicity in the drug business, and their specific criminal behaviors. This paper describes such data, collected during the second half of the 1980s as part of a broader study of drug use and serious delinquency in Miami, Florida.

Methods

In 1985, few people nationally had heard of crack, but it was already a problem in Miami (Inciardi 1987). Awareness of this permitted crack to be included in the drug-history section of a planned interview schedule for a street study of adolescent drug use and crime. The focus of the research was not crack per se, but was the drug-taking and drug-seeking behaviors of some 600 Miami youths who were "seriously delinquent," defined as having committed, in the prior twelve months, a minimum of ten FBI "index" offenses,[2] or 100 lesser crimes. Subjects were located through standard, multiple starting-point "snowball sampling" techniques (Inciardi 1986:119-122).

Preliminary analysis of the first interviews showed a surprisingly high prevalence and incidence of crack use. Of the first 308 youths interviewed, 95.5 percent reported having used crack at least once, and 87.3 percent reported current regular use—(i.e., in the ninety days prior to being interviewed, use three or more times a week). These unexpected figures motivated the design of a supplementary crack data instrument which was ultimately used during the last 254 interviews, from October 1986 through November 1987.

Findings

As indicated in Table 1, some 85 percent of the sample were males and 15 percent were females. In addition, 43.3 percent were whites, while 39.4 percent were blacks and 17.3 percent were Hispanics. While blacks (only 15 percent of the Miami-Dade population) are overrepresented in the sample, and Hispanics (44 percent of the population) areconsiderablyunderrepresented,thisrace/ethnic distribution in not unlike that found in other studies of the Miami drug scene (Inciardi 1986:123). These 254 youths had a median age of 14.7 years, with almost half in the 14-15-year-age cohort. Finally, although more than three-fourths were still attending school at the time of interview, almost all (89.4 percent) had been either expelled or suspended from school at least once, with such disciplinary actions often resulting from drug use or sales on school premises.

Table 1

Selected Characteristics of 254 Serious Delinquents Interviewed in Depth About Crack, Miami 1986-1987

		Number	Percent
Sex:	Males	216	85.0%
	Females	38	15.0%
Ethnicity:	Blacks	100	39.4%
	Whites	110	43.3%
	Hispanics	44	17.3%
Age:	12-13 years	62	24.4%
	14-15 years	107	42.1%
	16-17 years	85	33.5%
	Mean age	14.7 yrs.	-
School Status:			
Attending	grades 5-8	98	38.6%
	grades 9-10	79	31.1%
	grades 11-12	21	8.3%
Dropped out of school		56	22.0%
Mean Grades Completed		8.0 grades	-
Ever Expelled or Suspended from School:			
	For drug use	209	82.3%
	For drug sales	143	56.3%
	For other crime	91	35.8%
	For *any* reason	227	89.4%

Table 2

Drug Use Histories: Mean Age at Onset and Percent of Sample Involved

	Mean Age	Percent Involved
Alcohol		
First use	7.1	100.0%
First high	8.0	98.8%
First regular use	8.9	61.4%
Marijuana		
First use	9.9	100.0%
First regular use	11.0	100.0%
Cocaine		
First use	11.6	98.4%
First regular use	12.4	94.5%
Heroin		
First use	12.1	58.7%
First regular use	11.9	19.7%
Prescription Depressants		
First use	12.3	86.2%
First regular use	12.8	51.6%
Speed		
First use	12.4	50.0%
First regular use	12.7	4.7%
Crack		
First use	12.8	96.9%
First regular use	13.3	84.3%

Drug Use Histories

All of the juveniles interviewed had histories of multiple drug use with identifiable patterns of onset and progression. As illustrated by the mean ages reported in Table 2, they began their drug-using careers at age 7.1 years with alcohol experimentation and had been high by age 8. The majority (61.4 percent) proceeded to "regular use" (3+ times per week) of alcohol, at a mean age of 9 years. The onset of marijuana use began by age 10, followed by the regular use of the drug by age 11. Moreover, all of the youths reported having used marijuana "regularly." Cocaine use occurred next in the progression, with experimentation by

98.4 percent of the sample at age 11.6 years, followed by regular use less than a year later.

Experimentation with heroin, speed, and prescription depressants was clustered in the early part of these juveniles' twelfth year, with only half moving on to the regular use of depressants, 20 percent

reporting the regular use of heroin, and less than 5 percent using speed regularly. Some 96.9 percent reported experimentation with crack, however, at a mean age of 12.8 years, with the overwhelming majority of these moving on to the regular use of crack within but a few months.

Table 3
Current Drug Use by Crack-Business Involvement

| | Crack-Business Involvement | | | | Total |
| | *None* | *Minor* | *Dealer* | *Dealer+* | *Sample* |
	(N = 50)	(N = 20)	(N = 138)	(N = 46)	(N = 254)
Alcohol					
Daily	4.0%	5.0%	7.2%	8.7%	6.7%
Regular	14.0%	15.0%	39.9%	56.5%	35.8%
Occasional	78.8%	80.0%	48.6%	34.8%	54.3%
No use	4.0%	0.0%	4.3%	0.0%	3.1%
Marijuana					
Daily	66.0%	80.0%	91.3%	100.0%	87.0%
Regular	30.0%	20.0%	6.5%	0.0%	11.0%
Occasional	4.0%	0.0%	2.2%	0.0%	2.0%
Prescription-type Depressants					
Regular	2.0%	5.0%	32.6%	50.0%	27.6%
Occasional	56.0%	55.0%	52.9%	36.9%	50.8%
No use	42.0%	40.0%	14.5%	13.0%	21.7%
Cocaine Powder					
Daily	10.0%	15.0%	2.9%	0.0%	4.7%
Regular	44.0%	60.0%	21.0%	8.7%	26.4%
Occasional	36.0%	25.0%	76.1%	91.3%	66.9%
No use	10.0%	0.0%	0.0%	0.0%	2.0%
Crack					
Daily	2.0%	5.0%	70.3%	87.0%	54.7%
Regular	26.0%	50.0%	15.2%	6.5%	18.5%
Occasional	48.0%	45.0%	14.5%	6.5%	22.1%
No use	24.0%	0.0%	0.0%	0.0%	4.7%
All Forms of Cocaine*					
Daily	16.0%	30.0%	82.6%	95.7%	67.7%
Regular	58.0%	70.0%	17.4%	2.2%	26.8%
Occasional	16.0%	0.0%	0.0%	2.2%	3.5%
No use	10.0%	0.0%	0.0%	0.0%	2.0%

* Includes cocaine, crack, and/or basuco (coca paste).

Drug-Use and Crack-Business Involvement

Current drug-use rates were also high, but varied considerably, but varied considerably by degree of participation in the crack trade. Of the 254 youths under analysis here, all but 50 (19.7 percent) had some type of involvement in the crack business. Twenty subjects (7.9 percent) had only "minor" in-volvement, since they sold the drug only to their friends, worked for dealers as lookouts and spotters for dealers, or steered customers to one of Miami's approximately 700 crack houses. Most of the youths (138 or 54.3 percent) were crack "dealers," in-volved directly in the retail sale of crack. Finally, 46 subjects (18.1 percent) were designated as "dealer+," since they not only sold the drug, but also manufactured, smuggled, or wholesaled it.

Table 4
Drug Preferences and Bad Crack Highs for the 246 Youths Who Ever Tried Both Crack and Cocaine Powder

	Crack-Business Involvement				Total Ever Tried Crack And Cocaine
	None (N = 42)	Minor (N =20)	Dealer (N =138)	Dealer+ (N =46)	(N =246)
Two Most Preferred Drugs					
Cocaine (any form)	100.0%	100.0%	100.0%	100.0%	100.0%
Marijuana	95.2%	90.0%	94.2%	95.7%	94.3%
Alcohol	2.4%	5.0%	2.9%	4.3%	3.3%
Heroin	2.4%	5.0%	2.9%	0.0%	2.4%
Other	0.0%	0.0%	0.0%	0.0%	0.0%
Cocaine Preference					
Crack-cocaine	28.6%	55.0%	86.2%	93.5%	75.2%
Powdered cocaine	69.0%	30.0%	9.4%	4.3%	20.3%
No Preference	2.4%	15.0%	4.3%	2.2%	4.5%
Bad Highs on Crack					
Never	33.3%	40.0%	66.7%	71.7%	59.8%
Once or twice	45.2%	40.0%	29.7%	26.1%	32.5%
3+ times	21.4%	20.0%	3.6%	2.2%	7.7%

By examining drug use within the context of a youth's level of involvement with the crack busi-ness (none, minor, dealer, and dealer+), a num-ber of relationships quickly become evident. As indicated in Table 3, for example, the greater a youth's involvement in the crack business, the more likely was the daily or at least regular use of such drugs as marijuana, depressants, and crack. Whereas 66 percent of the youths with no busi-ness involvement were daily users of marijuana, this proportion increased to 80 percent for those with minor involvement, 91 percent for dealers, and 100 percent for those in the dealer+ group. The most pronounced differences were apparent with crack use, with the proportions using crack daily ranging from 2 percent of those with no crack-business involvement, to 87 percent of those in the dealer+ group.

When viewing all forms of cocaine collectively, the percentage of daily users increases from 16 percent of those with no involvement to 95.7 per-cent in the dealer+ group. These figures reflect total cocaine use, regardless of form, and hence include regular cocaine, crack, and *basuco*.

Basuco, also known as "susuko," "coca paste," "pasta basica de cocina," or just simply "pasta" (Jeri 1984), is an intermediate product in the trans-formation of coca leaves into cocaine. It is typically smoked straight, or in cigarettes mixed with tobacco or marijuana. The practice became popular in the coca-growing regions of South America, beginning in the early 1970s. Basuco was readily available, in-

Table 5

Getting Paid in Crack and Paying for Crack, Among Crack Users

	Crack-Business Involvement				Total Sample (N =242)
	None (N =38)	*Minor* (N =20)	*Dealer* (N =138)	*Dealer+* (N =46)	*Sample*
Paid in Crack for Dealing Last 12 Months					
Never	44.7%	10.0%	7.2%	2.2%	12.4%
Occasionally	39.5%	55.0%	8.0%	6.5%	16.5%
Often (6 + times)	15.8%	35.0%	84.8%	91.3%	71.1%
Money Spent on Crack for Personal Use, Last 90 Days					
$2400 or more	0.0%	0.0%	36.2%	52.2%	13.2%
$1000 or more	2.6%	0.0%	70.3%	93.5%	58.3%
Median amount	$75	$225	$2000	$2500	$1650

expensive, had a high cocaine content, and was absorbed rapidly when smoked. As the phenomenon was studied, it was quickly realized the smoking of basuco was likely far more dangerous than any other form of cocaine use. In addition to cocaine, basuco contains traces of all the chemicals used to initially process the coca leaves—kerosene, sulfuric acid, methanol, benzoic acid, and the oxidized products of these solvents, plus any number of other alkaloids that are present in the coca leaf (Almeida 1978). One analysis undertaken in Colombia in 1986 found, in addition to all of these chemicals, traces of various talcs, brick dust, ether, and leaded gasoline acid (Bogota *El Tiempo*, 19 June 1986:2D). In this sample, 10.6 percent (N=27) of the youths reported having some experience with the drug, and 3.1 percent (N=8) reported occasional use, during the 90-day period prior to interview.

The only data in Table 3 not following the same general trend of more frequent use, as involvement in the crack market increases, appears in the proportions of daily users of cocaine powder. None in the dealer+ group and only 2.9 percent of the dealers were daily users of this form of cocaine, and only 8.7 percent and 21 percent, respectively, were "regular" users. Consequently, there were considerably more daily and regular users of this drug among those having little or no involvement in the crack trade. One reason for this difference becomes clear in Table 4.

When the 246 youths who had some experience with both powder *and* crack cocaine were asked to indicate their two most preferred drugs, every one of them named cocaine, in one form or another; marijuana was almost as popular a choice. These preferences remained constant, regardless of level of involvement in the crack market. Differences clearly emerged, however, with preferences for crack versus cocaine powder—the greater one's involvement with the crack business, the greater the preference for crack over powder.

These differences can be explained in a number of ways. First, as shown in Table 4, some two-thirds of those with no crack-business involvement and three-fifths of those with minor involvement had bad experiences with crack. Almost the reverse was the case with those in the dealer and dealer+ groups. More importantly, however, market access determines a customer's ability to obtain a desired commodity, regardless of whether that commodity is diamonds, truffles, chocolate-covered grasshoppers, or crack-cocaine.

This access, furthermore, went beyond the obvious one of dealers having convenient opportunities to purchase crack for personal consumption. As Table 5 indicates, almost nine out of ten crack users actually received crack directly on at least an occasional basis, as part of their pay for drug sales. This was reported as a *frequent* occurrence by almost all (85 percent +) of the subjects in the two crack-

Table 6
Crime- and Arrest-Related Histories: Mean Age and Percent Involved

	Crack Business Involvement				Total
	None	Minor	Dealer	Dealer+	Sample
	(N = 50)	(N = 20)	(N = 138)	(N = 46)	(N = 254)
Drug Sale					
First marijuana	12.6	12.3	10.1	9.9	10.6
% ever	86.0%	100.0%	100.0%	100.0%	97.2%
First other	13.1	13.1	11.2	11.3	11.7
% ever	70.0%	100.0%	100.0%	100.0%	94.1%
Start regular	13.7	13.4	11.4	11.5	12.0
% ever	84.0%	100.0%	100.0%	100.0%	96.9%
Theft					
First time	12.0	12.6	10.8	10.7	11.2
% ever	94.0%	100.0%	100.0%	100.0%	98.8%
Start regular	13.4	13.5	11.7	11.7	12.0
% ever	74.0%	55.0%	89.9%	100.0%	85.8%
Crime (earliest)*					
First time	11.7	12.1	9.8	9.7	10.3
Start regular	13.2	13.2	11.2	11.2	11.7
% ever regular	100.0%	100.0%	100.0%	100.0%	100.0%
Arrest					
First	12.8	13.1	10.6	10.4	11.1
% ever	68.0%	100.0%	98.6%	93.5%	91.7%
Adjudication					
First arrest resulting in adjudication	14.1	14.6	10.9	10.9	11.3
% ever	20.0%	45.0%	84.8%	93.5%	70.5%
Incarceration					
First	14.2	15.0	12.6	12.8	12.8
% ever	12.0%	25.0%	61.6%	71.7%	50.8%
Treatment for Drug/Alcohol					
First entry	N/A	N/A	13.2	13.0	13.1
% ever	0.0%	0.0%	4.3%	8.7%	3.9%

* In each case (first, regular) age at time of first such occurrence, whether for drug sales, theft, prostitution, or robbery (the latter taken as "regular" at the tenth occurrence rather than at starting 3+ times/week).

dealer groups. Furthermore, the majority of crack users who had only minor or no crack business involvement were paid in crack at least sometimes, even though their dealing entailed some drug other than crack for all of the no-involvement group and unknown numbers of the minor-involvement group.

The last part of Table 5 shows, however, that being paid in crack for dealing was not sufficient to support the crack use patterns of most crack dealers. In fact, the greater the crack business involvement, the more money was spent buying crack for personal use. The money rarely came from legal sources, since only

Table 7
Involvement in Specific Crimes During the Twelve Months Prior to Interview

	Crack Business Involvement				Total
	None	Minor	Dealer	Dealer+	Sample
	(N = 50)	(N = 20)	(N = 138)	(N = 46)	(N = 254)
Major Felonies	44.0%	65.0%	87.7%	95.7%	78.7%
Robbery	12.0%	40.0%	66.7%	73.9%	55.1%
Assaults	4.0%	0.0%	8.0%	17.4%	8.3%
Burglary	24.0%	25.0%	70.3%	91.3%	61.4%
Motor Vehicle Theft	30.0%	35.0%	57.2%	73.9%	53.1%
Property Offenses	94.0%	95.0%	100.0%	100.0%	98.4%
Shoplifting	90.0%	95.0%	100.0%	100.0%	97.6%
Theft From Vehicle	34.0%	30.0%	75.4%	84.8%	65.4%
Pickpocketing	2.0%	5.0%	13.0%	10.9%	9.8%
Prostitute's Theft	8.0%	5.0%	20.3%	4.3%	13.8%
Other Larcenies	4.0%	0.0%	0.7%	0.0%	1.2%
Con Games	6.0%	5.0%	53.6%	63.0%	42.1%
Forgery (any)*	10.0%	5.0%	60.1%	73.9%	48.4%
Stolen Goods*	76.0%	85.0%	94.9%	97.8%	90.9%
Property Destruction*	16.0%	0.0%	35.5%	34.8%	28.7%
Other Crimes	0.0%	0.0%	0.7%	0.0%	0.4%
Vice Offenses	18.0%	5.0%	33.3%	17.4%	25.2%
Prostitution	18.0%	5.0%	22.5%	6.5%	17.3%
Procuring	4.0%	5.0%	30.4%	15.2%	20.5%
Drug Business (Any Drug)	86.0%	100.0%	100.0%	100.0%	97.2%

6.7 percent (N=17) of the 254 youths were employed at the time of interview. Rather, as the following section indicates, the primary source of this money was profit-making crime of all sorts.

Crack Business Involvement and Other Crime

Table 6 suggests a clear relationship between a youth's participation in the crack business and his or her overall crime and arrest history. It would appear, for example, that crack dealers, compared to youths with minor or no involvement in crack distribution, were markedly younger when they first committed a crime, and when first arrested, adjudicated, or incarcerated. Moreover, the greater the involvement in the crack business, the higher the likelihood of a youth's having been adjudicated, delinquent, or incarcerated at some time in his or her career.

In terms of the extent of criminal involvement during the twelve months prior to interview, once again, the greater the participation in crack distribution, the greater the level of other crime commission. Most notably, as indicated in Table 7, greater proportions of those closely tied to the crack business were involved in major felonies and property offenses than those more distant from the crack trade. The major exception to this pattern involved the vice offenses, due to the small percentage of females in the sample (15 percent), in combination with the fact that females accounted for the majority of these offenses. Overall, females were distributed in the crack business categories as follows: "None" (N=13), "Minor" (N=1), "Dealer" (N=22), and "Dealer+" (N=2). The distribution of vice involvement across the crack business categories thus reflects the number of females who happened to fall into each category.

In terms of absolute numbers, these 254 youths were responsible for a total of 223,439 criminal offenses during the twelve months prior to interview. Some 61.1 percent of these offenses were drug sales, 11.4 percent were vice offenses, 23.3 percent were property offenses, and 4.2 percent were major felonies, including robberies, assaults, burglaries,

and motor vehicle thefts. As indicated in Table 8, the relationship between crack-trade participation and level of other criminal involvement is quite clear. The mean number of crimes per subject during the twelve-month period ranges from 375.9, for those with no involvement in the crack business, to 1419.1 offenses, for those in the dealer+ category. Furthermore, although it did not hold for vice offenses, this pattern was apparent for major felonies, property crimes, and drug business offenses.

Table 8
Crimes and Arrests During the Twelve Months Prior to Interview

	Crack Business Involvement				Total
	None	Minor	Dealer	Dealer+	Sample
	(N = 50)	(N = 20)	(N = 138)	(N = 46)	(N = 254)
Number Done					
Major felonies	444	164	5,857	2,938	9,403
Property offenses	5,479	3,937	32,360	10,203	51,979
Drug business	9,785	6,630	70,365	49,766	136,546
Vice offenses	3,115	2,020	18,006	2,370	25,511
Total offenses	18,823	12,751	126,588	65,277	223,439
Mean Number per Subject					
Major felonies	8.9	8.2	42.4	63.9	37.0
Property offenses	109.6	196.9	234.5	221.8	204.6
Drug business	195.7	331.5	509.9	1081.9	537.6
Vice offenses	62.3	101.0	130.5	51.5	100.4
Total offenses	375.9	637.6	917.3	1419.1	879.6
% Arrested For					
Major felonies	6.0%	10.0%	17.4%	26.1%	16.1%
Property offenses	30.0%	25.0%	46.4%	32.6%	39.0%
Drug business	46.0%	90.0%	76.1%	58.7%	68.1%
Vice offenses	4.0%	5.0%	6.5%	2.2%	5.1%
Any Offense	64.0%	100.0%	94.9%	84.8%	87.4%

Table 8 also indicates that, although less than 1 percent of the 223,439 offenses resulted in arrest, some 87.4 percent of the sample were arrested during the twelve months prior to interview. The fact that the subjects were youths, that 358 (88.4 percent) of the 405 crimes resulting in arrest were either drug, vice, or petty property offenses, and that Miami-Dade has a seriously overburdened criminal justice system, explains why these youths

were still in the free community at the time of interview.

Discussion

Recent media reports appear to be correct in assessing youthful involvement in the crack business as a significant crime trend in some locales. If anything, media reports may underestimate its importance since the crack trade is related to not only heavier crack use but also more use of other drugs; young crack dealers commonly violate not merely drug laws but also those protecting persons and property; and the crack business appears criminogenic in ways that go beyond any potential it may have as a lure into crime.

This last point is particularly well illustrated by the sample described in this paper. For these youths, money to be made in the crack business was *not* the motive for initial criminal activities. Future research may show such cases, but as it happened, crack was not widely available until most of these subjects had been engaged in some sort of regular crime for at least a year or two. Due to this timing, most actually sold marijuana before ever using crack. This means that, crime initiation aside, the crack business is criminogenic in that it leads serious delinquents to become even more seriously involved in crime.

In particular, it should be noted that these data suggest that it is not drug sales in general but specifically the crack business which is so highly problematic. Tables 7 and 8 show that 86 percent of the no-crack-business group were selling *some* drug, averaging around 200 sales per year. But the involvement of this group in major felonies and petty property crime was distinctly lower than that of youths with even minor involvement in the crack business, let alone compared to that of crack dealers. At the other end of the scale, one might expect that more crack trade participation would lead to less time for, or less interest in, other crime. However, there is only a slight drop-off in petty property crime for the dealer+ group compared to other dealers, and for the most serious offenses—major felonies—the dealer+ group averaged nearly 50 percent more crimes per offender than other crack dealers, who in turn did nearly five times as many as subjects with minor or no crack trade participation.

So what explains the criminogenic effects of the crack trade? The general drugs-crime literature (Gandossey et al. 1980; Research Triangle Institute 1976) suggests that one factor is the interactive pattern typical of crime-drug relationships for addictive, expensive drugs: crime finances use, use encourages more use, more use encourages more crime. Crack certainly appears eligible for this general pattern, since it is highly addictive, and, although cheaper than other forms of cocaine use, it is expensive for unemployed users with anything more than a sporadic use pattern. At retail prices, a big crack habit—dozens or even scores of hits per day—can be at least as expensive as a big heroin habit, since the latter entails considerably fewer daily doses.

One major problem with the crack trade is that it facilitates crack addiction. Every single youth interviewed for this study who was involved in the crack business to even a minor degree was a crack user; of the crack dealers, over 70 percent used crack every day, while under 15 percent used it less than regularly. Furthermore, even though greater crack trade participation meant more crack earned directly, as payment for drug sales, it also meant heavier use patterns; so that crack dealers were paying an average of over $8,000 a year to purchase crack for personal use. The resemblance to the classic crime-drug interactive cycle seems clear: crack dealing finances crack use, crack use encourages more crack use, and more crack use requires more profit-making crimes of all sorts to support an ever-growing addictive use pattern.

To the degree that one driving force for this cycle is indeed crack use, one possibility for breaking the cycle is forced intervention into the addiction pattern. This requires that these youths be located, but the criminal justice system is, in fact, finding them: 92 percent of the total sample had been arrested at some time (true for almost 98 percent—199/204—of those with any crack business involvement at all). Moreover, over 87 percent had been arrested just within the twelve months prior to interview. This is a much higher percentage than that typical of young adult heroin users in street studies ten or twenty years ago. Although these youths have been located, intervention has not occurred. Fewer than 4 percent of this extremely drug-involved sample had *ever* been in drug treatment. This reflects not only an overburdened juvenile court system, but also inadequate treatment resources for adolescents. Both problems are commonplace across the nation.

An additional criminogenic aspect of the crack business—and another reason why compulsory intervention is required—is the crack trade's strong attractiveness as a lifestyle to the youths involved in it. This fascination is reminiscent of descriptions applied some years ago to the heroin-user subculture: the joys of hustling and "taking care of business," the thrills of a "cops and robbers" street life (Preble and Casey; Sutter 1969). Interviews with young crack dealers give the impression that the crack trade is, for them, not only all this but much more. Demand for crack makes dealing it remarkably easy and profitable—apparently much more so than selling heroin used to be. Further, crack business networks permit upward mobility, and therefore, a feeling of achievement; movement up the ranks is rare for heroin dealers. A likely additional factor is that the rewards for crack dealing include a drug that makes its users feel not merely unworried but omnipotent. Finally, the sheer youth of these young crack dealers means that dangers—street violence, arrest, overdose, and potential death—are perceived with particularly giddy enthusiasm as challenges to be outwitted and overcome. Participation in the crack trade, in short, provides its own kind of intoxication for the youths entangled in it.

In conclusion, the crack-crime dynamic, at least for adolescent crack dealers, represents an intensified version of the classic drug-crime relationship originally described for (adult) heroin users. Both patterns rest on addiction, but for crack, addiction onset appears to be more rapid, while maximum physiological intake—and thus financial requirements—seem more unlimited. For both, sales of the drug of choice are the most common criminal offense, but the rewards of the crack trade go well beyond those of "getting by" through heroin dealing. Finally, while both patterns ensnare youth in their formative years, young crack dealers are astonishingly more involved in a drugs-crime lifestyle at an alarmingly younger age.

* * *

James A. Inciardi and Anne E. Pottieger, "Kids, Crack, and Crime," *Journal of Drug Issues, 21* (Spring 1991), pp. 257-270. Copyright © 1991 by

Notes

1. See *New York Times*, 29 November 1985; *Newsweek*, 16 June 1986; *USA Today*, 16 June 1986; *Newsweek*, 30 June 1986; *New York Times*, 25 August 1986; *New York Times*, 24 November 1986; *Newsweek*, 27 April 1987; *New York Times*, 20 March 1988; *Miami Herald* ("Neighbors" supplement), 24 April 1988; *New York Times*, 23 June 1988; *Time*, 5 December 1988; *New York Doctor*, 10 April 1989; *U.S. News & World Report*, 10 April 1989.

2. "Index" offenses, in the FBI's *Uniform Crime Reports*, include homicide, forcible rape, aggravated assault, robbery, burglary, larceny/theft, motor vehicle theft, and arson.

References

Almeida, M. 1978. Contrabucion al Estudio de la Historia Natural de la Dependencia a la Pasta Basica de Cocina. *Revista de Neuro-Psiquiatria 41*:44-45.

Gandossey, R. P., J. R. Williams, J. Cohen, and H. J. Harwood. 1980. *Drugs and Crime; A Survey and Analysis of the Literature*. Washington, DC: National Institute of Justice.

Inciardi, J. A. 1986. *The War on Drugs: Heroin, Cocaine, Crime, and Public Policy*. Palo Alto, CA: Mayfield.

Inciardi, J. A. 1987. Beyond Cocaine: Basuco, Crack, and Other Coca Products. *Contemporary Drug Problems* Fall: 461-492.

Jeri, F. R. 1984. Coca-Paste Smoking in Some Latin American Countries: A Severe and Unabated Form of Addiction. *Bulletin on Narcotics* April-June: 15-31.

Preble, E. and J. J. Casey. 1969. Taking Care of Business: The Heroin User's Life on the Street. *International Journal of the Addictions 4*:1-24.

Research Triangle Institute (eds.). 1976. *Drug Use and Crime: Report of the Panel on Drug Use and Criminal Behavior*. Springfield, VA: National Technical Information Service.

Sutter, A. G. 1969. Worlds of Drug Use on the Street Scene. In *Delinquency, Crime, and Social Process*, Donald R. Cressey and David A. Ward (eds.). New York: Harper and Row. ✦

29. The Drugs/Violence Nexus: A Tripartite Conceptual Framework

Paul J. Goldstein

Most *of the research that addresses linkages between drug use and crime focuses on property crime. Less understood is the relationship between drugs and violence. In this regard, Paul J. Goldstein draws from existing research to propose a framework for considering the drugs/violence nexus. One linkage is psychopharmacological— drugs alter behavior by reducing inhibitions or instigating aggression. By contrast, economically compulsive violence occurs when individuals commit violent crimes in their efforts to secure funds to purchase drugs for self-use. Systemic violence is associated with the turf battles and struggles for control in the drug dealing and trafficking industries.*

Drug use, as well as the social context in which that use occurs, are etiological factors in a wide range of other social phenomena. Drug use is known to be causally related to a variety of physical and mental health problems, crime, poor school performance, family disruption, and the like. Previous research has also consistently found strong connections between drugs and violence.

For example, Zahn and Bencivengo (1974) reported that in Philadelphia, in 1972, homicide was the leading cause of death among drug users, higher even than deaths due to adverse effects of drugs; and drugs accounted for approximately 31 percent of the homicides in Philadelphia. Monforte and Spitz (1975), after studying autopsy and police reports in Michigan, suggested that drug use and distribution may be more strongly related to homicide than to property crime. Preble (1980) conducted an ethnographic study of heroin addicts in East Harlem between 1965 and 1967. About fifteen years later, in 1979 and 1980, he followed up the 78 participants and obtained detailed information about what had happened to them. He found that 28 had died. Eleven, 40 percent of the deaths, were the victims of homicide. The New York City Police Department (1983) classified about 24 percent of known homicides in 1981 as drug-related.

The drugs/violence nexus also appears consistently in newspaper headlines. For example, a seventeen-year-old boy who committed suicide by hanging himself in his jail cell had earlier confessed to committing a ritual stabbing and mutilation killing of another youth, because he believed the boy had stolen ten bags of PCP from him (*New York Times*, July 12, 1984). A New York City transit policeman was beaten with his own nightstick and his chin was nearly bitten off by a fare-beater who was high on angel dust (*New York Post*, September 19, 1984). A thirty-nine-year-old mother of three was killed by a stray bullet fired during a fight between drug dealers on the lower east side of Manhattan (*New York Post*, October 10, 1984). A front-page headline in the *New York Times* (October 29, 1984) claimed that "Increase in Gang Killings on Coast is Traced to Narcotics Trafficking." Less than a month later, another *New York Times* front-page headline announced that "Cocaine Traffickers Kill 17 in Peru Raid on Anti-Drug Team" (November 19, 1984). A Miami police official was quoted on television as saying that one-third of the homicides in Miami in 1984 were cocaine-related.

Even though the relationship between drugs and violence has been consistently documented in both the popular press and in social scientific research, it is only recently that attempts have been made to assess this problem on a national level. One such effort estimated that 10 percent of the homicides and assaults nationwide are the result of drug use (Harwood et al. 1984). Another recent report estimated that, in the United States in 1980, over 2,000 homicides were drug-related and, assuming an average life span of 65 years, resulted in the loss of about 70,000 years of life. This report further estimated that, in 1980, over 460,000 assaults were drug-related, and that, in about 140,000 of these assaults, the victims sustained physical injury, leading to about 50,000 days of hospitalization (Goldstein and Hunt 1984).

While the association between drugs and violence appears strong, and drug use and trafficking appear to be important etiological factors in the incidence of violence, there has been little effort to place this relationship into a conceptual framework to guide further empirical research. The purpose of this paper is to introduce such a framework.

Information for this report was gathered during the course of three separate empirical investigations. Sixty women were interviewed in 1976 and 1977 for a study of the relationship between prostitution and drugs (Goldstein 1979). Between 1978 and 1982, an ethnographic study was undertaken of the economic behavior of 201 street opiate users in Harlem.[1] Finally, in 1984, I began a study of the relationship between drugs and violence on the lower east side of Manhattan.[2] That study is guided by the conceptual framework presented below.

Drugs and violence are seen as being related in three possible ways: the psychopharmacological, the economically compulsive, and the systemic. Each of these models must be viewed, in a theoretical sense, as "ideal types," i.e., as hypothetically concrete ". . . devices intended to institute comparisons as precise as the stage of one's theory and the precision of one's instruments allow" (Martindale 1959:58-59). In fact, it will be shown below that there can be overlap between the three models. However, this overlap does not detract from the heuristic value of the tripartite conceptual framework.

Psychopharmacological Violence

The psychopharmacological model suggests that some individuals, as a result of short- or long-term ingestion of specific substances, may become excitable, irrational, and may exhibit violent behavior. The most relevant substances in this regard are probably alcohol, stimulants, barbiturates, and PCP. A lengthy literature exists, examining the relationship between these substances and violence (Tinklenberg 1973; Virkunnen 1974; Glaser, 1974; Gerson et al. 1979; Ellinswood 1971; Smith 1972; Asnis and Smith 1978; d'Orban 1976; Feldman et al. 1979).

Early reports which sought to employ a psychopharmacological model to attribute violent behavior to the use of opiates and marijuana have now been largely discredited (Finestone 1967; Inciardi and Chambers 1972; Kozel et al. 1972; Greenberg and Adler 1974; Schatzman 1975; Kramer 1976). In a classic statement of this point, Kolb argued the following.

> There is probably no more absurd fallacy prevalent than the notion that murders are committed and daylight robberies and holdups are carried out by men stimulated by large doses of cocaine or heroin which have temporarily distorted them into self-imagined heroes incapable of fear . . . violent crime would be much less prevalent if all habitual crimi-

nals were addicts who could obtain sufficient morphine or heroin to keep themselves fully charged with one of these drugs at all times. (Kolb 1925:78)

Kolb's point must be modified in one very important way. He is correct in claiming that ingestion of opiates is unlikely to lead to violence. However, the irritability associated with the withdrawal syndrome from opiates may indeed lead to violence. For example, in previous research on the relationship between drugs and prostitution, I found that heroin-using prostitutes often linked robbing and/or assaulting clients with the withdrawal experience (Goldstein 1979). These women reported that they preferred to talk a "trick" out of his money, but if they were feeling "sick," i.e., experiencing withdrawal symptoms, that they would be too irritable to engage in gentle conning. In such cases, they might attack the client, take his money, purchase sufficient heroin to "get straight," and then go back on the street. In a more relaxed physical and mental state, these women claimed that they could then behave like prostitutes rather than robbers.

Drug use may also have a reverse psychopharmacological effect and ameliorate violent tendencies. In such cases, persons who are prone to acting violently may engage in self-medication, in order to control their violent impulses. Several subjects have reported doing this. The drugs chosen for this function are typically heroin or tranquilizers.

Psychopharmacological violence may involve drug use by either offender or victim. In other words, drug use may contribute to a person behaving violently, or it may alter a person's behavior, in such a manner as to bring about that person's violent victimization. Previous research indicates relatively high frequencies of alcohol consumption in rape (Amir 1971; Rada 1975) and homicide victims (Shupe 1954; Wolfgang 1958). Public intoxication may invite a robbery or mugging. One study found that, in rapes where only the victim was intoxicated, she was significantly more likely to be physically injured (Johnson et al. 1973).

It is difficult to estimate the true rate of victim-precipitated psychopharmacological violence, because many such instances go unreported and, hence, unrecorded in official records. My own research in New York over the last decade indicated that many intoxicated victims do not report their victimization. Such victims say that they do not wish to talk to the police while drunk or "stoned." Further, since they are frequently confused about details of the event and, perhaps, unable to remember what their assailant looked like, they argue that reporting the event would be futile.

Assuming that the psychopharmacological violence is not precipitated by the victim, the victim can then be just about anybody. Psychopharmacological violence can erupt in the home and lead to spouse or child abuse. Psychopharmacological violence can occur in the workplace, on the streets, in bars, and so on. The incidence of psychopharmacological violence is impossible to assess at the present time, both because many instances go unreported and because when cases are reported, the psychopharmacological state of the offender is seldom recorded in official records.

Economic-Compulsive Violence

The economically compulsive model suggests that some drug users engage in economically-oriented violent crime, e.g., robbery, in order to support costly drug use. Heroin and cocaine, because they are expensive drugs typified by compulsive patterns of use, are the most relevant substances in this category. Economically compulsive actors are not primarily motivated by impulses to act out violently. Rather, their primary motivation is to obtain money to purchase drugs. Violence generally results from some factor in the social context in which the economic crime is perpetrated. Such factors include the perpetrator's own nervousness, the victim's reaction, weaponry (or the lack of it) carried by either offender or victim, the intercession of bystanders, and so on.

Research indicates that most heroin users avoid violent acquisitive crime, if viable non-violent alternatives exist (Preble and Casey 1969; Swezey 1973; Cushman 1974; Gould 1974; Goldstein and Duchaine 1980; Goldstein 1981, Johnson et al. 1985). This is because violent crime is more dangerous, embodies a greater threat of prison if one is apprehended, and because perpetrators may lack a basic orientation toward violent behavior. Bingham Dai reported similar findings nearly fifty years ago. His study of the criminal records of over one thousand opiate addicts in Chicago revealed that the most common offenses for which they were arrested were violations of the narcotics laws, followed by offenses against property.

... it is interesting to note that comparatively few of them resorted to violence in their criminal activities. The small percentage of addicts, committing such crimes as robbery, assault and battery, homicide, and others that involve the use of force, seems to discredit the view shared by many that the use of drugs has the effect of causing an individual to be a heartless criminal. On the contrary, our figures suggest that most of the crimes committed by addicts were of a peaceful nature that involve more the use of wit than that of force. (Dai 1937:69)

Victims of economic-compulsive violence, like those of psychopharmacological violence, can be anybody. Previous research (Goldstein and Johnson 1983; Johnson et al. 1985) indicates that the most common victims of this form of drug-related violence are people residing in the same neighborhoods as the offender. Frequently, the victims are engaged in illicit activities themselves. Other drug users, strangers coming into the neighborhood to buy drugs, numbers runners, and prostitutes are all common targets of economic-compulsive violence.

While research does indicate that most of the crimes committed by most of the drug users are of the non-violent variety, e.g., shoplifting, prostitution, drug selling, there are little data that indicate what proportion of violent economic crimes are committed for drug-related reasons. No national criminal justice data bases contain information on the motivations or drug-use pattern of offenders as they relate to specific crimes.

Systemic Violence

In the systemic model, violence is intrinsic to involvement with any illicit substance. Systemic violence refers to the traditionally aggressive patterns of interaction within the system of drug distribution and use. Some examples of systemic violence follow below:

1. disputes over territory between rival drug dealers.

2. assaults and homicides committed within dealing hierarchies as a means of enforcing normative codes.

3. robberies of drug dealers and the usually violent retaliation by the dealer or his/her bosses.

4. elimination of informers.

5. punishment for selling adulterated or phony drugs.

6. punishment for failing to pay one's debts.

7. disputes over drugs or drug paraphernalia.

8. robbery violence related to the social ecology of copping areas.

Substantial numbers of users of any drug become involved in drug distribution as their drug-using careers progress and, hence, increase their risk of becoming a victim or perpetrator of systemic violence. Examples of each type of systemic violence mentioned above are readily available.

We recently reported that much of the heroin in New York City is being distinctively packaged and sold under "brand names" (Goldstein et al. 1984). These labeling practices are frequently abused, and this abuse has led to violence. Among the more common abuses are the following: dealers mark an inferior-quality heroin with a currently popular brand name; users purchase the good heroin, use it, then repackage the bag with milk sugar for resale; the popular brand is purchased, the bag is "tapped," and further diluted for resale.

These practices get the real dealers of the popular brand very upset. Their heroin starts to get a bad reputation on the streets, and they lose sales. Purchasers of the phony bags may accost the real dealers, complaining about the poor quality and demanding their money back. The real dealers then seek out the purveyors of the phony bags. Threats, assaults, and/or homicides may ensue.

A common form of norm violation in the drug trade is known as "messing up the money." Basically, this involves a subordinate returning less money to his superior than is expected. For example, a street dealer is given a consignment of drugs to sell and is expected to return to his supplier or lieutenant with a specific amount of money. However, for any of a variety of reasons, he returns with too little money or fails to return at all. Some of the reasons why he might be short on his money are that he used some or all of the drugs himself; he sold all of the drugs, but then spent some or all of the money; he gave out too many "shorts," i.e., he sold the drugs for less than he should have; he was robbed, either of his drugs or of the money that he obtained from selling them.

When a street dealer fails to return sufficient money, his superior has several options. If only a small amount of money is involved, and the street dealer has few prior transgressions and a convincing justification for the current shortage, his superior is likely to give him another consignment and allow him to make up the shortage from his share of the new consignment. Other options include firing the street dealer, having him beaten up, or having him killed.

In a recent study, a lieutenant in a heroin dealing operation had been rather lax in supervising the six street dealers working under him. Just about everybody was "messing up the money," including himself. One day, the supplier and two "soldiers" picked up the lieutenant and took him for a ride in their car. The lieutenant was afraid that he was going to be killed. However, after cruising for a while, they spotted one of the street dealers who had been "messing up the money." The two soldiers jumped from the car and beat him with iron pipes. They positioned him in the street and drove the car over his legs, crippling him for life. The supplier then suggested to the lieutenant that he would be well-advised to run the operation more tightly in the future.

An interesting addendum to this discussion is that the "code of the streets" dictates that "blood cancels all debts." In other words, if a street dealer has "messed up the money" and is subsequently beaten up or wounded, then he no longer owes the money. The shedding of blood has canceled the debt.

The above account illustrates a direct punishment for a norm violation. Violence may also arise in the course of a dispute that stems from a norm violation. I was recently told of such an incident. A drug dealer operated out of an apartment in New York City. Prospective purchasers would line up in the hallway of the apartment house and give their money to a young Hispanic woman who worked for the dealer. The woman would then get the drugs from the dealer and give them to the buyers. Dealers seldom allow customers into the space where the drugs are actually kept.

One day, the line was long and three black men waited patiently to make their purchase. Finally, it was their turn. However, the woman bypassed them in favor of two Hispanic men who were at the back of the line. The Hispanic men made a large purchase, and the woman announced that the dealer had sold out for the day. The blacks were furious. An argument ensued, shots were fired, and one of the Hispanic men was killed. The norm violator in this case, the woman, was fired by the dealer.

A common precipitator of violence in the drug scene is the robbery of a dealer. No dealer who wishes to stay in business can allow himself or his associates to be robbed. Most dealers maintain an arsenal of weapons and a staff that knows how to use them. A subject in a recent study reported going with two friends to "take off" a neighborhood social club that was a narcotics distribution center. In the course of the hold-up, they shot one of the employees and beat up several other men and women. In retrospect, the subject admitted that they had probably used excessive force, but that at the time it had seemed justified because they were outnumbered about fifteen to three. One of the victims recognized one of the robbers. This robber was later shot to death in the street.

The Pulitzer Prize-winning study of narcotics trafficking, *The Heroin Trail*, documents many instances of systemic violence. One concerns Joseph Fucillo, a Brooklyn drug dealer who became a police informant in 1972.

> One day, as his wife watched from the window of their home in the Bensonhurst section of Brooklyn, Fucillo backed his car out of the driveway, and two men in ski masks walked up to it. Two guns fired rapidly and seven bullets went into Fucillo's head. He died. (*Newsday* Staff and Editors, 1974:226)

A pimp stated that he would never allow a "junkie broad" to work for him. One of his reasons was that an addicted woman might be easily turned into an informant by the police. When asked what he would do if one of his women did start to use narcotics, he replied that, if she didn't know too much about his activities, he would just fire her. However, if she did know too much, he would kill her (Goldstein 1979:107).

New York Magazine reported an event that was tragic both in its consequence and in the fact that it is so typical of the current drug scene.

> Sylvester, a sixteen-year-old boy, is stabbed in the chest . . . in the Crown Heights section of Brooklyn. He is taken to St. Mary's Hospital and dies a short time later. According to a witness, Sylvester sold marijuana to a group of adolescents a few days before the incident. His customers were apparently dissatisfied with its quality. Tonight, the teenagers, a group of about eight or ten, find Sylvester on the street and complain about the bad grass. The leader of the group, John Green, demands their money back. Sylvester then picks up a couple of bottles and throws them at the group, running away down the block. The teenagers chase Sylvester down Lincoln Place, where he picks up a stick and starts swinging. Knocking the stick out of his hand, John Green plunges a four-inch knife into Sylvester's chest.

> Green and the others escape from the scene. At one p.m. Sunday afternoon, in apparent retaliation for the Sylvester murder, John Green is shot once in the left rear side of the body. He too is taken to St. Mary's, where he too dies. (Goro 1977:31)

Violence associated with disputes over drugs have long been endemic in the drug world. Friends come to blows, because one refuses to give the other a "taste." A husband beats his wife, because she raided his "stash."

The current AIDS scare has led to an increasing amount of violence because of intravenous drug users' fear of contracting this fatal disease from contaminated "works." Some sellers of needles and syringes claim that the used works that they are trying to sell are actually new and unused. If discovered by would-be purchasers, violence may ensue. I was recently told of one incident that allegedly led to the death of two men. A heroin user kept a set of works in a "shooting gallery" that were for his exclusive use. One day, another man used these works. The owner of the works discovered what had happened and stabbed this man to death. He later stabbed a friend to death who was present when the stranger had used the works, had done nothing to stop him, and had failed to inform the owner of what had happened.

The social ecology of copping areas is generally well-suited for the perpetration of robbery violence. Most major copping areas in New York City are located in poor ghetto neighborhoods, such as Harlem. In these neighborhoods, drug users and dealers are frequent targets for robberies because they are known to be carrying something of value, and because they are unlikely to report their victimization. Dealers are sometimes forced to police their own blocks, so that customers may come and go in safety.

A subject in a current study earns money by copping drugs for other people. He stated that he was recently forced to protect one of his clients by fighting off two would-be robbers with a garbage-can lid. Interestingly, he knew the two attackers from the street, but he claimed to harbor no ill will towards them. He stated that they did what they had to do, and he did what he had to do.

Victims of systemic violence are usually those involved in drug use or trafficking. Occasionally, non-involved individuals become innocent victims. The case of a woman being killed by a stray bullet fired in a dispute between rival drug dealers was cited earlier. Several cases have been reported where whole families of drug dealers, including wives and young children, have perished in narcotics gang wars. However, the vast majority of victims of systemic violence are those who use drugs, who sell drugs, or are otherwise engaged in some aspect of the drug business.

Various sources have stressed the importance of what I have termed the systemic model in explaining drugs/violence relationships. Blum (1969) points out that, with the exception of alcohol, most drug users are not violent, but that this point does not apply to the typical dealer for whom there is strong evidence linking drugs and violence. Smith (1972), in his discussion of amphetamines and violence in San Francisco's Haight-Ashbury district, stated that the primary cause of violence on the streets was "burning," i.e., selling phony or adulterated drugs. Several sources suggest that studying the area of systemic violence may be more important than the study of the relationship of drug use to crime on the level of the individual user.

Racket-associated violence, a result of the intense competition for enormous profits involved in drugs, is flourishing. This is not the "crime in the streets" which is often associated with drugs, but an underworld in which ordinarily those people suffer from violence who in one way or another have become related to the traffic. (Fitzpatrick 1974:360)

Because these criminal entrepreneurs operate outside the law in their drug transactions, they are not bound by business etiquette in their competition with each other, in their collection of debts, or in their non-drug investments. Terror, violence, extortion, bribery, or any other expedient strategy is relied upon by these criminals. . . . (Glaser 1974:53)

Where a commodity is scarce and highly in demand (as may be the case with drugs), extreme measures of control, i.e., homicide, may be involved. Further, in areas of high scarcity and inelastic demand, bitter arguments centering on the commodity are likely to ensue. When such arguments take place in a subculture where violence is the modus operandi, and where implements of violence, e.g., guns, are readily available, homicide is likely to be the result. (Zahn 1975:409)

Zahn pointed out the importance of systemic violence in her recent study of homicide in twentieth-century United States. She showed that homicide rates peaked in the 1920s and early 1930s, declined and levelled off thereafter, began to rise in 1965,

and peaked again in 1974. This analysis led to the following conclusion:

> In terms of research directions, this historical review would suggest that closer attention be paid to the connection between markets for illegal goods and the overall rate of homicide violence. It seems possible, if not likely, that establishing and maintaining a market for illegal goods (booze in the 1920s and early 1930s; heroin and cocaine in the late 1960s and early 1970s) may involve controlling and/or reducing the competition, solving disputes between alternate suppliers or eliminating dissatisfied customers. . . . The use of guns in illegal markets may also be triggered by the constant fear of being caught either by a rival or by the police. Such fear may increase the perceived need for protection, i.e., a gun, thus may increase the arming of these populations and a resulting increased likelihood of use. For the overall society, this may mean a higher homicide rate. (Zahn 1980:128)

It was stated above that the three models of the drugs/violence nexus contained in the tripartite conceptual framework should be viewed as ideal types, and that overlap could occur between them. For example, a heroin user preparing to commit an act of economic-compulsive violence, e.g., a robbery, might ingest some alcohol or stimulants to give himself the courage to do the crime. This event now contains elements of both economic-compulsive and psychopharmacological violence. If the target of his robbery attempt was a drug dealer, the event would contain elements of all three types of drug-related violence.

The conceptual framework allows the event to be effectively analyzed and broken down into constituent parts and processes. The roles played in the event by different sorts of drugs can be explicated. In the above example, the need for money to purchase heroin was the primary motivation for the act. Alcohol and stimulants were ingested after the act was decided upon because of the robber's need for courage, and, presumably, because prior experience with these substances led the perpetrator to believe that they would serve that psychopharmacological function.

The choice of target, a drug dealer, is open for empirical investigation. It may turn out that the reason the heroin user needed to commit the robbery was because that dealer had cheated him earlier in the day on a drug purchase, perhaps selling him "dummy" bags. Our robber, needing to "get straight" and not having any more money, decides that robbing this unscrupulous dealer would be an appropriate revenge.

Several subjects in our studies reported committing economic-compulsive acts out of fear of becoming a victim of systemic violence. These were street dealers who had "messed up the money" and who were terrified of what their superiors might do to them. Some had already been threatened. This motivated them to do robberies as a quick way to obtain the money that they owed.

Thus, as the concepts are employed, a fuller understanding of the event emerges. The roles played by specific drugs become clearer. The actor's motivations and the process by which he undertakes to commit a robbery are elaborated upon.

If the above events were to be examined in official crime records, assuming they were reported, they would be listed as robberies. Victim-perpetrator relationships would probably be unknown, though they might be listed as "acquaintance" or "stranger." No mention of drugs would be made.

Victims of systemic violence frequently lie to the police about the circumstances of their victimization. Not a single research subject whom I have interviewed who was the victim of systemic violence and who was forced to give an account of his or her victimization to the police admitted that he or she had been assaulted because of owing a drug supplier money or selling somebody phony or adulterated drugs. All such victims simply claimed to have been robbed.

It would make little difference if the robbery were to develop into a homicide. The classification of the event would change from robbery to homicide, but victim-perpetrator relationship and nature of the homicide would remain unknown or be coded in such a broad fashion that the information would not be very useful. No mention of drugs would be made. Attention will now be focused on the quality of data available on the national level to elaborate on the drugs/violence nexus.

Quality of Data Available on Drugs/Violence Nexus

The drugs/violence nexus is one of the most important criminological and health issues, for which rigorously collected data is currently unavailable. While a variety of ethnographic studies focus on violent behavior of drug users, most of this material is not quantitative and does not allow national projec-

tions to be made. Official statistics collected in the criminal justice and health care systems do not link acts of criminal violence and resultant injuries or death to antecedent drug activity of victims or perpetrators. Broad recording categories make it virtually impossible to determine whether the offender or victim was a drug user or distributor, or whether the pharmacological status of either victim or offender was related to the specific event.

Uniform Crime Reports (UCR), collected by the Federal Bureau of Investigation, is the most visible source of crime data in the country. However, it is not very useful for an elaboration of the relationship between drugs and violence. UCR is a measure of crimes known to the police. Many crimes are not reported. The 1980 National Crime Survey found that the following proportions of violent victimizations were not reported to the police: 57 percent of the rapes; 41 percent of the robberies; 52 percent of the assaults (BJS 1982:71). UCR data on homicide, due to the presence of a body, is the most reliable crime-incidence category.

Reporting schedules, to which local law-enforcement agencies must adhere, frequently result in data being submitted to UCR before investigative work has been completed; and, hence, large numbers of unknowns usually appear in relevant categories. The New York City Police Department has addressed this issue by holding an annual debriefing of detective-squad commanders about all homicides that occurred in their precincts during the preceding year. It was in the context of these debriefings that the significance of drug-related homicides first emerged and became an important analytic category for the NYPD Crime Analysis Unit. The new data gathered during these debriefings have never been included in UCR, because no structure exists for their transmission. This has led to such curious statistical phenomena as New York City reporting more drug-related homicides for a given year than UCR reports for the nation as a whole, including New York City.

The major difficulty in using UCR to estimate drug-related violent crime is the lack of a descriptive component to supplement the quantitative presentation. The drug-relatedness of violent events is simply not coded. Therefore, it is not possible to link specific violent acts to antecedent drug activities of either victim or perpetrator.

An alternative data source is the National Crime Survey (NCS). This annual report issued by the Bureau of Justice Statistics (BJS) is based on data obtained from a stratified, multi-stage cluster sample. The basic sampling unit is the household. Respondents within households are asked for all instances of victimization in the past year. Projections are then made to the nation as a whole.

As was the case with UCR, the NCS is not very useful for elaborating on the drugs/violence nexus. Street drug users frequently are not part of a household, i.e., they may sleep in abandoned buildings, in subways, on park benches. Thus, a population that is posited to be at especially high risk for drug-related violence is likely to be underrepresented in this data. Also, victims may have difficulty recalling specific events or be reluctant to describe them to an interviewer.

> Research on the capacity of victims to recall specific kinds of crime . . . indicates that assault is the least well-recalled of the crimes measured by the NCS. This may stem in part from the observed tendency of victims not to report crimes committed by offenders known to them, especially if they are relatives. In addition, it is suspected that, among certain groups, crimes that contain the elements of assault are a part of everyday life and, thus, are simply forgotten or are not considered worth mentioning to a survey interviewer. Taken together, these recall problems may result in a substantial understatement of the "true" rate of victimization from assault. (BJS 1982:94)

A major problem with the NCS is that victims seldom know the motivation of offenders for committing acts of violence. Of course, this is less the case with systemic violence than it is with either psychopharmacological or economic-compulsive violence. With regard to psychopharmacological violence, victims may not be able to discern that assailants are "high" and, even if they could, it would be difficult to ascertain what substances are involved. Similarly, victims of economic-compulsive violence may not know that they are being robbed in order to finance a drug habit.

Summary and Conclusions

Drugs and violence were shown to be related in three possible ways: psychopharmacologically, economic-compulsively, and systemically. These different forms of drug-related violence were shown to be related to different types of substance use, different motivations of violent perpetrators, different types of victims, and differential influence by social con-

text. Current methods of collecting national-crime data were shown to be insensitive to the etiological role played by drug use and trafficking in creating violent crime.

No evidence currently exists as to the proportions of violence engaged in by drug users and traffickers that may be attributed to each of the three posited models. We need such data. My own impression, arising from research in New York, is that the area of systemic violence accounts for most of the violence perpetrated by, and directed at, drug users.

Systemic violence is normatively embedded in the social and economic networks of drug users and sellers. Drug use, the drug business, and the violence connected to both of these phenomena, are all aspects of the same general lifestyle. Individuals caught in this lifestyle value the experience of substance use, recognize the risks involved, and struggle for survival on a daily basis. That struggle is clearly a major contributor to the total volume of crime and violence in American society.

✳ ✳ ✳

For Discussion

The psychopharmacological linkage between drug use and violence assumes that some drug users have little control over their actions. Is it fair to punish these offenders in the same manner that we punish those users who engage in systemic violence?

Notes

1. This research was supported by the New York State Division of Substance Abuse Services by a Public Health Service Award from the National Institute on Drug Abuse (RO1-DA 01926); and by an interagency agreement between NIDA (RO1-DA 02355) and the Law Enforcement Assistance Administration (LEAA-J-IAA-005-8).

2. This research is being supported by the New York State Division of Substance Abuse Services and by a Public Health Service Award from the National Institute on Drug Abuse (RO1-DA 03182).

References

Amir, M. 1971. *Patterns in Forcible Rape*. Chicago: University of Chicago Press.

Asnis, S., and R. Smith. 1978. Amphetamine Abuse and Violence, *Journal of Psychedelic Drugs, 10*:317-377.

Biernacki, P. 1979. Junkie Work, Hustles, and Social Status Among Heroin Addicts, *Journal of Drug Issues, 9*:535-550.

Bureau of Justice Statistics. 1982. *Criminal Victimization in the United States, 1980*. Washington, DC: United States Department of Justice.

Cushman, P. 1974. Relationship between Narcotic Addiction and Crime, *Federal Probation, 38*:38-43.

Dai, B. 1937. *Opium Addiction in Chicago*. Montclair: Patterson Smith.

d'Orban, P. T. 1976. Barbiturate Abuse, *Journal of Medical Ethics, 2*:63-67.

Eckerman, W., J. Bates, J. Rachall, and W. Poole. 1971. *Drug Usage and Arrest Charges: A Study of Drug Usage and Arrest Charges among Arrestees in Six Metropolitan Areas of the United States*. Washington, DC: United States Department of Justice.

Ellinswood, E. 1971. Assault and Homicide Associated with Amphetamine Abuse, *American Journal of Psychiatry, 127*:1170-1175.

Feldman, H., M. H. Agar, and G. M. Beschner (eds.) 1979. *Angel Dust: An Ethnographic Study of PCP Users*. Lexington: Lexington Books.

Finestone, H. 1967. Narcotics and Criminality, *Law and Contemporary Problems, 22*:60-85.

Fink, L., and M. Hyatt. 1978. Drug Use and Violent Behavior, *Journal of Drug Education, 8*:139-149.

Fitzpatrick, J. P. 1974. Drugs, Alcohol, and Violent Crime, *Addictive Diseases, 1*:353-367.

Gerson, L. W., and D. A. Preston. 1979. Alcohol Consumption and the Incidence of Violent Crime, *Journal of Studies on Alcohol, 40*:307-312.

Glaser, D. 1974. Interlocking Dualities in Drug Use, Drug Control, and Crime, in Inciardi, J. A., and C. Chambers (eds.), *Drugs and the Criminal Justice System*. Beverly Hills: Sage Publications.

Goldstein, P. J. 1979. *Prostitution and Drugs*. Lexington: Lexington Books. 1981. Getting Over: Economic Alternatives to Predatory Crime Among Street Drug Users, in Inciardi, J. A. (ed.), *The Drugs/Crime Connection*. Beverly Hills: Sage Publications.

Goldstein, P. J., and N. Duchaine. 1980. Daily Criminal Activities of Street Drug Users, paper presented at annual meetings of the American Society of Criminology.

Goldstein, P. J., and B. D. Johnson. 1983. Robbery Among Heroin Users, presented at annual meetings of the Society for the Study of Social Problems.

Goldstein, P. J., and D. Hunt. 1984. Health Consequences of Drug Use, report to the Carter Center of Emory University and The Centers for Disease Control.

Goldstein, P. J., D. S. Lipton, E. Preble, I. Sobel, T. Miller, W. Abbott, W. Paige, and F. Soto. 1984. The Marketing of Street Heroin in New York City, *Journal of Drug Issues, 14*:553-566.

Goro, H. 1977. Saturday Night Dead, *New York Magazine, 10*:31.

Gould, L. 1974. Crime and the Addict: Beyond Common Sense, in Inciardi, J. A., and C. Chambers (eds.), *Drugs and the Criminal Justice System*. Beverly Hills: Sage Publications.

Greenberg, S., and F. Adler. 1974. Crime and Addiction: An Empirical Analysis of the Literature, 1920-1973, *Contemporary Drug Problems, 3*:221-270.

Harwood, H., D. Napolitano, P. Kristiansen, and J. Collins. 1984. *Economic Costs to Society of Alcohol and Drug Abuse and Mental Illness*. Final Report to the Alcohol, Drug Abuse and Mental Health Administration.

Inciardi, J. A., and C. Chambers. 1972. Unreported Criminal Involvement of Narcotic Addicts, *Journal of Drug Issues 2*:57-64.

Johnson, B. D., P. J. Goldstein, E. Preble, J. Schmeidler, D. S. Lipton, B. Spunt, and T. Mille. 1985. *Taking Care of Business: The Economics of Crime by Heroin Abusers*. Lexington: Lexington Books.

Johnson, S., L. Gibson, and R. Linden. 1976. Alcohol and Rape in Winnepeg: 1966-1975, *Journal of Studies on Alcohol 39*:1887-1894.

Klepfisz, A. and J. Racy. 1973. Homicide and LSD, *JAMA 223*:429-430.

Kolb, L.. 1925. Drug Addiction and its Relation to Crime, *Mental Hygiene, 9*:74-89.

Kozel, N., R. Dupont, and B. Brown. 1972. A Study of Narcotic Involvement in an Offender Population, *International Journal of the Addictions, 7*:443-450.

Kramer, J. C. 1976. From Demon to Ally—How Mythology Has and May Yet Alter National Drug Policy, *Journal of Drug Issues, 6*:390-406.

McBride, D. 1981. Drugs and Violence, in Inciardi, J. A. (ed.), *The Drugs/Crime Connection*. Beverly Hills: Sage Publication.

Martindale, D. 1959. Sociological Theory and the Ideal Type, in Gross, L. (ed.), *Symposium on Sociological Theory*. New York: Harper and Row.

Monforte, J. R., and W. U. Spitz. 1975. Narcotic Abuse Among Homicides in Detroit, *Journal of Forensic Sciences, 20*: 186-190.

Newsday Staff and Editors. 1974. *The Heroin Trail*. New York: Holt, Rinehart, and Winston.

New York City Police Department. 1983. *Homicide Analysis: 1981*.

Petersen, R., and R. Stillman (eds.). 1978. *Phencyclidine Abuse: An Appraisal*. Rockville, MD: National Institute on Drug Abuse.

Preble, E. 1980. El Barrio Revisited, paper presented at annual meetings of the Society for Applied Anthropology.

Preble, E., and J. Casey. 1969. Taking Care of Business: The Heroin Users Life on the Street, *International Journal of the Addictions, 4*:1-24.

Rada, R. 1975. Alcoholism and Forcible Rape, *American Journal of Psychiatry, 132*:444-446.

Schatzman, M. 1975. Cocaine and the Drug Problem, *Journal of Psychedelic Drugs*, 77-18.

Shupe, L. M. 1954. Alcohol and Crime: A Study of the Urine Alcohol Concentration Found in 882 Persons Arrested During or Immediately After the Commission of a Felony, *Journal of Criminal Law, Criminology, and Police Science, 44*:661-664.

Smith, R. 1972. Speed and Violence: Compulsive Methamphetamine Abuse and Criminality in the Haight-Ashbury District, in C. Zarsfonetis (ed.), *Drug Abuse: Proceedings of the International Conference*. Philadelphia: Lea and Febiger.

Swezey, R. 1973. Estimating Drug-Crime Relationships, *International Journal of the Addictions, 8*:701-721.

Tinklenberg, J. 1973. Drugs and Crime, in National Commission on Marijuana and Drug Abuse, Drug Use in America: Problems in Perspective. Appendix, Volume 1, Patterns and Consequences of Drug Use. Washington, DC: United States Government Printing Office.

Virkunnen, M. 1974. Alcohol as a Factor Precipitating Aggression and Conflict Behavior Leading to Homicide, British Journal of the Addictions, 69:149-154.

Wolfgang, M. E. 1958. Patterns in Criminal Homicide. Philadelphia: University of Philadelphia Press.

Zahn, M. A. 1975. The Female Homicide Victim, Criminology, 13:409. 1980. Homicide in the Twentieth Century United States, in Inciardi, J. A., and C. E. Faupel (eds.), History and Crime. Beverly Hills: Sage Publications.

Zahn, M. A., and M. Bencivengo. 1974. Violent Death: A Comparison between Drug Users and Non-Drug Users, Addictive Diseases, 1:283-296. ✦

Part VIII

AIDS and Drug Use

Acquired Immune Deficiency Syndrome (AIDS) was first described as a new and distinct clinical entity during the late spring and early summer of 1981. First, clinical investigators in Los Angeles reported five cases to the Centers for Disease Control (CDC) of *Pneumocystis carinii pneumonia* (PCP) among gay men. None of these patients had an underlying disease that might have been associated with PCP, or a history of treatment for a compromised immune system. All, however, had other clinical manifestations and laboratory evidence of immunosuppression. Second, and within a month, 26 cases of Kaposi's sarcoma (KS) were reported among gay men in New York and California.

What was so unusual was that prior to these reports, the appearance of both afflictions in populations of previously healthy young men was unprecedented. PCP is an infection caused by the parasite *P. carinii*, previously seen almost exclusively in cancer and transplant patients receiving immunosuppressive drugs. KS, a tumor of the blood vessel walls and often appearing as blue-violet to brownish skin blotches, had been quite rare in the United States—occurring primarily in elderly men, usually of Mediterranean origin. Like PCP, furthermore, KS had also been reported among organ-transplant recipients and others receiving immunosuppressive therapy. This quickly led to the hypothesis that the increased occurrences of the two disorders in gay men were due to some underlying immune-system dysfunction. This hypothesis was further supported by the incidence among homosexuals of "opportunistic infections"—infections caused by micro-organisms that rarely generate disease in persons with normal immune defense mechanisms. It is for this reason that the occurrence of KS, PCP, and/or other opportunistic infections in a person with unexplained immune dysfunction became known as the "acquired immune deficiency syndrome," or more simply, *AIDS*. With the recognition that the vast majority of the early cases of this new clinical syndrome involved gay and bisexual men, it seemed logical that the causes might be related to the lifestyle unique to that population. The sexual revolution of the 1960s and 1970s was accompanied not only by greater carnal permissiveness among both heterosexuals and gays, but also by a more positive social acceptance of homosexuality. The emergence of commercial bathhouses and other outlets for sexual contacts among gays further increased promiscuity, with certain segments of the male gay population viewing promiscuity as a facet of "gay liberation." In fact, among the early patients diagnosed with AIDS, their sexual recreation typically occurred within the anonymity of the bathhouses with similarly promiscuous men. Some had had as many as 20,000 sexual contacts and more than 1,100 sex partners. And to complicate matters, sexually active gay men with multiple sex partners were manifesting high rates of sexually transmitted diseases—gonorrhea, syphilis, genital herpes, anal warts, and hepatitis B.

Because of this, it is not surprising that such factors as frequent exposure to semen, rectal exposure to semen, the body's exposure to amyl nitrate and butyl nitrate (better known as "poppers" used to enhance sexual pleasure and performance), and/or a high prevalence of sexually transmitted diseases were themselves considered potential causes of AIDS. Yet while it was apparent that AIDS was a new disease, most of the gay lifestyle factors were *not* particularly new, having changed only in a relative sense. As such, it was difficult to immediately single out specific behaviors that might be related to the emerging epidemic. Within a brief period of time, however, the notion that AIDS was some form of "gay plague" was quickly extinguished. The disease was suddenly being reported in other populations, such as injection drug users,

265

blood transfusion patients, and hemophiliacs. And what these reports suggested to the scientific community was that an infectious etiology for AIDS had to be considered.

Almost immediately after the first cases of AIDS were reported in 1981, researchers at the Centers for Disease Control began tracking the disease backward in time to discover its origins. They ultimately determined that the first cases of AIDS in the United States probably occurred in 1977. By early 1982, AIDS had been reported in 15 states, the District of Columbia, and two foreign countries, but the total of cases remained extremely low—158 men and one woman. Although more than 90 percent of the men were either gay or bisexual, interviews with all of the patients failed to provide any definite clues about the origin of the disease.

Although it was suspected that AIDS might be transmitted through sexual relations among homosexually active men, the first strong evidence for the idea did not emerge until the completion of a case control study in June 1982 by epidemiologists at the Centers for Disease Control. In that investigation, data were obtained on the sexual partners of 13 of the first 19 cases of AIDS among homosexual men in the Los Angeles area. Within five years before the onset of their symptoms, nine had had sexual contact with people who later developed Kaposi's sarcoma or *P. carinii* pneumonia. The nine were also linked to another interconnected series of 40 AIDS cases in 10 different cities by one individual who had developed a number of the manifestations of AIDS and was later diagnosed with Kaposi's sarcoma. Overall, the investigation of these 40 cases indicated that 20 percent of the initial AIDS cases in the United States were linked through sexual contact—a statistical clustering that was extremely unlikely to have occurred by chance.

Yet even in the face of this evidence, there were those who doubted that AIDS was caused by some transmissible agent. However, when AIDS cases began to emerge in other populations—among individuals who had been injected with blood or blood products, but had no other expected risk factors—the transmission vectors for the disease became somewhat clearer. Such cases were confirmed first among people with hemophilia, followed by blood transfusion recipients and injection drug users who shared hypodermic needles, syringes, and other paraphernalia. Then, when there were documented cases of AIDS among the heterosexual partners of male injection drug users, it became increasingly evident that AIDS was a disease transmitted by the exchange of certain bodily fluids—primarily blood, blood products, and semen. "Sexual orientation" was not necessarily the only risk factor.

In 1983 and 1984, scientists at the Institute Pasteur in Paris and the National Institutes of Health in the United States identified and isolated the cause of AIDS—Human T-Cell Lymphotropic Virus, Type III (HTLV-III), or Lymphadenophy-Associated Virus (LAV). Later, this virus would be renamed human immunodeficiency virus, more commonly known as HIV. More specifically, HIV is a "retrovirus," a type of infectious agent that had previously been identified as causing many animal diseases. The designation of "retrovirus" derives from the backward, or "retro-" flow of genetic information from RNA to DNA, which reverses the normal flow of genetic messages. Subsequent studies demonstrated that HIV is transmitted when virus particles or infected cells gain direct access to the bloodstream. This can occur through all forms of sexual intercourse, the sharing of contaminated needles, blood, and blood products, and the passing of the virus from infected mothers to their unborn or newborn children. Within this context, AIDS involves a continuum of conditions associated with immune dysfunction, and is best described as a severe manifestation of infection with HIV.

With respect to the "AIDS/drugs connection," in 1987, the United States Public Health Service estimated that there were some 900,000 regular (at least weekly) injection drug users across the nation, 25 percent of whom were already infected with HIV. At the same time, the Centers for Disease Control was reporting that injection drug users, as already noted, were the second highest risk group for AIDS, representing 24 percent of all reported cases in the United States. By early 1988, drug injectors had come to represent 26 percent of known AIDS cases in the U.S., and by the 1990s the proportion exceeded 30 percent.

The ready transmission of HIV and AIDS among injection drug users is the result of the sharing of injection equipment, combined with the presence of "co-factors." Co-factors include any behavioral practices or microbiological agents that facilitate the transmission of HIV. For injecting heroin, cocaine, and amphetamine users, the blood transmission of HIV may occur as a result of using or sharing contaminated drug injection equipment. Of particular significance is "booting," a practice that increases the amount of residual blood left in drug paraphernalia. Booting involves the aspiration of venous blood back into a syringe for the purpose of mixing the drug with blood, while the needle remains inserted in the vein. The mixed blood/drug solution is then injected back into the vein. Most injection drug users believe that this "pre-mixing" enhances a drug's effects. Since injection users often share needles and syringes, particularly if they are administering the drugs in "shooting galleries"—places where users gather to take drugs—booting increases the probability that traces of HIV from an infected user will remain in a syringe to be passed on to the next user.

Additional risk factors in the AIDS/drug connection are prostitution and exchanges of sex for drugs. There is an extensive body of literature offering a strong empirical basis for the notion that prostitution is a major means of economic support for drug-using women. Moreover, it is well established that there is a high incidence of prostitution among women drug users. As such, the drug-injecting prostitute is not only at high risk for contracting HIV, but for transmitting it as well. Exchanges of sex for drugs, and particularly for crack, also represent risk factors for HIV and AIDS.

Drug users, in addition to being the second highest risk group for HIV and AIDS, also represent a population that appears difficult to impact with routine AIDS-prevention messages. The potential for HIV acquisition and transmission from infected paraphernalia and "unsafe" sex is likely known to most drug users. Yet most are accustomed to risking death (through overdose or the violence-prone nature of the illegal drug marketplace) and disease (hepatitis and other infections) on a daily basis, and these generally fail to eliminate their drug-taking behaviors. For these reasons, warnings that injection equipment sharing or unsafe sex may facilitate an infection that could cause death perhaps five or more years down the road have little meaning. It would appear that at least some IV drug users are willing to adjust a few behaviors related to the transmission of HIV, such as purchasing new needles, sterilizing used needles, and reducing the sharing of needles with others. However, the minimal research in this area has tended to be inconclusive, particularly since many of those who adjust their behaviors continue to share needles with friends, relatives, and others who appear healthy. In addition, prevention strategies have had little impact on sexual behaviors. In the three papers that follow, the range of AIDS-related drug-using practices are examined, as well as strategies for behavioral change. ✦

30. Kickin' Down to the Street Doc: Shooting Galleries in the San Francisco Bay Area

SHEIGLA MURPHY

AND

DAN WALDORF

"*Shooting galleries*" *serve a number of purposes for injection drug users (IDUs). First, these sites allow IDUs to inject drugs in an environment that is relatively safe from police intervention. Second, shooting galleries are often located near areas where drugs are purchased so that IDUs can inject shortly after obtaining their drugs. Third, IDUs can typically purchase or rent injection equipment from operators of shooting galleries. The following article by Sheigla Murphy and Dan Waldorf is a description of urban shooting galleries and their functions. The findings are based on interviews with 48 drug injectors in San Francisco. The authors report that shooting galleries can be classified as both informal or formal. These types are distinguished by hours of operation, paid gatekeepers, and the relationships among shooters.*

Needle sharing and the use of shooting galleries by intravenous drug users have received renewed attention with the advent of the AIDS epidemic. In the United States, homosexual males and IV drug users are considered the most high-risk groups to contract AIDS and ARC. Needle and syringe sharing are said to be the principal means by which HIV is spread among intravenous drug users (IVDU). Shooting galleries—places where drug users rent or use needles or syringes to inject illicit drugs—are said to contribute to the spread of HIV (Cohen et al. 1985; Weiss et al. 1985; Des Jarlais et al. 1986; Des Jarlais and Friedman 1987). At present, there is only limited information about needle sharing (Howard and Borges 1977; Des Jarlais and Friedman 1987; Friedman et al. 1987; Murphy 1987; Watters 1987; Battjes and Pickens 1988; Feldman and Biernacki 1988; Hopkins 1988; Power 1988; Waldorf et al. 1990), and even less is known about

the functions and utilization of shooting galleries (Des Jarlais et al. 1986; Waldorf et al. 1990). Some researchers have speculated that the geographic differences in the number of IV drug use-attributed AIDS cases in the United States, with greater percentages in Northeastern cities, as compared with Los Angeles and San Francisco, are due to greater utilization of shooting galleries in the Eastern cities.

This paper is a description of formal and informal shooting galleries in the San Francisco Bay Area. It reports the findings of 48 tape-recorded interviews conducted in 1988-1989 with methedrine, cocaine, and heroin injectors. The persons interviewed, long-term users of illicit drugs, were located by means of contacts with known intravenous users and chain-referral methods (Biernacki and Waldorf 1981). Many of the respondents have been in contact with one of the authors for a number of years as part of a long-term study of local policies about methadone maintenance. Interviews were conducted by one of the authors and by two ex-addicts trained to conduct focused interviews. All interviews were tape-recorded and transcribed for the analyses.

What Do You Call It?

When we first conceived the idea of doing interviews with habitues of shooting galleries, we were interested in whether the term "shooting gallery" was outmoded. We knew it was an old term, as we had heard people use it for years. Argot usually comes and goes in the drug world, and we assumed that some new terminology had replaced the "shooting gallery" or "drug house" designations. However, we were unable to discover any new names for public or private places where IVDUs gather to inject drugs. Respondents were not really comfortable with "shooting gallery," which many felt is not really in current use, but there are no other terms being used.

In response to the question, "What do you call a place where many people go to inject drugs?" several people answered, "My friend's house." Aside from its comic properties, this response is interesting from the point of view of the types of gathering places available to IVDUs when they need a place to inject drugs. Most shooting galleries in the San Francisco Bay Area seem to be organized around friendship groups. (Addicts are more comfortable with the term "associate." A common statement is, "I don't have many friends, just associates.") People who utilize Bay Area galleries are likely to be well-known to one another; consequently, users have a difficult time labeling these places as shooting galleries per se. From their perspective, these are the residences of their associates, running and shooting partners. They are also places where large groups of injectors regularly go to shoot drugs and share syringes, and where the resident(s) in a more or less regular fashion receives money and/or drugs for letting people use his/her place and injection and preparation equipment. For our purposes, places where these activities occur are shooting galleries.

What Do They Look Like?

Shooting galleries take a variety of forms. We have heard accounts that describe abandoned houses in a state of extreme dilapidation, hotel rooms, apartments, apartments in public-housing projects, and an old house trailer. We have also heard of an outdoor facility, under a bridge, where homeless drug users congregate and use drugs as well. But for the most part, Bay Area shooting galleries are located in users' homes, apartments, and hotel rooms.

One of the interviewers for the study went to visit a shooting gallery to meet a respondent who had agreed to do an interview, and described the place as follows:

> Before conducting this interview, I visited a local shooting gallery in the West Oakland housing project. It is located in a one-bedroom project apartment and run by an old junkie called Torchie. Inside the apartment were three people, and I was told that I had just missed the morning rush. The atmosphere was serious and not particularly friendly. Each of the visitors sat at a kitchen table, injected their drugs in my full view, and looked out the window. It seemed to be very matter of fact.

Here are three accounts by addicts interviewed for the study. The first is by a woman who had been using shooting galleries for 10 years. This gallery is also in the West Oakland neighborhood:

(I) So what kind of place was the gallery located in?

(R) In a ratty, condemned house up over an old-time nightclub.

(I) Can you describe it a little bit more?

(R) It was a whole house, but the house, the back part of the house has been burned out. And then the old guy who owned the house had a bunch of stuff piled up in it, where you couldn't pass the living room really. And they used two rooms, a room and a hallway. And there were folks everywhere.

(I) Did it have running water and stuff?

(R) Nope. It had lights, but no running water, and they just shit out the window. And the lights were hooked up from outside, you know, somebody else's shit.

The second account is of a gallery located in Hayward, an Alameda County suburb that has a large number of addicts.

(R) It's just a house, a house of a friend, or rather his parents' house. . . . The house is just totally gross. No one keeps it up, and the floor gots like pieces of wood all over it. When you step somewhere, you almost kill yourself. There was a bunch of people there, and he lets about five guys stay there. They hustle enough money to get about half a gram and barely make enough to get another one. In that house, there are so many people just hanging out, like about eleven people. Some have their own outfits, some don't. If you don't have an outfit and need a fix, whoever has an outfit is going to get a "kickdown" [a small portion of drugs in payment for outfit rental].

The last account is of an outdoor shooting gallery, known as 29 Bush:

(I) Okay, think about the very last shooting gallery you went to and tell me about it.

(R) It was this morning, and it was underneath a ramp where cars go over. I had to have somebody fix me, and I didn't want to walk all the way back to F_____. It was right at _____ Avenue, underneath a bridge, near the railroad tracks. It's underneath the bridge where the hobos sleep. There are cans and a chair there, and you fix right there. . . . It was dirty, there were dirty cushions there and cookers all over the ground and a bottle for water.

(I) Where do you think they got the water?

(R) I don't know, that's what I asked them. . . . He went around the side and come out of this bush with a Pepsi bottle of water. And it looked clean. Then I looked for a cooker on the ground and cleaned it up. It didn't really look that dirty, compared to the other ones.

(I) How many people were there at the time?

(R) Five people came while I was there.

Reasons for Using Shooting Galleries

The principal services provided to users in shooting galleries are: (a) provision of a relatively private place to inject their drugs; (b) syringes for rent and other materials to prepare the drugs for injection—water, cotton to filter the drug, matches, and a bottle cap to heat and dissolve the drugs; and (c) syringes for sale. In California, along with 11 other states, possession of syringes and other injection materials is illegal, and many addicts and other IVDUs are reluctant to carry their outfits on the street, and most particularly to and from their connections. The reluctance is understandable; they do not wish to risk being stopped and "jacked up" by the police for a paraphernalia offense.

People use shooting galleries because of their location, most importantly for their proximity to the connections or the places where people go to buy drugs. Just as a successful restaurateur would locate a lunch place near a high-density work area to ensure plenty of people needing a place to eat at noon, so do shooting galleries spring up near places where drugs are sold.

Proximity to the places where drugs are sold has implications that relate to shooting-gallery usage. Heroin addicts, especially sick or withdrawing heroin addicts, want to inject their heroin as quickly as possible. If the shooting gallery is two blocks away and their home two miles away from the source of drugs, the shooting gallery is where they will head, as soon as they have obtained their drugs. Drug injectors of all types do not want to have drugs in their possession while on the streets. The places where drug shooters go to buy their drugs are usually high-crime areas and are, therefore, heavily policed. The following respondent summed up these points, in answer to a question about the most important reasons to use shooting galleries:

To get down, to get fixed, to get it over with. Get it out of my possession and into my vein, so that I can not only feel good, but I will not be arrested.

Although small amounts of drugs are sometimes available in some shooting galleries, most operators do not sell drugs on a regular basis. Often, short-term business arrangements are formed between street dealers and shooting-gallery operators, whereby the seller is allowed to set up shop in the gallery, in exchange for supplying the operator with drugs for personal use. The following illustrates the business arrangements between street dealers and gallery operators:

Gloria is a self-described "sack spitter," or seller of heroin. The term "sack spitter" comes from street dealers' propensity to keep their balloons of drugs [usually heroin] for sale in their mouth for easy swallowing, in the event of a police encounter. Gloria spits sacks in Peaches' shooting gallery in return for supplying Peaches with heroin and sometimes rocks [crack cocaine] for her personal use. Peaches is a transvestite who runs a shooting gallery in East Oakland.

This arrangement is mutually beneficial, in that it brings in customers for both, but such arrangements are usually short-lived, because, as word spreads on the street, informants apprise the police as well. Arrests or fear of arrest usually cause the seller to move on. Another pressure on these tenuous mergers is the asymmetrical nature of the relationship between the seller and the shooting-gallery operator (i.e., one has the drugs, and the other wants increasingly larger amounts of those drugs), which often results in arguments and the eventual dissolution of their business arrangements.

Drug sellers often direct IVDUs to neighborhood shooting galleries, because they do not want their customers hanging out and fixing at their places. Or, if they sell on the street, they provide potential injection locations as an added service to their customers.

People also go to shooting galleries when they need help injecting drugs or purchasing drugs. Some drug shooters have a very difficult time injecting themselves, because they have deep or collapsed veins and have trouble getting a "register" (drops of blood in the syringe that let the injector know he/she is in a vein). Often, there are street "docs" adept at injecting, who sell their skills (for money or drugs) in shooting galleries. The following description of Franny, taken from field notes, illustrates well the role of the street "doc" in the world of drug injectors.

Franny is a male transvestite prostitute, or drag-queen hustler, who lives and works in the Tenderloin district in San Francisco. She [Franny always refers to herself with feminine pronouns, and so shall we] also works part-time as a street doc, operating out of her home. "I just sit around the house, [waiting for drug injectors to come by] and I'm more or less the doctor, you know, I hit a lot of people, you know. When I hit, that means I administer drugs." Like conventional medical doctors, Franny specializes; her specialty is injecting addicts in the neck. "Well, I'm really good in the neck area, and everybody, everybody . . . asks me to go [inject] in their neck."

Franny's interest in injecting in the neck was stimulated by her difficulties in injecting herself and by the amount of money she could make providing this needed service to others. The following is a description, in her own words, of Franny's street internship in 1975 as a neck shooter:

> I started my hormone therapy . . . in '68 . . . I noticed that all my veins, and . . . muscle tone had been just . . . knocked out of place, they didn't show that much anymore. 'Cause . . . the female hormones had just made them vanish. So, that make me hard to hit my drugs and, uh, I always take me an hour or 45 minutes to hit myself when I can hit 10 or 20 people in 15 minutes. . . . So I was kind of displeased with that . . . so I saw this young girl, she was hitting people in the neck. She was telling me, all you had to do is turn their neck and blow. . . . I never would see her . . . like putting the needle in the person's neck, when I blink my eye, she be saying . . . "Okay, get up, I'm through." And she would have two or three people lined up . . . she was go [inject] one okay, two, just like that. And I said, "My God, let her hit me" 'cause I wanted to learn how. . . . All I can do is watch the thing real close . . . [because] I asked her, "Would you show me how it hit?" She didn't want to show me, see now if she showed me how to do the neck, I could have took all her customers, and I didn't know that she was getting this kind of money. She was getting like from each person 10 sometimes 15, 20 dollars. It depends on how much money the individual had, and the littlest she was going was five dollars. And I said, "Shit." I said . . . most of them are making a killing out there.

> This young fellow came in, and he was in a hurry and he had to go back to work. So he was saying, ". . . I brought my own drugs, I already got it in the syringe, all I want you to do is . . . hit me in my neck." So I said, "How much you got to spend?" So he said, "I got 10 dollars." . . . Now, go into the bathroom. Now, I never done this before, but like I said, I had been watching . . . this other person do it . . . I had him turn . . . face-to-face me and turn his head, he turned his head . . . I knew this was where

it was. You're supposed to always go a little bit to the right, passage, the blood vessel up close, you know, because that way you won't hit . . . like, all over your body you have two veins . . . your ingoing and your outgoing . . . that's the clean blood, so you really want to get to the dirty blood, so you have to be looking for your right. I got that information from her. I went on, felt . . . the pressure point and I . . . inserted the needle and pulled back on the plunger, and the blood, it just took, and there it was, and I took the syringe and pulled it out, and that's all. So, I knew I had it in, from that day on I was doing it. . . . Yes, I've been hitting in the neck for about 13, 14 years. So, you know I'm good. Excellent now.

Franny takes a lot of professional pride in her work, even to the extent of using what she considers to be professional expressions to describe injecting drugs. She doesn't say she shoots or slams or hits drugs; she talks about "administering" drugs. Franny does have a number of regular "patients," who come by one or more times a day for her services. During the course of our seven days of interviews with her, she averaged five customers a day for her specialty shooting gallery.

Aside from those shooters who experience difficulty, there are a few IVDUs who do not know how to inject themselves and rely on others to inject them. For example, for two weeks prior to the interview, one of our female respondents was forced to use shooting galleries, while her husband was in jail. After three years of intravenous drug use, she did not know how to inject herself. Shooting galleries provide such services for people who need assistance or do not know how to inject drugs.

As we mentioned earlier, most shooting-gallery operators do not sell drugs with any regularity. However, shooting galleries are good places to find folks who will go and purchase drugs, in return for a portion of the drugs they purchase. So, shooting galleries also serve the purpose of providing sources of drugs.

Additionally, shooting galleries serve as clearinghouses of information important to drug users. To illustrate this point, one user said:

> It is easy and it's like a social hall, you know; you go there to see people you know and sit there and do drugs together, and you sit there and talk.

Drug users, like other people, exchange information about the things that are consequential in their everyday life. Who has the dope, what the dope is like, where the dope seller can be found, and how to get the money to buy the dope are the main topics of discussion. People check in on a daily basis to get messages, connect with running partners, hear the latest gossip. Who has been arrested, who has been released from jail, the latest fights and alliances, all are topics of conversation. It is important to know which areas are currently most heavily patrolled by the police, so they can be avoided if at all possible. It is also of paramount interest to know who the snitches or police informants are, for they too must be avoided. As one respondent told us very succinctly, there are both practical and social reasons for using shooting galleries: ". . . to get loaded, to bullshit."

Finally, perhaps the most obvious reason why injectors go to shooting galleries is that they have no other place to inject drugs. Homeless drug users use shooting galleries, because they have no other safe (from police) place to inject drugs. Young users who live with their parents and cannot inject drugs in their homes are likely to use shooting galleries. Drug injectors who live with partners who are either unaware or disapproving of drug use are also likely to use shooting galleries. Users who are hustling and using together still may not trust each other enough to let their running partner know where they live, so they use shooting galleries as meeting places. One respondent summed it up well:

> 'Cause not everybody got a hotel room or not everybody can bring drug-crazed people to their house. I don't bring nobody here.

Hanging out in shooting galleries is also a way to get some free dope. A user who is down on his or her luck may go to a shooting gallery and wait for an associate to arrive and ask for a "taste," a small amount of drugs. In fact, the presence of sick or withdrawing addicts or moochers is one of the most common reasons given for not wanting to use shooting galleries. Addicts feel uncomfortable turning down pleas for drugs from fellow users. Or even more problematic, from their perspective, is having to share their drugs. This comment from a 38-year-old white male heroin and methedrine shooter from the Tenderloin district illustrates this well:

> There's just a bunch of bums laying up in a room waiting for someone to come up and leave them some dope.

A black heroin and cocaine seller from Oakland responded succinctly to our question about whether people go to shooting galleries for companionship:

> Some of them . . . but the bottom line is they come there to get a free high. . . . Now, the excuse why they are coming is "to visit," but the bottom line is they're gonna get a hit or get some dope or whatever. They come for a good reason, and that is to get high.

Although some galleries are predominantly for heroin shooters, most respondents reported that habitués of shooting galleries use a variety of drugs by a variety of methods. Cocaine is both injected and smoked in the same shooting galleries. Not all shooting galleries serve as crack houses, but some respondents, especially blacks and Latinos from Oakland, reported that heroin users were including cocaine smoking in their daily drug-use patterns. The following is a description from field notes of a shooting gallery that also serves as a rock house:

> Mama is an old black woman in Oakland who is somewhere between 60 and 70 years old and runs a shooting gallery. She is known universally among her clients as Mama. A 27-year-old Hispanic female heroin shooter describes what addicts call "Mama's house":

> "Okay, at this shooting gallery, people smoke [crack] there, so it is real dark. There's people on the floor, the table, and standing around. Half of them are smoking, the other half are shooting up. People are in the bathroom. It's kind of dark, some of the windows are broken. It smells all stinky. And most of the people . . . some of them are kind of moody. It's a scary place to go, but they know me."

Mama presides over it all. Although she is not known for her housekeeping skills, she is famous for her ability to inject prodigious amounts of drugs and, therefore, prefers kick-downs to money in payment for using her gallery.

"Speedballing" (shooting a mixture of cocaine and heroin) is a long-standing practice of addicts and other IVDUs. Many of our respondents had begun using cocaine and heroin regularly in recent months, due to their decrease in price. Today, it is not uncommon for a user to shoot heroin with cocaine and then buy some rock and smoke that as well. The following is a respondent's description of a shooting gallery in Oakland where the regulars speedball and smoke:

Everybody who comes through the door, they'll shoot the dope and then they'll come back five or six times. [There are] . . . pipes, matches, broken pipes, whole pipes, broken outfits, whole outfits. . . . They know there are rocks there and that there is heroin there, powder coke there, there's nothing there that someone doesn't use, okay.

Types of Shooting Galleries

In the only published account of shooting galleries to date, Des Jarlais et al. (1986) offer a very detailed ethnographic description of a New York City gallery that is said to be typical. The description is of a rather well-organized, formal arrangement with a regular operator and an assistant, a price list on the wall for the services provided, and regular monetary exchanges for rental of works and assistance with injection. In order to explore shooting galleries in the Bay Area, we decided to ask a series of questions to determine what the galleries are like there and how they compare with New York galleries. These questions were utilized to establish how galleries in the Bay Area operate:

1. Was there a regular operator or someone in charge?

2. Were prices fixed for various services?

3. How were services paid for, and what were the prices of services?

4. When was the gallery open for business?

5. How many persons used the gallery?

6. Could strangers go there?

7. How long had the gallery been operating?

Answers to these questions revealed that there are two types of shooting galleries—formal and informal. Formal galleries are characterized by a recognized operator or permanent resident who runs the gallery. The gallery may also be the place where the operator and others live, but its primary function is that of a place of business. In most instances, the business of the shooting gallery, and payments the operator receives in cash or in "tastes" (small portions) of drugs, are his main hustle or income-generating activity. Several outfits are usually available for rent and sometimes for sale. Shooters pay in drugs and/or money to use the premises, the outfits, and the injection services. The gallery is usually open 24 hours a day, and strangers are allowed in, if they are not suspect or are accompanied by someone who is known to the

operator or customers. Very often, syringes can be bought directly from the operators. Large numbers of people use this type of gallery, as many as two and three hundred.

Many formal shooting galleries operate around the clock. If a person has money or drugs, he/she will be admitted, regardless of the hour. Strangers are likely to be admitted if they come with someone who is known and they have drugs and/or money. Sometimes, operators of shooting galleries are unwilling to sell outfits. As one respondent explained:

A lot of times people don't want to sell them, 'cause they want you to have to use theirs, so they say, "I ain't got one for sale, but I got one you can use." Lending needles is their weak hustle.

In many instances, the operator serves as a street "doctor," who helps drug users who, for a variety of reasons, need assistance to inject their drugs.

Interviews with 48 different addicts and IVDUs revealed four accounts of shooting galleries that we would consider to be formal. One was described as being clean and well-furnished, and the operator charged a five-dollar entrance fee. Another had an enforcer who stayed near the door with a gun to keep out thieves, strangers, and persons who had worn out their welcome at the facility. Most accounts by respondents were of informal arrangements.

An informal shooting gallery or drug house has no "paid staff," only a resident who is "kicked down"—given drugs or money out of courtesy. Generally, only people known to the resident are allowed to inject there. Of course, as in other kinds of social situations, consistently discourteous guests may not be allowed in. There may also be sets of works available for use for a "taste," if the borrower has enough to share. Informal galleries have more intermittent hours of operation, usually only when the resident/owner is home, awake, and interested in using. The operation of the informal shooting gallery is not the resident's main hustle, though it may serve to tide him or her over during lean periods. The space is primarily the operator's home and only secondarily serves as a hangout for users.

Who Uses Shooting Galleries?

By no means do all IVDUs frequent shooting galleries on a regular basis. Almost all of the respondents said that they preferred to inject drugs in the privacy of their own home. Shooting galleries can be and often are noisy, busy places with people laughing, talking, and arguing—lots of arguing over money and drugs, for the most part. Addicts with a lucrative hustle or a steady job are less likely to utilize shooting galleries regularly. The exigencies of the drug-using lifestyle deplete most users' resources at various times in their careers, so they tend to use shooting galleries during these periods. There are, of course, some addicts who are always poverty-stricken.

People use shooting galleries most frequently when they are temporarily without funds or a way to make money to buy drugs. If one's lifestyle consists of hustling then fixing, hustling then fixing, all day long, there may not be time to go home and fix and then go out to hustle. The following exchange between interviewer and interviewee describes this:

> (I) That's a good point you brought up. Would you say that it is normal that people will start using shooting galleries when they start hitting bottom [are at the end of their available resources]?

> (R) Yeah, sure. Because the reason for it is, you usually don't have the money and you're scooting to get the money and, if you have something else to do, you have to fit it into what you are doing. And, if you have to fit in what you're doing, you're cutting into your time. . . . I mean, you can't jump in and run home and fix. If you see a guy across the street, you're going to say, "Hey, gang, let's go do it." That's how that goes.

Several respondents told us there is one type of hustler more likely to be found in shooting galleries, and that is female prostitutes. Prostitutes working the streets are especially vulnerable to street searches and arrests. They are, therefore, understandably reluctant to carry injection equipment with them, while working. Drug-using prostitutes often work for drugs and need drugs to work (Rosenbaum 1981). Shooting galleries near prostitution areas have a high percentage of prostitutes among their clientele. A 35-year-old white male heroin and cocaine shooter describes the last shooting gallery he went to and in the process talks about prostitutes' usage of shooting galleries:

> It is always kind of loud and chaotic. Sometimes, the house would be just empty and real quiet. Then all of a sudden, all the prostitutes come back from making their money, and this guy comes in with his, and all of a sudden, it would be loud and chaotic. . . .

That's how it goes all day long; whores coming in and out after they make their money.

Shooting galleries, for the most part, are pretty well-integrated racially. Unlike other service facilities, race and ethnicity do not serve as barriers to entry. Respondents described a wide variety of types of users who go to shooting galleries. As one Latino male heroin addict explained, "Drugs have no barriers." Blacks, whites, and Latinos all were reported using the same shooting galleries. Different San Francisco neighborhoods would have a predominance of one ethnicity over another (Tenderloin, mostly white; the Mission, Latino; and Hunter's Point, blacks). But most respondents reported a mixture of ethnicities among shooting-gallery clienteles.

For the most part, injectors use shooting galleries sporadically over their entire drug-injecting careers. They are more likely to use shooting galleries when they are not doing very well financially. Although the galleries reflect the ethnicity of their geographic location, they are usually integrated, with multiple ethnicities represented among customers.

Needle Hygiene in Shooting Galleries

Needle hygiene was not an important priority in these drug users' lives, even though they all knew that bleach was a good antiseptic solution for HIV. Few respondents reported using bleach themselves or observing other injectors in shooting galleries using bleach. There was one noteworthy exception: the shooting gallery that was the most expensive, five dollars a visit, was also described as a place where bleach was used with some frequency. Other shooting galleries had bleach available, but our respondents reported that it was seldom used.

For the most part, respondents used only water to clean their needles and syringes. In many of the shooting galleries that were described to us, there was no on-site source of water. Shooting gallery operators would use outside garden taps or service-station restrooms for water sources and would store water in jugs or old soda bottles. Most often the water was not boiled, so there were, in fact, few sterilization practices. We would like to illustrate the lack of antiseptic practices with another quote about Mama's. Mama does not have bleach or alcohol available in her shooting gallery, and, if she has syringes, they are old and broken. The same Latino describes the condition of Mama's injection equipment:

> I'll ask her if she has got any alcohol or anything. She usually doesn't have nothing, and I just use water. But if she has got it, I'll use it. . . . Sometimes, she doesn't have any [syringes]. She never has any new ones, they're all old and dirty.

Interviewees were hard pressed to explain why they and fellow users were not using bleach, even on the occasions when it was available to them. Interviewers were struck by respondents' fatalism. Users often said, "I probably already have it" [AIDS]. Or when describing other users' practices, they would say they "just don't give a shit." Impoverished drug users have very little control or power over most areas of their lives, and health is no exception. They never know from one day to the next whether there will be drugs available or whether they will be able to come up with the money necessary to obtain them. They lead a chaotic and capricious lifestyle, where they may be jailed any day at any time and whatever possessions they have managed to accumulate will be lost. Chaos and fatalism permeate their world view. The idea that their own behavior can, in fact, protect them from sickness and suffering does not fit with their previous life experiences.

Summary

Shooting galleries in the Bay Area are numerous and take a variety of forms. Some resemble the formal and structured facilities described as operating in New York City (Des Jarlais, Friedman, and Strug 1986), but most are informal places developed by impoverished but experienced drug users as a "weak hustle," a way to earn small amounts of money and/or drugs by providing a basic service in considerable demand. Proprietors of shooting galleries have the following resources: space, a network of potential customers, some supply of syringes and outfits to inject drugs, and certain injection skills to assist individuals who have difficulties injecting their own drugs.

Formal shooting galleries are characterized by a primary orientation to business; they charge specific fees for services, primarily monetary exchanges; they are usually open 24 hours a day; they have an open policy as regards strangers; and gallery operation is the principal hustle of the operator. Informal galleries are more social and less business-like; operators (street docs) are usually paid in "kick-downs" of drugs, rather than in cash; strangers usually cannot use these facilities; the hours of operation are usually intermittent; and the operator usually does not conceive of his role as a regular money-generating activity, but rather as a "weak hustle" or short-term activity. If one were to operationalize the term "shooting gallery," one would have to consider the two types and the difference in their operations to make the term meaningful.

Shooting galleries serve several functions for intravenous drug users. First and foremost, they are relatively safe places to "get high," where syringes are available, if needed. They are usually convenient to copping areas and/or are located near drug sellers. Many customers use them as a temporary way station between their connection and home. Others use them, because they do not have a private place where they can inject themselves, or they lack the skill to do it effectively. They also serve social functions. Many addicts go to shooting galleries on a regular basis to meet friends and associates, to "bullshit," and to share information about their world.

Most persons who go to shooting galleries are intravenous drug users who are experiencing problems supporting their drug use and/or are relatively incompetent as hustlers. Very often, they go to solicit "tastes" from other users who have the drug. Other users go, because they do not have a private place to shoot drugs—they are homeless or are living with parents or with someone who disapproves of their drug use. Another group who use shooting galleries regularly are persons who do not know how to inject themselves, or are having difficulties doing it and need assistance from a street "doc." Prostitutes are also said to be regular users of shooting galleries.

Des Jarlais and his associates (1985, 1987) have stated that shooting galleries are an integral part of addict lifestyles in New York, but in the Bay Area they seem to be so for impoverished addicts, but not necessarily for capable or affluent addicts.

Shooting galleries, either formal or informal, are firmly entrenched in the world of impoverished and less affluent IVDUs. They serve important functions and services for users, most particularly so long as possession of needles is illegal and police often arrest addicts under paraphernalia laws. At the same time, they are also sites where HIV can be spread. Furthermore, very few of the galleries we discovered use antiseptic procedures or bleach.

* * *

Sheigla Murphy and Dan Waldorf, "Kickin' Down to the Street Doc: Shooting Galleries in the San Francisco Bay Area." Reprinted from *Contemporary Drug Problems* 18:9-29, 1991. Copyright © 1991 by *Contemporary Drug Problems*. All rights reserved. Reprinted by permission.

For Discussion

What would be the implications if local communities established major initiatives to eliminate shooting galleries?

References

Battjes, R. J., and Pickens, R. W. (eds.). 1988. "Introduction." *Needle Sharing Among Intravenous Drug Abusers: National and International Perspectives*, NIDA Research Monograph #80, Washington, DC: USGPO.

Biernacki, P., and Waldorf, D. 1981. "Snowball Sampling: Problems, Techniques, and Chain-Referral Sampling." *Sociological Methods and Research 10*(2):141-163.

Cohen, H., Marmor, M., and Des Jarlais, D. 1985. "Behavioral Risk Factors for HTLV-III/LAV Seropositivity Among Intravenous Drug Abusers." Paper presented at the International Conference on Acquired Immunodeficiency Syndrome (AIDS), Atlanta, GA: April 14-17.

Des Jarlais, D., Friedman, S., and Hopkins, W. 1985. "Risk Reduction for the Acquired Immunodeficiency Syndrome (AIDS) Among Intravenous Drug Users." *Annals of Internal Medicine 103*:755-759.

Des Jarlais, D., Friedman, S., and Strug, D. 1986. "AIDS and Needle Sharing Within the IV Drug-Use Subculture." In D. Feldman and T. Johnson (eds.), *The Social Dimensions of AIDS: Methods and Theory*. New York: Praeger: 141-160.

Des Jarlais, D., and Friedman, S. 1987. "HIV Infection Among Intravenous Drug Users: Epidemiology and Risk Reduction." *AIDS 1*(2):67-76.

Feldman, H., and Biernacki, P. 1988. "The Ethnography of Needle Sharing Among Intravenous Drug Users and Implications for Public Policies and Intervention Strategies." In R. J. Battjes and R. W. Pickens (eds.), *Needle Sharing Among Intravenous Drug Abusers: National and International Perspectives*, NIDA Research Monograph #80, Washington, DC: USGPO: 28-39.

Friedman, S., Des Jarlais, D., Sothran, J., Garber, J., Cohen, H., and Smith, D. 1987. "AIDS and Self-Organization Among Intravenous Drug Users." *International Journal of the Addictions 62*(3):201-219.

Hopkins, W. 1988. "Needle Sharing and Street Behavior in Response to AIDS in New York City." In R. J. Battjes and R. W. Pickens (eds.), *Needle Sharing Among Intravenous Drug Abusers National and International Perspectives*, NIDA Research Monograph #80, Washington, DC: USGPO: 18-27.

Howard, J., and Borges, P. 1977. "Needle Sharing in the Haight: Some Social and Psychological Functions." In D. Smith and G. Gay (eds.), *It's So Good Don't Even Try It Once: Heroin in Perspective*. Englewood Cliffs, NJ: Prentice-Hall, Inc.: 29-42.

Murphy, S. 1987. "Intravenous Drug Use and AIDS: Notes on the Social Economy of Needle Sharing." *Contemporary Drug Problems 14*(3):373-410.

Power, R. M. 1988. "The Influence of AIDS Upon Patterns of Intravenous Drug Use—Syringe and Needle Sharing—Among Illicit Drug Users in Britain." In R. J. Battjes and R. W. Pickens (eds.), *Needle Sharing Among Intravenous Drug Abusers: National and International Perspectives*, NIDA Research Monograph #80, Washington, DC: USGPO: 75-88.

Rosenbaum, M. 1981. *Women on Heroin*. New Brunswick, NJ: Rutgers University Press.

Waldorf, D., Murphy, S., Lauderbach, D., Reinarman, C., and Marotta, T. 1990. "Needle Sharing Among Male Prostitutes: Preliminary Findings of the Prospero Project." *Journal of Drug Issues 20*(2):309-334.

Watters, J. 1987. "Preventing Human Immunodeficiency Virus Contagion Among Intravenous Drug Users: The Impact of Street-Based Education on Risk-Reduction Behavior." Paper presented at the Third International Conference on AIDS, Washington, DC, June.

Weiss, S., Ginzburg, H., and Goedert, J. 1985. "Risk for HTLV-III Exposure and AIDS Among Parenteral Drug Abusers in New Jersey." Paper presented at the International Conference on the Acquired Immunodeficiency Syndrome (AIDS), Atlanta, GA, April 14-17. ✦

31. The Risk of Exposure to HIV-Contaminated Needles and Syringes in Shooting Galleries

JAMES A. INCIARDI,
J. BRYAN PAGE,
DUANE C. MCBRIDE,
DALE D. CHITWOOD,
CLYDE B. MCCOY,
H. VIRGINIA MCCOY,
AND
EDWARD TRAPIDO

The following study by James A. Inciardi and his colleagues in Miami combines a variety of data, including observations in shooting galleries and interviews with injection drug users. Most interestingly, the authors collected needles and syringes from three large shooting galleries in the Miami area. Laboratory analyses found many of the needle/syringe combinations to be infected with HIV. The authors estimated the probabilities of exposure to HIV-contaminated injection equipment, depending on the frequency of injection in shooting galleries, and found that the likelihood of exposure was quite high. Further, they discovered some contamination, even when needles and syringes appeared to be clean. Based on this study's findings, the authors suggest methods to facilitate risk reduction.

Background

Since it was first described in 1981, the acquired immune deficiency syndrome (AIDS) has been concentrated in the United States among people who engage in certain high-risk behaviors. Intravenous and other injection drug users (IDUs) represent the second highest risk group after gay and bisexual men (Centers for Disease Control 1993), and comprise an increasing percentage of all new AIDS cases. According to Centers for Disease Control (CDC) estimates, since October 1988, more than a fourth of all newly reported AIDS cases have been injection drug users. Furthermore, among blacks and Hispanics with AIDS, well over a third are IDUs. Epidemiologic studies have documented that the prevalence of antibodies to human immunodeficiency virus (HIV)—the causative agent of AIDS—among various populations of IDUs ranges as high as 70 percent, (Chaisson et al. 1987) and is likely increasing.

Although HIV is also sexually trasmitted among IDUs, the sharing and/or pooling of contaminated needles and other drug-related paraphernalia has been well-documented as a major mechanism of HIV transmission (Chitwood 1985; Chitwood et al. 1989; Chitwood et al. 1990). The intravenous administration of heroin, cocaine, and other drugs typically includes a practice known within drug subcultures as "booting." The practice involves the aspiration of venous blood back into a syringe for the purpose of mixing the drug with blood, while the needle remains inserted in the vein. The mixed blood/drug solution is then injected back into the vein. IDUs value the mixing of blood for various reasons: some repeated pumping and drawing back of the blood-drug mix allows the user to titrate the dose and avoid overdose or the full effects of drug contamination; the drawing of blood into the syringe also indicates that the needle has hit a usable vein; some believe that this "pre-mixing" enhances a drug's effects. Since IDUs often inject with needles and syringes previously used by others, particularly if they are administering the drugs in "shooting galleries" (places where drug users gather to take drugs), booting increases the probability that traces of HIV will remain in a syringe to be transmitted to the next user.

Research and clinical observation suggest that "booting," the use of shooting galleries, and the sharing of needles combine to explain the increasing proportion of IDUs infected with HIV (Chitwood et al. 1989; Curran et al. 1988). Little is known, however, about the prevalence of HIV antibodies in needle/syringe combinations utilized by IV drug users (Des Jarlais et al. 1985). Using the findings of Chitwood et al. (1990) as a framework, this paper computes an IDU's probability of selecting a needle contaminated with HIV when using needle/syringe combinations in the shooting galleries studied. Ethnographic findings about patterns of needle use taken from field observations (cf. Page et al. 1990; Page, Smith, and Kane 1990) and open ended interviews elaborate on the likelihood of contaminated exposure in Miami "get-offs" (shooting galleries).

Currently Florida is considered a "high prevalence" state in terms of the cumulative numbers of the disease reported to the CDC since 1981. Almost one-third of these cases were diagnosed in the Miami-Dade SMSA. In addition, Miami is well known as the drug "import capital" of North America, a situation that has resulted in high rates of drug use in general, and injection drug use in particular (Gould et al. 1974; Hanson et al. 1985; Inciardi 1987; Inciardi 1979).

In most urban locales where rates of injection drug use are high, common sites for injecting drugs (and sometimes purchasing drugs) are known in street jargon as neighborhood get-off houses. After purchasing heroin, cocaine, amphetamines, or some other injectable substance in a local "copping" (drug selling) area, users are faced with three logistical problems (cf. Agar 1973): how to get off the street quickly to avoid arrest for possession of drugs, where to obtain a set of "works" (drug paraphernalia) with which to administer the drugs, and where to find a safe place to "get off" (inject the drugs). As such, get-off houses occupy a functional niche in the world of IV drug abuse, where for a fee of two or three dollars users can rent a set of "works" and relax while "getting off" (Inciardi and Pottieger 1986). After using a syringe and needle the user generally returns them to a central storage place in the get-off house where they are held until someone else rents them. The abundance of disposable syringes at get-off houses in South Florida has resulted in more pooling (where each user is given a syringe by the manager, or "house man" and the works are rotated from a central storage container) and less sharing (passing works from one user to another).

Methods

Information presented here comes from three basic sources; direct observations of needle using behavior in Miami get-offs, 40 open-ended interviews with active IDUs, and laboratory analyses of needles collected from three get-offs for presence of HIV antibody. The first source required field observers to gain entry into local get-off houses with the help of a cultural guide, usually a participant in a longitudinal ethnographic study of active IDUs. As observers, the field ethnographers who visited get-offs paid standard entry fees (not more than $5 per person) for the privilege of being allowed to observe injection behavior. They explained the purpose of their visit, and assured confidentiality of what they were to witness. If a client raised objections to their presence, the observers left without making observations.

The second source of information comes from 40 open-ended interviews on needle use conducted with active IDUs. The research team recruited interviewees from 230 participants in a longitudinal study of active IDUs (cf. Page et al. 1990). The purpose of the interviews was to explore the system of values and thought processes underlying intravenous drug use with relation to the individual's interaction with the needle during the course of his/her life. The investigators attempted in selecting interviewees to cover the range of variation in the study population, choosing half males and half females, half baseline HIV seropositive (hereafter, Ab+) and half seronegative, and as wide a range as possible of lifestyles and shooting patterns (from regularly employed once-a-week shooters to unemployed, ten-a-day shooters). Since these interviews were intended to provide descriptive information on a variation of shooting patterns and the values and beliefs that underlie them, they were not subjected to statistical analysis of responses.

Both the observations and the interviews were tape recorded and transcribed verbatim into word processing files. The field observers coded these materials for retrievability and indexed them for quick scanning with the help of Zyindex software. Scanning capabilities allowed rapid search for specific content areas that could then be arrayed and inspected for patterns. Results of some of these analyses appear in Page (1990).

The third source of information, laboratory analysis of syringe/needle sets collected from Miami get-offs, is material reported in Chitwood et al. (1990). A single street outreach worker collected all sets from all sites, and was able to do so based on a combination of his own established rapport with house proprietors as an ex-shooter and the rapport established by the other field workers in the course of the longitudinal project. The tests conducted in the laboratory were only possible on still usable syringes, and they detected only the presence of traces of blood with HIV antibody.

Study Sites

Based on the investigators' knowledge of the Miami-Dade drug scene and the mapping of get-off locations through interviews with IDUs recruited for a variety of research projects, three particular get-offs were selected for collection of needles. All three were popular galleries in different geographical sectors of Miami.

Site 1 was a three bedroom house operated as a shooting gallery since 1982 and as a "base house" for the sale and smoking of crack-cocaine since 1985. *Site 2* was a one bedroom apartment in a two-family structure operated as a shooting gallery continuously since 1973. *Site 3* was a single room apartment in a 14-unit complex established only recently as both a shooting gallery and base house.

The three sites were located along a 15-mile arc, stretching from the vicinity of downtown Miami to the city's northwestern edge. Furthermore, the houses were located in areas having the county's highest rates of both drug use and crime (Inciardi 1979). According to U.S. Bureau of Census data, these areas were also characterized by high rates of unemployment, poor housing, infant mortality, teenage pregnancy, and low educational attainment. While a complete listing of Miami's get-offs was not available for a random selection of study sites, the location and neighborhood contexts of those chosen reflected settings typical of those described by sociologists and anthropologists in their discussions of street drug use (Inciardi and Pottieger 1986; Jackson et al. 1988; Jain et al. 1988).

Evidence of HIV infection is usually determined indirectly through standard tests for the presence of antibodies to HIV. An antibody is a protein in the blood produced in response to exposure to specific foreign molecules. The presence of any given antibodies in the blood against viruses that cause acute diseases indicates that a previous infection registered on the body's immune system, or that a vaccine elicited an appropriate antibody response. The Chitwood et al. (1990) study looked for the presence of HIV antibodies as evidence of infection.

Although the number of customers frequenting these galleries tended to vary from one day to the next, Table I demonstrates that there were no apparent directions in seropositivity rates detected in syringe/needle sets by day of the week.

Discussion

In Miami-Dade and elsewhere, get-offs have never been systematically studied. Nevertheless, based on the investigators' observations combined with reports from a variety of ethnographic and other research studies in drug communities in several parts of the United States (Inciardi and Pottieger 1986; Jackson et al. 1988; Jain et al. 1988; Johnson et al. 1985; Lowenstein et al. 1988;

McBride and McCoy 1981) their more obvious roles and characteristics can be described.

Table I
Seropositivity Rates by Day of the Week

Day	Total Cases	% Seropositive
Sunday	16	12.5
Monday	7	14.3
Tuesday	19	10.5
Wednesday	32	9.4
Thursday	29	10.3
Friday	26	7.7
Saturday	19	5.3

$x2 = 1.1$
p .98
$V = .09$

Get-offs and the Injection Drug User

Get-offs are situated in basements and backrooms in the rundown sections of cities where drug use rates are high. Typically, they are only sparsely furnished and cleanliness is absent. Moreover, they are run by drug dealers, drug users, and user-dealers. Neighborhood heroin and/or cocaine dealers may operate get-offs as a service to customers—providing them with a nearby location to safely "shoot up" for just a few dollars. More often, however, gallery operators are drug users who provide a service for a small fee or a "taste" of someone else's drugs.

For the majority of IDUs, get-offs are considered to be the least desirable places to patronize. Most prefer to use their own homes or apartments or those of drug-using friends. These are considered safer than galleries, and there are few users who appreciate having to pay a fee to use someone else's drug paraphernalia. Yet for a minority of hard core IV users, there is the matter of personal hygiene. As one heroin user summed it up:

> Galleries ain't where it's at. We wasn't brought up like that. They be definitely hardcore junkies and they don't give a damn no more about how their appearance is or nothing like that. Ain't nobody want to give another two dollars. Their works . . . all dirty, man. An' people be shootin' blood all over you. (Jackson et al. 1988)

Nevertheless, for many IDUs, the use of get-offs is routine and commonplace. Moreover, there are repeated occasions in the lives of all IDUs, including the most hygienically fastidious types, when get-offs become necessary. If they have no "works" of their own, or if friends or other "running partners" have no works, then a neighborhood gallery is the only recourse. Similarly, users who purchase drugs far from home also gravitate toward get-offs. This tendency is based on the heightened risk of arrest when carrying drugs and drug paraphernalia over long stretches. The gallery operator also often serves as a middleman between drug user and drug dealer, thus making the "get-off" house the locus of exchange. For example, as one Miami heroin user explained it in 1988:

> OK, let's say I'm white, but the only place I can "cop" some "smack" [heroin] is in the black neighborhoods, but I'm afraid that I'll be "ripped off" [robbed] there. But then there's this gallery an' I know the man there, he's "right" [trusted] by the buyers and sellers. So I go there an' he "cops" for me for a few dollars and maybe a "taste." For another $3 I can use his "works" and house to lay up in for a little while. (Page and Smith 1990)

And finally, there are a few IDUs who actually *prefer* local galleries because of the opportunities they provide to socialize with other drug users. In short, despite their unsavory character, get-offs occupy a functional niche in the street worlds of intravenous drug-taking and drug-seeking.

Get-offs and HIV Contagion

Within this context, it would appear that given the findings of this study, get-offs represent a significant health problem as far as the spread of the HIV infection is concerned. The operators of the galleries studied here reported that each serviced an average of 125 IDUs per week, with many of the clients visiting more than once.

In a further attempt to understand the potential health risk of using needles and syringes in get-offs, data are presented in Table 2 suggesting the probability of encountering an Ab+ needle/syringe, given a 10.1 percent seropositivity rate and when "shooting up" one to five times a day. These probabilities must be examined with caution, however, for they were computed on the basis of two assumptions:

1. an equal distribution of a 10.1 percent positivity rate across sites and days of the week (since Tables 1 and 2 indicated no significant differences by site or day of week); and,

2. a user's random selection of needles and syringes at the shooting gallery.

On the latter assumption, although there are no studies reported in the literature describing needle selection patterns, observations by members of the research team combined with reports from IDUs in the Miami area suggest that for the most part the process is indeed random. In some cases "works" are kept in a bucket or lying on a table at some convenient location in the gallery. Under these circumstances, the user has some opportunity for examining a needle/syringe, but the typical selection is based on sharpness rather than cleanliness. As a 24-year-old cocaine user commented early in 1989:

> Most don't really care what the needle looks like. If it's sharp and the plunger moves, that's all they care about.

In other situations the "gimmick" is handed out by the gallery operator, and hence, the observation, examination, and selection of the gallery's full stock of needles and syringes is difficult. Observations and reports underscore that an initially selected or provided needle may be replaced by another if it appears dull or clogged. As such, the assumption of pure mathematical randomness may be unreasonable here, but for the sake of providing baseline data it was made for the first set of probabilities.

Not only for these assumptions must the data be interpreted with caution, but in addition, research has not as yet demonstrated the precise relationship between using an HIV-contaminated needle and becoming infected. The presence of the virus itself or its condition were not analyzed—*only the presence of antibodies*. Nevertheless, it appears important to examine the implications of the base rate of seropositivity for risk of exposure in attempting to understand the high seropositivity rates among IV drug users.

Table II
Number of Days Before There Is a 90 Percent Probability of a Seropositive Needle/Syringe Encounter at Varying Frequencies of Injection

1x per day	22 days
2x per day	11 days
3x per day	7 days
4x per day	5 days
5x per day	4 days

The data in Table II are derived from a calculation of the probability term $(1 - p)^n$ where $1 - p$ is the likelihood of *not* encountering an HIV contaminated on a single injection experience, and n is the number of times the behavior is repeated. The data indicate that given the assumptions of randomness and a 10.1 percent likelihood of needle/syringe contamination, a user shooting up just once a day in a gallery would have a 90 percent chance of encountering an HIV contaminated needle/syringe (or 10 percent likelihood of *not* encountering one) within 22 days. Shooting up three times a day in a gallery (and using a different needle each time) reduces the number of days to seven, and shooting up five times a day further reduces the time for a seropositive encounter to within four days. We should point out that, depending on the drug used and the personal schedule of the user, those who shoot more than once a day could be using the same needle more than once a day. A cocaine shooter, for example, may come in for three quick hits on a single occasion, using the same house-issued needle all three times.

Table III

Number of Days Before There Is a 90 Percent Probability of a Seropositive Needle/Syringe Encounter at Varying Frequencies of Injection when Selecting Drug Paraphernalia with "No Visible Blood"

1x per day	44 days
2x per day	22 days
3x per day	15 days
4x per day	11 days
5x per day	9 days

The data reported by Chitwood et al. (1990) indicated a significant relationship between the visual appearance of the needle/syringe and the presence of HIV antibodies. Only five percent of the "clean-appearing" needles were positive for HIV antibodies (Chitwood et al. 1990). Within this context, the probabilities reported in Table 2 were recomputed, based on the assumption that a cautious user might select only those "works" appearing to be "clean" (having *no visible blood* or dirt). As indicated in Table III, these computations demonstrate that even when choosing an apparently "safe" needle/syringe, the 90 percent probability of an encounter with traces of HIV Ab+ blood occurs within 44 days for

those one-a-day shooters shooting up in get-offs. As such, even the choice of the apparently "lowest risk" needle/syringe yields a high probability of encountering the human immunodeficiency virus within a relatively short period of time.

Comment

The 10.1 percent seropositivity rate and the high probability of encountering an HIV-contaminated needle/syringe in a shooting gallery may help to understand the high rates of HIV infection among IDUs being reported in the literature (Chaisson et al. 1987; Chitwood 1985; Chitwood et al. 1989; Chitwood et al. 1990). But the existence of get-offs across the urban landscape combined with the drug-taking behaviors of intravenous drug users poses a dilemma. Although virtually all IDUs are aware of AIDS and the risk of infection through needle sharing, there is a substantial group of IDUs among whom the prevention messages are either not being heard or are not listened to.

The problem is that heroin and cocaine are highly involving drugs. For those dependent on them, heroin and cocaine become life consuming. They become mother, father, spouse, lover, counselor, confessor, and confidant. Since they are short-acting drugs, they must be taken regularly and repeatedly. Because there is a more rapid onset and a more powerful euphoric "high" when taken by injection, most heroin users and a growing number of cocaine users inject their drugs. Collectively, these attributes result in a majority of chronic users more concerned with drug-taking and drug-seeking than with any other aspect of their existence. As such, it would appear that altering the risky needle-using behaviors of drug consumers might be difficult. Or as one IV cocaine-using prostitute summed it up to a member of the research team at the close of 1988:

> Every day I risk my health, and my life for that matter, when I shoot up. Every time I go out to "cop" [buy drugs] I risk getting "cut" [stabbed] or even killed. Every time I'm "strolling" [walking the streets soliciting clients] at night, there are all kinds of crazies, geeks, thugs, and death freaks out there just waiting to carve up my ass. Now they say that if I use some dirty needle I can get sick, even die in a few years. So I care? I'm probably *already* dead. Why should I care?

In other words, it is difficult to prevent behavior that may cause sickness and death in two or five years or more when the injection drug user is confronted with violence, sickness, and death almost every day; it is difficult to motivate behaviors aimed at preventing death in the future within a population already at high risk of imminent death.

The finding that HIV antibodies were present in 10.1 percent of the needle/syringe combinations tends to be at odds with contentions about needle-cleaning by the operators of the three galleries studied. *All* claimed that *all* of their needles and syringes were cleaned after each use. At Sites 1 and 3, cleaning was reportedly accomplished by running water through each needle and syringe, then bleach, and then water. At Site 2 the same method was used but with isopropyl alcohol instead of bleach. Upon further inquiry, however, it was found that the cleaning process at all three locations was unsystematic. On some occasions the gallery operators cleaned the paraphernalia, while on others customers were provided with a "taste" or a place to sleep in return for a day's worth of needle cleaning. Most of the time, however, cleaning was the responsibility of each client after his or her use of a set of "works." Invariably, the needle cleaning process was either abbreviated or ignored. House men are widely variable in their approach to enforcing cleaning rules. In one observed site, people were "skeeting" rinse water into the jar designated for drug mixing ("clean water"). In another house, the house man required clients to use new syringes and break them when they were finished.

All of this suggests that AIDS risk reduction among IV drug users is an intractable problem that cannot be dealt with effectively through conventional AIDS prevention messages. Nevertheless, several studies (Kaplan, Morival, and Sterk 1986; Ljungsburg et al. 1988; Robertson, Skidmore, and Roberts 1988; Stimson 1989) have indicated that IDUs are receptive to efforts to modify self injection behaviors. These studies relied heavily on self report of changing attitudes, however, and they also lacked (with the exception of Robertson, Skidmore and Roberts 1988) longitudinal perspective. Ethnographic perspective on risk behaviors involving needle use in get-offs indicates that there may be discrepancies between attitude and practice (Page, Smith, and Kane 1990; Rettig et al. 1977). Risk reduction must therefore involve vigorous outreach (i.e. monetary inducements for participation in HIV testing and counseling programs, contact of IDUs through street based networks of active drug users, and culturally sensitive approaches to intervention)

into the IV drug using community combined with strategies for making the needle cleaning process an integral part of intravenous drug taking in the places where it is practiced (Robert-Guroff et al. 1986).

✳ ✳ ✳

References

Agar, Michael 1973. Ripping and Running. New York: Viking Press.

Centers for Disease Control 1993. HIV/AIDS Surveillance. Center for Disease Control, September.

Chaisson, Richard, A. Moss, R. Onishi, D. Osmond, and J. Carlson 1987. Human Immunodeficiency Virus Infection in Heterosexual Intravenous Drug Users in San Francisco. American Journal Public Health 77:169-172.

Chitwood, Dale D. 1985. Patterns and Consequences of Cocaine Use. In Cocaine Use in America: Epidemiologic and Clinical Perspectives. Kozel MS, Adams EH, eds. Pp. 111-129. Maryland: National Institute on Drug Abuse.

Chitwood, Dale, Clyde B. McCoy, James Inciardi, Duane McBride, Mary Comerford, Edward Trapido, H. Virginia McCoy, J. Bryan Page, James Griffin, Mary Ann Fletcher and Margarita Ashman 1990. HIV Seropositivity of Needles from Shooting Galleries in South Florida. American Journal Public Health 80:1-3.

Curran, J., H. Jaffe, A. Hardy, W. Morgan, R. Selik, and T. Dondero 1988. Epidemiology of HIV infection and AIDS in the United States. Science 239:610-616.

Des Jarlais, Don C., Samuel Friedman, and Wayne Hopkins 1985. Risk Reduction for Acquired Immunodeficiency Syndrome Among Intravenous Drug Users. Annals Internal Medicine 103:755-759.

Fiddle, S. 1967. Portraits from a Shooting Gallery. New York: Harper and Row.

Gould, L., A. Walker, L. Crane, and C. Lidz 1974. Connections: Notes from the Heroin World. New Haven: Yale University Press.

Hanson, B., G. Beschner, J. Watters, and E. Boville1985. Life With Heroin: Voices from the Inner City. Massachusetts: D.C. Heath.

Inciardi, James A.1987. Beyond Cocaine: Basuco, Crack and other Coca Products. Contemporary Drug Problems 14:461-492.

Inciardi, James A. 1979. Heroin Use and Street Crime. Crime and Delinquency 25: 335-346.

Inciardi, James A., and A. Pottieger 1986. Drug Use and Crime Among Two Cohorts of Women Narcotics Users: An Empirical Assessment. Journal Drug Issues 16:91-106.

Jackson, J., L. Rothkiewitz, D. Wells 1988. IVDU AIDS Knowledge and Behavioral Change. Presentation at the IV International Conference on AIDS. Stockholm: Sweden Abstract # 8007.

Jain, Unita, N. Flynn, V. Bailey, R. Anderson, S. Harper, B. Siegel, and N. Levi 1988. IV Drug Users and AIDS: Changing Attitudes and Behavior. Presentation at the IV International Conference on AIDS. Stockholm: Sweden Abstract #8003.

Johnson, Bruce, P. Goldstein, E. Preble, J. Schmeidler, D. Lipton, B. Spunt, and T. Miller 1985. Taking Care of Business: The Economics of Crime by Heroin Users. Massachusetts: D.C. Heath.

Ljungberg Bjorn, B. Andersson, B. Christensson 1988. Distribution of Sterile Equipment to IV Drug Abusers as Part of an HIV Prevention Program. IV International Conference on AIDS, Stockholm, June.

Stimson, George V. 1989. Syringe-exchange Programmes for Injecting Drug Users. AIDS 3:253:260.

Kaplan, Charles D., M. Morival, C. Sterk 1986. Needle-exchange, IV Drug Users and Street IV Drug Users: A Comparison of Background Characteristics, Needle and Sex Practices, and AIDS Attitudes. NIDA, Community Epidemiology Work Group Proceedings.

Robertson, Roy, C. Skidmore, J.J.K. Roberts 1988. HIV Infection in Intravenous Drug Users: A follow-up Study Indicating Changes in Risk Taking Behavior. British Journal of the Addictions 83:387-391.

Lowenstein, William, H. Durand, M. Stern, J. Tourani, and P. Even 1988. Changes of Behaviors in French IV Drug Addicts (IVDA). Presentation at the IV International Conference on AIDS. Stockholm: Abstract #8009.

McBride, Duane C., and Clyde McCoy 1981. Crime and Drug Using Behavior: An Area Analysis. Criminology 19:281-302.

Page, J. Bryan 1990. Shooting Scenarios. American Behavioral Scientist 33(4):478-490

Page, J. Bryan, Prince C. Smith, and Normie Kane 1990. Shooting Galleries, their Proprietors, and Implications for Prevention of HIV Infection. Drugs and Society 5(1/2):69-85.

Page, J. Bryan, and Prince C. Smith 1990. Venous Envy: The Importance of Having Usable Veins. Journal of Drug Issues 20(2):291-308.

Page, J. Bryan, Dale D. Chitwood, Prince C. Smith, Normie Kane, and Duane C. McBride 1990. Intravenous Drug Use and HIV Infection in Miami. Medical Anthropology Quarterly 4:56-72.

1988 Personal Communication, Miami, Florida.

Rettig, R.P., M. Torres, and G. Garrett 1977. Manny: A Criminal Addict's Story. Boston: Houghton Mifflin Press.

Robert-Guroff, M., J. Giron, A. Jennings, H. Ginzburg, I. Margolis, W. Blattner, and R. Gallo 1986. Prevalence of Antibodies to HTLV-I, -II, and -III in Intravenous Drug Abusers from an AIDS Endemic Region. Journal of American Medical Association 255:3133-3137. ✦

32. Needle Access as an AIDS-Prevention Strategy for IV Drug Users: A Research Perspective

MERRILL SINGER,
RAY IRIZARRY,
AND
JEAN J. SCHENSUL

The following article by Merrill Singer, Ray Irizarry, and Jean J. Schensul is a description of needle-exchange programs and the benefits associated with such an AIDS-risk reduction strategy. The authors review various studies on needle sharing among intravenous drug users, noting that the practice is extensive, and cite evidence that needle-exchange programs can work to decrease needle sharing among drug injectors. Further, according to the results of one study, needle-exchange programs did not result in an increase in new users. Describing community attitudes about exchange programs, the authors conclude that local residents might be more willing to approve of needle exchange as their knowledge of AIDS increases.

Needle exchange and needle distribution as AIDS-prevention strategies have attracted considerable attention over the last five years. Consideration of these approaches was especially emphasized at the Fifth International Conference on AIDS in Montreal (Des Jarlais et al. 1989; Hagan, Des Jarlais et al. 1989; Hagan, Reid et al. 1989; Hartgers et al. 1989; Purchase et al. 1989). In the absence of an effective treatment or preventive vaccine for HIV infection, and in response to an alarming rise in the rate of AIDS cases among IV drug users (CDC 1989), prevention workers have been forced to consider options that they recognize are emotionally loaded and highly controversial. Consideration of needle access emerges from the realization that our ability to slow the AIDS epidemic "lies in breaking the link between substance abuse and HIV infection" (Joseph and Des Jarlais 1989:5). Interest in needle access has been especially sharp in Australia, the United Kingdom, the U.S., and in Scandinavia. Private companies in both Norway and the Netherlands have produced and are field-testing syringe-exchange vending machines (Buning et al. 1989; Stimson 1989; Stimson et al. 1990). In assessing the appropriateness of making clean syringes and needles available to IV drug users (IVDUs) as a means of preventing the transmission of HIV infection, several questions emerge:

1. How common is needle sharing among IVDUs?
2. If needle access existed in any given city, would IVDUs make use of it?
3. What is the attitude of the wider non-IV drug-user community: is needle access a socially acceptable AIDS-prevention strategy?
4. Will needle access contribute to the recruitment of new IVDUs or increased IV injection among current users?
5. Will needle access contribute to a drop in needle sharing and HIV incidence among IVDUs?

All of these are *research questions*, and should be answered through accepted procedures of scientific inquiry. It is in light of the findings of such research that we can develop informed opinions about needle access. Separate from such research, however, we have only a variety of conflicting uninformed attitudes, necessarily limited personal experiences, ideologically rooted biases, and personal preferences. Given the gravity of the AIDS situation in this country, especially among IVDUs, their sexual partners, and children, the time has come to move the issue of needle exchange out of the realm of emotionalism and into the realm of empiricism. We will do so on the basis of our own research in Hartford, as well as through a review of other studies by drug and AIDS researchers. While thus far we have available limited "policy-relevant research" (van Willigen 1986:146) concerning the aforementioned questions, there is a discernable trend in the findings of existing studies. Following a discussion of ongoing AIDS-related research efforts in Hartford, findings that relate to each of the above questions will be reviewed in turn.

AIDS Research in Hartford

Social-science AIDS research in Hartford is rooted in the community-action model (J. Schensul 1985; J. Schensul et al. 1987; S. Schensul 1973, 1974, 1985; S. Schensul and J. Schensul 1978;

Singer 1989). As summarized recently (Barger and Reza 1989:258):

> With this approach, the social scientist may provide many of the same functions as with policy science, such as research and expert information, but there are two principles which distinguish this model from others. First, it is the needs and goals of a particular community-based group which are being served, and it is this "target group" which has the initiative in seeking changes. Second, the applied scientist takes a clear value position and an active involvement in change events. A primary value is that democratic self-determination is the most effective and constructive means of change, both for the community group concerned and for the larger society.

This is the approach adopted by medical anthropology researchers affiliated with both the Hispanic Health Council and the Institute for Community Research, the two community-based research institutions that collaborate together and with other community organizations in much of the ongoing AIDS research in Hartford (Singer et al. 1991).

This work began in the mid-1980s, in response to recognition that AIDS-prevention efforts had been hampered by a lack of empirical information on public knowledge and beliefs about AIDS, the contemporary distribution of sexual-risk behaviors, and the extent and distribution of IV drug use, especially in ethnic minority populations known to have markedly disproportionate rates of AIDS and HIV infection (Singer, Castillo et al. 1990; Singer, Flores et al. 1990). To overcome these gaps in existing knowledge, researchers at the Institute for Community Research and the Hispanic Health Council helped to organize a consortium of community-based organizations. Known as the AIDS Community Research Group (ACRG), this consortium has undertaken two studies. The first was designed to locate and interview an ethnically stratified random sample of 290 individuals living in a clearly delineated neighborhood that reflected the ethnic and socioeconomic diversity found citywide (ACRG 1988; J. Schensul et al. 1988). In addition, a number of groups engaged in high-risk behaviors, namely sex professionals, IVDUs, and gay males, were known from previous research to be living in the neighborhood. Interviews were conducted in respondents' homes, using a structured instrument developed by the research team. The second study, employing the same methodology, interviewed 416 individuals in three ethnically homogeneous neighborhoods (Latino, African American, and Italian/Polish, respectively) and in several city-housing projects (ACRG 1989; Singer, Flores et al. 1990).

The Hispanic Health Council also is part of a second consortium, known as the Northeast Hispanic AIDS Consortium. This group is conducting a 13-city AIDS research project that employs a focus-group design targeted to selected at-risk sectors of the Latino community (e.g., IVDUs) (Singer and Castillo 1989). Participants are recruited to an opportunistic sample, using community advertising and existing community networks. Focus groups are guided by a facilitator to respond to a structured list of topics and questions. Issues and understandings raised during the course of the group discussion are recorded by a trained observer. The objective of this research is to gain deeper comprehension of community beliefs and attitudes concerning AIDS, and the relationship of AIDS-related beliefs and behaviors to core values and understandings.

The largest social-scientific AIDS research effort in Hartford is a community demonstration initiative entitled Project COPE. This project is a consortium effort that includes the Institute for Community Research, the Hispanic Health Council, Latino/as Contra SIDA, the Urban League, the Hartford Dispensary, and the City Health Department. Project COPE is designed to study rates of HIV infection, AIDS risk, AIDS knowledge, and culturally appropriate risk reduction for IVDUs and their sexual partners citywide. Using nationally standardized interview instruments at intake and at two points of follow-up (six months and 12 months), as well a locally generated, supplemental-interview component during follow-up, Project COPE assesses drug use, safer needle-injection patterns, and safer sex practices in its target populations. Following the initial interview, participants are assigned randomly to one of three AIDS education and prevention programs, a community-based, culturally appropriate intervention program for Latinos, a community-based, culturally appropriate program for African Americans, or a multi-cultural program based in a drug-treatment center. Although the approach varies across interventions, all three provide AIDS 101 education, one-on-one or group counseling, and advocated referral for additional social or medical services. Since it began in October of 1988, Project COPE has interviewed over 900 individuals who are either IVDUs or their sexual partners (or both). During the planning phase of this project, the lead author also conducted in-depth, open-ended interviews and focus-group interviews with a dozen active IVDUs or IVDUs in treatment. These interviews were tape-recorded and provide illustrative material on IVDU experiences and attitudes concerning AIDS risk and response to the AIDS crisis.

Needle-Sharing Patterns Among IV Drug Users

It is clear to all observers of the contemporary drug scene that needle sharing is a common behavior among IVDUs (Battjes and Pickens 1988); however, it is equally certain that some types of individuals are much more likely to share than others, some social contexts promote needle sharing more than others, and the users of some drugs administered intravenously are more likely to share than the users of other types of drugs. Among the first 200 participants in Project COPE, we found that men are more likely to report needle sharing than women (76 percent and 48 percent, respectively), while women are more likely to engage in needle cleaning (41 percent and 28 percent, respectively). Research by Selwyn and co-workers found that the most common reason (46 percent of persistent needle-sharers) given by IVDUs for continued needle sharing, despite awareness of the inherent AIDS risk, was "the need to inject drugs, with no clean needle available" (Selwyn 1988:102). Similarly, Magura et al. (1989), in a study of methadone patients who reported current IV drug use, found that the variables directly associated with needle sharing included inability to afford new needles and not owning a set of "works" (syringes and related paraphernalia), in addition to attitudes conducive to sharing (e.g., tolerance of withdrawal symptoms, concern about insulting friends, fatalistic beliefs). In the National Institute on Drug Abuse-sponsored national AIDS demonstration outreach projects (NADR), of 10,174 IVDUs interviewed, as of September 30, 1989, 40 percent indicated that they had shared a needle with a sex partner in the last six months, 54 percent had shared needles with a close friend, and 24 percent had shared needles with a stranger (NOVA 1989). In this study, use of unclean needles is equally common among white, African American, and Latino IVDUs.

This last finding is significant, because higher rates of HIV prevalence among African American and Latino IVDUs, compared to white addicts, has lead to the assumption that minority IVDUs are more involved in needle sharing. According to the Centers for Disease Control (1989), approximately 78 percent of known AIDS cases among heterosexual IVDUs are black or Latino. Studies that have examined needle-sharing patterns across ethnic and racial groups have produced conflicting results, with some studies suggesting greater concern with using clean needles among white IVDUs and other studies finding that whites have higher rates of needle sharing than African American and Latino "shooters" (Schilling et al. 1989). Based on their research in Texas, Dolan et al. (1987) concluded that, compared to IVDUs who do not share needles, those who do (1) tend to combine multiple drugs, such as heroin and cocaine, or amphetamine and methamphetamine in a single injection; (2) are more likely to shoot up in a shooting gallery; and (3) are more deeply involved in drug use. However, needle sharing was found to be (1) not peculiar to a particular racial or ethnic group; (2) not associated with a user's level of education; and (3) not characteristic of a particular personality profile (Dolan et al. 1987). Chaisson et al. (1987:93) conclude that, "While needle sharing is no more prevalent among blacks and Latinos than among whites, the risk of infection is clearly greater for individuals who share needles with minority group members due to the higher prevalence of infection in this group." Moreover, it may be that, while needle sharing and use of unclean needles occurs among a large percentage of street IVDUs, regardless of race or ethnicity, African Americans and Latinos may be forced more frequently to adopt these behaviors. As Rogers and Williams (1987:91) suggest, "Sterile needles may be more available to whites, and whites may be more able to afford them."

Dolan's finding of a relationship between shooting galleries and needle sharing is of special pertinence to the assessment of needle exchange (also see Des Jarlais, Friedman, and Strug 1986; Marmor et al. 1987). Shooting galleries or "get-off houses," as they are known in some regions, have become a cottage industry in the drug subculture, not only because they provide a comparatively safe place to inject drugs and, if necessary, access to needles and syringes, but because they offer an arena for socialization among fellow users and a degree of protection in case of a drug overdose. Still, most IVDUs avoid galleries, if they can, because "no user likes to part with the fee" (Walters 1985:43) charged by the owner. About 40 percent of the IVDUs in the national NIDA sample, nonetheless, reported using shooting galleries at least some of the time. The character of needle-sharing behavior in shooting galleries is seen in the following account by the former operator of a gallery interviewed by the lead author in Hartford in 1988:

> Every day, people would come to my house. They would cop [buy drugs] and do their drugs right there in my house. If they stay in my house to get high, they would have to give me some. A lot of people would come to my house. . . . Sometimes I'd go for four days without sleeping. Word got around that it was a place you could get high. I would charge them. Some guys would give me $10 for using works, plus they got to give me a high. I'd buy a bundle of works from people who were diabetic. . . . We shared works. If one would clog up, someone would use another works to clean it out without washing it. We didn't care, we only cared about the high. . . . Usually, ten to twelve people would come to the house every day, twenty-four hours a day. . . . I had two bedrooms that I would use to rent to guys who did drugs. Some guy might go in their with a girlfriend to get laid. I'd rent him the room for the money and the drugs.

This man, who is now HIV positive, reported driving to New York City several times a week to purchase drugs. Interviews with other addicts in Hartford indicate that this is a common practice and that generally customers will "shoot up for the trip home" with rented and/or shared needles. This pattern, promoted by the illegality of needle possession without a prescription in Connecticut, has contributed to the rapid diffusion of HIV infection among the state's IVDUs.

A study of shooting gallery behavior among 125 IVDUs by Friedman and co-workers (Friedman et al. 1989a) in New York found that IV cocaine users are less likely than IV heroin users to share needles in shooting galleries because cocaine users "shoot up" much more frequently and, thus, like to hang on to their own needles. Friedman also suggests that cocaine tends to engender a greater sense of mistrust which also interferes with needle sharing. Friedman and co-workers (Friedman, Des Jarlais et al. 1989b), moreover, found that increased use of crack and the inhalation of heroin (a practice called "chasing the dragon") have not led to any measurable decrease in intravenous drug use. Since awareness of AIDS and its routes of transmission are now widespread among IVDUs in New York, it does not appear that this population is switching to alternative means of drug consumption to avoid the risk of HIV infection.

In a street ethnography project in New York, Hopkins (1988) reports the following findings: (1) illicit needle sellers make profits of 50 to 100 percent from the sale or rental of needles; (2) needles are commonly purchased with forged prescriptions stolen from hospital emergency rooms, and purchased from diabetics with prescriptions; and (3) about half of illicit needle sellers report repackaging and reselling used, unsterilized needles. These findings indicate there is a strong demand among IVDUs for clean needles, and this demand produces behaviors that put users at risk for both infection and arrest.

Finally, over 30,000 IVDUs in the U.S. already have been diagnosed with AIDS (CDC 1990). Among active street IVDUs in Hartford, Project COPE (Flores et al. 1989; Singer, Owens, and Reyes 1989) found an HIV-positivity rate in the first 900 program participants of about 40 percent. In New Jersey, IVDUs now account for 54 percent of reported AIDS cases (CDC 1989), while in Puerto Rico they comprise 60 percent of AIDS cases among men (ARS 1990). A study of IVDUs in methadone treatment in New York by Selwyn et al. (1989) found a threefold increase in deaths due to AIDS, with mortality related to AIDS growing from 3.6 per 1000 in 1984 to 13.6 per 1000 in 1987. Needless to say, this is a disturbing rate of increase. Moreover, HIV infection is not equally distributed among IVDUs. Cross-tabulations of data from the first 200 participants in Project COPE showed that individuals who reported always "shooting up" at home, were significantly more likely to be HIV negative (i.e., uninfected) than individuals who never or only sometimes shoot up at home ($p = 0.026$). Conversely, IVDUs who have injected drugs in a shooting gallery were significantly more likely to be infected than those who reported never using galleries ($p = 0.035$). Also, respondents who reported that they at least sometimes gave their needle to a friend immediately after injecting drugs (i.e., needle sharers) were significantly more likely to be infected than those who never gave their equipment to friends to use ($p = 0.031$).

In short, sharing needles and injecting drugs in places where needle sharing is more likely, especially in the northeast sector of the U.S., are risky practices and will likely lead to exposure to the virus that causes AIDS, unless it is carried out in a closed circle of uninfected needle sharers or is accompanied by rigid adherence to effective needle-cleaning procedures. Unfortunately, many IVDUs do not regularly follow recognized needle-cleaning guidelines. Consequently, all of the studies we have cited point to the need for further action to prevent the spread of HIV infection among IVDUs. Lacking many other viable alternatives, increasingly, interest has been expressed among researchers and service/treatment workers both in the U.S. and in Europe in clean-needle exchange to combat the spread of HIV infection. But, as indicated, several critical questions emerge with regard to this option.

IV Drug-User Response to the AIDS Epidemic

The standard conception of an IV drug user (a view, by the way, that is shared by some active and some ex-users) is that of an individual who is so preoccupied with shooting up and avoiding "getting sick" (undergoing drug withdrawal) that s/he couldn't care less about viral infection. As Becker and Joseph (1988:403) note, "There is a general impression that IVDUs are incapable of (or disinterested in) changing their behavior, while IVDUs view public-health authorities with suspicion and distrust." If one embraces this view of the IVDU, then needle exchange by definition is a dead-end approach, because it is assumed that IVDUs will not go to the trouble of getting clean needles from a distribution program. There are problems with this understanding of the IVDU, however, as there is consistent evidence showing that IVDUs can and do change their behavior in response to the threat of HIV infection. Over half of IVDUs interviewed in New York in several different studies report behavioral changes to reduce the risk of infection (Selwyn et al. 1986; Des Jarlais et al. 1988). The two most commonly reported changes in this regard are (1) increased use of (illicitly acquired) sterile needles, and (2) reduction in the number of partners with whom an individual shares needles. The demand for sterile needles has already been felt among illicit needle suppliers in New York (Des Jarlais et al. 1985). Research in San Francisco has shown that an IVDU street-education program, that included the distribution of bottles of 2.5 percent bleach solution, produced a marked increase in needle-cleaning behavior among addicts. In 1985, only 6 percent of needle sharers interviewed in San Francisco reported that they usually or always sterilized their needles with bleach; by 1987, this figure had jumped to 47 percent, while the percentage of indi-

viduals who maintained that they never used bleach dropped from 76 percent to 36 percent (Chaisson et al. 1987). In the national NIDA study mentioned above, of the first 570 individuals who were exposed to AIDS education and counseling as part of the study, 22 percent had not "shot up" again six months after their first interview; among the remaining individuals who were still using drugs intravenously, 28 percent decreased the number of people they shared needles with, 20 percent increased the number of individuals they shared needles with, and 52 percent reported no change in needle sharing behavior (Sowder 1989). Among the active "shooters," 15 percent reported that they had stopped renting or borrowing needles, 13 percent started renting or borrowing needles, and 73 percent reported no change in this behavior. Finally, 28 percent reported switching to safer needle practices, such as using new or bleach-cleaned needles, 11 percent changed to less safe needle practices, and 61 percent reported no changes in needle practices. A New York study by Kleinman and colleagues (cited in Friedman, Des Jarlais et al. 1989) found that 16 percent of IVDUs who had been injecting for under two years, 29 percent of individuals who had been injecting for three to five years, and 33 percent of individuals who had been injecting from six to ten years, reported taking deliberate steps to reduce exposure to the human immunodeficiency virus. These changing attitudes and patterns are reflected in the following comments of a respondent in Project COPE:

> Very few people are going to stop using drugs. I don't do as much. If I became a 1st- and 16th-of-the-month junkie, that's an improvement. I have bleach signs up in my house. . . . You have to assume that everyone has [the virus].

What these data suggest is that some IV drug users, especially those who have longer drug-injection histories, are changing their behaviors to prevent HIV infection. This finding supports the needle-exchange strategy in two ways: (1) some IVDUs would decide to make use of needle exchange as an AIDS-prevention strategy, because they are open to behavioral change; and (2) existing prevention strategies for IVDUs, that do not include a needle-exchange component, are insufficient to prevent exposure to viral infection.

A final piece of evidence that should be mentioned in this regard is the view of IVDUs toward the needle-exchange concept. The generally shared atti-

tude of IVDUs who participated in the Northeast Hispanic AIDS Consortium focus groups was that the
illegality of needle possession in Hartford contributed to needle sharing, because of the legal risk to
individuals of carrying their own injection equipment. One ex-addict described in some detail the
conditions IVDUs are willing to put up with at shooting galleries to avoid the threat of arrest for the
possession of drug paraphernalia:

> If you don't have any works, they come out with a
> bag of the most disgusting, vile-looking tools [syr-
> inges] you ever saw. They're so old, the numbers
> are worn off of them, the needles are so dull, it feels
> like you're poking through leather to get a hit, but
> that's what people use. I've seen people use needles
> that were ready to bust in half, I know plenty of peo-
> ple that have had them bust off in their arm. The
> reasons that people went to shooting galleries is be-
> cause people didn't like to carry works on them.
> You got caught with works, you were busted.

Another ex-addict with AIDS affirmed, "To stop
the spread of AIDS, the main thing is education and
loosening up the legal restrictions on works." These
attitudes are not unique. Beginning in November
1988, during their first follow-up interview, IVDUs
in Project COPE were asked whether they would participate in a needle-exchange program if it was available in Hartford. Of the first 54 respondents interviewed, 87 percent indicated that they would participate in the program. The primary reasons given by
these individuals for supporting an NEP program
were: (1) reducing risk of infection; (2) gaining access to free needles; and (3) increasing the convenience of getting needles when needed.

Community Attitudes Concerning Needle Exchange

There is also the issue of community attitudes.
For example, Congressman Charles B. Rangel,
chairman of the House Select Committee on Narcotics Abuse and Control, a number of police agencies,
and several prominent ministers have complained
either that needle access will promote drug use or
that it will be used as a cheap substitute for the
effective drug-treatment programs that are so sorely
needed in inner-city areas. Needle exchange is seen
by opponents as "sending the wrong message" to
current IVDUs and others at risk for drug involvement, and it is viewed as cruel abandonment of
these individuals to the tortures of drug addiction.

As a staff member of Project COPE in Hartford
stated, "I refuse to give my brother a needle to stick
in his arm."

Moreover, there is a concern in African American
and Latino communities that needle access reflects
a racist disregard for the heavy toll drugs and drug-
related behavior take on people of color in this
country. Consequently, needle exchange has been
seen as genocidal by some of its opponents. In the
words of Rev. Reginald Williams of the Addicts Rehabilitation Center in East Harlem:

> . . . there will never be a needle-exchange program
> here. I think the communities and neighborhoods
> will rise up in opposition. . . . Why must we again
> be the guinea pigs in this genocidal mentality?
> (quoted in Marriott 1988:8)

Additionally, in the view of some individuals from
minority communities, drug use only became a national concern when white, middle-class youth began to show up in the drug statistics. Further, the
idea exists that the ready availability of drugs in
many African American and Latino communities is
not an accident, but rather part of a governmental
plan for the exploitation and social control of minorities. As a participant in the Heroin Lifestyles
Study asserted:

> A black man has no control what goes down in this
> world. Not in America. There's no heroin where the
> white boys hang out at. They don't let it up in their
> neighborhoods. They send it down to where the poor
> black boys hang out at. . . . No black man could have
> brought that kind of shit [heroin] into this country,
> they just don't allow that, they don't allow that.
> (Beschner and Brower 1985:19-20)

In an insightful summation of African American
response to the AIDS epidemic, Dalton (1989:219)
asks of needle-exchange advocates:

> You say that making drug use safer [by giving away
> bleach or distributing clean needles] won't make it
> more attractive to our children or our neighbor's
> children. But what if you are wrong? What if, as a
> result, we have even more addicts to contend with?
> Will you be around to help us then, especially if the
> link between addiction and AIDS has been severed?
> Why do you offer addicts free needles but not free
> health care? Why do you show them how to clean
> their works but not how to clean up their lives?

In fact, none of these concerns can be dismissed
out of hand. While heroin use became widespread

among African American and Latino youth in the 1950s, it was not until 1970, *after the emergence of a middle-class youth drug subculture*, that the Nixon administration began to implement a federal treatment program (Chein et al. 1964; Hanson et al. 1985). In his study of the governmental response to the drug problem, Epstein (1977) demonstrates the exclusive role of political, as opposed to public, health considerations in directing federal efforts. For example, the Harrison Narcotic Act of 1914, that outlawed the use of heroin and related drugs and insured, thereby, the creation of an underground drug use and needle-sharing subculture, was not motivated by public health concerns but rather by a Congressional interest in "restricting British dominance of the opium trade to China" (Partridge 1978:356-357). Also, we do not know yet if needle exchange, if it proved effective in preventing the spread of HIV infection, would come to be seen as a low-budget, cost-cutting approach for keeping AIDS out of the white heterosexual population. Financial considerations, rather than research and treatment needs, certainly dominated federal response to the AIDS crisis during the Reagan administration (Shilts 1987). And there have been various reports that intelligence branches of the federal government have been involved with groups active in drug smuggling, both during the Vietnam War and more recently in Afghanistan and Central America (McCoy 1972). What is clear is that community concerns about needle exchange, and the meaning such programs have for oppressed communities, must be taken into consideration in the needle-exchange debate. Community resistance to needle access could doom such programs, even if they proved to be effective in AIDS prevention (e.g., Podolefsky 1985).

To help assess community attitudes, the AIDS Community Research Group studies in Hartford included data collection on the "cultural feasibility" (van Willigen 1986) of needle exchange. In the first study, 41 percent of the respondents stated that they supported government-sponsored NEPs for IV drug users as an AIDS-prevention approach. Support was highest among African American respondents, with 49 percent saying needle exchange should be initiated, while the lowest percentage of supporters was found among Latino respondents, with only 37 percent supporting this strategy (ACRG 1988). In the second study, 67 percent of the respondents supported needle exchange, with 67 percent of African Americans, 63 percent of Latinos, and 72 percent of whites supporting this strategy (ACRG 1989). In both studies, it should be noted, community support was higher for distribution of condoms and bleach for needle cleaning than for distribution of sterile needles. And in both studies, Latinos were the least enthusiastic about needle exchange. Nonetheless, these data suggest that, while there is considerable community concern about NEPs, a perhaps growing percentage of people of all major ethnic backgrounds in Hartford would support the initiation of a government-sponsored NEP. This interpretation rests on the assumption that the differences in the findings between the two studies reflect a mounting receptivity to the idea of needle exchange in Hartford, perhaps as a result of growing public awareness and understanding of AIDS. This interpretation is supported by the fact that participants in the second study were better informed about the disease and its prevention than were participants in the first study. Moreover, there has been increasing mass-media attention to the issue of needle exchange, so that the initial unfamiliarity and discomfort with the practice may be waning. The possibility also exists that different attitudes toward needle access exist in different parts of the city and that neighborhood demographics or experience, rather than the passage of time between the two studies, explains the ACRG findings.

The Impact of Needle Exchange on IV Drug Use

There also is serious concern that NEPs will lead to increased drug use, while not effectively promoting decreased needle sharing. Existing evidence, however, suggests these concerns are not warranted. One of the most publicized NEPs has been going on in the Netherlands since 1984. By 1987, 700,000 needles had been distributed through existing social agencies and treatment facilities, and needle exchange is now ongoing in 40 municipalities in the Netherlands. In a recently reported longitudinal study of the Amsterdam program, van den Hoek and co-workers (1989:1359) report that they found "no evidence that the non-intravenous drug users in [their] study started intravenous use, in spite of the availability of clean needles and syringes." This finding is supported by a parallel study in the southern part of the Netherlands (Buning et al. 1989; Buning 1990). Also of note is a NEP in Liverpool, England, run by the municipal drug-dependency clinic. During the initial months of this program, addicts returned 2,949 needles in exchange for a sterile replacement, indicating that IVDUs will bring in used needles, if clean needles are made available. Users of the Liverpool needle exchange are also supplied condoms (Marks and Parry 1987).

There are over half a dozen public or underground NEPs going on in the U.S. The Tacoma Syringe Exchange, with support from the Tacoma-Pierce County Board of Health, is distributing 1,400 needles per week. The AIDS Prevention Project needle exchange in Seattle is giving out about 4,000 syringes a month. The Prevention Point, an underground program in San Francisco, has recorded a rate of 450 exchanges each evening since it began in November 1988. The ACEs program, an underground effort in New Haven, CT, distributes 200 needles and bleach kits each week. The Project Exchange in Boulder, CO, run by the county health department, also has recently began distributing needles. Until it was discontinued by the mayor, there was, in addition, the Pilot Needle Exchange in New York City (AIDS Community Educators 1989; Buning et al. 1989; McGough 1989; New York City Department of Health 1989; Prevention Point 1989; Strickland 1989). Finally, in its 1990 legislative session, the Connecticut State Legislature became the first state government in the nation to approve a NEP pilot program (for New Haven), followed shortly thereafter by Hawaii. Organizers of many of these programs came together in 1989 at a public forum sponsored by the San Francisco AIDS Foundation. As Buning et al. (1989:11) point out, the overriding conclusion of forum participants was that "such programs did not increase drug use. . . ." In the view of Samuel Friedman of the Narcotic and Drug Research, Inc., who participated in the San Francisco forum (Des Jarlais et al. 1988:171):

> Barring a dramatic breakthrough with respect to increased use of proper sterilization techniques, IV drug users must have access to non-contaminated injection equipment, if the spread of HIV among continuing IV drug users . . . is to be contained. . . . Based on current data from . . . face-to-face education programs, there appears to be no contradiction between teaching IV drug users how to sterilize drug injection equipment and reducing IV drug use. . . . [N]on-judgmental programs for AIDS risk reduction—programs that do not tell an IV drug user that he or she must stop injecting drugs—appear to be

"discouraging" rather than "encouraging" IV drug use.

These conclusions were affirmed by participants at the first North American Syringe Exchange Convention, held in Tacoma in October 1990.

Needle Exchange and Needle Sharing

But do needle exchange programs produce less needle sharing among active IVDUs? An examination of several of the existing programs suggests that they do. The Seattle program, for example, began in March 1989 as a project of the local branch of Act Up, a grassroots activist organization that has been highly critical of government foot-dragging in response to the AIDS crisis. In April of 1989, at the urging of AIDS Prevention Project staff, the Seattle-King County Board of Health approved needle exchange. The AIDS Prevention Project subsequently began to staff the exchange program, while Act Up members continued to provide volunteer support. Needles are exchanged in a section of town known for its high rate of drug trafficking, as well as police surveillance. Nonetheless, 40 syringes are exchanged each hour, two to four hours a day, six days a week. New syringes are marked for identification and are counted upon return. Participants in the program can exchange up to ten needles at a time, and they are not required to provide I.D. About 70 percent of the needles turned in to the program in exchange for new ones bear the project's identifying mark. In other words, a yet to be determined number of IVDUs in Seattle are making regular and repeated use of the exchange program for the purpose of AIDS prevention. In addition to sterile needles, the project also provides participants with bleach, condoms, AIDS educational materials, and referral for drug treatment, health, and social needs. Plans are underway for a well-designed evaluation of the project (McGough 1989).

In September and October 1988, a pilot survey was conducted of the Tacoma needle-exchange program begun by David Purchase (Hagan, Des Jarlais et al. 1989; Hagan, Reid et al. 1989). During the survey, every third individual who brought in a needle for exchange was approached about participating in an interview, concerning needle-use practices, before and after first use of the exchange program. Sixty-six of the 75 individuals who were approached agreed to participate in the study. Of these, 57 percent were male, their mean age was

32.4 years, and the largest percentage (49 percent) were white, with 21 percent being African American and 15 percent being Latino. The majority (66 percent) of the respondents reported that they had been injecting drugs for more than five years, while 54 percent had not been in drug treatment during the last year. Most (67 percent) were "speedballers" (combiners of heroin and cocaine). Participants averaged 150 IV injects per month, or about five per day, prior to and following their involvement with the NEP. In other words, the program is serving established IVDUs, rather than users attracted to IV drug use by the existence of the NEP. Seventy-one percent reported engaging in needle sharing prior to visiting the needle-exchange program, while 37 percent shared needles after visiting the program. Bleach was used for needle cleaning by 51 percent of those who shared needles before visiting the program, compared to 75 percent of those who engaged in needle sharing afterward (Hagan, Des Jarlais et al. 1989; Hagan, Reid et al. 1989). Ninety percent of the respondents reported that, after visiting the program, they either did not share needles or else shared them but almost always used bleach or boiling for sterilization, compared to 66 percent prior to exchanging needles. All of the respondents who had been to the needle exchange six or more times reported these safer needle practices.

In the U.K., changes in needle-sharing patterns have been measured through a repeat interview design over a three-month period.

> Clients who continued to attend reported a gross improvement in behavior, so that in three months of attendance, the basic rate of sharing was reduced from 34 to 27 percent. In other words, at Time 2, 73 percent were not sharing, to which can be added a further 6 percent who continued to share, but at a reduced level of risk behavior. Overall, a total of 79 percent sustained low-risk injecting behavior, adopted low-risk injecting behavior, or reduced their level of risk behavior. This rate of sharing is the lowest recorded in U.K. literature. (Stimson 1989:257)

Additionally, the U.K. data indicate that needle exchange in England has tended to reach lower-risk IVDUs. In comparison with the 34 percent of program users who report needle sharing in the four-week period prior to their first exchange, needle sharing rates of as high as 60 percent have been found in the U.K. among IVDUs not using the program (Donoghoe et al. 1989).

Finally, van den Hoek et al. (1989) report that among participants in the Amsterdam study, the proportion of individuals who obtained their injection equipment exclusively through the exchange program rose from 31.2 percent at the first visit to 52.3 percent by the user's third visit to the program. Associated with this drop was a reduction in the borrowing and lending of needles among program participants. While 55.6 percent of participants reported borrowing and 50.9 percent reporting lending during the first phase of the program (the program was divided into 207-day intake periods), these figures had dropped to 46.9 percent and 34.4 percent by the fourth phase. These changes occurred in both women and men, among Dutch, German, and other participants, and regardless of awareness of serostatus. The authors conclude, "The results of this follow-up study clearly show that IV drug users are able to reduce their sharing of needles/syringes" (van den Hoek et al. 1989:1356). However, the authors acknowledge that results were not uniformly encouraging: "Borrowing used needles and syringes—at least once in the prior six months—was as often reported by those who entered our study at the end in 1988 as it was in 1986" (van den Hoek 1989:1357). In a recent review of needle-exchange programs throughout the U.K. and Europe, Stimson (1989:258) concludes, "The evidence so far is that syringe exchange reaches injectors who are not in touch with other services, does this at reasonable cost, is delivered in a way that is acceptable to most clients, helps some drug injectors maintain low-risk behaviors, and helps some others to adopt them."

Van den Hoek et al. (1989) assert that, to achieve maximum results in needle-exchange programs, there must be concomitant, intensive counseling for IV drug users. In other words, they reject an either/or approach to needle exchange vs. drug counseling, and instead view these as compatible components of comprehensive AIDS-prevention efforts for IVDUs. Similar conclusions have been drawn in the Tacoma needle-exchange program. In fact, in Tacoma, needle exchange has proven to be an effective outreach and trust-building device that can be the first step in moving participants into drug treatment (Strickland 1989). Charles Eaton, coordinator of the New York City NEP during its ten-month existence, a program that especially was effective both in advocating for the opening of new treatment slots and in moving program participants into those slots, has commented:

I have been involved in drug treatment for 29 years and see no contradiction between what I am doing now and my drug-treatment work. The one thing I never learned in 29 years in drug treatment is how to rehabilitate a dead drug addict. (Eaton 1989)

Studies of needle-exchange programs have been criticized on two grounds. Most of the studies have been based on the self-report of IVDUs and control groups generally have not been built into the study design. Needless to say, the special circumstance under which needle exchange takes place does not lend itself easily to sophisticated research designs. Further, designs that are too intrusive on program users may tend to discourage participation (Joseph and Des Jarlais 1989; Stimson et al. 1989). Nonetheless, in response to criticisms, exchange programs are attempting to improve their evaluation methodology. The pilot needle-exchange study in New York, for example, specifically was developed to address the control-group problem. In the study, a sample of IVDUs received sterile syringes in exchange for used injection equipment, as well as drug counseling and intensive AIDS education. A control group, recruited from the IV drug-using patients at a private medical practice in the South Bronx, received counseling and AIDS education but did not participate in the exchange component. Both groups were recruited for drug treatment. The purposes of the study were (1) to test whether needle exchange helps to keep IVDUs on often protracted waiting lists for drug treatment; and (2) to see if needle-exchange programs create an environment that fosters effective AIDS-risk reduction (New York City Department of Health 1988). The Portland NEP, run by the Outside Inn, an agency that provides health services for low-income populations, also is maintaining a control group of IVDUs who receive AIDS prevention education but not needle exchange. To avoid providing needles to individuals who are not currently IVDUs, participants in the Portland program are required to show visual evidence of "tracks" (scarification of veins, due to intravenous drug injection). In addition to sterile needles, participants are provided a safety kit that includes AIDS prevention information, bleach, condoms, a clean "cooker" (bottle cap for "cooking down" or dissolving drugs), and a fresh cotton ball (used to filter drugs to avoid clogging the needle). These last two items are offered to participants because of the risk of HIV transmission through shared cookers and cotton, a type of infection risk

that is not addressed through either bleach or syringe distribution. In the Boulder Exchange, participants may receive five needles for the first needle they bring in, but must exchange on a one-for-one basis thereafter. In this program, needles are packaged with a label that indicates they are sterile needles for AIDS prevention. Labels are designed so that they come off when removed from the package, so that the needles cannot be used and repacked for sale with the sterile-needle label. In Boulder, sterile needles can be obtained 24 hours a day through a drug-detoxification program.

As the foregoing discussion suggests, there is a movement toward more sophisticated NEP research that does not rely on participant self-report, including blood or saliva testing of program participants and analysis of returned needles for evidence of both sharing (e.g., residue of multiple blood types) and seroconversion among program participants. Three studies from outside of the U.S.—London, England, Lund, Sweden, and Sydney, Australia— each using a different methodology, have explicitly tested for seroconversion. All three found comparatively low rates of conversion to HIV antibody positivity among program participants (Hart et al. 1989; Ljungberg, Tunving, and Andersson 1989; Wolk, Wodak, and Guinan 1988). In the New York NEP, over 150 needles were tested for multiple blood types; "the vast majority showed no blood residue or were inconclusive, demonstrating that addicts can and will learn to clean their works" (Joseph and Des Jarlais 1989:6). However, in a small number of the tested syringes, multiple-blood types were found, indicating that not all exchange-program users immediately change their needle-sharing patterns (New York City Department of Health 1989).

Beyond critiques of the research efforts intended to evaluate their effectiveness, exchange programs face difficulty on a number of other fronts as well. The Tacoma program, for example, is threatened with closure, because the city attorney decided in July 1989 that needle exchange is illegal. This decision is being tested in the courts by the county health department and may well lead to a ruling that could have ramifications on all exchange programs now in existence, as well as those being considered by local health officials. Other projects, like the Portland NEP, have encountered difficulties with liability insurance, although in this instance, financial aid from the county health department helped to overcome the problem. In Glasgow, England, local residents picketed the local program for six months (Stimson et al. 1989). Lack of support outside the health department cost the New York NEP its community-based sites, making access to the program difficult for participants (Eaton 1989).

> Due to community opposition, a mayoral mandate precluded any site for needle exchange located within 1000 feet of a school. The only available site was a former X-ray clinic on the first floor of . . . the central office of the Department of Health. This setting, surrounded by criminal-justice facilities and personnel, and far from the residential neighborhoods where addicts live, was not the user-friendly site that had been planned. (New York City Department of Health 1989:7)

A problem reported for exchange programs in both the U.K. and in New York is a high turnover of clients. In his evaluation of British NEPs, Stimson (1989) found that only 33 percent returned for as many as five exchanges. Similarly, in New York, the number of revisits during the first ten months ranged between one and 15 with a mean of 2.2 (New York City Department of Health 1989). There are a number of reasons, positive and negative, for the high turnover rate, including entrance into drug treatment, cessation of IV drug use, a decision not to participate following counseling, imprisonment, and death. Finally, a number of programs have not been particularly successful in attracting younger IVDUs and women (Stimson 1989). However, in the New York program, one-third of the participants were women. The mean age of participants in New York was 33.4 years, which compares with a mean age of 40.7 for IV drug users recruited for the comparison group (New York City Department of Health 1989). Despite the problems they encounter, new NEPs continue to appear. For example, approval has been granted recently for programs in Victoria and Vancouver, B.C.

Conclusion

Ten years before the first AIDS patient was diagnosed, Edward Brecher (1972:524) prophetically warned that the criminalization of the sale or possession of hypodermic needles without a prescription "leads to the use of non-sterile needles, to the sharing of needles, and to epidemics of hepatitis and other crippling, sometimes fatal, needle-borne diseases." Failure to heed this warning has contributed to the contemporary AIDS crisis. The dimension and toll of the AIDS epidemic demand a reconceptualization of societal response to intravenous drug users. Needle exchange is one of a number of controversial strategies that have appeared in recent years (widespread street distribution of condoms and bleach for needle cleaning are others) in an effort to halt the spread of AIDS to the drug-using sector of the population.

The stance taken by individuals and institutions with regard to needle exchange often has been influenced by emotional, political, or other factors, in the absence of a serious consideration of existing research. For example, Louis Sullivan, Secretary of Health and Human Services, stated in March 1989 that he would be very supportive of experimental needle-exchange trials. However, following President Bush's July 1989 statement that he opposed needle exchange "under any circumstance" (Ginzburg 1989:1351), Sullivan denounced clean-needle programs as inconsistent with administration policy (Strickland 1989).

The existing research, however, suggests that needle exchange should not be ruled out as an AIDS-prevention strategy. There is no evidence to suggest that needle exchange leads to the production of new IV drug users or more IV drug use, while there is evidence indicating that at least some IVDUs do change their behaviors to avoid HIV infection, do make use of existing needle-distribution programs, do decrease their needle-sharing behaviors when provided access to a ready supply of clean needles, and will use needle exchange as a gateway to drug treatment, if it is available. Needle-exchange programs also provide a mechanism for the safe disposal of potentially contaminated needles, reducing thereby the risk of accidental exposure through contact with a discarded needle. In other words, in a narrowly defined cost/benefit analysis, with increased drug use being the potential cost and prevention of AIDS transmission being the potential benefit, needle exchange, especially when combined with AIDS counseling/education and implemented as a gateway to drug treatment, appears to have merit (Joseph and Des Jarlais 1989; Stimson 1989; Stimson et al. 1988).

But human affairs, including health promotion and disease-prevention efforts, are never decided in such restricted terms. Issues of social relationship and power, as well as community understandings and interpretation, always influence the development of health policy, the implementation of health programs, and community response to both. In Partridge's (1978:371) apt phrase, the "formation of policy is a political process. . . ." Thus, Partridge points to Willner's (1973:550) caution that:

> Politicians and the policy makers they appoint are not likely to be influenced by knowledge, unless it is politically convenient or personally congenial. And politically convenient information can always be found to buttress political decisions.

A notable example of this pattern was the impact of the "culture of poverty" notion on public policy. In Valentine's (1971:193) estimation, "Few ideas put forward by social scientists in recent years have been so widely accepted or so influential in practical affairs as the 'culture of poverty' concept propounded by Oscar Lewis." The appeal of this concept is not hard to find. As Hicks and Handler (1978:322) note:

> The massive War on Poverty mounted by the federal government in the 1960s was based, according to Gladwin, "upon a definition of poverty as a way of life" (Gladwin 1967:26). The entire series of programs—VISTA, Job Corps, Head Start, and so on—aimed at changing attitudes, beliefs, and values, rather than on redistributing wealth and power.

Policies based on political convenience have produced cynicism and distrust in minority communities. These attitudes are magnified by community awareness of past abuses in the health field, including the use of Puerto Rico for clinical trials of oral contraceptives during the 1950s and 1960s (Vaughan 1972), and the withholding of medical treatment from 600 African American syphilis patients for 40 years in the Tuskegee Study of the long-term biological effects of venereal disease (Heller 1972). As Benjamin Ward, New York City's Police Commissioner, stated on a television call-in program, "As a black person, [I] have a particular sensitivity to doctors conducting experiments, and they too frequently seem to be conducted against blacks" (quoted in Marriott 1988:8). At present, there are very strong and very understandable concerns in minority communities about the ultimate purposes and effects of needle-exchange programs.

However, continued research findings like those reported in this paper might help to create a broad public consensus for federally or state-funded needle-exchange trials. As noted, our research in Hartford suggests the possibility that community resistance to needle exchange may lessen, as AIDS knowledge increases. Community-based organizations working in AIDS prevention can play an im-

portant role in this regard. In San Francisco, for example, a number of minority organizations, including the Black Coalition on AIDS, the Latino AIDS Coalition, and the Third World AIDS Advisory Task Force, have come out in support of needle exchange (Buning et al. 1989). In Connecticut in 1989, the Hispanic Leadership Council passed a resolution that called for a legalization of needle sales and possession, initiation of a pilot needle-exchange program, and increased availability of drug treatment in the state. The needle-exchange concept was also endorsed by the board of directors of the Hispanic Health Council in Hartford. NEPs that are implemented by or in collaboration with community-based organizations and consortiums, especially programs that have the support of experienced community AIDS-prevention workers, have the greatest chance of winning community support. Further, as most organizers of NEPs maintain, needle exchange must be accompanied by and connected to other interventions, including AIDS education and counseling, active referral for drug treatment and social services, and advocacy on behalf of the health, treatment, job training, and related needs of IV drug users and their families.

It is now estimated that between one and one and a half million individuals in the U.S. are infected with the virus that causes AIDS. Approximately 50 individuals die of AIDS each day in the U.S. African American and Latino populations, groups that already suffer from disproportionate rates of poverty and related health and social problems, comprise about 40 percent of known AIDS cases, although they constitute only about 18 percent of the total U.S. population. IV drug use has become a dominant source of new infection, especially in ethnic minority communities (Singer, Flores et al. 1990). While needle exchange will continue to have vocal opponents in high places, especially among those who fear it represents a trial balloon for the decriminalization of drug use, already the AIDS crisis has produced several heretofore unexpected changes in government health policy (e.g., the early release of experimental AIDS drugs), clinical interest in previously unthinkable treatment options (e.g., the payment of IVDUs to enter and remain in treatment), and public acceptance of formerly unmentionable topics (e.g., condom use, sexual practices). Clearly existing approaches to both the drug problem and the spread of HIV infection among IVDUs have not led to significant improvements. For example, failure of the Reagan's 1982

War on Drugs (primarily cocaine) did not lead to any notable innovations in Bush's War on Drugs. Similarly, the last three governors of New York have launched aggressive though ineffective campaigns to stop drug use by catching and punishing suppliers (Peele 1985). Perhaps the time has come for radical alternatives.

* * *

Merrill Singer, Ray Irizarry, and Jean J. Schensul, "Needle Access as an AIDS-Prevention Strategy for IV Drug Users: A Research Perspective." Reproduced by permission of the Society for Applied Anthropology from *Human Organization*, *50* (2) (1991), pp. 142-153. Copyright © 1991 by Society for Applied Anthropology.

For Discussion

The United States government does not attempt to prohibit alcoholics from frequenting drinking establishments. Why then are most U.S. communities so hesitant to initiate needle exchange programs?

References

AIDS Community Educators. 1989. *A Report From the Underground: A Report on the Current Status of the Unauthorized Needle-Exchange Program in New Haven, CT.* New Haven: AIDS Community Educators.

AIDS Community Research Group (ACRG). 1988. *AIDS: Knowledge, Attitudes, and Behavior in an Ethnically Mixed Urban Neighborhood*. Hartford: Connecticut State Department of Health Services. 1989. *AIDS: Knowledge, Attitudes, and Behavior in Hartford's Neighborhoods*. Hartford: Connecticut State Department of Health Services.

AIDS Reporting System. 1990. Acquired Immunodeficiency Syndrome (AIDS). *Surveillance Report*, August. San Juan, Puerto Rico.

Barger, W. K, and Ernesto Reza. 1989. Policy and Community-Action Research: The Farm Labor Movement in California. In *Making Our Research Useful: Case Studies in the Utilization of Anthropological Knowledge*. John van Willigen, Barbara Rylko-Bauer, and Ann McElroy, eds., pp. 257-282. Boulder, CO: Westview Press.

Battjes, Ralph, and Roy Pickens. 1988. *Needle Sharing among Intravenous Drug Abusers: National and International Perspectives*. Rockville, MD: National Institute on Drug Abuse.

Becker, Marshal, and Jill Joseph. 1988. AIDS and Behavioral Change to Reduce Risk: A Review. *American Journal of Public Health* 78:394-410.

Beschner, George, and William Brower. 1985. The Scene. In *Life with Heroin*. Bill Hanson, George Beschner, James Walters, and Elliot Bovelle, eds., pp. 19-30. Lexington, MA: Lexington Books.

Brecher, Edward. 1972. *Licit and Illicit Drugs*. Boston: Little, Brown.

Buning, Ernst, Terry Reid, and Les Pappas. 1989. Needle Exchange V: Update on the Netherlands and the United States. *The Newsletter of the International Working Group on AIDS and IV Drug Use* 4(2):9-11.

Buning, Ernst. 1990. The Role of Harm-Reduction Programs in Curbing the Spread of HIV by Drug Injectors. In *AIDS and Drug Misuse*. John Strang and Gerry Stimson, eds., pp. 153-161. London: Routledge.

Centers for Disease Control (CDC). 1989. *Acquired Immunodeficiency Syndrome (AIDS) Monthly Surveillance Report* (August). Atlanta: Centers for Disease Control. 1990. *HIV/AIDS Surveillance: U.S. AIDS Cases Reported Through July 1990*. Atlanta: Centers for Disease Control.

Chaisson, R., A. Moss, R. Onishi, D. Osmond, and J. Carlson. 1987. Human Immunodeficiency Virus Infection in Heterosexual Intravenous Drug Users in San Francisco. *American Journal of Public Health* 77:169-172.

Chein, I., D. Gerald, R. Lee, and E. Rosenfeld. 1964. *The Road to H: Narcotics, Delinquency, and Social Policy*. New York: Basic Books.

Dalton, Harlon. 1989. AIDS in Blackface. *Daedalus 118*:205-227.

Des Jarlais, Don, Samuel Friedman, and William Hopkins. 1985. Risk Reduction for the Acquired Immunodeficiency Syndrome among Intravenous Drug Users. *Annuals of Internal Medicine 103*:755-759.

Des Jarlais, Don, Samuel Friedman, and David Strug. 1986. AIDS and Needle Sharing within the IV Drug Use Subculture. In *The Social Dimensions of AIDS*. Doug Feldman and Tom Johnson, eds., pp. 111-125. New York: Praeger.

Des Jarlais, Don, Samuel Friedman, Jo Sotheran, and Randy Stoneburner. 1988. The Sharing of Drug Injection Equipment and the AIDS Epidemic in New York City: The First Decade. In *Needle Sharing among Intravenous Drug Abusers: National and International Perspectives*. Robert Battjes, Roy Pickens, eds., pp. 1160-1175. Rockville, MD: National Institute on Drug Abuse.

Des Jarlais, Don, Holly Hagan, David Purchase, Terry Reid, and Samuel Friedman. 1989. *Safer Injection among Participants in the First Non-American Syringe Exchange Program*. Paper presented at the Fifth International Conference on AIDS. Montreal, Canada.

Dolan, Michael, John Black, Horace Deford, John Skinner, and Ralph Robinowitz. 1987. Characteristics of Drug Abusers that Discriminate Needle Sharers. *Public Health Reports 102*:395-398.

Donoghoe, Martin, Gerry Stimson, Kate Dolan, and L. Alldritt. 1989. Changes in HIV Risk Behavior in Clients of Syringe Exchange Schemes in England and Scotland. *AIDS 3*:267-272.

Eaton, Charles. 1989. Remarks at the Hartford Health Department Public Forum on Needle Access. Hartford: University of Hartford.

Epstein, E. 1977. *Agency of Fear: Opiates and Political Power in America*. New York: Putnam.

Flores, Candida, Merrill Singer, Jean Schensul, Paul McLaughlin, Regina Dyton, and Clara Acosta-Glynn. 1989. *Project COPE: AIDS Research and Outreach Project*. Paper presented at the Society for Applied Anthropology Annual Meeting. Santa Fe, NM.

Friedman, Samuel, Claire Sterk, Meryl Sufian, and Don Des Jarlais. 1989a. Will Bleach Decontaminate Needles During Cocaine Binges in Shooting Galleries? Letters. *Journal of the American Medical Association 262*:1467.

Friedman, Samuel, Don Des Jarlais, Alan Neaigus, A. Abdul-Quader, Jo Sotheran, Meryl Sufian, M. Tross, S., and Doug Goldsmith. 1989b. AIDS and the New Drug Injector. *Nature 339*:333-334.

Ginzburg, Harold. 1989. Needle Exchange Programs: A Medical or Policy Dilemma? *American Journal of Public Health 79*:1350-1351.

Gladwin, Thomas. 1967. *Poverty U.S.A.* Boston: Little, Brown.

Hagan, Holly, Don Des Jarlais, David Purchase, Terry Reid, and Samuel Friedman. 1989. *Drug Use Trends among Participants in the Tacoma Syringe Exchange*. Paper presented at the Fifth International Conference on AIDS. Montreal, Canada.

Hagan, Holly, Terry Reid, David Purchase, Harry Jensen, Joycelyn Woods, Samuel Friedman, and Don Des Jarlais. 1989. *Needle Exchange in Tacoma, Washington: Initial Results*. Paper presented at the Fifth International Conference on AIDS. Montreal, Canada.

Hanson, Bill, George Beschner, James Walters, and Elliot Bovelle. 1985. *Life with Heroin*. Lexington, MA: Lexington Books.

Hart, G., A. Carvell, and N. Woodward. 1989. Evaluation of Needle Exchange in Central London: Behavior Change and Anti-HIV Status Over One Year. *AIDS 3*:261-265.

Hartgers, Christina, Ernst Buning, and R. Coutinho. 1989. *Evaluation of the Needle Exchange Program in Amsterdam*. Paper presented at the Fifth International Conference on AIDS. Montreal, Canada.

Heller, Jean. 1972. Syphilis Victims in U.S. Study Went Untreated for 40 Years. *New York Times*, pp. 1, 8, July 26.

Hicks, George, and Mark Handler. 1978. Ethnicity, Public Policy, and Anthropologists. In *Applied Anthropology in America*. Elizabeth Eddy and William Partridge, eds., pp. 292-325. New York: Columbia University Press.

Hopkins, William. 1988. Needle Sharing and Street Behavior in Response to AIDS in New York. In *Needle Sharing among Intravenous Drug Abusers: National and International Perspectives*. Robert Battjes and Roy Pickens, eds., pp. 18-27. Rockville, MD: National Institute on Drug Abuse.

Joseph, Stephen, and Don Des Jarlais. 1989. Needle and Syringe Exchange as a Method of AIDS Epidemic Control. *AIDS Updates 2*:1-8.

Ljungberg, B., K. Tunving, and B. Anderson. 1989. *Rena Sprutor till Narkomaner HIV-förebyggande Åtgärder Enligt Lundamodellen* (Clean Needles for Drug Users, The Lund Model for HIV Prevention). Lund, Sweden: Studentlitteratur.

Magura, Stephen, Joel Grossman, Douglas Lipton. Qudsia Siddiqi, Janet Shapiro, Ira Marion, and Kenneth Amann. 1989. Determinants of Needle Sharing among Intravenous Drug Users. *American Journal of Public Health 79*:459-462.

Marks, I., and A. Parry. 1987. Syringe Exchange Program for Drug Addicts. *Lancet 1*:691-692.

Marmor, M., Don Des Jarlais, and H. Cohen. 1987. Risk Factors for Infections with Human Immunodeficiency Virus among Intravenous Drug Abusers in New York City. *AIDS 1*:39-44.

Marriott, Michel. 1988. Needle Exchange Angers Many Minorities. *New York Times*, pp. 1, 8. November 7.

McCoy, Alfred. 1972. *The Politics of Heroin in Southeast Asia*. New York: Harper and Row.

McGough, James. 1989. *The Needle Exchange Program in Seattle, Washington*. Paper presented at the First Annual NADR National Meeting. Washington, DC.

New York City Department of Health. 1988. *The Pilot Needle Exchange Study in New York: A Bridge to Treatment*. New York: Department of Health. 1989. *The Pilot Needle-Exchange Study in New York: A Bridge to Treatment. A Report on the First Ten Months of Operation*. New York: Department of Health.

NOVA. 1989. Quarterly Report on NADR National Data, as of 9/30/89. Rockville, MD: NOVA Research Group.

Partridge, William. 1978. Uses and Non-Uses of Anthropological Data on Drug Abuse. In *Applied Anthropology in America*. Elizabeth Eddy and William Partridge, eds., pp. 350-372. New York: Columbia University Press.

Peele, Stanton. 1985. *The Meaning of Drug Addiction*. Lexington, MA: Lexington Books.

Podolefsky, Aaron. 1985. Rejecting Crime Prevention Programs: The Dynamics of Program Implementation in High-Need Communities. *Human Organization 44*:41-49.

Prevention Point. 1989. *Questions and Answers About Needle Exchange in San Francisco-Prevention Point: The Next Step in AIDS Prevention*. San Francisco: Prevention Point.

Purchase, David, Holly Hagan, Don Des Jarlais, and Terry Reed. 1989. *Historical Account of the Tacoma Syringe Exchange*. Poster presentation, Fifth International Conference on AIDS. Montreal, Canada.

Rogers, Martha, and Walter Williams. 1987. AIDS in Blacks and Hispanics: Implications for Prevention. *Issues in Science and Technology 3*:89-96.

Schensul, Jean J. 1985. Systems Consistency in Field Research, Dissemination, and Social Change. *American Behavioral Scientist 29*:186-204.

Schensul, Jean, Donna Denelli-Hess, Maria Borrero, and Ma Prem Bhavati. 1987. Urban Comadronas: Maternal and Child Health Research and Policy Formulation. In *Collaborative Research and Social Change*. Don Stull and Jean Schensul, eds., pp. 9-33. Boulder, CO: Westview Press.

Schensul, Jean, Miriam Torres, Georgine Burke, Merrill Singer, and Candida Flores. 1988. *AIDS Knowledge, Attitudes, and Behaviors in an Ethnically Mixed Neighborhood*. Paper presented at the Society for Applied Anthropology meeting. Tampa, FL.

Schensul, Stephen. 1973. Action Research: The Applied Anthropologist in a Community Mental Health Program. In *Anthropology Beyond the University*. Alden Redfield, ed., pp. 106-119. Athens: University of Georgia Press. 1974. Skills Needed in Action Anthropology: Lessons from El Centro de La Causa. *Human Organization 33*:203-208. 1985. Science, Theory, and Application in Anthropology. *American Behavioral Scientist 29*:164-185.

Schensul, Stephen, and Jean J. Schensul. 1978. Advocacy and Applied Anthropology. In *Social Scientists as Advocates: Views from the Applied Disciplines*. George Weber and George McCall, eds., pp. 121-165. Beverly Hills, CA: Sage Publications.

Schilling, Robert, Steven Schinke, Stuart Nichols, Luis Zayas, Samuel Miller, Mario Orlando, and Gilbert Botvin. 1989. Developing Strategies for AIDS Prevention Research with Black and Hispanic Drug Users. *Public Health Reports 104*:2-11.

Selwyn, Peter. 1988. Sterile Needles and the Epidemic of Acquired Immunodeficiency Syndrome: Issues for Drug Treatment and Public Health. *Advances in Alcohol and Substance Abuse* 7:99-105.

Selwyn, Peter, C. Cox, C. Feiner, C. Lipshutz, and R. Cohen. 1986. *Knowledge About AIDS and High-Risk Behavior among Intravenous Drug Abusers in New York City*. Paper presented at the Second International Conference on AIDS. Paris, France.

Selwyn, Peter, Diana Hanel, William Wasserman, and Ernest Drucker. 1989. Impact of AIDS Epidemic on Morbidity and Mortality among Intravenous Drug Users in a New York City Methadone Maintenance Program. *American Journal of Public Health* 79:1358-1362.

Shilts, Randy. 1987. *And the Band Played On*. New York: St. Martin's Press.

Singer, Merrill. 1989. *Knowledge for Use: Anthropology and Community-Centered Substance Abuse Research*. Paper presented at the American Anthropological Association Meeting. Washington, DC.

Singer, Merrill, and Zaida Castillo. 1989. *Northeast Hispanic AIDS Consortium, Report of First Year Findings: Hartford Subsample*. Hartford: Hispanic Health Council.

Singer, Merrill, Zaida Castillo, Lani Davison, and Candida Flores. 1990. Owning AIDS: Latino Organizations and the AIDS Epidemic. *Hispanic Journal of Behavioral Sciences* 12:196-210.

Singer, Merrill, Candida Flores, Lani Davison, Georgine Burke, and Zaida Castillo. 1991. Puerto Rican Community Mobilizing in Response to the AIDS Crisis. *Human Organization* 50:73-81.

Singer, Merrill, Candida Flores, Lani Davison, Georgine Burke, Zaida Castillo, Kelley Scanlon, and Migdalia Rivera. 1990. SIDA: The Economic, Social, and Cultural Context of AIDS among Latinos. *Medical Anthropology Quarterly* 4:73-117.

Singer, Merrill, Peggy Owens, and Lydia Reyes. 1989. *Culturally Appropriate AIDS Prevention for IV Drug Users and Their Sexual Partners*. Paper presented at the First Annual NADR National Meeting. Washington, DC.

Sowder, Barbara. 1989. *A Preliminary Look at National AFA-Reported Behavior Change*. Paper presented at the First Annual NADR National Meeting. Washington, DC.

Stimson, Gerry. 1989. Syringe Exchange Programs for Injecting Drug Users. *AIDS* 3:253-260.

Stimson, Gerry, L. Alldritt, Kate Dolan, Martin Donoghoe, Rachel Lart. 1988. *Injecting Equipment Exchange Schemes: Final Report, Monitoring Research Group*. London: Goldsmith's College.

Stimson, Gerry, Kate Dolan, Martin Donoghoe, Rachel Lart, Andrew Johns, David Nurco, Colin Drummond, and Reginald Smart. 1989. Syringe Exchange Schemes: a Report and Some Commentaries. *British Journal of Addictions* 84:1283-1290.

Stimson, Gerry, Kate Dolan, Martin Donoghoe, and Rachel Lart. 1990. Distributing Sterile Needles and Syringes to People Who Inject Drugs: The Syringe-Exchange Experiment. In *AIDS and Drug Misuse*. John Strang and Gerry Stimson, eds., pp. 222-231. London: Routledge.

Strickland, David. 1989. Needle Swap Can Lead to Care. *Medical World News*, p. 58, August 28.

Valentine, Charles. 1971. The "Culture of Poverty": Its Scientific Significance and its Implications for Action. In *The Culture of Poverty: A Critique*. Eleanor Leacock, ed., pp. 193-225. New York: Simon and Schuster.

van den Hoek, J., H. van Haastrecht, and R. Coutinho. 1989. Risk Reduction among Intravenous Drug Users in Amsterdam under the Influence of AIDS. *American Journal of Public Health* 79:1355-1358.

van Willigen, John. 1986. *Applied Anthropology*. South Hadley, MA: Bergin and Garvey.

Vaughan, R. 1972. *The Pill on Trial*. New York: Penguin Books.

Walters, James. 1985. "Taking Care of Business" Updated: A Fresh Look at the Daily Routine of Heroin Users. In *Life with Heroin*. Bill Hanson, George Beschner, James Walters, and Elliot Bovelle, eds., pp. 31-48. Lexington, MA: Lexington Books.

Willner, Dorothy. 1973. Anthropology: Vocation or Commodity. *Current Anthropology* 14:547-555.

Wolk, J., A. Wodak, and J. Guinan. 1988. *HIV Seroprevalence in Syringes of Intravenous Drug Users Using Syringe Exchanges in Sydney, Australia, 1987*. Poster presentation, Fourth International Conference on AIDS. Stockholm, Sweden. ✦

Part IX

Treatment

Aconsiderable body of literature describes and documents the effectiveness of five major modalities of substance abuse/addiction treatment: chemical detoxification, methadone maintenance, drug-free outpatient treatment, self-help groups, and residential therapeutic communities. Each has its own particular view of substance abuse/addiction, and each impacts the client in different ways.

Chemical Detoxification

Designed for persons dependent on narcotic drugs, chemical detoxification programs are typically situated in inpatient settings and endure for seven to 21 days. The rationale for detoxification as a treatment approach is grounded in two basic principles. The first is a conception of "addiction" as drug-craving, accompanied by physical dependence that motivates continued usage, resulting in a tolerance to the drug's effects and a syndrome of identifiable physical and psychological symptoms when the drug is abruptly withdrawn. The second is that the negative aspects of the abstinence syndrome discourages many addicts from attempting withdrawal and, hence, influences them to continue using drugs. Given this, the aim of chemical detoxification is the elimination of physiological dependence through a medically supervised procedure.

Methadone, a synthetic narcotic, is the drug of choice for detoxification. Generally, a starting dose of the drug is gradually reduced in small increments until the body adjusts to the drug-free state. While many detoxification programs address only the addict's physical dependence, some provide individual and/or group counseling in an attempt to address the problems associated with drug abuse. A few refer clients to other, longer-term treatments.

Almost all narcotics addicts have been in a chemical detoxification program at least once. Studies document, however, that virtually all relapse.

Nevertheless, detoxification is a temporary treatment which provides addicts with the opportunity for reducing their drug intake; for many, this means that the criminal activity associated with their drug-taking and drug-seeking is interrupted. Finally, given the association between injection drug use and HIV/AIDS, detoxification also provides counseling to reduce AIDS-related risk behaviors.

Methadone Maintenance

Since the 1960s, methadone has been in common use for the treatment of heroin addiction. Methadone-maintenance programs take advantage of its unique properties as a narcotic and its cross-dependence with heroin. As such, it is a substitute narcotic that prevents withdrawal. More importantly, however, methadone is orally effective, making intravenous use unnecessary. In addition, it is longer acting than heroin, with one oral dose lasting up to 24 hours. These properties have made methadone useful in the management of chronic narcotic addiction. During the first phase of methadone treatment, the patient is detoxified from heroin on dosages of methadone sufficient to prevent withdrawal without either euphoria or sedation. During the maintenance phase, the patient is stabilized on a dose of methadone high enough to eliminate the craving for heroin. Although this process would appear to substitute one narcotic for another, the rationale behind methadone maintenance is to stabilize the patient on a less debilitating drug and make counseling and other treatment services available.

Studies have demonstrated that, while few methadone maintenance patients have remained drug-free after treatment, those who remain on methadone have highly favorable outcomes in terms of employment and no arrests. As such, methadone maintenance is effective for blocking heroin dependency. However, methadone is also a primary drug of abuse among some narcotic addicts, resulting in a small street market for the drug. Most illegal methadone is diverted from legitimate maintenance programs by methadone patients. Hence, illegal supplies of the drug are typically available only where such programs exist.

Drug-Free Outpatient Treatment

Drug-free outpatient treatment encompasses a variety of non-residential programs that do not employ methadone or other pharmacotherapeutic agents. Most are based on a mental-health perspective, and the primary services include individual and group therapy, while some offer family therapy and relapse prevention support. An increasing number of drug-free outpatient programs are including case-management services as adjuncts to counseling. The basic case-management approach is to assist clients in obtaining needed services in a timely and coordinated manner. The key components of this approach are assessing, planning, linking, monitoring, and advocating for clients within the existing nexus of treatment and social services.

Evaluating the effectiveness of drug-free outpatient treatment is difficult since programs vary widely—from drop-in "rap" centers to highly structured arrangements that offer counseling or psychotherapy as the treatment mainstay. A number of studies have found that outpatient treatment has been moderately successful in reducing daily drug use and criminal activity. However, the approach appears to be inappropriate for the most troubled and antisocial users.

Self-Help Groups

Self-help groups, also known as 12-step programs, are composed of individuals who meet regularly to stabilize and facilitate their recovery from substance abuse. The best known is Alcoholics Anonymous (AA), in which sobriety is based on fellowship and adhering to the "Twelve Steps" of recovery. The twelve steps stress faith, confession of wrongdoing, and passivity in the hands of a "higher power." They progress group members from an admission of powerlessness over drugs and alcohol to a resolution that they will carry the message of help to others and will practice the principles learned in all affairs.

In addition to AA, other popular self-help groups are Narcotics Anonymous (NA), Cocaine Anony-

mous (CA), and Drugs Anonymous (DA), all of which follow the twelve-step model. All such organizations operate as stand-alone fellowship programs, but are used as well as adjuncts to other modalities. Although few evaluation studies of self-help groups have been carried out, the weight of clinical and observational data suggest that they are crucial to facilitating recovery.

Residential Therapeutic Communities

The therapeutic community, or TC, is a total treatment environment in which the primary clinical staff are typically former substance abusers— "recovering addicts"—who themselves were rehabilitated in therapeutic communities. The treatment perspective of the TC is that drug abuse is a disorder of the whole person—that the problem is the *person* and not the drug, that addiction is a *symptom* and not the essence of the disorder. In the TC's view of recovery, the primary goal is to change the negative patterns of behavior, thinking, and feeling that predispose drug use. As such, the overall goal is a responsible drug-free lifestyle. Recovery through the TC process depends on positive and negative pressures to change, and this is brought about through a self-help process in which relationships of mutual responsibility to every resident in the program are built.

In addition to individual and group counseling, the TC process has a system of explicit rewards that reinforce the value of earned achievement. As such, privileges are *earned*. In addition, TCs have their own specific rules and regulations that guide the behavior of residents and the management of their facilities. Their purposes are to maintain the safety and health of the community and to train and teach residents through the use of discipline. TC rules and regulations are numerous, the most conspicuous of which are total prohibitions against violence, theft, and drug use. Violation of these cardinal rules typically results in immediate expulsion from a TC. Therapeutic communities have been in existence for decades, and their successes have been well documented.

In the essays that follow, three modalities are examined in detail—the therapeutic community, methadone maintenance, and Alcoholics Anonymous. ✦

33. The Therapeutic Community for Substance Abuse: Perspective and Approach

GEORGE DE LEON

The therapeutic community (TC) is a drug-treatment modality that uses a holistic design for creating lifestyle changes. It is characterized by a democratic philosophy with foundations in social learning theory. In this article, George De Leon describes the methods by which TCs operate. Generally, the TC functions as a multi-stage process in which individuals are assessed by attitudinal and behavioral changes. The traditional TC is a residential program with highly structured activities. Participants may gain or lose status, depending on their productivity, work, and achievements. The TC is viewed as a community where the role of peers functions as an integral part of rehabilitation. Individual therapy is often part of treatment although TCs are more often characterized by group counseling that features encounter or confrontational therapy.

Since the 1960s, the spectrum of drug abusers has widened. Differences among users in drug-abuse patterns, lifestyle, and motivation for change are addressed by four major treatment modalities—detoxification, methadone maintenance, drug-free outpatient and drug-free residential therapeutic communities (TCs). Each modality has its view of substance abuse and each impacts the drug abuser in different ways.

The TC views drug abuse as a deviant behavior, reflecting impeded personality development and/or chronic deficits in social, educational, and economic skills. Its antecedents lie in socio-economic disadvantage, poor family effectiveness, and in psychological factors. Thus, the principal aim of the therapeutic community is a global change in lifestyle; abstinence from illicit substances, elimination of anti-social activity, employability, pro-social attitudes and values. The rehabilitative approach requires multi-dimensional influence and training which for most can only occur in a 24-hour residential setting.

The therapeutic community can be distinguished from other major drug-treatment modalities in two fundamental ways. *First*, the primary "therapist" and teacher in the TC is the community itself, consisting of peers and staff who, as role models of successful personal change, serve as guides in the recovery process. Thus, the community provides a 24-hour learning experience, in which individual changes in conduct, attitudes, and emotions are monitored and mutually reinforced in the daily regime.

Second, unlike other modalities, TCs offer a systematic approach to achieve its main rehabilitative objective which is guided by an explicit perspective on the drug-abuse disorder, the client, and recovery.

This paper outlines the therapeutic community approach to rehabilitation. The initial section provides an overview of the TC, its background and perspective on rehabilitation. The second section draws a picture of the TC approach, in terms of its basic elements and the stages of treatment.

Overview

Background

Therapeutic communities for substance abuse appeared a decade later than did therapeutic communities in psychiatric settings pioneered by Jones and others in the United Kingdom.

The two models evolved in parallel independence, reflecting differences in their philosophy, social organization, clients served, and therapeutic processes. Jones explains that the therapeutic community referred to a movement which originated in psychiatry in the United Kingdom at the end of World War II. It was "an attempt to establish a democratic system in hospitals, where the domination of the doctors in a traditional hierarchy system was replaced by open communication, information sharing, decision-making by consensus, and problem-solving sharing, as far as possible, with all patients and staff" (Jones 1953). The name therapeutic community evolved in these settings.

The therapeutic community for substance abuse emerged in the 1960s as a self-help alternative to existing conventional treatments. Unhelped by the medical and correctional establishments, recovering alcoholics and drug addicts were its first participant-developers. Though its modern antecedents can be traced to Alcoholics Anonymous and Synanon, the TC prototype is ancient, existing in all forms of communal healing and support. Today, the term "therapeutic community" is generic, describing a variety of drug-free residential programs. About a quarter of these conform to the traditional long-term model. These have made the greatest impact upon rehabilitating substance abusers.

The Traditional TC

Traditional therapeutic communities are similar in planned duration of stay (15-24 months), structure, staffing pattern, perspective, and in rehabilitative regime, although they differ in size (30-600 beds) and client demographics. Staff are a mixture of TC-trained clinicians and human-service professionals. Primary clinical staff are usually former substance abusers who themselves were rehabilitated in TC programs. Ancillary staff consist of professionals in mental-health vocational, educational, family counseling, fiscal, administration, and legal services.

TCs accommodate a broad spectrum of drug abusers. Although it originally attracted narcotic addicts, a majority of their client populations are non-opioid abusers. Thus, this modality has responded to the changing trend in drug use patterns, treating clients with drug problems of varying severity, different lifestyles, and various social, economic, and ethnic backgrounds.

Clients in traditional programs are usually male (75 percent) and in their mid-twenties (50 percent). TCs are almost all racially mixed, and most are age-integrated, with 25 percent of their clients under 21, although a few TCs have separate facilities for adolescents. About half of all admissions are from broken homes or ineffective families, and more than three quarters have been arrested at some time in their lives.

The TC Perspective

Full accounts of the TC perspective are described elsewhere (Deitch and Zweben 1976, 1979; De Leon 1981, 1984a, 1985; De Leon and Beschner 1977; De Leon and Rosenthal 1979; Kaufman and De Leon 1978). Although expressed in a social-psychological idiom, this perspective evolved directly from the experience of recovering participants in therapeutic communities.

Drug abuse is viewed as a disorder of the whole person, affecting some or all areas of functioning. Cognitive and behavioral problems appear, as do mood disturbances. Thinking may be unrealistic or disorganized; values are confused, non-existent, or anti-social. Frequently, there are deficits in verbal, reading, writing, and marketable skills. And, whether couched in existential or psychological terms, moral or even spiritual issues are apparent.

Abuse of any substance is viewed as over-determined behavior. Physiological dependency is secondary to the wide range of influences which control the individual's drug-use behavior. Invariably, problems and situations associated with discomfort become regular signals for resorting to drug use. For some abusers, physiological factors may be important, but for most these remain minor relative to the functional deficits which accumulate with continued substance abuse. Physical addiction or dependency must be seen in the wider context of the individual's life.

Thus, the problem is the person, not the drug. Addiction is a symptom, not the essence of the disorder. In the TC, chemical detoxification is a condition of entry, not a goal of treatment. Rehabilitation focuses upon maintaining a drug-free existence.

Rather than drug-use patterns, individuals are distinguished along dimensions of psychological dysfunction and social deficits. Many clients have never acquired conventional lifestyles. Vocational and educational problems are marked; middle-class mainstream values are either missing or unachievable. Usually, these clients emerge from a socially disadvantaged sector, where drug abuse is more a social response than a psychological disturbance. Their TC experience is better termed habilitation, the development of a socially productive, conventional lifestyle for the first time in their lives.

Among clients from more advantaged backgrounds, drug abuse is more directly expressive of psychological disorder or existential malaise, and the word rehabilitation is more suitable, emphasizing a return to a lifestyle previously lived, known, and perhaps rejected.

Nevertheless, substance abusers in TCs share important similarities. Either as cause or consequence of their drug abuse, all reveal features of personality disturbance and/or impeded social function. Thus, all residents in the TC follow the same regime. Individual differences are recognized in specific treatment plans that modify the emphasis, not the course, of their experience in the therapeutic community.

In the TC's view of recovery, the aim of rehabilitation is global. The primary psychological goal is to change the negative patterns of behavior, thinking, and feeling that predispose drug use; the main social goal is to develop a responsible drug-free lifestyle. Stable recovery, however, depends upon a successful integration of these social and psychological goals. For example, healthy behavioral alternatives to drug use are reinforced by commitment to the values of abstinence; acquiring vocational or educational skills and social productivity is motivated by the values of achievement and self-reliance. Behavioral change is unstable without insight, and insight is insufficient without felt experience. Thus, conduct, emotions, skills, attitudes, and values must be integrated to insure enduring change.

The rehabilitative regime is shaped by several broad assumptions about recovery.

Motivation

Recovery depends upon positive and negative pressures to change. Some clients seek help, driven by stressful external pressures; others are moved by more intrinsic factors. For all, however, remaining in treatment requires continued motivation to change. Thus, elements of the rehabilitation approach are designed to sustain motivation, or detect early signs of premature termination.

Self-Help

Although the influence of treatment depends upon the person's motivation and readiness, change does not occur in a vacuum. The individual must permit the impact of treatment or learning to occur. Thus, rehabilitation unfolds as an interaction between the client and the therapeutic environment.

Social Learning

A lifestyle change occurs in a social context. Negative patterns, attitudes, and roles were not acquired in isolation, nor can they be altered in isolation. Thus, recovery depends not only upon what has been learned, but how and where learning occurs. This assumption is the basis for the community itself, serving as teacher. Learning is active, by doing and participating. A socially responsible role is acquired by acting the role. What is learned is identified with the people involved in the learning process, with peer support and staff, as credible role models. Because newly acquired ways of coping are threatened by isolation and its potential for relapse, a perspective on self, society, and life must be affirmed by a network of others.

Treatment as an Episode

Residency is a relatively brief period in an individual's life, and its influence must compete with the influence of the years before and after treatment. For this reason, unhealthy "outside" influences are minimized, until the individuals are better prepared to engage these on their own and the treatment regime is designed for high impact. Thus, life in the TC is necessarily intense, its daily regime demanding, its therapeutic confrontations unmoderated.

The TC Approach

A. TC Structure

TCs are stratified communities composed of peer groups that hold memberships in wider aggregates that are led by individual staff. Together, they constitute the community, or family, in a residential facility. This peer-to-community structure strengthens the individual's identification with a perceived, ordered network of others. More importantly, it arranges relationships of mutual responsibility to others at various levels of the program.

The operation of the community itself is the task of the residents, working under staff supervision. Work assignments, called job functions, are arranged in a hierarchy, according to seniority, individual progress, and productivity. The new client enters a setting of upward mobility. Job assignments begin with the most menial tasks (e.g., mopping the floor) and lead vertically to levels of coordination and management. Indeed, clients come in as patients and can leave as staff. This social organization reflects the fundamental aspects of the rehabilitative approach, mutual self-help, work as therapy, peers as role models, and staff as rational authorities.

Mutual Self-Help

The essential dynamic in the TC is mutual self-help. Thus, the day-to-day activities of a therapeutic community are conducted by the residents themselves. In their jobs, groups, meetings, recreation, personal and social time, it is residents who continually transmit to each other the main messages and expectations of the community.

The extent of the self-help process in the TC is evident in the broad range of resident job assignments. These include conducting all house services (e.g., cooking, cleaning, kitchen service, minor repair), serving as apprentices and running all departments, conducting meetings and peer encounter groups.

The TC is managed as an autocracy, with staff serving as rational authorities. Their psychological relationship with the residents is as role models and parental surrogates who foster the self-help developmental process through managerial and clinical means. They monitor and evaluate client status, supervise resident groups, assign and supervise resident job functions, and oversee house operations. Clinically, staff conduct all therapeutic groups, provide individual counseling, organize social and recreational projects, and confer with significant others. They decide matters of resident status, discipline, promotion, transfers, discharges, furloughs, and treatment planning.

Work as Education and Therapy

In the TC, work mediates essential educational and therapeutic effects. Vertical job movements carry the obvious rewards of status and privilege. However, lateral job changes are more frequent, providing exposure to all aspects of the community. Typically, residents experience many lateral job changes that enable them to learn new skills and to negotiate the system. This increased involvement also heightens their sense of belonging and affirms their commitment to the community.

Job changes in the TC are singularly effective therapeutic tools, providing both measures of, and incentives for, behavioral and attitudinal change. In the vertical structure of the TC, ascendancy marks how well the client has assimilated what the community teaches and expects; hence, the job promotion is an explicit measure of the resident's improvement and growth.

Conversely, lateral or downward job movements also create situations that require demonstrations of personal growth. A resident may be removed from one job to a lateral position in another department or dropped back to a lower status position for clinical reasons. These movements are designed to teach new ways of coping with reversals and change that appear to be unfair or arbitrary.

Peers as Role Models

People are the essential ingredient in the therapeutic community. Peers as role models and staff as role models and rational authorities are the primary mediators of the recovery process.

Indeed, the strength of the community as a context for social learning relates to the number and quality of its role models. All members of the community are expected to be role models—roommates, older and younger residents, junior, senior, and directorial staff. TCs require these multiple-role models to maintain the integrity of the community and assure the spread of social-learning effects.

Residents who demonstrate the expected behaviors and reflect the values and teachings of the community are viewed as role models. This is illustrated in two main attributes.

Role models "act as if." They behave as the person they should be, rather than as the person they have been. Despite resistance, perceptions, or feelings to the contrary, they engage in the expected behavior and consistently maintain the attitudes and values of the community. These induce self-motivation, commitment to work and striving, positive regard for staff as authority, and an optimistic outlook toward the future.

In the TC's view, "acting as if" has significance beyond conformity. It is an essential mechanism for more complete psychological change. Feelings, insights, and altered self-perceptions often follow, rather than precede, behavior change.

Role models display responsible concern. This concept is closely akin to the notion of, "I am my brother's keeper." Showing responsible concern involves willingness to confront others whose behavior is not in keeping with the rules of the TC, the spirit of the community, or the knowledge which is consistent with growth and rehabilitation. Role models are obligated to be aware of the appearance, attitude, moods, and performances of their peers, and confront negative signs in these. In particular, role models are aware of their own behavior in the overall community and the process prescribed for personal growth.

Staff as Rational Authorities

TC clients often have had difficulties with authorities who have not been trusted or perceived as guides and teachers. Thus, they need a successful experience with a rational authority who is credible (recovered), supportive, correcting, and protecting, in order to gain authority over themselves (personal autonomy). Implicit in their role as rational authorities, staff provide the reasons for their decisions and the meaning of consequences. They exercise their powers to train and guide, facilitate and correct, rather than punish, control, or exploit.

B. Daily Regime: Basic Elements

The daily regime is full and varied. Although designed to facilitate the management of the community, its scope and schedule reflect an understanding of the conditions of drug abuse. It provides an orderly environment for many who customarily have lived in chaotic or disruptive settings; it reduces boredom and distracts from negative preoccupations which have, in the past, been associated with drug use; and it offers opportunity to achieve satisfaction from a busy schedule and the completion of daily chores.

The typical day in a therapeutic community is highly structured, beginning with a 7 a.m. wake-up and ending at 11 p.m. in the evening. It includes a variety of meetings, job functions (work therapy), therapeutic groups, recreation, and individual counseling. These activities contribute to the TC process and may be grouped into three main elements, community enhancement, therapeutic-educative, community and clinical management.

Community Enhancement Element

These activities, which facilitate assimilation into the community, include the four main facility-wide meetings: the morning meeting, seminar and house meeting, held each day, and the general meeting, which is called when needed.

Morning meeting: all residents of the facility and the staff on premises assemble after breakfast, usually for 30 to 45 minutes. The purpose is to initiate the daily activities with a positive attitude, motivate residents, and strengthen unity. This meeting is particularly important, in that most residents of TCs have never adapted to the routine of an ordinary day.

Seminars convene every afternoon, usually for 1 to 1-1/2 hours. The seminar collects all the residents together at least once during the working day. Thus, staff observation of the entire facility is regularized, since the seminar in the afternoon complements the daily morning meetings, and the house meeting in the evening. A clinical aim of the seminar, however, is to balance the individual's emotional and cognitive experience. Of the various meetings and group processes in the TC, the seminar is unique in its emphasis upon listening, speaking, and conceptual behavior.

House meetings convene nightly, after dinner, usually for one hour. The main aim of these meetings is to transact community business, although they also have a clinical objective. In this forum, social pressure is judiciously employed to facilitate individual change through public acknowledgement of positive or negative behaviors among certain individuals or subgroups.

General meetings convene only when needed to address negative behavior, attitudes, or incidents in the facility. All residents and staff (including those not on duty) are assembled at any time and for indefinite duration. These meetings, conducted by staff, are designed to identify problem people or conditions, to reaffirm motivation, and reinforce positive behavior and attitudes. A variety of techniques may be employed, e.g., special sessions to relieve guilt, staff lecturing and testimony, dispensing sanctions for individuals or groups.

Therapeutic-Educative Element

These activities consist of various groups and staff counseling. This element focuses on individual issues. It provides an exclusive setting for expressing feelings for resolution of personal and business issues in the evening. It trains communication and interpersonal relating skills; examines and confronts the behaviors and attitudes displayed in the various roles of the clients; offers instruction in alternate modes of behavior.

There are four main forms of group activity in the TC: encounters, probes, marathons, and tutorials. These differ somewhat in format, aims, and methods, but all attempt to foster trust and peer solidarity, in order to facilitate personal disclosure, insight, and therapeutic change.

Peer encounter is the cornerstone of group process in the TC. The term "encounter" is generic, describing a variety of forms which utilize confrontational procedures as their main approach. Encounter groups meet at least three times weekly, usually in the evening, for two hours. Although its process is intense, its aim is modest: to heighten the individual's awareness of the images, attitudes, and conduct that should be modified.

Probes meet as needed, usually in the early months of residency. These groups, which last 4 to 8 hours, aim to strengthen trust and identification with others; and to increase the staff's understanding of important background of the person.

Marathons are extended group sessions that meet as needed, usually for 24 to 30 hours, to initiate a process of resolution of life experiences that have impeded the individual's growth or development. Marathons make liberal use of dramatic, visual, auditory, and environmental props to facilitate a "working through" of deeper emotional experiences.

Tutorial groups meet regularly and are primarily directed toward training or teaching. Three major themes of tutorials are personal growth concepts, (e.g., self reliance, independence, relationships); job-skill training, (e.g., managing a department or the reception desk); clinical-skills training (e.g., use of the encounter tools).

The important differences across these groups are in leadership, objectives, material used, and approach. All but the encounter groups are led by staff, with the help of senior residents.

The focus of the encounter is behavioral, its approach is confrontational; its material draws upon peer and staff observation of the individual's daily conduct. Probes go much beyond the here-and-now behavioral incident, which is the primary material of the encounter, to the events and experiences of the individual's history. Although certain encounter tools are utilized, (e.g., identification, prodding), the main techniques of the probe are conversational but may include role playing or other methods to reduce defensiveness and resistance to strong emotional memories. Rather than confrontation, the probe emphasizes the use of support, understanding, and empathy. The main distinctions between the probe and the marathon are length, intensity of therapeutic intervention, and goals. The probe may be employed as a regular clinical intervention or to prepare the individual for the marathon. Another difference lies in the range of techniques and paraphernalia which are used. Tutorials emphasize teaching, which contrasts with the confrontation of the encounter to correct behavior or the methods in probes and marathons to facilitate emotional catharsis and insight.

The four basic groups are supplemented by others that convene as needed. These vary in focus, format, and composition. For example, gender, ethnic, or age-specific groups may utilize encounter, tutorial, or probe formats; dormitory, room, or departmental encounters will address issues of daily community living.

Counseling. One-to-one counseling further balances the needs of the individual with those of the community. Peer exchange is ongoing, frequent, and constitutes the most consistent counseling in TCs. However, staff-counseling sessions are conducted on an as-needed basis, usually informally. The staff counseling method in the TC is not traditional, evident in its main features: interpersonal sharing, direct support, minimal interpretation, didactic instruction, and encounter.

Community-Clinical Management Element

The objective of these activities is to protect the community as a whole and to strengthen it as a context for social learning. The main activities consist of privileges and disciplinary sanctions.

Privilege. In the TC, privileges are explicit rewards that reinforce the value of earned achievement. Privileges are accorded by behavior, attitude change, job performance, and overall clinical progress in the program. Displays of inappropriate behavior or negative attitude can result in loss of some or all privileges, offering the resident the opportunity to earn them back by showing improvement.

Privileges acquire their importance, because they are earned. The earning process requires investment of time, energy, self-modification, risk of failure, and disappointment. Thus, the earning process establishes the value of privileges, and hence their potency as social reinforcements.

The type of privilege is related to clinical progress and time in program, ranging from phone and letter writing in early treatment to overnight furloughs in later treatment. Successful movement through each stage earns privileges that grant wider personal latitude and increased self-responsibility.

Discipline and Sanctions. Therapeutic communities have their own specific rules and regulations that guide the behavior of residents and the management of facilities. Their explicit purpose is to ensure the safety and health of the community; their implicit aim is to train and teach residents through the use of discipline.

In the TC, social and physical safety are prerequisites for psychological trust. Thus, sanctions are invoked against any behavior which threatens the safety of the therapeutic environment. For example, breaking the TC's cardinal rules—no violence or the threat of violence, verbal or gestural—can bring immediate expulsion. Even minor house rules are addressed, such as stealing mundane sundries (toothbrushes, books, etc.).

The choice of sanction depends upon the severity of the infraction, time in the program, and history of infractions. For example, verbal reprimands, loss of privileges, or speaking bans may be selected for less severe infractions; job demotions, loss of residential time, or expulsion may be invoked for more serious infractions. These measures (contracts) vary in duration from 3 to perhaps 21 days and are re-evaluated by staff and peers in terms of their efficacy.

Though often perceived as punitive, the basic purpose of contracts is to provide a learning experience through compelling residents to attend to their own conduct, to reflect on their own motivation, to feel some consequence of their behavior, and to consider alternate forms of acting under similar situations.

Contracts also have important community functions. The entire facility is made aware of disciplinary actions that have been taken with any resident. Thus, contracts act as deterrents against violations; they provide vicarious learning experiences in others; and as symbols of safety and integrity, they strengthen community cohesiveness.

C. The TC Process

Rehabilitation in the TC unfolds as a developmental process occurring in a social-learning context. Values, conducts, emotions, and cognitive understanding (insight) must be integrated in the evolution of a socially responsible, personally autonomous individual.

The developmental process itself can be understood as a passage through three main stages of incremental learning; the learning which occurs at each stage facilitates change at the next, and each change reflects increased maturity and personal autonomy.

Stage I (Induction—0 to 60 days)

The main goals of this initial phase of residency are assessment of individual needs and orientation to the TC. Important differences among clients generally do not appear, until they experience some reduction in the circumstantial stress usually present at entry and have had some interaction with the treatment regime. Thus, observation of the individual continues during the initial residential period to identify special problems in their adaptation to the TC.

The goal of orientation in the initial phase of residency is to assimilate the individual into the community through full participation and involvement in all of its activities. Rapid assimilation is crucial at this point, when clients are most ambivalent about the long tenure of residency. Thus, the new resident is immediately involved in the daily residential regime. Emphasis, however, is placed not upon treatment but upon education and role induction into the community process. Therapeutic and educational activities focus on the TC perspective, its approach, and the rationale for long-term residential treatment.

Stage II (Primary Treatment—2 to 12 Months)

During this state, main TC objectives of socialization, personal growth, and psychological awareness are pursued through all of the therapeutic and community activities. Primary treatment actually consists of three phases separated by natural landmarks in the socialization-developmental process. Phases roughly correlate with time in program (1 to 4 months, 5 to 8 months, and 9 to 12 months). These periods are marked by plateaus of stable behavior, which signal further change.

In each phase, the daily regime of meetings, work, recreation, and therapeutic groups remains the same. However, progress is reflected in the client's profile at the end of each phase, which can be typified in terms of three interrelated dimensions, community status, developmental and psychological change. Community status describes the degree to which residents have acquired the attributes of the role model, measured mainly in their job functions and privileges. The developmental dimension describes the degree to which residents have altered their drug-involved profile, in conduct, language, attitude, and outlook. This is mainly reflected in the extent to which they have internalized the TC's perspective and commitment to change. The psychological dimension describes the degree to which residents reveal personal growth, e.g., maturity, openness, insight-self-awareness, emotional stability, and self-esteem.

Stage III (Re-Entry—13 to 24 Months)

Re-entry is the stage at which the client must strengthen skills for autonomous decision-making and the capacity for self-management with less reliance on rational authorities or a well-formed peer network. There are two phases of the re-entry stage.

Early Re-Entry (13 to 18 Months)

The main goal of this phase, during which clients continue to live in the facility, is preparation for healthy separation from the community.

Emphasis upon rational authority decreases, under the assumption that the client has acquired a sufficient degree of self-management. This is reflected in more individual decision-making about privileges, social plans, and life design. The group process involves fewer leaders at this stage, fewer encounters, and more shared decision-making. Particular emphasis is placed upon life-skills seminars which provide didactic training for life outside the community. Attendance is mandated for sessions on budgeting, job seeking, use of alcohol, sexuality, parenting, use of leisure time, etc.

During this stage, individual plans are a collective task of the client, a key staff member, and peers. These plans are actually blueprints of educational and vocational programs which include goal attainment schedules, methods of improving interpersonal and family relationships, as well as social and sexual behavior. Clients may be attending school or holding full-time jobs either within or outside the TC at this point. Still, they are expected to participate in house activities when possible and carry some community responsibilities (e.g., facility coverage at night).

Late Re-Entry (18 to 24 Months)

The goal of this phase is to complete a successful separation from residency. Clients are on "live-out" status, involved in full-time jobs or education, maintaining their own households, usually with live-out peers. They may attend such after-care services as A.A., N.A., or take part in family or individual therapy. This phase is viewed as the end of residency, but not of program participation. Contact with the program is frequent at first and only gradually reduced to weekly phone calls and monthly visits with a primary counselor.

Completion marks the end of active program involvement. Graduation itself, however, is an annual event conducted in the facility, for completees at least a year beyond their residency.

Thus, the therapeutic community experience is preparation rather than cure. Residence in the program facilitates a process of change that must continue throughout life, and what is learned in treatment are the tools to guide the individual on a steady path of continued change. Completion, or graduation, therefore, is not an end, but a beginning.

* * *

For Discussion

Therapeutic communities were designed initially for opiate users. Are they an effective treatment approach for cocaine users? Why or why not? ✦

34. Methadone Maintenance: A Theoretical Perspective

VINCENT P. DOLE

AND

MARIE NYSWANDER

While therapeutic communities view drug addiction as an underlying symptom of other life problems, methadone maintenance treatment sees addiction as a disease rather than an expression of a character or psychological disorder.

When administered orally, methadone serves to "block" the euphoric effects of heroin. That is, when an individual is given sufficient doses of methadone, he or she will be unable to "get high" from heroin. Vincent P. Dole and Marie Nyswander were the first to introduce methadone as a treatment for heroin addiction. In this article, these investigators discuss issues related to methadone treatment. Their study of methadone clients found that criminal activity decreased greatly when addicts were enrolled in maintenance programs. This finding, they argue, suggests that antisocial behavior, such as criminal activity, occurs as a result rather than a cause of drug addiction.

The Methadone Maintenance Research Program (Dole and Nyswander 1965, 1966; Dole et al. 1966) began in 1963 with pharmacological studies conducted on the metabolic ward of the Rockefeller University Hospital. Only six addict patients were treated during the first year, but the results of this work were sufficiently impressive to justify a trial of maintenance treatment of heroin addicts admitted to open medical wards of general hospitals in the city.

The dramatic improvements in social status of patients on this program exceeded expectations. The study started with the hope that heroin-seeking behavior would be stopped by a narcotic blockade, but it certainly was not expected that we would be able to retain more than 90 percent of the patients and that almost three-fourths would be socially productive and living as normal citizens in the commu-

nity after only six months of treatment. Prior to admission, almost all of the patients had supported their heroin habits by theft or other anti-social activities. Further handicapped by the ostracism of the community, slum backgrounds, minority group status, school dropout status, prison records, and anti-social companions, they had seemed poor prospects for social rehabilitation.

The unexpected response of these patients to a simple medical program forced us to reexamine some of the assumptions that we brought to the study. Either the patients that we admitted to treatment were quite exceptional, or we had been misled by the traditional theories of addiction (Terry and Pellens 1928). If, as is generally assumed, our patients' long-standing addiction to heroin had been based on weaknesses of character—either a self-indulgent quest for euphoria or a need to escape reality—it was difficult to understand why they so consistently accepted a program that blocked the euphoric action of heroin and other narcotic drugs, or how they could overcome the frustrations and anxieties of competitive society to hold responsible jobs.

Implicit in the maintenance programs is an assumption that heroin addiction is a metabolic disease, rather than a psychological problem. Although the reasons for taking the initial doses of heroin may be considered psychological—adolescent curiosity or neurotic anxiety—the drug, for whatever reason it is first taken, leaves its imprint on the nervous system. This phenomenon is clearly seen in animal studies: a rat, if addicted to morphine by repeated injections at one to two months of age and then detoxified, will show a residual tolerance and abnormalities in brain waves in response to challenge doses of morphine for months, perhaps for the rest of its life. Simply stopping the drug does not restore the nervous system of this animal to its normal, pre-addiction condition. Since all studies to date have shown a close association between tolerance and physical dependence, and since the discomfort of physical dependence leads to drug-seeking activity, a persistence of physical dependence would explain why both animals and humans tend to relapse to use of narcotics after detoxification. This metabolic theory of relapse obviously has different implications for treatment than the traditional theory that relapse is due to moral weakness.

Whatever the theory, all treatment should be measured by results. The main issue, in our opinion, is whether the treatment can enable addicts to become normal, responsible members of society; and, if medication contributes to this result, it should be regarded as useful chemotherapy. Methadone, like sulfanilamide of the early antibiotic days, undoubtedly will be supplanted by better medications, but the success of methadone maintenance programs has at least established the principle of treating addicts medically.

The efficacy of methadone as a medication must be judged by its ability or failure to achieve the pharmacological effect that is intended—namely, elimination of heroin hunger and heroin-seeking behavior, and blockade against the euphoriant actions of heroin. The goal of social rehabilitation of criminal addicts by a treatment program is a much broader objective: it includes the stopping of heroin abuse, but is not limited to this pharmacological effect. Failures in rehabilitation programs, therefore, must be analyzed to determine whether they are due to failures of the medicine, or to inability of the therapists to rehabilitate patients who have stopped heroin use. Individuals who have stopped heroin use with methadone treatment but who continue to steal, drink excessively, or abuse non-narcotic drugs, or are otherwise anti-social, are failures of the rehabilitation program but not of the medication.

When the Food and Drug Administration asks for proof of efficacy of a new drug, it is the pharmacological efficacy that is in question. For example, diphenylhydantoin is accepted as an efficacious drug for prevention of epileptic seizures. Whether or not the treated epileptics obtain employment, or otherwise lead socially useful lives, is not relevant to the evaluation of this drug as an efficacious drug for prevention of epileptic seizures or as an anti-convulsant; similarly with methadone.

With thousands of patients now living socially acceptable lives with methadone blockade, and with many more street addicts waiting for admission, the question as to whether these patients are exceptional is no longer a practical issue. The theoretical question, however, remains: is addiction caused by an antecedent character defect, and does the maintenance treatment merely mask the symptoms of an addictive personality? The psychogenic theory of addiction would say so. This theory has a long history—at least 100 years (Terry and Pellens 1928)—and is accepted as axiomatic by many people. What, then, is the evidence for it?

Review of the literature discloses two arguments to support the psychogenic, or character defect, theory: the sociopathic behavior and attitude of addicts and the inability of addicts to control their drug-using impulse. Of these arguments, the first is the most telling. Even a sympathetic observer must concede that addicts are self-centered and indifferent to the needs of others. To the family and the community, the addict is irresponsible, a thief, and a liar. These traits, which are quite consistently associated with addiction, have been interpreted as showing a specific psychopathology. What is lacking in this argument is proof that the sociopathic traits preceded addiction.

It is important to distinguish the causes from the consequences of addiction. The decisive proof of a psychogenic theory would be a demonstration that potential addicts could be identified by psychiatric examination before drug usage had distorted behavior and metabolic functions. However, a careful search of the literature has failed to disclose any study in which a characteristic psychopathology or "addictive personality" has been recognized in a number of individuals prior to addiction. Retrospective studies, in which a record of delinquency before addiction is taken as evidence of sociopathic tendencies, fail to provide the comparative data needed for diagnosis of deviant personality. Most of the street addicts in large cities come from the slums, where family structure is broken and drugs are available. Both juvenile delinquency and drug use are common. Some delinquents become addicted to narcotic drugs under these conditions, whereas others do not. There is no known way to identify the future addicts among the delinquents. No study has shown a consistent difference in behavior or pattern of delinquency of adolescents who later become addicts and those who do not.

Theft is the means by which most street addicts obtain money to buy heroin and, therefore, is nearly an inevitable consequence of addiction. For the majority, this is the only way that they can support an expensive heroin habit. The crime statistics show both the force of drug hunger and its specificity; almost all of the crimes committed by addicts relate to the procurement of drugs. The rapid disappearance of theft and anti-social behavior in patients on the methadone maintenance program strongly supports the hypothesis that the crimes that they had previously committed as addicts were a consequence of drug hunger, not the expression of some more basic psychopathology. The so-called sociopathic personality was no longer evident in our patients.

The second argument, that of deficient self-control, is more complicated, because it involves the personal experience of the critic as well as that of the patient. Moralists generally assume that opiates are dangerously pleasant drugs that can be resisted only by strength of character. The pharmacology is somewhat more complicated than this. For most normal persons morphine and heroin are not enjoyable drugs—at least not in the initial exposures. Given to a post-operative patient, these analgesics provide a welcome relief of pain, but addiction from such medical use is uncommon. When given to an average pain-free subject, morphine produces nausea and sedation, but rarely euphoria. What, then, is the temptation to become an addict? So far as can be judged from the histories of addicts, many of them found the first trials of a narcotic in some sense pleasurable or tranquilizing, even though the drug also caused nausea and vomiting. Perhaps their reaction to the drug was abnormal, even on the first exposure. However this may be, with repeated use and development of tolerance to side effects, the euphoric action evolved and the subjects became established addicts.

Drug-seeking behavior, like theft, is observed after addiction is established and the narcotic drug has become euphorigenic. The question as to whether this abnormality in reaction stems from a basic weakness of character or is a consequence of drug usage is best studied when drug hunger is relieved. Patients on the methadone maintenance program, blockaded against the euphorigenic action of heroin, turn their energies to schoolwork and jobs. It would be easy for them to become passive, to live indefinitely on public support, and claim that they had done enough in winning the fight against heroin. Why they do not yield to this temptation is unclear, but in general they do not. Their struggles to become self-supporting members of the community should impress the critics who had considered them self-indulgent when drug-hungry addicts. When drug hunger is blocked without production of narcotic effects, the drug-seeking behavior ends.

So far as can be judged from retrospective data, narcotic drugs have been quite freely available in some areas of New York City, and experimentation by adolescents is common. The psychological and metabolic theories diverge somewhat in interpreting this fact; the first postulates preexisting emotional problems and a need to seek drugs for escape from reality, whereas the alternative is that trial of drugs, like smoking the first cigarette, may be a result of a normal adolescent curiosity and not of psychopathology (Wikler and Rasor 1953). As to the most important point—the reasons for continuation of drug use in some cases and not in others—there is no definitive information, either psychological or metabolic. This is obviously a crucial gap in knowledge. Systematic study of young adolescents in areas with high addiction rates is needed to define the process of becoming addicted and to open the way for prevention.

The other extreme—the cured addict—involves a controversy as to the goal of therapy. Those of us who are primarily concerned with the social productivity of our patients define success in terms of behavior—the ability of the patients to live as normal citizens in the community—whereas, other groups seek total abstinence, even if it means confinement of the subjects to an institution. This confusion of goals has barred effective comparison of treatment results.

Actually, the questions to be answered are straightforward and of great practical importance. Do the abstinent patients in the psychological programs have a residual metabolic defect that requires continued group pressure and institutionalization to enforce the abstinence? Conversely, do the patients who are blockaded with methadone exhibit any residual psychopathology? No evidence is available to answer the first question. As to the latter point, we can state that the evidence, so far, is negative. The attitudes, moods, and intellectual and social performance of patients are under continuous observation by a team of psychiatrists, internists, nurses, counselors, social workers, and psychologists. No consistent psychopathology has been noted by these observers or by the social agencies, to which we have referred patients for vocational placement. The good records of employment and school work further document the patients' capacity to win acceptance as normal citizens in the community.

The real revolution of the methadone era was its emphasis on rehabilitation, rather than on detoxification. This reversed the traditional approach to addiction, which had been based on the assumption that abstinence must come first. According to the old theory, rehabilitation is impossible while a person is taking drugs of any kind, including methadone. The success of methadone programs in rehabilitating addicts who had already failed in abstinence programs decisively refuted this old theory. Indeed, nowhere in the history of treatment has a program with the abstinence approach achieved even a fraction of the retention rate and social rehabilitation now seen in the average methadone clinic. This statement includes all of the abstinence-oriented programs of governmental institutions, therapeutic communities, and religious groups for which any data are available (Brecher 1972; Glasscote 1972).

We believe that it is a serious mistake for programs to put a higher value on abstinence than on the patient's ability to function as a normal member of society. After the patient has arrived at a stable way of life with a job, a home, a position of respect in his community, and a sense of worth, it may or may not be best to discontinue methadone, but at least he can consider this option without pressure. The pharmacologic symptoms of withdrawal will be the same, whether or not the addict is socially rehabilitated; but with a job and family there is much more to lose if relapse occurs, and, therefore, the motivation to resist a return to heroin will be strong. The time spent in maintenance treatment does not make detoxification more difficult. It has proved very easy to withdraw methadone from patients who have been maintained for one to eight years when the reduction in dose has been gradual and the patient free from anxiety.

As with heroin, the real problems begin after withdrawal. The secondary abstinence syndrome, first described by Himmelsbach, Martin, Wikler, and colleagues at the United States Public Health Hospital, Lexington, Kentucky, in patients detoxified from morphine and heroin, reflects the persistence of metabolic and autonomic disturbances in the post-narcotic withdrawal period (Himmelsbach 1942; Martin et al. 1963; Martin and Jasinski 1969): these persistent abnormalities in metabolism are clearly pharmacologic, since they occur also in experimental animals addicted to narcotics and then detoxified. Follow-up studies of abstinent ex-addicts have emphasized the frequency of alcoholism and functional deterioration (Brecher 1972).

An unfortunate consequence of the early enthusiasm for methadone treatment is today's general disenchantment with chemotherapy for addicts. What was not anticipated at the onset was the nearly universal reaction against the concept of substituting one drug for another, even when the second drug enabled the addict to function normally. Statistics, showing improved health and social rehabilitation of the patients receiving methadone, failed to meet this fundamental objection. The analogous

long-term use of other medications, such as insulin and digitalis, in medical practice has not been considered relevant.

Perhaps the limitations of medical treatment for complex medical-social problems were not sufficiently stressed. No medicine can rehabilitate persons. Methadone maintenance makes possible a first step toward social rehabilitation by stabilizing the pharmacological condition of addicts who have been living as criminals on the fringe of society. But to succeed in bringing disadvantaged addicts to a productive way of life, a treatment program must enable its patients to feel pride and hope and to accept responsibility. This is often not achieved in present-day treatment programs. Without mutual respect, an adversary relationship develops between patients and staff, reinforced by arbitrary rules and the indifference of persons in authority. Patients held in contempt by the staff continue to act like addicts, and the overcrowded facility becomes a public nuisance. Understandably, methadone maintenance programs today have little appeal to the communities or to the majority of heroin addicts on the street.

Methadone maintenance, as part of a supportive program, facilitates social rehabilitation; but methadone treatment clearly does not prevent opiate abuse after it is discontinued, nor does social rehabilitation guarantee freedom from relapse.

For the previously intractable heroin addict with a pretreatment history of several years of addiction and social problems, the most conservative course, in our opinion, is to emphasize social rehabilitation and encourage continued maintenance. On the other hand, for patients with shorter histories of heroin use, especially the young ones, a trial of withdrawal with a systematic follow-up is indicated when physician and patient feel ready for the test, and when they understand the potential problems after detoxification. The first step of withdrawing methadone is relatively easy and can be achieved with a variety of schedules, none of which have been shown to have any specific effect on the long-range outcome. The real issue is how well the patient does in the years after termination of maintenance.

* * *

Vicent P. Dole and Marie Nyswander, "Methadone Maintenance: A Theoretical Perspective," in Dan J. Lettieri, Mollie Sayers, and Helen Wallenstein Pearson (eds.), Theories on Drug Abuse (Rockville, MD:

National Institute on Drug Abuse, 1980), pp. 256-261.

For Discussion

1. Experts on methadone maintenance often believe that some heroin users should be treated with methadone periodically throughout their lives. Who should fund life treatment and is it cost effective?

2. In the first section of this book, Lindesmith argues that individuals continue to use opiates to eliminate the pain associated with withdrawal. Is the philosophy of methadone treatment consistent with Lindesmith's theory of addiction? If so, how? ✦

35. *Alcoholics Anonymous*

Karen McElrath

Alcoholics Anonymous (AA) is perhaps the best known of treatment approaches for alcoholics and problem drinkers. In this first essay, Karen McElrath briefly describes the AA approach, its "Twelve Steps" and "Twelve Traditions," and what occurs at AA meetings. Since only minimal research data are available on AA, little is known about its actual effectiveness.

> "My name is Carol G. and I am an alcoholic. Twice I've been admitted to emergency rooms for delirium tremens. Twice I've almost died. I knew I hit rock bottom when my drinking caused me to miss numerous work days and resulted in my failure to meet job deadlines. I was fired after having worked for that company for 16 years."

The above statement represents one of several "stories" recounted by an alcoholics during a meeting of Alcoholics Anonymous (AA). Disclosures are anonymous, hence, the name "Carol G." AA members always begin their stories with the self-identified label, "I am an alcoholic" because recognition of the illness is viewed as the first stage of recovery. These testimonials often include the tremendous consequences of alcoholism whereby members disclose the manner by which alcoholism has affected their personal and professional lives. Such disclosures might normally result in disapproval and negative sanctions in everyday social interactions; yet, during AA meetings, this dialogue is viewed with compassion, empathy, and support (Denzin 1987). The underlying philosophy of AA is that alcoholism is a disease for which no cure is available. Sobriety, rather than controlled drinking, is the goal of the program. Subsequent use of alcohol or relapse is not considered failure, however, nor are persons who relapse treated with disdain by other members.

AA is perhaps the largest and most popular treatment modality for addressing alcoholism. AA is described often as a self-help group because involvement is voluntary, in theory. The program might be better described as a collective-help group because reciprocal support among members is believed to significantly aid in the recovery process. For many members, AA provides an important social network through which members learn appropriate behaviors and coping skills in drinking situations and become involved in various (non-drinking) leisure activities with other recovering alcoholics.

Meetings are categorized as open or closed. Open meetings consist of participants interested in the program or interested in alcoholism. During open meetings, the audience might include both alcoholics and nonalcoholics. Closed meetings involve alcoholics only. Generally, anonymity is stressed more during open meetings, at the start of which members are often reminded of their anonymity.

There are no formal admission criteria for AA. Individuals become members by attending meetings and by the self-recognition that one is an alcoholic. Many members attend several times per week. Some attend only after drinking binges. AA philosophy assumes, "Once an alcoholic, always an alcoholic"; therefore, many members attend meetings throughout their lives, even after years of abstinence.

The Twelve Steps

The backbone of the program features the Twelve Steps to recovery (see Table 1). These tenets are designed to help individuals in the recovery process. Six of these principles specifically mention or make reference to God, which reflect the spiritual foundation of the program. Further, meetings often open with the "Serenity Prayer" and close with the "Lord's Prayer" (Denzin 1987). Since some individuals have objected to these spiritual references, Steps 3 and 11 now include the words "God as we understood Him" (Trice 1958).

Table 1
The Twelve Steps

1. We admitted we were powerless over alcohol—that our lives had become unmanageable.

2. We came to believe that a Power greater than ourselves could restore us to sanity.

3. We made a decision to turn our will and our lives over to the care of God as we understood Him.

4. We made a searching and fearless moral inventory of ourselves.

5. We admitted to God, to ourselves, and to another human being the exact nature of our wrongs.

6. We were entirely ready to have God remove all these defects of character.

7. We humbly asked Him to remove our shortcomings.

8. We made a list of all persons we have harmed, and became willing to make amends to them all.

9. We made direct amends to such people, wherever possible, except when to do so would injure them or others.

10. We continued to take personal inventory and when we were wrong, promptly admitted it.

11. We sought through prayer and meditation to improve our conscious contact with God as we understood Him, praying only for knowledge of his Will for us and the power to carry that out.

12. Having had a spiritual awakening as the result of these steps, we tried to carry this message to alcoholics and practice these principles in all our affairs.

Step 12 refers to the "Slogan of Responsibility," the pledge to help other alcoholics and to show them the benefits of AA. Thus, AA members serve as major sources of recruitment and referral. Most members purchase a copy of the "Big Book," which outlines methods to achieve goals of abstinence through the Twelve Steps.

Local Meetings

The first AA meeting occurred in 1935 when two alcoholics, Bill W. and Bob S., met in Akron, Ohio. It is perhaps no coincidence that this first meeting occurred two years after prohibition was repealed. There were approximately 100 members by 1938 and by 1944 an estimated 10,000 individuals claimed membership. This dramatic increase in membership was fueled in part by an article about the program that appeared in the *Saturday Evening Post* in 1941 (Trice 1958). Today, international membership in AA is over one million, with several hundred thousand members in the United States. In some large metropolitan areas there are hundreds of meetings per week.

Once known as a group serving primarily middle-class white males, AA meetings are increasingly diverse in their membership. Robertson (1988) notes that program aspects have changed little since its beginnings; however, member profiles have changed over the years. For example, females now comprise a larger proportion of membership and virtually all ethnic groups are represented. These changes more accurately reflect use of alcohol in the larger society; a behavior that cuts across all demographic and socioeconomic groups. In the tradition of the first meeting between Bill W. and Bob S., an AA group meeting consists of two or more persons. Some reports indicate that newcomers enjoy a temporary yet special status and that it is customary for members to recount their stories for the newcomer (Denzin 1987). Other studies report that in some groups, the newcomer is often ignored (Trice 1958).

The Twelve Traditions

Local AA groups typically follow the Twelve Traditions (See Table 2). The Twelve Traditions emphasize the importance of maintaining spiritual unity. These serve as a guide for local groups, and few groups depart from the Traditions. Local autonomy is emphasized in Traditions 2, 4, and 11. There is no bureaucratic governing body which determines local agendas. Each local group elects a representative, referred to as a General Services Representative (GSR). This representative serves as liaison between the local group and AA. One representative from a given geographic area is then elected for a one or two year term to attend the national General Service Conference.

Table 2
The Twelve Traditions

1. Our common welfare should come first—personal recovery depends on AA unity.

2. For our group purpose, there is but one ultimate authority—a loving God as he may express Himself in our group conscience. Our leaders are but trusted servants; they do not govern.

3. The only requirement for AA membership is a desire to stop drinking.

4. Each group should be autonomous, except in matters affecting other groups or AA as a whole.

5. Each group has but one primary purpose—to carry its message to the alcoholic who still suffers.

6. An AA group ought never endorse, finance, or lend the AA name to any related facility or outside enterprise, lest problems of money, prop-

erty, and prestige divert us from our primary purpose.

7. Every AA group ought to be fully self-supporting, declining outside contributions.

8. Alcoholics Anonymous should remain forever nonprofessional, but our service centers may employ special workers.

9. AA, as such, ought never be organized; but we may create service boards or committees directly responsible for those they serve.

10. Alcoholics Anonymous has no opinion on outside issues; hence, the AA name ought never be drawn into public controversy.

11. Our public-relations policy is based on attraction rather than promotion; we need always maintain personal autonomy at the level of press, radio, and films.

12. Anonymity is the spiritual foundation of our traditions, ever reminding us to place principles before personalities.

Unlike most substance abuse-treatment programs, local meetings require little funding. There are no staff to pay, no drugs to purchase. Members are not asked to pay dues, but those in attendance often donate a few dollars to pay for refreshments and meeting space. Charitable donations and gifts are not generally accepted, although member donations in amounts of $1000 or less a year are accepted. It is believed that larger donations will compromise the goal of AA, allowing contributors to dictate or influence national and local decisions. Local groups do contribute a proportion of funds to the national body, but the millions of dollars raised each year stems mostly from sales of AA literature purchased by members, libraries, professionals, and other interested parties.

Denzin (1987) describes the rituals that characterize local meetings. Many of these rituals promote kinship and group solidarity. Meetings often open with a verbal history of AA. The Preamble is read, along with the "Thought for the Day." Everyone is allowed to speak, to provide his or her "story." There are no interruptions during the oral histories of the members. The meeting Chair often determines the order of the speeches—left to right or right to left. Extrinsic rewards for sobriety include the presentation of medallions and "birthday" cakes with candles marking the number of years of abstinence. The AA handshake is customary at the close of meetings. During the recital of the "Lord's Prayer," members often join hands, a latent symbol of collective strength.

AA *Effectiveness*

To date, we have little scientific knowledge about the effectiveness of AA. Tournier (1979) notes the limitations that inhibit research evaluations of AA. First, there are no shared research definitions of recovery; that is, studies differ regarding the ways in which successes and failures are measured. Many investigators measure recovery in terms of whether or not the client is drinking. This definition may be too simplistic but is consistent with the AA goal of total abstinence. Similarly, although the term "alcoholism" was first described in 1852, one review of the literature disclosed more than 200 definitions of the disorder (Jellinek 1960). Lacking clear definitions of these terms, it is difficult to compare results across studies. Tournier notes also that the requirement of anonymity of members and lack of recordkeeping make it difficult for researchers to identify AA members. A review of the research on AA finds that most studies fail to compare the treatment group (AA members) with appropriate control groups, so it is not often known about the behaviors of non-members. Also, studies rely greatly on volunteer research subjects, so that investigators know little about drinkers who do not participate in studies. Further, random assignment is often not feasible, because AA is largely a volunteer organization. Without random assignment, it is impossible to demonstrate whether individuals might have abstained from alcohol use had they not been exposed to the program. Additionally, the drop-out rate has been estimated at 40 percent (Robertson 1988), and it is not often known whether drop outs maintain sobriety. Another impediment to AA research is that studies rely greatly on self-reported alcohol use among members. Despite these limitations, however, there is considerable anecdotal evidence that provides support for the effectiveness of AA as a treatment option. Many people have abstained from alcohol use for years and attribute recovery to their participation in AA. Success of AA is demonstrated also by similar programs that have adopted the Twelve Step philosophy, e.g., Alateen, Alanon, Narcotics Anonymous, Cocaine Anonymous.

In recent years, much has been written about matching client needs with the appropriate treatment. No treatment works for everyone, and AA is no exception. AA might be better suited for members who drink to cope with loneliness because of the social support that AA provides (Tournier 1979).

In some instances, individuals are forced to attend AA meetings as a result of their criminal-justice involvement. Judicially-coerced referrals are antithetical to the philosophy of AA as a volunteer program. Studies of legally-mandated methadone treatment have shown recently that chronic heroin addicts who are forced into treatment do not differ in post-treatment behaviors from volunteer treatment subjects (Anglin, Brecht, and Maddahian 1989). This finding has yet to be replicated among AA members. In fact, a study by Brandsma, Maultsby, and Welsh (1980) found that among judicially-referred subjects, those assigned to AA had lower retention rates than subjects assigned to other treatment modalities.

Conclusion

Alcoholics Anonymous is an important treatment modality for addressing alcoholism. Through AA, members share similar experiences and gain social support. The program provides both intrinsic and extrinsic rewards and offers few negative sanctions. Unlike many treatment modalities, operating costs are minimal. At present, it is not known whether AA is more effective than other treatment options; research is inhibited most often as a result of program aspects. Few researchers can deny, however, that AA has helped numerous alcoholics and the program is likely to assist many others.

*　*　*

For Discussion

Should judges have the authority to coerce offenders to participate in AA programs? Why or why not?

References

Anglin, M. D., Brecht, M., and E. Maddahian (1989). Pretreatment characteristics and treatment performance of legally coerced versus voluntary methadone maintenance admissions. *Criminology* 27: 537-557.

Brandsma, J. M., M. C. Maultsby, and R. J. Walsh (1980). *Outpatient Treatment of Alcoholism: A Review and Comparative Study*. Baltimore: University Park.

Denzin, N. K. (1987). *The Recovering Alcoholic*. Newbury Park, CA: Sage.

Jellinek, E. M. (1960). *The Disease Concept of Alcoholism*. New Haven, CT: College and University Press.

Robertson, N. (1988). The changing world of Alcoholics Anonymous. *The New York Times Magazine* (February 21), pp. 40, 42-44, 47, 92.

Tournier, R. E. (1979). Alcoholics Anonymous as treatment and as ideology. *Journal of Studies on Alcohol* 40:230-239.

Trice, H. (1958). Alcoholics Anonymous. *The Annals of the American Academy of Political and Social Science* 315:109-123. ✦

Part X
Policy

The federal approach to drug abuse and drug control has included a variety of avenues for reducing both the *supply of*, and the *demand for*, illicit drugs. Historically, the supply-and-demand reduction strategies were grounded in the classic deterrence model: through legislation and criminal penalties, individuals would be discouraged from using drugs; by setting an example of traffickers, the government would force potential dealers to seek out other economic pursuits. In time, other components were then added: treatment for the user; education and prevention for the would-be user; and research to determine how to best develop and implement plans for treatment, education, and prevention.

By the early 1970s, when it appeared that the war on drugs had won few, if any, battles, new avenues for supply-and-demand reduction were added. There were the federal interdiction initiatives: the Coast Guard, Customs, and Drug Enforcement Administration operatives were charged with intercepting drug shipments coming to the United States from foreign ports; in the international sector, there were attempts to eradicate drug-yielding crops at their source. On the surface, none of these strategies seemed to have any effect, and illicit drug use continued to spread.

The problems were many. Legislation and enforcement alone were not enough, and early-education programs of the "scare" variety quickly lost their credibility. Moreover, for most social scientists and clinicians, treating drug abuse as a medical problem seemed to be the logical answer. But treatment programs didn't seem to be working too well, most likely because the course of treatment just wasn't long enough to have any significant impact.

Given the perceived inadequacy of the traditional approaches to drug-abuse control, during the late 1970s federal authorities began drawing plans for a more concerted assault on drugs, both legislative and technological. It began with the RICO (Racketeer-Influenced and Corrupt Organizations) and CCE (Continuing Criminal Enterprise) statutes. What RICO and CCE accomplish is the forfeiture of the fruits of criminal activities. Their intent is to eliminate the rights of traffickers to their personal assets, whether these be cash, bank accounts, real estate, automobiles, jewelry and art, equity in businesses, directorships in companies, or any kind of goods or entitlements that are obtained in or used for a criminal enterprise.

Added to the perceived strength offered by RICO and CCE was a new extradition treaty between the United States and the Republic of Colombia, signed on September 14, 1979 and entered into force on March 4, 1982. The treaty was notable, in that it added to the list of extraditable crimes a whole variety of offenses related to drug trafficking, aircraft hijacking, obstruction of justice, and bribery. In addition, Article 8 of the treaty was a considerable innovation in international affairs, in that it imposed an obligation on the government of Colombia to extradite *all* persons, *including its nationals*, when the offense was a punishable act in both countries and was intended to be consummated in the United States.

The new, evolving federal drug strategy considered it crucial to include the U.S. military in its war on drugs. In 1982, the Department of Defense Authorization Act was signed into law, making the entire war chest of U.S. military power available to law enforcement—for training, intelligence gathering, and detection. Beginning in 1982, the "war on drugs" had a new look. Put into force was the Bell 209 assault helicopter, more popularly known as the Cobra. There was none in the military arsenal that was faster, and in its gunship mode it could destroy a tank. In addition, there was the awesome Sikorsky Black Hawk assault helicopter, assigned for operation by U.S. Customs Service pilots. Customs also had the Cessna Citation, a jet aircraft equipped with radar originally designed for F-16 fighters. There was the Navy's EC-2, an aircraft equipped with a radar disk capable of detecting other aircraft from as far as 300 miles away. There were "Fat Albert" and his pals—aerostat surveillance balloons 175 feet in length equipped with sophisticated radar and listening devices. Fat Albert could not only pick up communications from Cuba and Soviet satellites but also detect traffic in "Smugglers' Alley," a wide band of Caribbean sky that is virtually invisible to land-based radar systems. There were NASA satellites to spy on drug operations as far apart as California and Colombia, airborne infrared sensing and imaging equipment that could detect human body heat in the thickest underbrush of Florida's Everglades, plus a host of other high-technology devices. In all, drug enforcement appeared well-equipped for battle.

The final component added to the drug-war armamentarium was "zero-tolerance," a 1988 White House anti-drug policy based on a number of premises: 1) that if there were no drug abusers there would be no drug problem; 2) that the market for drugs is created not only by availability, but also by demand; 3) that drug abuse starts with a willful act; 4) that the perception that drug users are powerless to act against the influences of drug availability and peer pressure is an erroneous one; 5) that most illegal drug users can choose to stop their drug-taking behaviors and must be held accountable if they do not; 6) that individual freedom does not include the right to self and societal destruction; and, 7) that public tolerance for drug abuse must be reduced to *zero*. As such, the zero-tolerance policy expanded the war on drugs from suppliers and dealers to users as well—especially casual users—and meant that planes, vessels, and vehicles could be confiscated for carrying even the smallest amount of a controlled substance.

By 1988, well after the newest "war on drugs" had been declared and put into operation, it had long since been decided by numerous observers that the 74 years of federal prohibition since the passage of the Harrison Act of 1914 were not only a costly and abject failure, but represented a totally doomed effort as well. It was argued that drug laws and drug enforcement had served mainly to create enormous profits for drug dealers and traffickers, overcrowded jails, police and other government corruption, a distorted foreign policy, predatory street crime carried on by users in search of the funds necessary to purchase black-market drugs, and urban areas harassed by street-level drug dealers and terrorized by violent drug gangs.

Much of what these observers were remarking about had been the case. And there were other problems: the continued use of illegal drugs, with many cities seemingly overwhelmed with crack-cocaine; violence in the inner cities and elsewhere, as drug-trafficking gangs competed for distribution territories; street crime, committed by users for the sake of supporting their drug habits; and corruption in law enforcement and other branches of government, brought on by the considerable economic opportunities for those involved in drug distribution.

Within the context of the concerns, 1988 also marked the onset of renewed calls for the *decriminalization*, if not the outright *legalization*, of most or all illicit drugs. The arguments posed by the supporters of legalization seem all too logical. *First*, they argue, the drug laws have created evils far worse than the drugs themselves—corruption, violence, street crime, and disrespect for the law. *Second*, legislation passed to control drugs has failed to reduce demand. *Third*, you cannot render illegal that which a significant segment of the population in any society is committed to doing. You simply cannot arrest, prosecute, and punish such large numbers of people, particularly in a democracy. And specifically in this behalf, in a liberal democracy, the government must not interfere with *personal* behavior, if liberty is to be maintained. *Fourth*, they added, if marijuana, cocaine, crack, heroin, and other drugs were legalized, a number of very positive things would happen:

1. drug prices would fall;

2. users could obtain their drugs at low, government-regulated prices and would no longer be forced to engage in prostitution and street crime to support their habits;

3. the fact that the levels of drug-related crime would significantly decline would result in less crowded courts, jails, and prisons, and free law-enforcement personnel to focus their energies on the "real criminals" in society;

4. drug production, distribution, and sale would be removed from the criminal arena; no longer would it be within the province of organized crime, and as such, such criminal syndicates as the Medellin Cartel and the Jamaican posses

would be decapitalized, and the violence associated with drug-distribution rivalries would be eliminated;

5. government corruption and intimidation by traffickers, as well as drug-based foreign policies, would be effectively reduced, if not eliminated entirely; and,

6. the often draconian measures undertaken by police to enforce the drug laws would be curtailed, thus restoring to the American public many of its hard-won civil liberties.

Those opposed to legalizing drugs argued a counter position, suggesting that making heroin, cocaine, and other illicit drugs more available would create a public health problem of massive proportions. In the three papers that follow, the arguments for and against legalizing drugs are thoroughly examined, as are alternative policy choices. ✦

36. Drug Prohibition in the United States: Costs, Consequences, and Alternatives

Ethan A. Nadelmann

Ethan A. Nadelmann argues that "drug legalization" merits serious consideration as a policy alternative in the United States. Criminal justice approaches to the drug problem have been of limited value in curtailing drug abuse, and they have been both costly and counterproductive. Nadelmann suggests that a drug legalization policy that is wisely implemented can minimize the risks of legalization, dramatically reduce the costs of current policies, and directly address the problems of drug abuse.

As frustrations with the drug problem and current drug policies rise daily, growing numbers of political leaders, law-enforcement officials, drug-abuse experts, and common citizens are insisting that a radical alternative to current policies be fairly considered: the controlled legalization (or decriminalization) of drugs.[1]

Just as "Repeal Prohibition" became a catch phrase that swept together the diverse objections to Prohibition, so "Legalize (or Decriminalize) Drugs" has become a catch phrase that means many things to many people. The policy analyst views legalization as a model for critically examining the costs and benefits of drug-prohibition policies. Libertarians, both civil and economic, view it as a policy alternative that eliminates criminal sanctions on the use and sale of drugs that are costly in terms of both individual liberty and economic freedom. Others see it simply as a means to "take the crime out of the drug business." In its broadest sense, however, legalization incorporates the many arguments and growing sentiment for de-emphasizing our traditional reliance on criminal-justice resources to deal with drug abuse, and for emphasizing instead drug abuse, prevention, treatment, and education, as well as non-criminal restrictions on the availability and use of psychoactive substances and positive inducements to abstain from drug abuse.

There is no one legalization option. At one extreme, some libertarians advocate the removal of all criminal sanctions and taxes on the production and sale of all psychoactive substances—with the possible exception of restrictions on sales to children. The alternative extremes are more varied. Some would limit legalization to one of the safest (relatively speaking) of all illicit substances: marijuana. Others prefer a "medical" oversight model similar to today's methadone maintenance programs. The middle ground combines legal availability of some or all illicit drugs with vigorous efforts to restrict consumption by means other than resorting to criminal sanctions. Many supporters of this dual approach simultaneously advocate greater efforts to limit tobacco consumption and the abuse of alcohol, as well as a transfer of government resources from law enforcement to drug prevention and treatment. Indeed, the best model for this view of drug legalization is precisely the tobacco-control model advocated by those who want to do everything possible to discourage tobacco consumption, short of criminalizing the production, sale, and use of tobacco.

Clearly, neither drug legalization nor enforcement of anti-drug laws promises to "solve" the drug problem. Nor is there any question that legalization presents certain risks. Legalization would almost certainly increase the availability of drugs, decrease their price, and remove the deterrent power of the criminal sanction, all of which invite increases in drug use and abuse. There are at least three reasons, however, why these risks are worth taking. First, drug-control strategies that rely primarily on criminal-justice measures are significantly and inherently limited in their capacity to curtail drug abuse. Second, many law-enforcement efforts are not only of limited value but also highly costly and counter-productive; indeed, many of the drug-related evils that most people identify as part and parcel of "the drug problem" are, in fact, the costs of drug-prohibition policies. Third, the risks of legalization may well be less than most people assume, particularly if intelligent alternative measures are implemented.

The Limits of Drug-Prohibition Policies

Few law-enforcement officials any longer contend that their efforts can do much more than they are already doing to reduce drug abuse in the

United States. This is true of international drug-enforcement efforts, interdiction, and both high-level and street-level, domestic drug-enforcement efforts.

The United States seeks to limit the export of illicit drugs to this country by a combination of crop-eradication and crop-substitution programs, financial inducements to growers to abstain from the illicit business, and punitive measures against producers, traffickers, and others involved in the drug traffic. These efforts have met with scant success in the past and show few indications of succeeding in the future. The obstacles are many: marijuana and opium can be grown in a wide variety of locales and even the coca plant "can be grown in virtually any subtropical region of the world which gets between 40 and 240 inches of rain per year, where it never freezes, and where the land is not so swampy as to be waterlogged. In South America, this comes to [approximately] 2,500,000 square miles," of which less than 700 square miles are currently being used to cultivate coca.[2] Producers in many countries have reacted to crop eradication programs by engaging in "guerrilla" farming methods, cultivating their crops in relatively inaccessible hinterlands, and camouflaging them with legitimate crops. Some illicit drug-producing regions are controlled not by the central government but by drug-trafficking gangs or political insurgents, thereby rendering eradication efforts even more difficult and hazardous.

Even where eradication efforts prove relatively successful in an individual country, other countries will emerge as new producers, as has occurred with both the international marijuana and heroin markets during the past two decades and can be expected to follow from planned coca-eradication programs. The foreign-export price of illicit drugs is such a tiny fraction of the retail price in the United States [approximately 4 percent with cocaine, 1 percent with marijuana, and much less than 1 percent with heroin][3] that international drug-control efforts are not even successful in raising the cost of illicit drugs to U.S. consumers.

U.S. efforts to control drugs overseas also confront substantial and, in some cases, well-organized political opposition in foreign countries.[4] Major drug traffickers retain the power to bribe and intimidate government officials into ignoring or even cooperating with their enterprises.[5] Particularly in many Latin American and Asian countries, the illicit drug traffic is an important source of income and employment, bringing in billions of dollars in hard currency each year and providing liveable wages for many hundreds of thousands. The illicit drug business has been described—not entirely in jest—as the best means ever devised by the United States for exporting the capitalist ethic to potentially revolutionary Third World peasants. By contrast, United States-sponsored eradication efforts risk depriving those same peasants of their livelihoods, thereby stimulating support for communist insurgencies, ranging from Peru's Shining Path[6] to the variety of ethnic and communist organizations active in drug-producing countries, such as Colombia and Burma. Moreover, many of those involved in producing illicit drugs overseas do not perceive their moral obligation as preventing decadent gringos from consuming cocaine or heroin; rather, it is to earn the best living possible for themselves and their families. In the final analysis, there is little the U.S. government can do to change this perception.

Interdiction efforts have shown little success in stemming the flow of cocaine and heroin into the United States.[7] Indeed, during the past decade, the wholesale price of a kilo of cocaine has dropped by 80 percent, even as the retail purity of a gram of cocaine has quintupled from 12 to about 60 percent; the trend with heroin over the past few years has been similar, if less dramatic.[8] Easily transported in a variety of large and small aircraft and sea vessels, carried across the Mexican border by legal and illegal border crossers, hidden in everything from furniture, flowers, and automobiles to private body parts and cadavers, heroin and cocaine shipments are extraordinarily difficult to detect. Despite powerful congressional support for dramatically increasing the role of the military in drug interdiction, military leaders insist that they can do little to make a difference. The Coast Guard and U.S. Customs continue to expand their efforts in this area, but they too concede that they will never seize more than a small percentage of total shipments. Because cocaine and heroin are worth more than their weight in gold, the incentives to transport these drugs to the United States are so great that we can safely assume that there will never be a shortage of those willing to take the risk.

The one success that interdiction efforts can claim concerns marijuana. Because marijuana is far bulkier per dollar of value than either cocaine or heroin, it is harder to conceal and easier to detect. Stepped-up interdiction efforts in recent years appear to have reduced the flow of marijuana into the

United States and to have increased its price to the American consumer.[8] The unintended consequences of this success are twofold: the United States has emerged as one of the world's leading producers of marijuana; indeed, U.S. producers are now believed to produce among the finest strains in the world;[8] and many international drug traffickers appear to have redirected their efforts from marijuana to cocaine. The principal consequence of U.S. drug interdictions efforts, many would contend, has been a glut of increasingly potent cocaine and a shortage of comparatively benign marijuana.

Domestic law-enforcement efforts have proven increasingly successful in apprehending and imprisoning rapidly growing numbers of illicit drug merchants, ranging from the most sophisticated international traffickers to the most common street-level drug dealers. The principal benefit of law-enforcement efforts directed at major drug-trafficking organizations is probably the rapidly rising value of drug-trafficker assets forfeited to the government. There is, however, little indication that such efforts have any significant impact on the price or availability of illicit drugs. Intensive and highly costly street-level law-enforcement efforts, such as those mounted by many urban police departments in recent years, have resulted in the arrests of thousands of low-level drug dealers and users and helped improve the quality of life in targeted neighborhoods.[9] In most large urban centers, however, these efforts have had little impact on the overall availability of illicit drugs.

The logical conclusion of the foregoing analysis is not that criminal-justice efforts to stop drug trafficking do not work at all; rather, it is that even substantial fluctuations in those efforts have little effect on the price, availability, and consumption of illicit drugs. The mere existence of criminal laws, combined with minimal levels of enforcement, is sufficient to deter many potential users and to reduce the availability and increase the price of drugs. Law-enforcement officials acknowledge that they alone cannot solve the drug problem, but contend that their role is nonetheless essential to the overall effort to reduce illicit drug use and abuse. What they are less ready to acknowledge, however, is that the very criminalization of the drug market has proven highly costly and counter-productive in much the same way that the national prohibition of alcohol did 60 years ago.

The Costs and Consequences of Drug-Prohibition Policies

Total government expenditures devoted to enforcement of drug laws amounted to a minimum of $10 billion in 1987. Between 1981 and 1987, federal expenditures on anti-drug law enforcement more than tripled, from less than $1 billion per year to about $3 billion.[10] State and local law-enforcement agencies spent an estimated $5 billion, amounting to about one-fifth of their total investigative resources, on drug-enforcement activities in 1986.[11] Drug law violators currently account for approximately 10 percent of the roughly 550,000 inmates in state prisons, more than one-third of the 50,000 federal prison inmates, and a significant (albeit undetermined) proportion of the approximately 300,000 individuals confined in municipal jails.[12] The U.S. Sentencing Commission has predicted that in 15 years the federal prison population will total 100,000 to 150,000 inmates, of whom one-half will be incarcerated for drug law violations.[13] Among the 40,000 inmates in New York State prisons, drug-law violations surpassed first-degree robbery in 1987 as the number-one cause of incarceration, accounting for 20 percent of the total prison population.[14] In Florida, the 8,506 drug-law violators admitted to state prisons in fiscal 1987-88 represented a 525 percent increase from fiscal 1983-84 and 27.8 percent of all new admissions to prison in 1987-88.[15] Nationwide, drug-trafficking and drug-possession offenses accounted for approximately 135,000 (23 percent) of the 583,000 individuals convicted of felonies in state courts in 1986.[16] State and local governments spent a minimum of $2 billion last year to incarcerate drug offenders. The direct costs of building and maintaining enough prisons to house this growing population are rising at an astronomical rate. The costs, in terms of alternative social expenditures foregone and other types of criminals not imprisoned, are perhaps even more severe.[17]

Police have made about 750,000 arrests for violations of the drug laws during each of the last few years.[18] Slightly more than three-quarters of these have been not for manufacturing or dealing drugs but solely for possession of an illicit drug, typically marijuana.[19] [Those arrested, it is worth noting, represent less than 2 percent of the 35 to 40 million Americans estimated to have illegally consumed a drug during each of the past years.][20] On the one hand, these arrests have clogged many urban criminal-justice systems: in New York City, drug-law violations in 1987 accounted for more than 40 percent of all felony indictments, up from 25 percent in 1985;[21] in Washington, D.C., the figure was 52 percent in 1986, up from 13 percent in 1981.[22] On the other hand, they have distracted criminal-justice officials from concentrating greater resources on violent offenses and property crimes. In many cities, urban law enforcement has become virtually synonymous with drug enforcement.

The greatest beneficiaries of the drug laws are organized and unorganized drug traffickers. The criminalization of the drug market effectively imposes a *de facto* value-added tax that is enforced and occasionally augmented by the law-enforcement establishment and collected by the drug traffickers. More than half of all organized-crime revenues are believed to derive from the illicit drug business; estimates of the dollar value range between $10 and $50 billion per year.[23] By contrast, annual revenues from cigarette bootlegging, which persists principally because of differences among states in their cigarette tax rates, are estimated at between $200 million and $400 million.[23] If the marijuana, cocaine, and heroin markets were legal, state and federal governments would collect billions of dollars annually in tax revenues. Instead, they expend billions in what amounts to a subsidy of organized criminals.

The connection between drugs and crime is one that continues to resist coherent analysis, both because cause and effect are so difficult to distinguish and because the role of the drug-prohibition laws in causing and labeling "drug-related crime" is so often ignored. There are five possible connections between drugs and crime, at least three of which would be much diminished, if the drug-prohibition laws were repealed. First, the production, sale, purchase, and possession of marijuana, cocaine, heroin, and other strictly controlled and banned substances are crimes in and of themselves, which occur billions of times each year in the United States alone. In the absence of drug-prohibition laws, these activities would largely cease to be considered crimes. Selling drugs to children would, of course, continue to be criminalized, and other evasions of government regulation of a legal market would continue to be prosecuted, but, by and large, the connection between drugs and crime that now accounts for all of the criminal-justice costs noted above would be severed.

Second, many illicit drug users commit crimes, such as robbery and burglary, as well as other vice crimes, such as drug dealing, prostitution, and numbers running, to earn enough money to purchase cocaine, heroin, and other illicit drugs— drugs that cost far more than alcohol and tobacco, not because they cost much more to produce, but because they are illegal.[24] Because legalization would inevitably lead to a reduction in the cost of the drugs that are now illicit, it would also invite a significant reduction in this drug-crime connection. At the same time, current methadone-maintenance programs represent a limited form of drug legalization that attempts to break this connection between drugs and crime, by providing an addictive opiate at little or no cost to addicts who might otherwise steal to support their illicit heroin habits. Despite their many limitations, such programs have proven effective in reducing the criminal behavior and improving the lives of thousands of illicit drug addicts;[25] they need to be made more available, in part by adapting the types of outreach programs for addicts devised in the Netherlands.[26] Another alternative, the British system of prescribing not just oral methadone but also injectable heroin and methadone to addicts who take drugs intravenously, persists on a small scale even today, despite continuing pressures against prescribing injectables. This too merits adoption in the United States, particularly if one accepts the assumption that the primary objective of drug policy should be to minimize the harms that drug abusers do to others.[27]

The third connection between drugs and crime is more coincidental than causal in nature. Although most illicit drug users do not engage in crime aside from their drug use, and although many criminals do not use or abuse illicit drugs or alcohol, substance abuse clearly is much higher among criminals than among non-criminals. A 1986 survey of state prison inmates found that 43 percent were using illegal drugs on a daily or near-daily basis in the month before they committed the crime for which they were incarcerated; it also found that roughly one-half of the inmates who had used an illicit drug did not do so until after their first arrest.[28] Perhaps many of the same factors that lead individuals into lives of crime also push them in the direction of substance abuse. It is possible that legalization would diminish this connection by removing from the criminal subculture the lucrative opportunities that now derive from the illegality of the drug market. But it is also safe to assume that the criminal milieu will continue to claim a dispro-portionately large share of drug abusers, regardless of whether or not drugs are legalized.

The fourth link between drugs and crime is the commission of violent and other crimes by people under the influence of illicit drugs. It is this connec-tion that seems to most infect the popular imagina-tion. Clearly, some drugs do "cause" some people to commit crimes, by reducing normal inhibitions, unleashing aggressive and other asocial tendencies, and lessening senses of responsibility. Cocaine, par-ticularly in the form of "crack," has gained such a reputation in recent years, just as heroin did in the 1960s and 1970s, and marijuana did in the years before that. Crack cocaine's reputation for inspiring violent behavior may well be more deserved than were those of marijuana and heroin, although the evidence has yet to substantiate media depictions.[29] No illicit drug, however, is as strongly associated with violent behavior as is alcohol. According to Jus-tice Department statistics, 54 percent of all jail in-mates convicted of violent crimes in 1983 reported having used alcohol just prior to committing their offense.[30] A 1986 survey of state prison inmates similarly found that most of those convicted of ar-son, as well as violent crimes, such as murder, in-voluntary manslaughter, and rape, were far more likely to be have been under the influence of alco-hol, or both alcohol and illicit drugs, than under the influence of illicit drugs alone.[31] The impact of drug legalization on this aspect of the drug-crime con-nection is the most difficult to assess, largely be-cause changes in the overall level and nature of drug consumption are so difficult to predict.

The fifth connection is the violent, intimidating, and corrupting behavior of the drug traffickers. In many Latin American countries, most notably Co-lombia, this connection virtually defines the "drug problem." But even within the United States drug-trafficker violence is rapidly becoming a major con-cern of criminal-justice officials and the public at large. The connection is not difficult to explain. Ille-gal markets tend to breed violence, both because they attract criminally minded and violent individu-als and because participants in the market have no resort to legal institutions to resolve their dis-putes.[32] During Prohibition, violent struggles be-tween bootlegging gangs and hijackings of booze-laden trucks and sea vessels were frequent and no-torious occurrences. Today's equivalents are the booby traps that surround some marijuana fields, the pirates of the Caribbean looking to rob drug-

laden vessels en route to the shores of the United States, the machine-gun battles and executions of the more sordid drug gangs, and the generally high levels of violence that attend many illicit drug rela-tionships; the victims include not just drug dealers but witnesses, bystanders, and law-enforcement of-ficials. Most law-enforcement authorities agree that the dramatic increases in urban murder rates dur-ing the past few years can be explained almost en-tirely by the rise in drug-dealer killings, mostly of one another.[33] At the same time, the powerful allure of illicit drug dollars is responsible for rising levels of corruption not just in Latin America and the Car-ibbean but also in federal, state, and local criminal-justice systems throughout the United States.[34] A drug-legalization strategy would certainly deal a se-vere blow to this link between drugs and crime.

Perhaps the most unfortunate victims of the drug-prohibition policies have been the poor and law-abiding residents of urban ghettos. Those poli-cies have proven largely futile in deterring large numbers of ghetto dwellers from becoming drug abusers, but they do account for much of what ghetto residents identify as the drug problem. In many neighborhoods, it often seems to be the ag-gressive, gun-toting drug dealers who upset law-abiding residents far more than the addicts nodding out in doorways.[35] Other residents, however, per-ceive the drug dealers as heroes and successful role models. In impoverished neighborhoods, from Medellín and Rio de Janeiro to many leading U.S. cities, they often stand out as symbols of success to children who see no other options. At the same time, the increasingly harsh criminal penalties im-posed on adult drug dealers have led to the wide-spread recruiting of juveniles by drug traffickers.[36] Where once children started dealing drugs only af-ter they had been using them for a few years, today the sequence is often reversed. Many children start to use illegal drugs now only after they have worked for older drug dealers for a while. And the juvenile-justice system offers no realistic options for dealing with this growing problem.

Perhaps the most difficult costs to evaluate are those that relate to the widespread defiance of the drug-prohibition laws: the effects of labeling as criminals the tens of millions of people who use drugs illegally, subjecting them to the risks of crimi-nal sanction, and obliging many of those same peo-ple to enter into relationships with drug dealers (who may be criminals in many more senses of the word) in order to purchase their drugs; the cynicism that such laws generate toward other laws and the law in general; and the sense of hostility and suspicion that many otherwise law-abiding individuals feel toward law-enforcement officials. It was costs such as these that strongly influenced many of Prohibition's more conservative opponents.

Among the most dangerous consequences of the drug laws are the harms that stem from the unregulated nature of illicit drug production and sale.[37] Many marijuana smokers are worse off for having smoked cannabis that was grown with dangerous fertilizers, sprayed with the herbicide paraquat, or mixed with more dangerous substances. Consumers of heroin and the various synthetic substances sold on the street face even more severe consequences, including fatal overdoses and poisonings from unexpectedly potent or impure drug supplies. In short, nothing resembling an underground Food and Drug Administration has arisen to impose quality control on the illegal drug market and provide users with accurate information on the drugs they consume. More often than not, the quality of a drug addict's life depends greatly on his or her access to reliable supplies. Drug-enforcement operations that succeed in temporarily disrupting supply networks are thus a double-edged sword: they encourage some addicts to seek admission into drug-treatment programs, but they oblige others to seek out new and hence less reliable suppliers, with the result that more, not fewer, drug-related emergencies and deaths occur.

Today, about 25 percent of all acquired immunodeficiency syndrome (AIDS) cases in the United States and Europe, as well as the large majority of human immunodeficiency virus (HIV)-infected heterosexuals, children, and infants, are believed to have contracted the dreaded disease directly or indirectly from illegal intravenous (IV) drug use.[38] In the New York metropolitan area, the prevalence of a seropositive test for HIV among illicit IV drug users is over 50 percent.[39] Reports have emerged of drug dealers beginning to provide clean syringes together with their illegal drugs.[40] In England, recent increases in the number of HIV-infected drug users have led to renewed support among drug-treatment clinicians for providing IV heroin addicts with free supplies of injectable methadone and heroin; this reversal of the strong preference among many drug-treatment clinicians, since the early 1970s for oral methadone maintenance has been spearheaded by Philip Connell, chairman of the Home Office Advisory Committee on the Misuse of Drugs.[41] But even

as governments in England, Scotland, Sweden, Switzerland, Australia, the Netherlands, and elsewhere actively attempt to limit the spread of AIDS by and among drug users by removing restrictions on the sale of syringes and instituting free syringe-exchange programs,[42] state and municipal governments in the United States have resisted following suit, arguing, despite mounting evidence to the contrary,[43] that to do so would "encourage" or "condone" the use of illegal drugs.[44] Only in late 1988, did needle-exchange programs begin emerging in U.S. cities, typically at the initiative of non-governmental organizations. By mid-1989, programs were under way or close to being implemented in New York City; Tacoma, Washington; Boulder, Colorado; and Portland, Oregon.[45] At the same time, drug-treatment programs remain notoriously underfunded, turning away tens of thousands of addicts seeking help, even as increasing billions of dollars are spent to arrest, prosecute, and imprison illegal drug sellers and users.

Other costs of current drug-prohibition policies include the restrictions on using the illicit drugs for legitimate medical purposes.[46] Marijuana has proven useful in alleviating pain in some victims of multiple sclerosis, is particularly effective in reducing the nausea that accompanies chemotherapy, and may well prove effective in the treatment of glaucoma;[47-49] in September 1988, the administrative law judge of the Drug Enforcement Administration accordingly recommended that marijuana be made legally available for such purposes,[49] although the agency head has yet to approve the change. Heroin has proven highly effective in helping patients to deal with severe pain; some researchers have found it more effective than morphine and other opiates in treating pain in some patients.[50] It is legally prescribed for such purposes in Britain[50] and Canada.[51] The same may be true of cocaine, which continues to be used by some doctors in the United States to treat pain, despite recently imposed bans.[52] The psychedelic drugs, such as LSD (*d*-lysergic acid diethylamide), peyote, and MDMA (known as Ecstasy) have shown promise in aiding psychotherapy and in reducing tension, depression, pain, and fear of death in the terminally ill;[53] they also have demonstrated some potential, as yet unconfirmed, to aid in the treatment of alcoholism.[47,53] Current drug laws and policies, however, greatly hamper the efforts of researchers to investigate these and other potential medical uses of illegal drugs; they make it virtually impossible for any of the illegal drugs, particularly those in Schedule I, to be legally provided to those who would benefit from them; and they contribute strongly to the widely acknowledged undertreatment of pain by the medical profession in the United States.[54]

Among the strongest arguments in favor of legalization are the moral ones. On the one hand, the standard refrain regarding the immorality of drug use crumbles in the face of most Americans' tolerance for alcohol and tobacco use. Only the Mormons and a few other like-minded sects who regard as immoral any intake of substances to alter one's state of consciousness or otherwise cause pleasure are consistent in this respect; they eschew not just the illicit drugs but also alcohol, tobacco, caffeinated coffee and tea, and even chocolate. "Moral" condemnation by the majority of Americans of some substances and not others is little more than a transient prejudice in favor of some drugs and against others.

On the other hand, drug enforcement involves its own immoralities. Because drug-law violations do not create victims with an interest in notifying the police, drug-enforcement agents must rely heavily on undercover operations, electronic surveillance, and information provided by informants. In 1986, almost half of the 754 court-authorized orders for wiretaps in the United States involved drug-trafficking investigations.[55] These techniques are certainly indispensable to effective law enforcement, but they are also among the least desirable of the tools available to police. The same is true of drug testing. It may be useful and even necessary for determining liability in accidents, but it also threatens and undermines the right of privacy to which many Americans believe they are morally and constitutionally entitled. There are good reasons for requiring that such measures be used sparingly.

Equally disturbing are the increasingly vocal calls for people to inform not just on drug dealers but on neighbors, friends, and even family members who use illicit drugs. Intolerance of illicit drug use and users is heralded not merely as an indispensable ingredient in the war against drugs but as a mark of good citizenship. Certainly, every society requires citizens to assist in the enforcement of criminal laws. But societies, particularly democratic and pluralistic ones, also rely strongly on an ethic of tolerance toward those who are different but do no harm to others. Overzealous enforcement of the drug laws risks undermining that ethic and propagating in its place a society of informants. Indeed,

enforcement of drug laws makes a mockery of an essential principle of a free society, that those who do no harm to others should not be harmed by others, and particularly not by the state. Most of the nearly 40 million Americans who illegally consume drugs each year do no direct harm to anyone else; indeed, most do relatively little harm even to themselves. Directing criminal and other sanctions at them, and rationalizing the justice of such sanctions, may well represent the greatest societal cost of our current drug-prohibition system.

Alternatives to Drug-Prohibition Policies

Repealing the drug-prohibition laws clearly promises tremendous advantages. Between reduced government expenditures on enforcing drug laws and new tax revenue from legal drug production and sales, public treasuries would enjoy a net benefit of at least $10 billion per year and possibly much more; thus, billions in new revenues would be available, and ideally targeted, for funding much-needed drug-treatment programs, as well as the types of social and educational programs that often prove most effective in creating incentives for children not to abuse drugs. The quality of urban life would rise significantly. Homicide rates would decline. So would robbery and burglary rates. Organized criminal groups, particularly the up-and-coming ones that have yet to diversify into non-drug areas, would be dealt a devastating setback. The police, prosecutors, and courts would focus their resources on combating the types of crimes that people cannot walk away from. More ghetto residents would turn their backs on criminal careers and seek out legitimate opportunities instead. And the health and quality of life of many drug users and even drug abusers would improve significantly. Internationally, U.S. foreign policymakers would get on with more important and realistic objectives, and foreign governments would reclaim the authority that they have lost to the drug traffickers.

All the benefits of legalization would be for naught, however, if millions more people were to become drug abusers. Our experience with alcohol and tobacco provides ample warnings. Today, alcohol is consumed by 140 million Americans and tobacco by 50 million. All of the health costs associated with abuse of the illicit drugs pale in comparison with those resulting from tobacco and alcohol abuse. In 1986, for instance, alcohol was identified as a contributing factor in 10 percent of work-related injuries, 40 percent of suicide attempts, and about 40 percent of the approximately 46,000 annual traffic deaths in 1983. An estimated 18 million Americans are reported to be either alcoholics or alcohol abusers. The total cost of alcohol abuse to American society is estimated at over $100 billion annually.[56] Estimates of the number of deaths linked directly and indirectly to alcohol use vary from a low of 50,000 to a high of 200,000 per year.[57] The health costs of tobacco use are different but of similar magnitude. In the United States alone, an estimated 320,000 people die prematurely each year as a consequence of their consumption of tobacco. By comparison, the National Council on Alcoholism reported that only 3,562 people were known to have died in 1985 from use of all illegal drugs combined.[58] Even if we assume that thousands more deaths were related in one way or another to illicit drug use but not reported as such, we still are left with the conclusion that all of the health costs of marijuana, cocaine, and heroin combined amount to only a small fraction of those caused by either of the two licit substances. At the very least, this contrast emphasizes the need for a comprehensive approach to psychoactive substances, involving much greater efforts to discourage tobacco and alcohol abuse.

The impact of legalization on the nature and level of consumption of those drugs that are currently illegal is impossible to predict with any accuracy. On the one hand, legalization implies greater availability, lower prices, and the elimination (particularly for adults) of the deterrent power of the criminal sanction—all of which would suggest higher levels of use. Indeed, some fear that the extent of drug abuse and its attendant costs would rise to those currently associated with alcohol and tobacco.[59] On the other hand, there are many reasons to doubt that a well-designed and implemented policy of controlled drug legalization would yield such costly consequences.

The logic of legalization depends in part upon two assumptions: that most illegal drugs are not as dangerous as is commonly believed; and that those types of drugs and methods of consumption that are most risky are unlikely to prove appealing to many people, precisely because they are so obviously dangerous. Consider marijuana. Among the roughly 60 million Americans who have smoked marijuana, not one has died from a marijuana overdose,[49] a striking contrast with alcohol, which is involved in approximately 10,000 overdose deaths annually, half in combination with other drugs.[57] Although there are good health reasons for people not to smoke marijuana daily, and for children, pregnant women, and some others not to smoke at all, there still appears to be little evidence that occasional marijuana consumption does much harm at all. Certainly, it is not healthy to inhale marijuana smoke into one's lungs; indeed, the National Institute on Drug Abuse (NIDA) has declared that "marijuana smoke contains more cancer-causing agents than is found in tobacco smoke."[60] On the other hand, the number of "joints" smoked by all but a very small percentage of marijuana smokers is a tiny fraction of the 20 cigarettes a day smoked by the average cigarette smoker; indeed, the average may be closer to one or two joints per week than one or two per day. Note that the NIDA defines a "heavy" marijuana smoker as one who consumes at least two joints "daily." A heavy tobacco smoker, by contrast, smokes about 40 cigarettes per day.

Nor is marijuana strongly identified as a dependence-causing substance. A 1982 survey of marijuana use by young adults (18 to 25 years) found that 64 percent had tried marijuana at least once, that 42 percent had used it at least ten times, and that 27 percent had smoked in the last month. It also found that 21 percent had passed through a period during which they smoked "daily" (defined as 20 or more days per month) but that only one-third of those currently smoked daily and only one-fifth (or about 4 percent of all young adults) could be described as heavy daily users (averaging two or more joints per day).[61] This suggests in part that daily marijuana use is typically a phase through which people pass, after which their use becomes more moderate. By contrast, almost 20 percent of high-school seniors smoke cigarettes daily.

The dangers associated with cocaine, heroin, the hallucinogens, and other illicit substances are greater than those posed by marijuana, but not nearly so great as many people seem to think. Consider the case of cocaine. In 1986, NIDA reported that over 20 million Americans had tried cocaine, that 12.2 million had consumed it at least once during 1985, and that nearly 5.8 million had used it within the past month. Among 18- to 25-year-olds, 8.2 million had tried cocaine; 5.3 million had used it within the past year; 2.5 million had used it within the past month; and 250,000 had used it on the average weekly.[20] One could extrapolate from these figures that a quarter of a million young

Americans are potential problem users. But one could also conclude that only 3 percent of those 18- to 25-year-olds who had ever tried the drug fell into that category, and that only 10 percent of those who had used cocaine monthly were at risk. (The NIDA survey did not, it should be noted, include persons residing in military or student dormitories, prison inmates, or the homeless.)

All of this is not to say that cocaine is not a potentially dangerous drug, especially when it is injected, smoked in the form of "crack," or consumed in tandem with other powerful substances. Clearly, many tens of thousands of Americans have suffered severely from their abuse of cocaine and a tiny fraction have died. But there is also overwhelming evidence that most users of cocaine do not get into trouble with the drug. So much of the media attention has focused on the relatively small percentage of cocaine users who become addicted that the popular perception of how most people use cocaine has become badly distorted. In one survey of high-school seniors' drug use, the researchers questioned those who had used cocaine recently whether they had ever tried to stop using cocaine and found that they could not stop. Only 3.8 percent responded affirmatively, in contrast to the almost 7 percent of marijuana smokers who said they had tried to stop and found they could not, and the 18 percent of cigarette smokers who answered similarly.[62] Although a survey of crack users and cocaine injectors surely would reveal a higher proportion of addicts, evidence such as this suggests that only a small percentage of people who snort cocaine end up having a problem with it. In this respect, most people differ from captive monkeys, who have demonstrated in tests that they will starve themselves to death, if provided with unlimited cocaine.[63]

With respect to the hallucinogens, such as LSD and psilocybic mushrooms, their potential for addiction is virtually nil. The dangers arise primarily from using them irresponsibly on individual occasions.[53] Although many of those who have used hallucinogens have experienced "bad trips," far more have reported positive experiences and very few have suffered any long-term harm.[53] As for the great assortment of stimulants, depressants, and tranquilizers produced illegally or diverted from licit channels, each evidences varying capacities to create addiction, harm the user, or be used safely.

Until recently, no drugs were regarded with as much horror as the opiates, and in particular heroin. As with most drugs, it can be eaten, snorted,

smoked, or injected. The custom among most Americans, unfortunately, is the last of these options, although the growing fear of AIDS appears to be causing a shift among younger addicts toward intranasal ingestion.[64] There is no question that heroin is potentially highly addictive, perhaps as addictive as nicotine. But despite the popular association of heroin use with the most down-and-out inhabitants of urban ghettos, heroin causes relatively little physical harm to the human body. Consumed on an occasional or regular basis under sanitary conditions, its worst side effect, apart from the fact of being addicted, is constipation.[65] That is one reason why many doctors in early 20th-century America saw opiate addiction as preferable to alcoholism and prescribed the former as treatment for the latter, where abstinence did not seem a realistic option.[66,67]

It is both insightful and important to think about the illicit drugs as we do about alcohol and tobacco. Like tobacco, some illicit substances are highly addictive but can be consumed on a regular basis for decades without any demonstrable harm. Like alcohol, many of the substances can be, and are, used by most consumers in moderation, with little in the way of harmful effects; but, like alcohol, they also lend themselves to abuse by a minority of users who become addicted or otherwise harm themselves or others as a consequence. And, like both the legal substances, the psychoactive effects of each of the illegal drugs vary greatly from one person to another. To be sure, the pharmacology of the substance is important, as is its purity and the manner in which it is consumed. But much also depends upon not just the physiology and psychology of the consumer but his expectations regarding the drug, his social milieu, and the broader cultural environment, what Harvard University psychiatrist Norman Zinberg called the "set and setting" of the drug.[68] It is factors such as these that might change dramatically, albeit in indeterminate ways, were the illicit drugs made legally available.

It is thus impossible to predict whether or not legalization would lead to much greater levels of drug abuse. The lessons that can be drawn from other societies are mixed. China's experience with the British opium pushers of the 19th century, when millions reportedly became addicted to the drug, offers one worst-case scenario. The devastation of many native American tribes by alcohol presents another. On the other hand, the decriminalization of marijuana by 11 states in the United States during the mid-1970s does not appear to have led to increases in marijuana consumption.[69] In the Netherlands, which went even further in decriminalizing cannabis during the 1970s, consumption has actually declined significantly; in 1976, 3 percent of 15- and 16-year-olds and 10 percent of 17- and 18-year-olds used cannabis occasionally; by 1985, the percentages had declined to 2 and 6 percent, respectively.[70] The policy has succeeded, as the government intended, "in making drug use boring." Finally, late 19th-century America is an example of a society, in which there were almost no drug laws or even drug regulations, but levels of drug use were about what they are today.[71] Drug abuse was regarded as a relatively serious problem, but the criminal-justice system was not regarded as part of the solution.[72]

There are, however, strong reasons to believe that none of the currently illicit substances would become as popular as alcohol or tobacco, even if they were legalized. Alcohol has long been the principal intoxicant in most societies, including many in which other substances have been legally available. Presumably, its diverse properties account for its popularity: it quenches thirst, goes well with food, often pleases the palate, promotes appetite as well as sociability, and so on. The widespread use of tobacco probably stems not just from its powerful addictive qualities but from the fact that its psychoactive effects are sufficiently subtle that cigarettes can be integrated with most other human activities. None of the illicit substances now popular in the United States share either of these qualities to the same extent, nor is it likely that they would acquire them if they were legalized. Moreover, none of the illicit substances can compete with alcohol's special place in American culture and history, one that it retained even during Prohibition.

Much of the damage caused by illegal drugs today stems from their consumption in particularly potent and dangerous ways. There is good reason to doubt that many Americans would inject cocaine or heroin into their veins, even if given the chance to do so legally. And just as the dramatic growth in the heroin-consuming population during the 1960s leveled off, for reasons apparently having little to do with law enforcement, so we can expect, if it has not already occurred, a leveling off in the number of people smoking crack.

Perhaps the most reassuring reason for believing that repeal of the drug-prohibition laws will not lead to tremendous increases in drug-abuse levels is the fact that we have learned something from our past experiences with alcohol and tobacco abuse. We now know, for instance, that consumption taxes are an effective method for limiting consumption rates and related costs, especially among young people.[73] Substantial evidence also suggests that restrictions and bans on advertising, as well as promotion of negative advertising, can make a difference.[74] The same seems to be true of other government measures, including restrictions on time and place of sale,[75] bans on vending machines, prohibitions of consumption in public places, packaging requirements, mandated adjustments in insurance policies, crackdowns on driving while under the influence,[76] and laws holding bartenders and hosts responsible for the drinking of customers and guests. There is even some evidence that some education programs about the dangers of cigarette smoking have deterred many children from beginning to smoke.[77] At the same time, we also have come to recognize the great harms that can result when drug-control policies are undermined by powerful lobbies, such as those that now block efforts to lessen the harms caused by abuse of alcohol and tobacco.

Legalization, thus, affords far greater opportunities to control drug use and abuse than do current criminalization policies. The current strategy is one in which the type, price, purity, and potency of illicit drugs, as well as the participants in the business, are largely determined by drug dealers, the peculiar competitive dynamics of an illicit market, and the perverse interplay of drug-enforcement strategies and drug-trafficking tactics. During the past decade, for instance, the average retail purities of cocaine and heroin has increased dramatically, the wholesale prices have dropped greatly, the number of children involved in drug-dealing has risen, and crack has become readily and cheaply available in a growing number of American cities.[8] By contrast, marijuana has become relatively scarcer and more expensive, in part because it is far more vulnerable to drug-enforcement efforts than are cocaine or heroin; the result has been to induce both dealers and users away from the relatively safer marijuana and toward the relatively more dangerous cocaine.[8] Also by contrast, while the average potency of most illicit substances has increased during the 1980s, that of most legal psychoactive substances has been declining. Motivated in good part by health concerns, Americans are switching from hard liquor to beer and wine, from high tar and nicotine cigarettes to lower tar and nicotine cigarettes, as well as smoke-less tobaccos and nicotine chewing gums, and even from caffeinated to decaffeinated coffees, teas, and sodas. It is quite possible that these diverging trends are less a reflection of the nature of the drugs than of their legal status.

A drug-control policy, based predominantly on approaches other than criminal justice, thus offers a number of significant advantages over the current criminal-justice focus in controlling drug use and abuse. It shifts control of production, distribution, and, to a lesser extent, consumption out of the hands of criminals and into the hands of government and government licensees. It affords consumers the opportunity to make far more informed decisions about the drugs they buy than is currently the case. It dramatically lessens the likelihood that drug consumers will be harmed by impure, unexpectedly potent, or misidentified drugs. It corrects the hypocritical and dangerous message that alcohol and tobacco are somehow safer than many illicit drugs. It reduces by billions of dollars annually government expenditures on drug enforcement and simultaneously raises additional billions in tax revenues. And it allows government the opportunity to shape consumption patterns toward relatively safer psychoactive substances and modes of consumption.

Toward the end of the 1920s, when the debate over repealing Prohibition rapidly gained momentum, numerous scholars, journalists, and private and government commissions undertook thorough evaluations of Prohibition and the potential alternatives. Prominent among these were the Wickersham Commission appointed by President Herbert Hoover and the study of alcohol regulation abroad, directed by the leading police scholar in the United States, Raymond Fosdick, and commissioned by John D. Rockefeller.[78] These efforts examined the successes and failings of Prohibition in the United States and evaluated the wide array of alternative regimes for controlling the distribution and use of beer, wine, and liquor. They played a major role in stimulating the public reevaluation of Prohibition and in envisioning alternatives. Precisely the same sorts of efforts are required today.

The controlled drug-legalization option is not an all-or-nothing alternative to current policies. Indeed, political realities ensure that any shift toward legalization will evolve gradually, with ample opportunity to halt, reevaluate, and redirect drug policies that begin to prove too costly or counter-productive.

The federal government need not play the leading role in devising alternatives; it need only clear the way to allow state and local governments the legal power to implement their own drug-legalization policies. The first steps are relatively risk-free: legalization of marijuana, easier availability of illegal and strictly controlled drugs for treatment of pain and other medical purposes, tougher tobacco- and alcohol-control policies, and a broader and more available array of drug-treatment programs.

Remedying the drug-related ills of America's ghettos requires more radical steps. The risks of a more far-reaching policy of controlled drug legalization—increased availability, lower prices, and removal of the deterrent power of the criminal sanction—are relatively less in the ghettos than in most other parts of the United States, in good part because drug availability is already so high, prices so low, and the criminal sanction so ineffective in deterring illicit drug use that legalization can hardly worsen the situation. On the other hand, legalization would yield its greatest benefits in the ghettos, where it would sever much of the drug-crime connection, seize the market away from criminals, deglorify involvement in the illicit drug business, help redirect the work ethic from illegitimate to legitimate employment opportunities, help stem the transmission of AIDS by IV drug users, and significantly improve the safety, health, and well-being of those who do use and abuse drugs. Simply stated, legalizing cocaine, heroin, and other relatively dangerous drugs may well be the only way to reverse the destructive impact of drugs and current drug policies in the ghettos.

There is no question that legalization is a risky policy, one that may indeed lead to an increase in the number of people who abuse drugs. But that risk is by no means a certainty. At the same time, current drug-control policies are showing little progress, and new proposals promise only to be more costly and more repressive. We know that repealing the drug-prohibition laws would eliminate or greatly reduce many of the ills that people commonly identify as part and parcel of the "drug problem." Yet that option is repeatedly and vociferously dismissed without any attempt to evaluate it openly and objectively. The past 20 years have demonstrated that a drug policy shaped by rhetoric and fear-mongering can only lead to our current disaster. Unless we are willing to honestly evaluate all our options, including various legalization strategies, there is a good chance that we will never identify the best solutions for our drug problems.

* * *

Ethan A. Nadelmann, "Drug Prohibition in the United States: Costs, Consquences, and Alternatives," From *Science* (245) (September 1, 1989), pp. 939-47. Copyright © 1989 by the AAAS. Reprinted by permission.

For Discussion

1. Although marijuana may not be totally harmless, most studies have found that the drug does not present serious problems for users. Why then does the government and perhaps the American people insist on keeping marijuana illegal?

2. Nadelmann argues that drug violators have placed a tremendous burden on criminal justice resources. Indeed, the "War on Drugs" is in part responsible for the substantial increases in state prison populations. Why have legislators and citizens failed to recognize the impact of current drug policies on criminal justice resources?

3. What drugs should be legalized? What criteria should be used in determining whether a drug should be illegal or legal?

Notes

1. The terms "legalization" and "decriminalization" are used interchangeably here. Some interpret the latter term as a more limited form of legalization, involving the removal of criminal sanctions against users but not against producers and sellers.

2. Statement by Senator D. P. Moynihan, citing a U.S. Department of Agriculture report, in *Congr. Rec. 134* (no. 77), p. S7049 (27 May 1988).

3. Drug Enforcement Administration, Department of Justice, *Intell. Trends 14* (no. 3), 1 (1987).

4. See, for example, K. Healy, *J. Interam. Stud. World Aff. 30* (no. 213), 105 (summer/fall 1988).

5. E. A. Nadelmann, *ibid. 29* (no. 4), 1 (winter 1987-88).

6. C. McClintock, *ibid. 30* (no. 2/3), 127 (summer/fall 1988); J. Kawell, *Report on the Americas 22* (no. 6), 13 (March 1989).

7. P. Reuta, *Public Interest* (no. 92), 51 (summer 1988).

8. See the annual reports of the National Narcotics Intelligence Consumers Committee, edited by the Drug Enforcement Administration, Department of Justice, Washington, DC.

9. *Street-Level Drug Enforcement: Examining the Issues*, M. R. Chaiken, ed. (National Institute of Justice, Department of Justice, Washington, DC, September 1988).

10. National Drug Enforcement Policy Board, *National and International Drug Law Enforcement Strategy* (Department of Justice, Washington, DC, 1987).

11. *Anti-Drug Law Enforcement Efforts and Their Impact* (report prepared for the U.S. Customs Service by Wharton Econometric Forecasting Associates, Washington, DC, 1987), pp. 2, 38-46.

12. *Sourcebook of Criminal Justice Statistics, 1987* (Bureau of Justice Statistics, Department of Justice, Washington, DC, 1988), pp. 490, 494, 518; "Prisoners in 1987," *Bur. Justice Stat. Bull. 24* (April 1988).

13. U.S. Sentencing Commission, *Supplementary Report on the Initial Sentencing Guidelines and Policy Statements* (U.S. Sentencing Commission, Washington, DC, 18 June 1987), pp. 71-75.

14. R. D. McFadden, *New York Times*, 5 January 1988, p. B1.

15. *Annual Report, 1987-88* (Florida Department of Corrections, Tallahassee, FL, 1988), pp. 26, 50, 51.

16. "Felony sentences in state courts, 1986," *Bur. Justice Stat. Bull.* (February 1989).

17. The numbers cited do not, it should be emphasized, include the many inmates sentenced for drug-related crimes, such as violent crimes committed by drug dealers, typically against one another, and robberies committed to earn the money needed to pay for illegal drugs.

18. See the annual editions of *Sourcebook of Criminal Justice Statistics* (Bureau of Justice Statistics, Department of Justice, Washington, DC).

19. *Sourcebook of Criminal Justice Statistics, 1987* (Bureau of Justice Statistics, Department of Justice, Washington, DC, 1988), pp. 400-401.

20. *Data from the 1985 National Household Survey on Drug Abuse* (National Institute on Drug Abuse, Rockville, MD, 1987).

21. S. Raab, *New York Times*, 7 June 1987, p. A38.

22. *Drug Use and Drug Programs in the Washington Metropolitan Area: An Assessment* (Greater Washington Research Center, Washington, DC, 1988), pp. 16-17.

23. Wharton Econometric Forecasting Associates, *The Impact: Organized Crime Today* (President's Commission on Organized Crime, Washington, DC, 1986), pp. 413-494.

24. B. D. Johnson et al., *Taking Care of Business: The Economics of Crime By Heroin Abusers* (Lexington Books, Lexington, MA, 1985).

25. B. D. Johnson, D. Lipton, E. Wish, *Facts About the Criminality of Heroin and Cocaine Abusers and Some New Alternatives to Incarceration* (Narcotic and Drug Research, New York, 1986), p. 30.

26. G. F. van de Wijngart, *Am. J. Drug Alcohol Abuse 14* (no. 1), 125 (1988).

27. A controlled trial, in which 96 confirmed heroin addicts, requesting a heroin-maintenance prescription, were randomly allocated to treatment with injectable heroin or oral methadone showed that "refusal [by doctors] to prescribe heroin is . . . associated with a considerably higher abstinence rate, but at the expense of an increased arrest rate and a higher level of illicit drug involvement and criminal activity

among those who did not become abstinent." R. L. Hartnoll et al., *Arch. Gen. Psychiatry 37*, 877 (1980).

28. "Drug use and crime," *Bur. Justice Stat. Spec. Rep.* (July 1988).

29. See the discussion in P. J. Goldstein, P. A. Bellucci, B. J. Spunt, T. Miller, "Frequency of Cocaine Use and Violence: A Comparison Between Men and Women" [in *NIDA* (National Institute on Drug Abuse) *Res. Monogr. Ser.*, in press].

30. *Sourcebook of Criminal Justice Statistics, 1986* (Bureau of Justice Statistics, Department of Justice, Washington, DC, 1987), p. 398.

31. *Sourcebook of Criminal Justice Statistics, 1987* (Bureau of Justice Statistics, Department of Justice, Washington, DC, 1988), p. 497.

32. P. J. Goldstein, in *Pathways to Criminal Violence*, N. A. Weiner and M. E. Wolfgang, eds. (Sage: Newbury Park, CA, 1989), pp. 16-48.

33. "A tide of drug killing," *Newsweek*, 16 January 1989, p. 44.

34. P. Shenon, *New York Times*, 11 April 1988, p. A1.

35. W. Nobles, L. Goddard, W. Cavil, P. George, *The Culture of Drugs in the Black Community* (Institute for the Advanced Study of Black Family Life and Culture, Oakland, CA, 1987).

36. T. Mieczowski, *Criminology 24*, 645 (1986).

37. C. L. Renfroe and T. A. Messinger, *Semin. Adolescent Med. 1* (no. 4), 247 (1985).

38. D. C. Des Jarlais and S. R. Friedman, *J. AIDS 1*, 267 (1988).

39. D. C. Des Jarlais et al. *J. Am. Med. Assoc. 261*, 1008 (1989).

40. S. R. Friedman et al. *Int. J. Addict. 22* (no. 3), 201 (1987).

41. T. Bennett, *Law Contemp. Prob. 51*, 310 (1988).

42. R. J. Battjes and R. W. Pickens, eds., *NIDA Res. Monogr. Ser. 80* (1988).

43. D. C. Des Jarlais and S. R. Friedman, *AIDS 2* (suppl. 1), S65 (1988).

44. M. Marriot, *New York Times*, 7 November 1988, p. B1; *ibid.*, 30 January 1989, p. A1.

45. *Int. Work. Group AIDS IV Drug Use Newsl. 3*, 3 (December 1988).

46. See, for example, P. Fitzgerald, *St. Louis Univ. Public Law Rev. 6*, 371 (1987).

47. L. Grinspoon and J. B. Bakalar, in *Dealing with Drugs: Consequences of Government Control*, R. Hamowy, ed. (Lexington Books, Lexington, MA, 1987), pp. 183-219.

48. T. H. Mikuriya, ed., *Marijuana: Medical Papers, 1839-1972* (Medi-Comp Press, Oakland, CA, 1973).

49. *In the Matter of Marijuana Rescheduling Petition*, Docket No. 86-22, 6 September 1988, Drug Enforcement Administration, Department of Justice.

50. A. S. Trebach, *The Heroin Solution* (Yale Univ. Press, New Haven, CT, 1982), pp. 59-84.

51. L. Appleby, *Saturday Night* (November 1985), p. 13.

52. F. R. Lee, *New York Times*, 10 February 1989, p. B3; F. Barre, *Headache 22*, 69 (1982).

53. L. Grinspoon and J. B. Bakalar, *Psychedelic Drugs Reconsidered* (Basic Books, New York, 1979).

54. M. Donovan, P. Dillon, L. McGuire, *Pain 30*, 69 (1987); D. E. Weissman, *Narc Officer 5* (no. 1), 47 (January 1989); D. Goleman, *New York Times*, 31 December 1987, p. B5. The

Controlled Substances Act, 21 U.S.C. Sec. 801, *et seq.*, defines a Schedule I drug as one that: (i) has a high potential for abuse; (ii) has no currently accepted medical use in treatment in the United States; and (iii) for which there is a lack of accepted safety for use under medical supervision. It is contrary to federal law for physicians to prescribe Schedule I drugs to patients for therapeutic purposes.

55. *Sourcebook of Criminal Justice Statistics, 1987* (Bureau of Justice Statistics, Department of Justice, Washington, DC, 1988), p. 417.

56. "Toward a national plan to combat alcohol abuse and alcoholism: A report to the United States Congress" (Department of Health and Human Services, Washington, DC, September 1986).

57. D. R. Gerstein, in *Alcohol and Public Policy: Beyond the Shadow of Prohibition*, M. H. Moore and D. R. Gerstein, eds. (National Academy Press, Washington, DC, 1981), pp. 182-224.

58. Cited in T. Wicker, *New York Times*, 13 May 1987, p. A27.

59. M. M. Kondracke, *New Repub. 198* (no. 26), 16 (27 June 1988).

60. "Marijuana" (National Institute on Drug Abuse, Washington, DC, 1983).

61. J. D. Miller and I. H. Cisin, *Highlights from the National Survey on Drug Abuse, 1982* (National Institute on Drug Abuse, Washington, DC, 1983), pp. 1-10.

62. P. M. O'Malley, L. D. Johnston, J. G. Bachman, *NIDA Monogr. Ser. 61* (1985), pp. 50-75.

63. T. G. Aigner and R. L. Balster, *Science 201*, 534 (1978); C. E. Johanson, *NIDA Monogr. Ser. 50* (1984), pp. 54-71.

64. J. F. French and J. Safford, *Lancet 1*, 1082 (1989); D. C. Des Jarlais, S. R. Friedman, C. Casriel, A. Kott, *Psychol. Health 1*, 179 (1987).

65. J. Kaplan, *The Hardest Drug: Heroin and Public Policy* (Univ. of Chicago Press, Chicago, IL, 1983), p. 127.

66. S. Siegel, *Res. Adv. Alcohol Drug Probl. 9*, 279 (1986).

67. J. A. O'Donnell, *Narcotics Addicts in Kentucky* (Public Health Service Publ. 1881, National Institute of Mental Health, Chevy Chase, MD, 1969), discussed in *Licit and Illicit Drugs* [E. M. Brecher and the Editors of Consumer Reports (Little, Brown, Boston, 1972), pp. 8-103].

68. See N. Zinberg, *Drug, Set, and Setting: The Basis for Controlled Intoxicant Use* (Yale Univ. Press, New Haven, CT, 1984).

69. L. D. Johnston, J. G. Bachman, P. M. O'Malley, "Marijuana decriminalization: the impact on youth, 1975-1980" (Monitoring the Future, *Occasional Paper 13*, Univ. Of Michigan Institute for Social Research, Ann Arbor, MI, 1981).

70. "Policy on drug users" (Ministry of Welfare, Health, and Cultural Affairs, Rijswijk, the Netherlands, 1985).

71. D. Courtright, *Dark Paradise: Opiate Addiction in America Before 1940* (Harvard Univ. Press, Cambridge, MA, 1982).

72. E. M. Brecher and the Editors of Consumer Reports, *Licit and Illicit Drugs* (Little, Brown, Boston, 1972), pp. 1-41.

73. See P. J. Cook, in *Alcohol and Public Policy: Beyond the Shadow of Prohibition*, M. H. Moore and D. R. Gerstein, eds. (National Academy Press, Washington, DC, 1981), pp. 255-285; D. Coate and M. Grossman, *J. Law Econ. 31*, 145

(1988); also see K. E. Warner, in *The Cigarette Excise Tax* (Harvard Univ. Institute for the Study of Smoking Behavior and Policy, Cambridge, MA, 1985), pp. 88-105.

74. J. B. Tye, K. E. Warner, S. A. Glantz, *J. Public Health Policy* 8, 492 (1987).

75. O. Olsson and P. O. H. Wikstrom, *Contemp. Drug Problem* 11, 325 (fall 1982); M. Terris, *Am. J. Public Health* 57, 2085 (1967).

76. M. D. Laurence, J. R. Snortum, F. E. Zimring, eds., *Social Control of the Drinking Driver* (Univ. of Chicago Press, Chicago, IL, 1988).

77. J. M. Polich, P. L. Ellickson, P. Rueter, J. P. Kahan, *Strategies for Controlling Adolescent Drug Use* (RAND, Santa Monica, CA, 1984), pp. 145-152.

78. R. B. Fosdick and A. L. Scott, *Toward Liquor Control* (Harper, New York, 1933). ✦

37. Against the Legalization of Drugs

JAMES Q. WILSON

In contrast to Ethan Nadelmann's position, James Q. Wilson offers a number of arguments against legalizing drugs, especially heroin and cocaine. Wilson claims that because heroin has been illegal for so many years, the actual number of users has remained relatively stable since the early 1970s. Heroin is costly and difficult to obtain, and these factors deter individuals from using it. Cocaine, and especially "crack" cocaine, is a far more serious drug, and, if legalized, a major public health problem might ensue.

In 1972, the President appointed me chairman of the National Advisory Council for Drug Abuse Prevention. Created by Congress, the Council was charged with providing guidance on how best to coordinate the national war on drugs. (Yes, we called it a war then, too.) In those days, the drug we were chiefly concerned with was heroin. When I took office, heroin use had been increasing dramatically. Everybody was worried that this increase would continue. Such phrases as "heroin epidemic" were commonplace.

That same year, the eminent economist Milton Friedman published an essay in *Newsweek*, in which he called for legalizing heroin. His argument was on two grounds: as a matter of ethics, the government has no right to tell people not to use heroin (or to drink or to commit suicide); as a matter of economics, the prohibition of drug use imposes costs on society that far exceed the benefits. Others, such as the psychoanalyst Thomas Szasz, made the same argument.

We did not take Friedman's advice. (Government commissions rarely do.) I do not recall that we even discussed legalizing heroin, though we did discuss (but did not take action on) legalizing a drug, cocaine, that many people then argued was benign. Our marching orders were to figure out how to win the war on heroin, not to run up the white flag of surrender.

That was 1972. Today, we have the same number of heroin addicts that we had then—half a million, give or take a few thousand. Having that many heroin addicts is no trivial matter; these people deserve our attention. But not having had an increase in that number for over fifteen years is also something that deserves our attention. What happened to the "heroin epidemic" that many people once thought would overwhelm us?

The facts are clear: a more or less stable pool of heroin addicts has been getting older, with relatively few new recruits. In 1976, the average age of heroin users who appeared in hospital emergency rooms was about twenty-seven; ten years later, it was thirty-two. More than two-thirds of all heroin users appearing in emergency rooms are now over the age of thirty. Back in the early 1970s when heroin got onto the national political agenda, the typical heroin addict was much younger, often a teenager. Household surveys show the same thing—the rate of opiate use (which includes heroin) has been flat for the better part of two decades. More fine-grained studies of inner-city neighborhoods confirm this. John Boyle and Ann Brunswick found that the percentage of young blacks in Harlem who used heroin fell from 8 percent in 1970-71 to about 3 percent in 1975-76.

Why did heroin lose its appeal for young people? When the young blacks in Harlem were asked why they stopped, more than half mentioned "trouble with the law" or "high cost" (and high cost is, of course, directly the result of law enforcement). Two-thirds said that heroin hurt their health; nearly all said they had had a bad experience with it. We need not rely, however, simply on what they said. In New York City in 1973-75, the street price of heroin rose dramatically and its purity sharply declined, probably as a result of the heroin shortage caused by the success of the Turkish government in reducing the supply of opium base and of the French government in closing down heroin-processing laboratories located in and around Marseilles. These were short-lived gains, for, just as Friedman predicted, alternative sources of supply—mostly in Mexico—quickly emerged. But the three-year heroin shortage interrupted the easy recruitment of new users.

Health and related problems were no doubt part of the reason for the reduced flow of recruits. Over the preceding years, Harlem youth had watched as more and more heroin users died of overdoses, were poisoned by adulterated doses, or acquired hepatitis from dirty needles. The word got around: heroin can kill you. By 1974, new hepatitis cases and drug-overdose deaths had dropped to a fraction of what they had been in 1970.

Alas, treatment did not seem to explain much of the cessation in drug use. Treatment programs can and do help heroin addicts, but treatment did not explain the drop in the number of *new* users (who, by definition, had never been in treatment) nor even much of the reduction in the number of experienced users.

No one knows how much of the decline to attribute to personal observation, as opposed to high prices or reduced supply. But other evidence suggests strongly that price and supply played a large role. In 1972, the National Advisory Council was especially worried by the prospect that U.S. servicemen returning to this country from Vietnam would bring their heroin habits with them. Fortunately, a brilliant study by Lee Robins of Washington University in St. Louis put that fear to rest. She measured drug use of Vietnam veterans shortly after they had returned home. Though many had used heroin regularly while in Southeast Asia, most gave up the habit when back in the United States. The reason: here, heroin was less available and sanctions on its use were more pronounced. Of course, if a veteran had been willing to pay enough—which might have meant traveling to another city and would certainly have meant making an illegal contact with a disreputable dealer in a threatening neighborhood in order to acquire a (possibly) dangerous dose—he could have sustained his drug habit. Most veterans were unwilling to pay this price, and so their drug use declined or disappeared.

Reliving the Past

Suppose we had taken Friedman's advice in 1972. What would have happened? We cannot be entirely certain, but at a minimum we would have placed the young heroin addicts (and, above all, the prospective addicts) in a very different position from the one in which they actually found themselves. Heroin would have been legal. Its price would have been reduced by 95 percent (minus whatever we chose to recover in taxes.) Now that it could be sold by the same people who make aspirin, its quality would have been assured—no poisons, no adulterants. Sterile hypodermic needles would have been readily available at the neighborhood drugstore, probably at the same counter where the heroin was sold. No need to travel to big cities or unfamiliar neighborhood—heroin could have been purchased anywhere, perhaps by mail order.

There would no longer have been any financial or medical reason to avoid heroin use. Anybody could have afforded it. We might have tried to prevent children from buying it, but as we have learned from our efforts to prevent minors from buying alcohol and tobacco, young people have a way of penetrating markets theoretically reserved for adults. Returning Vietnam veterans would have discovered that Omaha and Raleigh had been converted into the pharmaceutical equivalent of Saigon.

Under these circumstances, can we doubt for a moment that heroin use would have grown exponentially? Or that a vastly larger supply of new users would have been recruited? Professor Friedman is a Nobel Prize-winning economist whose understanding of market forces is profound. What did he think would happen to consumption under his legalized regime? Here are his words: "Legalizing drugs might increase the number of addicts, but it is not clear that it would. Forbidden fruit is attractive, particularly to the young."

Really? I suppose that we should expect no increase in Porsche sales if we cut the price by 95 percent, no increase in whiskey sales if we cut the price by a comparable amount—because young people only want fast cars and strong liquor when they are "forbidden." Perhaps Friedman's uncharacteristic lapse from the obvious implications of price theory can be explained by a misunderstanding of how drug users are recruited. In his 1972 essay, he said that "drug addicts are deliberately made by pushers, who give likely prospects their first few doses free." If drugs were legal, it would not pay anybody to produce addicts, because everybody would buy from the cheapest source. But as every drug expert knows, pushers do not produce addicts. Friends or acquaintances do. In fact, pushers are usually reluctant to deal with non-users, because a non-user could be an undercover cop. Drug use spreads in the same way any fad or fashion spreads: somebody who is already a user urges his friends to try, or simply shows already eager friends how to do it.

But we need not rely on speculation, however plausible, that lowered prices and more abundant supplies would have increased heroin usage. Great Britain once followed such a policy and with almost exactly those results. Until the mid-1960s, British physicians were allowed to prescribe heroin to certain classes of addicts. (Possessing these drugs without a doctor's prescription remained a criminal offense.) For many years, this policy worked well enough because the addict patients were typically middle-class people who had become dependent on opiate painkillers while undergoing hospital treatment. There was no drug culture. The British system worked for many years, not because it prevented drug abuse, but because there was no problem of drug abuse that would test the system.

All that changed in the 1960s. A few unscrupulous doctors began passing out heroin in wholesale amounts. One doctor prescribed almost 600,000 heroin tablets—that is, over thirteen pounds—in just one year. A youthful drug culture emerged with a demand for drugs far different from that of the older addicts. As a result, the British government required doctors to refer users to government-run clinics to receive their heroin.

But the shift to clinics did not curtail the growth in heroin use. Throughout the 1960s, the number of addicts increased—the late John Kaplan of Stanford estimated by fivefold—in part as a result of the diversion of heroin from clinic patients to new users on the streets. An addict would bargain with the clinic doctor over how big a dose he would receive. The patient wanted as much as he could get; the doctor wanted to give as little as was needed. The patient had an advantage in this conflict, because the doctor could not be certain how much was really needed. Many patients would use some of their "maintenance" dose and sell the remaining part to friends, thereby recruiting new addicts. As the clinics learned of this, they began to shift their treatment away from heroin and toward methadone, an addictive drug that, when taken orally, does not produce a "high" but will block the withdrawal pains associated with heroin abstinence.

Whether what happened in England in the 1960s was a mini-epidemic or an epidemic depends on whether one looks at numbers or at rates of change. Compared to the United States, the numbers were small. In 1960, there were 68 heroin addicts known to the British government; by 1968, there were 2,000 in treatment and many more who refused treatment. (They would refuse, in part because they did not want to get methadone at a clinic, if they could get heroin on the street.) Richard Hartnoll estimates that the actual number of addicts in England is five times the number officially registered. At a minimum, the number of British addicts increased by thirtyfold in ten years; the actual increase may have been much larger.

In the early 1980s, the numbers began to rise again, and this time nobody doubted that a real epidemic was at hand. The increase was estimated to be 40 percent a year. By 1982, there were thought to be 20,000 heroin users in London alone. Geoffrey Pearson reports that many cities—Glasgow, Liverpool, Manchester, and Sheffield among them—were now experiencing a drug problem that once had been largely confined to London. The problem, again, was supply. The country was being flooded with cheap, high-quality heroin, first from Iran and then from Southeast Asia.

The United States began the 1960s with a much larger number of heroin addicts and probably a bigger at-risk population than was the case in Great Britain. Even though it would be foolhardy to suppose that the British system, if installed here, would have worked the same way or with the same results, it would be equally foolhardy to suppose that a combination of heroin available from leaky clinics and from street dealers who faced only minimal law-enforcement risks would not have produced a much greater increase in heroin use than we actually experienced. My guess is that, if we had allowed either doctors or clinics to prescribe heroin, we would have had far worse results than were produced in Britain, if for no other reason than the vastly larger number of addicts with which we began. We would have had to find some way to police thousands (not scores) of physicians and hundreds (not dozens) of clinics. If the British civil service found it difficult to keep heroin in the hands of addicts and out of the hands of recruits when it was dealing with a few hundred people, how well would the American civil service have accomplished the same tasks when dealing with tens of thousands of people?

Back to the Future

Now cocaine, especially in its potent form, crack, is the focus of attention. Now, as in 1972, the government is trying to reduce its use. Now, as then, some people are advocating legalization. Is there any more reason to yield to those arguments today than there was almost two decades ago?[1]

I think not. If we had yielded in 1972, we almost certainly would have had today a permanent population of several million, not several hundred thousand, heroin addicts. If we yield now, we will have a far more serious problem with cocaine.

Crack is worse than heroin by almost any measure. Heroin produces a pleasant drowsiness and, if hygienically administered, has only the physical side effects of constipation and sexual impotence. Regular heroin use incapacitates many users, especially poor ones, for any productive work or social responsibility. They will sit nodding on a street corner, helpless but at least harmless. By contrast, regular cocaine use leaves the user neither helpless nor harmless. When smoked (as with crack) or injected, cocaine produces instant, intense, and short-lived euphoria. The experience generates a powerful desire to repeat it. If the drug is readily available, repeat use will occur. Those people who progress to "bingeing" on cocaine become devoted to the drug and its effects, to the exclusion of almost all other considerations—job, family, children, sleep, food, even sex. Dr. Frank Gawin at Yale and Dr. Everett Ellinwood at Duke report that a substantial percentage of all high-dose, binge users become uninhibited, impulsive, hypersexual, compulsive, irritable, and hyperactive. Their moods vacillate dramatically, leading at times to violence and homicide.

Women are much more likely to use crack than heroin, and, if they are pregnant, the effects on their babies are tragic. Douglas Besharov, who has been following the effects of drugs on infants for twenty years, writes that nothing he learned about heroin prepared him for the devastation of cocaine. Cocaine harms the fetus and can lead to physical deformities or neurological damage. Some crack babies have, for all practical purposes, suffered a disabling stroke while still in the womb. The long-term consequences of this brain damage are lowered cognitive ability and the onset of mood disorders. Besharov estimates that about 30,000 to 50,000 such babies are born every year, about 7,000 in New York City alone. There may be ways to treat such infants, but from everything we now know, the treatment will be long, difficult, and expensive. Worse, the mothers who are most likely to produce crack babies are precisely the ones who, because of poverty or temperament, are least able and willing to obtain such treatment. In fact, anecdotal evidence suggests that crack mothers are likely to abuse their infants.

The notion that abusing drugs such as cocaine is a "victimless crime" is not only absurd but dangerous. Even ignoring the fetal drug syndrome, crack-dependent people are, like heroin addicts, individuals who regularly victimize their children by neglect, their spouses by improvidence, their employers by lethargy, and their co-workers by carelessness. Society is not and could never be a collection of autonomous individuals. We all have a stake in ensuring that each of us displays a minimal level of dignity, responsibility, and empathy. We cannot, of course, coerce people into goodness, but we can and should insist that some standards must be met if society itself—on which the very existence of the human personality depends—is to persist. Drawing the line that defines those standards is difficult and contentious, but if crack and heroin use do not fall below it, what does?

The advocates of legalization will respond by suggesting that my picture is overdrawn. Ethan Nadelmann of Princeton argues that the risk of legalization is less than most people suppose. Over 20 million Americans between the ages of eighteen and twenty-five have tried cocaine (according to a government survey), but only a quarter million use it daily. From this, Nadelmann concludes that at most 3 percent of all young people who try cocaine develop a problem with it. The implication is clear: make the drug legal, and we only have to worry about 3 percent of our youth.

The implication rests on a logical fallacy and a factual error. The fallacy is this: the percentage of occasional cocaine users who become binge users when the drug is illegal (and thus expensive and hard to find) tells us nothing about the percentage who will become dependent when the drug is legal (and thus cheap and abundant). Drs. Gawin and Ellinwood report, in common with several other researchers, that controlled or occasional use of cocaine changes to compulsive and frequent use "when access to the drug increases," or when the user switches from snorting to smoking. More cocaine more potently administered alters, perhaps sharply, the proportion of "controlled" users who become heavy users. The factual error is this: the federal survey Nadelmann quotes was done in 1985, before crack had become common. Thus, the probability of becoming dependent on cocaine was derived from the responses of users who snorted the drug. The speed and potency of cocaine's action increases dramatically when it is smoked. We do not yet know how greatly the advent of crack increases the risk of dependency, but all the clinical evidence suggests that the increase is likely to be large.

It is possible that some people will not become heavy users, even when the drug is readily available in its most potent form. So far, there are no scientific grounds for predicting who will and who will not become dependent. Neither socio-economic background nor personality traits differentiate between casual and intensive users. Thus, the only way to settle the question of who is correct about the effect of easy availability on drug use, Nadelmann or Gawin and Ellinwood, is to try it and see.

But that social experiment is so risky as to be no experiment at all; for, if cocaine is legalized, and if the rate of its abusive use increases dramatically, there is no way to put the genie back in the bottle, and it is not a kindly genie.

Have We Lost?

Many people who agree that there are risks in legalizing cocaine or heroin still favor it, because, they think, we have lost the war on drugs. "Nothing we have done has worked," and the current federal policy is just "more of the same." Whatever the costs of greater drug use, surely they would be less than the costs of our present, failed efforts. That is exactly what I was told in 1972—and heroin is not quite as bad a drug as cocaine. We did not surrender, and we did not lose. We did not win, either. What the nation accomplished then was what most efforts to save people from themselves accomplish: the problem was contained and the number of victims minimized, all at a considerable cost in law enforcement and increased crime. Was the cost worth it? I think so, but others may disagree. What are the lives of would-be addicts worth? I recall some people saying to me then, "Let them kill themselves." I was appalled. Happily, such views did not prevail.

Have we lost today? Not at all. High-rate cocaine use is not commonplace. The National Institute of Drug Abuse (NIDA) reports that less than 5 percent of high-school seniors used cocaine within the last thirty days. Of course, this survey misses young people who have dropped out of school and miscounts those who lie on the questionnaire, but even if we inflate the NIDA estimate by some plausible percentage, it is still not much above 5 percent. Medical examiners reported in 1987 that about 1,500 died from cocaine use; hospital emergency rooms reported about 30,000 admissions related to cocaine abuse.

These are not small numbers, but neither are they evidence of a nationwide plague that threatens to engulf us all. Moreover, cities vary greatly in the proportion of people who are involved with cocaine. To get city-level data, we need to turn to drug tests carried out on arrested persons, who obviously are more likely to be drug users than the average citizen. The National Institute of Justice, through its Drug Use Forecasting (DUF) project, collects urinalysis data on arrestees in 22 cities. As we have already seen, opiate (chiefly heroin) use has been flat or declining in most of these cities over the last decade. Cocaine use has gone up sharply, but with great variation among cities. New York, Philadelphia, and Washington, D.C., all report that two-thirds or more of their arrestees tested positive for cocaine, but in Portland, San Antonio, and Indianapolis, the percentage was one-third or less.

In some neighborhoods, of course, matters have reached crisis proportions. Gangs control the streets, shootings terrorize residents, and drug-dealing occurs in plain view. The police seem barely able to contain matters. But in these neighborhoods—unlike at Palo Alto cocktail parties—the people are not calling for legalization, they are calling for help. And often, not much help has come. Many cities are willing to do almost anything about the drug problem except spend more money on it. The federal government cannot change that; only local voters and politicians can. It is not clear that they will.

It took about ten years to contain heroin. We have had experience with crack for only about three or four years. Each year, we spend perhaps $11 billion on law enforcement (and some of that goes to deal with marijuana) and perhaps $2 billion on treatment. Large sums, but not sums that should lead anyone to say, "We just can't afford this anymore."

The illegality of drugs increases crime, partly because some users turn to crime to pay for their habits, partly because some users are stimulated by certain drugs (such as crack or PCP) to act more violently or ruthlessly than they otherwise would, and partly because criminal organizations, seeking to control drug supplies, use force to manage their markets. These also are serious costs, but no one knows how much they would be reduced, if drugs were legalized. Addicts would no longer steal to pay black-market prices for drugs, a real gain. But some, perhaps a great deal, of that gain would be offset by the great increase in the number of addicts. These people, nodding on heroin or living in the delusion-ridden high of cocaine, would hardly be ideal employees. Many would steal simply to support themselves, since snatch-and-grab, opportunistic crime can be managed even by people unable to hold a regular job or plan an elaborate crime. Those British addicts who get their supplies from government clinics are not models of law-abiding decency. Most are in crime, and, though their per-capita rate of criminality may be lower thanks to the cheapness of their drugs, the total volume of crime they produce may be quite large. Of course, society could decide to support all unemployable addicts on welfare, but that would mean that gains from lowered rates of crime would have to be offset by large increases in welfare budgets.

Proponents of legalization claim that the costs of having more addicts around would be largely, if not entirely, offset by having more money available with which to treat and care for them. The money would come from taxes levied on the sale of heroin and cocaine.

To obtain this fiscal dividend, however, legalization's supporters must first solve an economic dilemma. If they want to raise a lot of money to pay for welfare and treatment, the tax rate on the drugs will have to be quite high. Even if they themselves do not want a high rate, the politicians' love of "sin taxes" would probably guarantee that it would be high anyway. But the higher the tax, the higher the price of the drug; and the higher the price, the greater the likelihood that addicts will turn to crime to find the money for it, and that criminal organizations will be formed to sell tax-free drugs at below-market rates. If we managed to keep taxes (and thus prices) low, we would get that much less money to pay for welfare and treatment, and more people could afford to become addicts. There may be an optimal tax rate for drugs that maximizes revenue, while minimizing crime, bootlegging, and the recruitment of new addicts; but our experience with alcohol does not suggest that we know how to find it.

The Benefits of Illegality

The advocates of legalization find nothing to be said in favor of the current system except, possibly, that it keeps the number of addicts smaller than it would otherwise be. In fact, the benefits are more substantial than that.

First, treatment. All the talk about providing "treatment on demand" implies that there is a demand for treatment. That is not quite right. There are some drug-dependent people who genuinely want treatment and will remain in it, if offered; they should receive it. But there are far more who want only short-term help after a bad crash; once stabilized and bathed, they are back on the street again, hustling. And even many of the addicts who enroll in a program, honestly wanting help, drop out after a short while when they discover that help takes time and commitment. Drug-dependent people have very short time horizons and a weak capacity for commitment. These two groups—those looking

for a quick fix and those unable to stick with a long-term fix—are not easily helped. Even if we increase the number of treatment slots—as we should—we would have to do something to make treatment more effective.

One thing that can often make it more effective is compulsion. Douglas Anglin of UCLA, in common with many other researchers, has found that the longer one stays in a treatment program, the better the chances of a reduction in drug dependency. But he, again like most other researchers, has found that drop-out rates are high. He has also found, however, that patients who enter treatment under legal compulsion stay in the program longer than those not subject to such pressure. His research on the California civil-commitment program, for example, found that heroin users involved with its required drug-testing program had, over the long term, a lower rate of heroin use than similar addicts who were free of such constraints. If for many addicts compulsion is a useful component of treatment, it is not clear how compulsion could be achieved in a society in which purchasing, possessing, and using the drug were legal. It could be managed, I suppose, but I would not want to have to answer the challenge from the American Civil Liberties Union that it is wrong to compel a person to undergo treatment for consuming a legal commodity.

Next, education. We are not investing substantially in drug-education programs in the schools. Though we do not yet know for certain what will work, there are some promising leads. But I wonder how credible such programs would be, if they were aimed at dissuading children from doing something perfectly legal. We could, of course, treat drug education like smoking education: inhaling crack and inhaling tobacco are both legal, but you should not do it, because it is bad for you. That tobacco is bad for you is easily shown; the Surgeon General has seen to that. But what do we say about crack? It is pleasurable, but devoting yourself to so much pleasure is not a good idea (though perfectly legal)? Unlike tobacco, cocaine will not give you cancer or emphysema, but it will lead you to neglect your duties to family, job, and neighborhood? Everybody is doing cocaine, but you should not?

Again, it might be possible under a legalized regime to have effective drug-prevention programs, but their effectiveness would depend heavily, I think, on first having decided that cocaine use, like tobacco use, is purely a matter of practical consequences; no fundamental moral significance attaches to either. But if we believe—as I do—that dependency on certain mind-altering drugs *is* a moral issue, and that their illegality rests in part on their immorality, then legalizing them undercuts, if it does not eliminate altogether, the moral message.

That message is at the root of the distinction we now make between nicotine and cocaine. Both are highly addictive; both have harmful physical effects. But we treat the two drugs differently, not simply because nicotine is so widely used as to be beyond the reach of effective prohibition, but because its use does not destroy the user's essential humanity. Tobacco shortens one's life, cocaine debases it. Nicotine alters one's habits, cocaine alters one's soul. The heavy use of crack, unlike the heavy use of tobacco, corrodes those natural sentiments of sympathy and duty that constitute our human nature and make possible our social life. To say, as does Nadelmann, that distinguishing morally between tobacco and cocaine is "little more than a transient prejudice" is close to saying that morality itself is but a prejudice.

The Alcohol Problem

Now we have arrived where many arguments about legalizing drugs begin: is there any reason to treat heroin and cocaine differently from the way we treat alcohol?

There is no easy answer to that question, because, as with so many human problems, one cannot decide simply on the basis either of moral principles or of individual consequences; one has to temper any policy by a common-sense judgment of what is possible. Alcohol, like heroin, cocaine, PCP, and marijuana, is a drug—that is, a mood-altering substance—and, consumed to excess, it certainly has harmful consequences: auto accidents, barroom fights, bedroom shootings. It is also, for some people, addictive. We cannot confidently compare the addictive powers of these drugs, but the best evidence suggests that crack and heroin are much more addictive than alcohol.

Many people, Nadelmann included, argue that, since the health and financial costs of alcohol abuse are so much higher than those of cocaine and heroin abuse, it is hypocritical folly to devote our efforts to preventing cocaine or drug use. But, as Mark Kleiman of Harvard has pointed out, this comparison is quite misleading. What Nadelmann is doing is showing that a *legalized* drug (alcohol) produces greater social harm than *illegal* ones (cocaine and heroin). But of course. Suppose that in the 1920s

we had made heroin and cocaine legal and alcohol illegal. Can anyone doubt that Nadelmann would now be writing that it is folly to continue our ban on alcohol, because cocaine and heroin are so much more harmful?

And let there be no doubt about it—widespread heroin and cocaine use are associated with all manner of ills. Thomas Bewley found that the mortality rate of British heroin addicts in 1968 was 28 times as high as the death rate of the same age group of non-addicts, even though in England at the time an addict could obtain free or low-cost heroin and clean needles from British clinics. Perform the following mental experiment: suppose we legalized heroin and cocaine in this country. In what proportion of auto fatalities would the state police report that the driver was nodding off on heroin or recklessly driving on a coke high? In what proportion of spouse-assault and child-abuse cases would the local police report that crack was involved? In what proportion of industrial accidents would safety investigators report that the forklift or drill-press operator was in a drug-induced stupor or frenzy? We do not know exactly what the proportion would be, but anyone who asserts that it would not be much higher than it is now would have to believe that these drugs have little appeal, except when they are illegal. And that is nonsense.

An advocate of legalization might concede that social harm—perhaps harm equivalent to that already produced by alcohol—would follow from making cocaine and heroin generally available. But at least, he might add, we would have the problem "out in the open," where it could be treated as a matter of "public health." That is well and good, *if* we knew how to treat—that is, cure—heroin and cocaine abuse. But we do not know how to do it for all the people who would need such help. We are having only limited success in coping with chronic alcoholics. Addictive behavior is immensely difficult to change, and the best methods for changing it—living in drug-free therapeutic communities, becoming faithful members of Alcoholics Anonymous or Narcotics Anonymous—require great personal commitment, a quality that is, alas, in short supply among the very persons—young people, disadvantaged people—who are often most at risk for addiction.

Suppose that today we had, not 15 million alcohol abusers, but half a million. Suppose that we already knew what we have learned from our long experience with the widespread use of alcohol.

Would we make whiskey legal? I do not know, but I suspect there would be a lively debate. The Surgeon General would remind us of the risks alcohol poses to pregnant women. The National Highway Traffic Safety Administration would point to the likelihood of more highway fatalities caused by drunk drivers. The Food and Drug Administration might find that there is a non-trivial increase in cancer associated with alcohol consumption. At the same time, the police would report great difficulty in keeping illegal whiskey out of our cities, officers being corrupted by bootleggers, and alcohol addicts often resorting to crime to feed their habit. Libertarians, for their part, would argue that every citizen has a right to drink anything he wishes and that drinking is, in any event, a "victimless crime."

However the debate might turn out, the central fact would be that the problem was still, at that point, a small one. The government cannot legislate away the addictive tendencies in all of us, nor can it remove completely even the most dangerous addictive substances. But it can cope with harms when the harms are still manageable.

Science and Addiction

One advantage of containing a problem, while it is still containable, is that it buys time for science to learn more about it and perhaps to discover a cure. Almost unnoticed in the current debate over legalized drugs is that basic science has made rapid strides in identifying the underlying neurological processes involved in some forms of addiction. Stimulants, such as cocaine and amphetamines, alter the way certain brain cells communicate with one another. That alteration is complex and not entirely understood, but in simplified form it involves modifying the way in which a neurotransmitter called dopamine sends signals from one cell to another.

When dopamine crosses the synapse between two cells, it is in effect carrying a message from the first cell to activate the second one. In certain parts of the brain, that message is experienced as pleasure. After the message is delivered, the dopamine returns to the first cell. Cocaine apparently blocks this return, or "reuptake," so that the excited cell and others nearby continue to send pleasure messages. When the exaggerated high produced by cocaine-influenced dopamine finally ends, the brain cells may (in ways that are still a matter of dispute) suffer from an extreme lack of dopamine, thereby making the individual unable to experience any

pleasure at all. This would explain why cocaine users often feel so depressed after enjoying the drug. Stimulants may also affect the way in which other neurotransmitters, such as serotonin and noradrenaline, operate.

Whatever the exact mechanism may be, once it is identified, it becomes possible to use drugs to block either the effect of cocaine or its tendency to produce dependency. There have already been experiments, using desipramine, imipramine, bromocriptine, carbamazepine, and other chemicals. There are some promising results.

Tragically, we spend very little on such research, and the agencies funding it have not in the past occupied very influential or visible posts in the federal bureaucracy. If there is one aspect of the "war on drugs" metaphor that I dislike, it is its tendency to focus attention almost exclusively on the troops in the trenches, whether engaged in enforcement or treatment, and away from the research-and-development efforts back on the home front, where the war may ultimately be decided.

I believe that the prospects of scientists in controlling addiction will be strongly influenced by the size and character of the problem they face. If the problem is a few hundred thousand chronic, high-dose users of an illegal product, the chances of making a difference at a reasonable cost will be much greater than if the problem is a few million chronic users of legal substances. Once a drug is legal, not only will its use increase but many of those who then use it will prefer the drug to the treatment: they will want the pleasure, whatever the cost to themselves or their families, and they will resist—probably successfully—any effort to wean them away from experiencing the high that comes from inhaling a legal substance.

If I Am Wrong . . .

No one can know what our society would be like, if we changed the law to make access to cocaine, heroin, and PCP easier. I believe, for reasons given, that the result would be a sharp increase in use, a more widespread degradation of the human personality, and a greater rate of accidents and violence.

I may be wrong. If I am, then we will needlessly have incurred heavy costs in law enforcement and some forms of criminality. But if I am right, and the legalizers prevail anyway, then we will have consigned millions of people, hundreds of thousands of infants, and hundreds of neighborhoods to a life of oblivion and disease. To the lives and families destroyed by alcohol, we will have added countless more destroyed by cocaine, heroin, PCP, and whatever else a basement scientist can invent.

Human character is formed by society; indeed, human character is inconceivable without society, and good character is less likely in a bad society. Will we, in the name of an abstract doctrine of radical individualism, and with the false comfort of suspect predictions, decide to take the chance that somehow individual decency can survive amid a more general level of degradation?

I think not. The American people are too wise for that, whatever the academic essayists and cocktail-party pundits may say. But if Americans today are less wise than I suppose, then Americans at some future time will look back on us now and wonder, what kind of people were they that they could have done such a thing?

✳ ✳ ✳

James Q. Wilson, "Against the Legalization of Drugs," from *Commentary*, February 1990. Reprinted by permission of James Q. Wilson and of *Commentary*; all rights reserved. Copyright © 1990 by James Q. Wilson.

For Discussion

Wilson argues that the number of heroin users has remained stable over the years because it is costly and difficult to obtain. Can this argument explain heroin use among individuals from middle and upper income backgrounds? Why or why not?

Notes

1. I do not here take up the question of marijuana. For a variety of reasons—its widespread use and its lesser tendency to addict—it presents a different problem from cocaine or heroin. For a penetrating analysis, see Mark Kleiman, *Marijuana: Costs of Abuse, Costs of Control* (Greenwood Press, 217 pp.). ✦

38. Hawks Ascendant: The Punitive Trend of American Drug Policy

PETER REUTER

Peter Reuter of the RAND Corporation provides a framework for organizing three alternative views for addressing the illegal drug problem. The "Hawks'" supply-side perspective sees drug prohibition as a necessity—the value systems of drug users do not coincide with mainstream culture; drug treatment is often ineffective; and because the drug users commit many crimes, enforcement should be the primary means of control. According to the "Doves," individuals use drugs for pleasure, and the negative consequences of drug use occur largely because the drugs are illegal. Doves advocate a legalization of drugs. The "Owls" believe that current drug policies have failed and advocate prohibition, but with greater emphasis on treatment and prevention than in the past. Reuter suggests that current drug policies reflect the philosophy of the Hawks. Government budgets designated for controlling drug use emphasize enforcement rather than treatment. Drug testing is used for punitive purposes rather than referrals for treatment. Finally, the author discusses the negative aspects of the Hawks' perspective that are embedded in social and legal policy.

Drug policy has generated two debates. The more elevated one concerns the retention of our current prohibitions, the legalization debate. Though it has occasionally impinged on the rhetoric of political discussion, as in the attack against legalization in the introduction to the first *National Drug Strategy*, this debate remains largely a parlor sport for intellectuals, divorced from the policy-making process. The more consequential, albeit less lofty, debate has been that between what are usually called the supply-side advocates and the demand-side advocates. The supply-siders, with former National Drug Control Director William Bennett as their most articulate spokesman, seek continued expansion of the nation's effort to imprison drug sellers and detect and punish (in various ways) drug users, while denying that they are slighting demand-side

considerations.[1] The demand-side advocates, led by Senator Joseph Biden, while generally accepting the need for "vigorous enforcement," argue that current resource commitments to programs directly aimed at demand (prevention and treatment) are grossly underfunded and should be massively increased, even if this is at the expense of enforcement.[2]

Neither debate is satisfactory. The legalization debate is too focused on extremes, excluding the possibility of compromise. It is strident, with both sides casting aspersion on the values of the other. On the other hand, the debate between the supply- and demand-siders is too narrow, allowing only minor programmatic tinkering.

Borrowing liberally from the classic essay of Nye, Allison, and Carnesale on approaches to preventing nuclear war,[3] I propose to combine the two debates on drug policy into a three-sided discussion among hawks (supply-side advocates), doves (legalizers), and owls (bold demand-side advocates) about the nature of the drug problem and the consequences of different approaches to controlling it.[4]

Drug-policy debates have been conducted largely in terms of images. The hawks point to the immediacy of the problems in the streets (particularly the carnage surrounding drug distribution) and reasonably (though in intemperate tones) ask whether efforts at drug prevention or treatment offer any reasonable hope for controlling those markets and associated violence in the near future. They note the apparently low success rates of drug-treatment programs; many programs show relapse rates of more than 60 percent.[5] Prevention programs aimed at seventh graders (the most commonly targeted grade) will reduce the number of adult drug addicts only with a five-to-ten-year lag. Finally, they argue that effective prevention and treatment require intense enforcement, both to make drugs difficult to obtain (driving users into treatment) and to make drug use appear legally risky (reinforcing prevention messages).[6]

The doves' message is even clearer than that of the hawks. After defending themselves from the charge that they condone the use of drugs by asserting that society should strive to reduce use of all dangerous psychoactive drugs,[7] including alcohol and cigarettes, they go on to argue that most of the current evils associated with drugs arise from the prohibitions and enforcement of those prohibitions. The violence, overdoses, and massive illegal incomes that are such a prominent part of our current concerns with psychoactive drugs are not consequences of the nature of the drugs themselves, but rather of the conditions of use that society has created. Doves are strong on critiques of the current regime,[8] but rather weak in describing their preferred alternatives. However, they are clear that criminal prohibitions should play no role in society's efforts to keep use of psychoactive drugs to a minimum.[9]

The current owls are less eloquent. They argue that drug enforcement has proven a failure. The intensification of enforcement throughout the 1980s failed to stem a massive growth in the nation's drug problems. Enforcement does not go to the root of the problem; with a loss of faith in source-country control programs (such as crop eradication and crop substitution),[10] the root of the problem is now seen to be the initiation of new users in the United States and the failure to provide good-quality treatment for addicts. Prevention and treatment receive a derisory share of what the nation spends to control its drug problems. Public treatment programs, faced with the most difficult clients, have far fewer resources to spend on those clients than do private treatment programs.[11] Success in reducing the nation's drug problem requires a change in spending priorities. *Sotto voce*, at most, they also suggest that intense drug enforcement increases crime and may exacerbate health problems related to drug use; however, they believe in the value of the criminal prohibition and significant enforcement against drug dealers.

This essay has two goals. The first is to describe the increasing success of the hawks. To an extraordinary degree, they have taken control of drug policy and given it a distinctively punitive hew. The second goal is the more difficult one, namely to suggest that the hawks may have gone too far. The punishment is expensive, not so much in money terms (though the sums are no longer trivial, even in an inflation-adjusted Everett Dircksen sense) as in terms of the human costs of locking up many people for relatively minor offenses and not locking up many others for more serious offenses. Intense enforcement also increases the harms caused by drug users to themselves and others. I believe that we might well be better off, if we simply punished drug dealers less aggressively; I believe that matters would be still further improved, if some of the money saved by reduced punishment were spent on better-quality treatment of the drug dependent. But the emphasis should be on "believe"; I cannot

claim to have shown the consequences of shifting to a less punitive regime. I hope, however, that the reader will be persuaded that the question of "excessive punitiveness" is worth considering.

This is clearly the essay of an owl,[12] but of one that feels that his current representatives fail to present the position strongly enough. The concession that enforcement must be maintained at its current level importantly limits the domain of policy options, particularly at a time when federal drug-control budgets have stopped growing in real terms and when the corresponding state and local budgets are likely to shrink. I shall suggest that more aggressive owlishness, derived from the European "harm reduction" movement, is appropriate.

The differences among the three positions (summarized very crudely in Table 1, borrowed again from Nye, Allison, and Carnesale) in part come from different views of what constitutes the drug problem and the sources of that problem. For hawks, the heart of the matter is the threat to youth and to American values; drug use means an abandoning of concern with others, and focusing on short-term pleasures for oneself. It is a lack of clarity about values in society and a failure to ensure that drug use is punished that leads to so many young people becoming regular users of psychoactives. The violence and health damage are merely the visible emblems of a more fundamental problem. The first *National Drug Control Strategy* says it eloquently: for "most drug users," use is the result of a "human flaw" that leads them to pursue "a hollow, degrading, and deceptive pleasure." What is required is "a firm moral stand that using drugs is wrong and should be resisted." If values are the heart of the matter, then all institutions of society must join in the fight; the 1992 *Strategy* says, "[T]he family, neighborhood, community, church, school, and workplace must be very active in this effort. If they are not, they implicitly signal to young people that drug use is not to be taken seriously, at least not seriously enough to do anything about it."

Doves believe that individuals use psychoactive substances because they provide pleasure, and that society should minimize the harm that results from the use of such substances, without criminalizing the choice of a particular substance. Psychoactive drugs can harm individuals, and society has a responsibility to inform adolescents about the consequences of choosing drugs and to help those who become dependent deal with the problem. But the criminal law makes those tasks more difficult, as well as imposing direct costs on society.

Owls focus on the damage arising from heavy drug use by a relatively small number of those who become dependent. The health consequences are given considerable weight. Again, drug use is regarded as evil in and of itself but, in my preferred version, attention is given to the evils created by enforcement. Criminal law may be an important tool for minimizing the damage done by dangerous and attractive psychoactives in a world of imperfect decisionmakers, but enforcement is a not a good in itself; indeed, one wants the lowest level of enforcement compatible with keeping initiation down and encouraging the dependent to seek treatment.[13] Drug control is also not the only goal, and higher drug use may be accepted in return for better performance with respect to some other social goal, such as reduced spread of HIV infection.

Table 1
Drug War Strategies: Hawks, Owls, and Doves

Position	Nature of Drug Problem	Explanation for Drug Use	Policy Emphasis	Consequence of Failure
HAWKS	Amorality of Drug Users and Sellers	Selfishness, Lack of Clear Social Values	Tough Enforcement	Violence, Repression
OWLS	Addiction, Disease	Adverse Social Conditions	Prevention, Treatment, Prohibition	Continuation of Present Problems
DOVES	The Bad Effects of Prohibition	Pleasures from Drugs	Legalize, Inform	Large Increase in Drug Abuse

There is much truth in the descriptive statements of all three groups. Indeed, I suspect that they are all true. However, none of them provide much help in working out what our drug policy should be. No one can describe, even very roughly, the consequences of doubling the number of treatment slots available for addicts without insurance coverage for such treatment, or what would happen if we were to increase the number of drug arrests by 25 percent. Over five years, would these result in declines of 20 percent in the extent of heroin addiction or in drug-related homicides? What else might occur as a consequence, positive or negative, of these actions? The doves may be correct that many of the current evils are the consequence of prohibition, but they have little basis for suggesting the consequence of the removal of those prohibitions on either the extent of use or the way that users would behave in a legalized regime.[14]

The research-minded reader at this stage may object that recent experiences ought to allow us to examine the effects of at least some policy variation. Cities differ in the extent of treatment availability and stringency of enforcement. Surely, that should provide the basis for determining whether tougher enforcement reduces drug use. Unfortunately, the data available at the local level are so sparse and inconsistent that research on the consequences of local variation is still in its infancy.[15]

An alternative source of insight might be the experiences of other countries, at least other developed nations. Again, the research effort in this area is barely nascent, but I will briefly show that some Western European nations have adopted much less punitive approaches and have fared no worse than the United States in terms of controlling drug use and its related harms.

But whatever the shakiness of the arguments and evidence of the various positions, the simple truth is that the hawks have prevailed; indeed, their ascendance still seems to be increasing. Thus, the next section deals mainly with their position, describing the many dimensions of their success. The section entitled "Changing Patterns of Drug Use and Related Problems" summarizes what has happened to the drug problem since 1980, pointing to the mixed record of success of American drug policy. A later section presents what we can reasonably claim to know about "the consequences of toughness," both good and bad. It also includes a brief survey of the experiences of Western Europe, to show what other approaches are possible. The concluding section begins with a short excursion into the political dynamics of the drug issue, explaining why the hawks almost always win, and then speculates about the likely future of U.S. drug policy.

The Triumph of the Hawks

Many have noted that American drug policy has traditionally been heavily dependent on criminal law when compared to most other Western societies. Particularly in the last decade, the hawks have been in soaring ascendance. Though they grumble about the lack of severity in punishment of drug users and dealers, they have managed to massively increase funding for such punishment, to expand the scope of efforts to detect drug users in many settings, and to intensify the severity of penalties imposed on those convicted of selling or using drugs.

Budgets, Legislation, and Programs

Budget allocations help make the point. The federal budget for drug control has increased substantially over the last decade; in constant dollars, it has risen from $1.5 billion in fiscal year 1980 to $6.7 billion in fiscal year 1990. Throughout that period, it has been dominated by enforcement programs; the share going to such programs never fell below 70 percent and rose as high as 80 percent. The federal drug control budget in 1990 allocated only 29 percent of total expenditures to treatment and prevention.

Even this understates the extent of the hawks' budgetary dominance. State and local governments spend more in total than the federal government (even eliminating federal pass-throughs) but allocate a still smaller share to treatment and prevention programs. It is difficult to assemble a national drug-control budget, since most state and local drug enforcement is carried out by non-specialized law-enforcement agencies, and the allocation of their budgets to drug control has a very judgmental element. My own estimate is that, in 1990, state and local governments spent roughly $18 billion on drug control and 80 percent of that went for enforcement.[16] This suggests a 1990 national drug control budget of $28 billion for all levels of government, with 75 percent going to enforcement.[17] Less than $5 billion went to treatment, compared to over $20 billion spent on enforcement of various kinds, mostly at the local level. Indeed, the treatment figure may have been only $3 billion, though there may be another $2 billion of private funding through health insurance.

Budget allocation is, of course, only one measure of the hawks' triumph. Legislatures throughout the country, with the U.S. Congress very much in the vanguard, have dramatically increased the sentences for drug offenses, though prison overcrowding has undercut the effectiveness of these sentencing statutes. For example, in the 1988 Anti-Drug Abuse Control Act, Congress raised the mandatory sentence for selling 50 grams of crack to five years. The state of Michigan has imposed mandatory life imprisonment without parole for those convicted of selling 650 grams of cocaine. Congress has required that states impose various penalties, such as loss of drivers' licenses, for persons convicted of drug offenses, including simple possession of marijuana; federal highway funds are to be withheld from states that do not impose such penalties.

Drug-testing programs have become almost ubiquitous in many institutional settings, with an emphasis on penalty rather than treatment for those who test positive. For example, many of the new Intensively Supervised Probation programs require frequent drug testing, though providing few of their clients with access to drug treatment.[18] The federal government has imposed drug testing on much of its civilian work force, while perhaps half of large corporations test job applicants for drug use.

I include the recent decisions by the Drug Enforcement Administration (DEA) and by the Public Health Service (PHS) to disallow use of marijuana for medical purposes, even on an experimental basis, as reflecting the hawkishness of current policies. DEA is responsible for the scheduling of drugs; marijuana is currently classified as Schedule I (high abuse potential, no currently accepted medical use in treatment). A number of organizations initiated a suit in 1972, seeking to have the drug reclassified as Schedule II, allowing it to be prescribed. They claimed that marijuana can alleviate nausea associated with chemotherapy, as well as relieve glaucoma; it now also appears that marijuana can improve the appetite of AIDS patients. The PHS has, for the last year, allowed "compassionate" approval of marijuana prescriptions, produced on the government's marijuana farm in Mississippi, for thirteen patients.

In March 1992, the head of DEA once again refused to reschedule marijuana, and the PHS announced the end of the compassionate exemption program. Both agencies deny that they had any concern with the symbolic effect of allowing marijuana to be used for therapeutic purposes.[19] On the basis of conversations with various government officials and other observers, I disbelieve that claim, though I can offer no documentary backing for this. The official argument asserts that there is no credible evidence that marijuana, as opposed to synthetic drugs containing some of its active ingredients, has greater therapeutic value. In large part, this reflects the lack of research on the topic. The PHS rejection flew in the face of a survey of oncologists that found a majority who believed that marijuana should be available on prescription.[20] Indeed, that survey found that almost half of the oncologists responding currently advised their patients to use marijuana, even though the drug was not legally available. The DEA Administrator's decision reversed a remarkably strongly worded decision by the administrative law judge that the Schedule I classification was "unreasonable, arbitrary, and capricious." The head of the Public Health Service did suggest that it would send a "wrong signal" to hand out a drug that can cloud judgment with respect to automobile driving or sexual behaviors.[21]

The rejection of experimentation with marijuana for therapeutic purposes has an earlier parallel in the rejection of heroin for treatment of pain. In many other nations, heroin is routinely provided for relief of pain in terminal cancer patients; here, it remains on Schedule I, not allowed for any medicinal use in treatment. There is a genuine controversy about whether other synthetic opiates might not be more effective in each of the possible circumstances that heroin is a candidate pain reliever. However, the evidence for the effectiveness of heroin is strong enough that it might be left to the individual physician to decide; leakage to the illicit market is likely to provide only a negligible supplement to existing supplies.

Marijuana's "signal" value has also been emphasized by the concerted effort to reverse the decriminalization statutes that were passed in thirteen states in the 1970s. William Bennett appeared before a number of state legislatures to argue for recriminalization and was successful in Alaska in 1990.

Increasing Punitiveness

One symbol of the hawks' success is that they have managed to sustain the belief that drug sellers and users are at low risk from law enforcement, a belief that has helped promote more stringent sentencing statutes. They have emphasized stories about arrested drug sellers returning to the streets more rapidly than the police who arrested them and not getting jailed until they have been convicted numerous times. The truth is more complicated. By contemporary American standards, drug selling has become quite risky and drug use may be very risky for certain classes of users.

All this depends on a great deal of speculative arithmetic which is only summarized here.[22] Enforcement intensity is a function not simply of the total number of arrests or imprisonments for drug offenses, but of the ratio of such figures to the number of drug offenses. It is hard to find good measures of the number of such offenses but, if the rise in illicit drug episodes, in Drug Abuse Warning Network (DAWN), is taken as a surrogate, then it rose faster than arrests or imprisonments from 1980 to 1985 but not as rapidly from 1985 to 1990. Moreover, most drug arrests probably did not lead to serious penal sanction in the first period; but in the second half of the 1980s aggressive arrest policies at last led to large increases in the number of incarcerations. Thus, it is likely that the intensity of enforcement decreased, at least for cocaine offenses, in the first half of the 1980s, but then rose in the second half of that decade.

Table 2
Disposition of California Felony Drug Arrests 1980, 1985, 1990

	1980	**1985**	**1990**
Felony Arrests	40,451	63,766	84,538
Disposed of Number			
Convicted	18,800	30,100	53,200
(percent of arrests)	(45)	(48)	(63)
Number to State			
Prisons	921	3,366	10,494
(percent of convicted)	(5)	(11)	(20)
Number to Jail	9,700	22,500	33,900
(percent of convicted)	(52)	(75)	(64)

Source: Unpublished tabulations, California Bureau of Criminal Statistics.

So far, I have not made much of differences among drugs. Law and policy appropriately make such distinctions, though not necessarily in appropriate ways. Enforcement has been quite drug-specific, and the impacts differ by drugs. Most attention in this section will be given to cocaine, but it is worth noting marijuana enforcement patterns as well. In contrast to cocaine, marijuana enforcement became more stringent throughout the decade as usage dropped.

Enforcement has increased massively in absolute terms. The number of state and local arrests for drug offenses increased rapidly, from 581,000 in 1980 to 1,090,000 in 1990. The composition of these arrests changed in an important way over the same period. Whereas, the 1980 total was dominated by arrests for marijuana (70 percent) and possession (82 percent) offenses, in 1990 heroin/cocaine[23] arrests had come to exceed the number for marijuana (591,000 versus 391,000) and distribution arrests now accounted for a much larger share than in 1980 (27 percent versus 18 percent). In effect, the average seriousness of arrest offense has increased sharply.

Arrest is only the first step in the criminal justice process; it is conviction and sentence that provide the principal punishment, though arrest itself can lead to seizure of drugs and other assets. At the national level, we cannot systematically trace through the disposition of arrests prior to 1986. We

have to rely on fragments of data collected for a few states on an occasional basis to get a sense of how many drug offenders were imprisoned during the earlier years.

The best data cover felony drug arrests in California; Table 2 shows the disposition of these arrests in 1980, 1985, and 1990.

The number of felony drug arrests disposed of increased by about 21,000 in each half of the decade. What changed dramatically was the position of those arrests. The percentage convicted rose, particularly after 1985, and the percentage of convictions resulting in prison sentence went up dramatically. The total number of persons sent to prison for drug offenses rose threefold between 1980 and 1985 and tripled again in the following five years; over the entire decade, the figure rose from less than 1,000 to over 10,000. A focus simply on the number of drug arrests fails to capture the increasing stringency of enforcement.

Nationally, the only available data on the sentencing for felony drug convictions cover 1986 and 1988.[24] In that two year period, there was a very sharp increase (from 135,000 to 225,000, approximately a 70-percent rise) in the number of persons convicted of felony drug trafficking or possession charges.[25] The number receiving state prison sentences (i.e., more than twelve months) rose from 49,900 to 92,500, though there was a modest decline in their expected time served from twenty-two months to twenty months.[26] In 1988, drug offenses accounted for approximately one-third of all felony convictions in state courts.[27]

The most recent year, for which available data permit rough estimates of prison and jail years meted out for drug felonies by state courts, is 1988. About 90,000 persons were sentenced to prison, and another 65,000 were sentenced to local jails. The federal court system also imposes punishment on drug dealers. Though federal drug convictions constitute a small share of the total, the average time served for those incarcerated is much higher than for state-sentenced offenders, reflecting mandatory penalties for many drug-selling offenses of ten years or more and no parole. In 1988, federal courts generated an estimated 50,000 years of expected prison time for drug dealers, compared to only one-tenth that amount in 1980. That reflected increasing numbers of convictions, rising sentence length and, most significantly, a rise in the share of sentences that the inmate expected to serve; this last was the result of the imposition of sentencing guidelines and the abolition of federal parole. The total of federal and state incarceration figures for 1988 was about 200,000 cell years; this is perhaps ten times the 1980 figure.

The Penal Risks of the Drug Trade

One way to assess what this punishment represents is to consider the risks of arrest faced by users, and the risk of imprisonment faced by sellers, of cocaine and marijuana.

To calculate roughly the 1990 absolute risks-per-user year for the two drugs, we need estimates of the total number of current users. If there were 15 million marijuana users, a relatively generous figure based on the survey data,[28] then they faced an average risk of 2 percent of arrest in that year; though this seems low, note that in steady state that amounted to a one in five chance of being arrested in a ten-year using career. For cocaine, with a much smaller user base (no more than perhaps 5 million, ignoring those who use less than once per month), the annual arrest risk was 6 percent. The risk in a ten-year using career might then be as high as 60 percent.

These are, of course, very aggregate calculations. Not all users are at the same risk of apprehension. Those who use frequently might be expected to be at much higher risk, because they engage in more of the risky transaction of purchase. But there are other characteristics that seem to be associated with risk of arrest for drug possession, in particular race and gender. In the District of Columbia, of those residents arrested for drug possession between 1985 and 1987, 96 percent were African-American; 82 percent were male. No reasonable estimate of the prevalence of drug use in different populations would suggest that this represented the share of African-Americans or males in the drug-using population. These percentages probably reflect the fact that many possession arrests are failed sales arrests; a seller is caught with drugs but not in the act of selling, and the seller population in exposed situations (i.e., selling on the street and in crack houses) seems to be predominantly male and (in the District of Columbia) African-American.

In summary, some user groups may be at very high risk of apprehension, others at quite modest risk. That is not a casual observation, since I shall suggest later that it appears that the big declines in drug use have occurred among the groups at low risk of arrest.

For sellers, the arrest risks differed even more substantially for the two drugs. Using the same assumptions as Reuter and Kleiman[29], concerning the ratio of buyers to sellers for each drug, marijuana sellers may have faced not much more than a 10-percent probability of being arrested in the course of a year of selling; the comparable figure for cocaine might be as high as 40 percent.

I estimate that the total cell years in 1988 for marijuana sellers was about 40,000 and for cocaine sellers about 110,000. The ratio of marijuana to cocaine is surprising in light of the great concern attached to cocaine use. But the federal courts, which provide clearly separated figures for the different drugs, show a similar ratio. The cell-year calculations are more speculative than those for arrests, but 110,000 cell years for a population of perhaps 350,000 cocaine dealers suggests that, by 1988, that activity had indeed become a risky one. A study of drug dealers in Washington, D.C., in the late 1980s[30] estimated that street sellers of drugs faced about a 22-percent probability of imprisonment in the course of a year's selling and that, given expected time served, they spent one-third of their selling career in prison.

Does this make drug selling appropriately risky? One-third of one's time in prison strikes me as a lot. On the other hand, the risk per selling transaction is extraordinarily low; a seller who works two days per week at this trade may make 1,000 transactions in the course of a year. His imprisonment risk per transaction is only about 1 in 4,500; by that metric, it is a great deal lower than the risks associated with other crimes, such as burglary and robbery. Another way of expressing the risk is that a dealer may spend a day imprisoned for each ten sales transactions.

In many ways, these figures mirror the realities for property crimes. Most robberies and burglaries result in no arrest; yet, those who engage frequently in robbery or burglary are likely to spend a significant portion of their criminal careers incarcerated. So, it appears to be for those who are regular drug sellers, at least in exposed settings.

Changing Patterns of Drug Use and Related Problems

By historic and international standards, use of illegal psychoactive drugs in the United States in the early 1990s is extraordinarily high.[31] Moreover, that drug use is associated with more severe and diverse problems than those associated with illegal drugs in other periods or societies. It is almost certain, nevertheless, that the prevalence of drug use has declined sharply from the dizzying heights of the early to mid-1980s and is likely to continue to decline. These two discordant facts present a dilemma in assessing the effectiveness of current policies. Should we focus on the high absolute levels, and conclude that these policies have failed, or on the declines and conclude that they are finally succeeding?

In any assessment, it is important to note that the levels of drug use and drug problems (as well as their declines) are far from uniform across population groups. Drug abuse or dependence[32] is increasingly concentrated in inner-city populations and appears to be disproportionately a problem for the minority community, particularly inner-city, young, African-American males. Drug use apart, inner-city communities have been much more affected by the violence and disorder surrounding drug distribution. This skewing of adversities has had an important influence on the politics of drug policies. For most of the nation, the drug problem is lessening, but for many poorer communities there are few, if any, signs of relief; this exacerbates the growing sense of a division within society, the emergence of a hardening into "Two Nations."

The Prevalence of Drug Use

The broad population surveys, of the household population and of high school seniors, tell a consistent story.[33] Initiation into drug use (as measured, for example, by the percentage of successive cohorts of 18 year olds reporting use in past year) escalated rapidly in the late 1970s and early 1980s, and then began to decline by 1986 or slightly earlier. The peaks were alarming; in 1978, 11 percent of high-school seniors reported using marijuana on a daily basis in the previous month. Every number is now down sharply from its peak; for example, by 1991 less than 2 percent of seniors reported daily use in the previous month.

The declines, as reported in the surveys, have been surprisingly evenly spread across age/race/sex groups. The surveys also have shown a complex and changing relationship between education and drug use. In 1985, prevalence rates among males born between 1959 and 1964 were very similar for high-school graduates and for dropouts; indeed, the former showed slightly higher rates for both recent use (past thirty days) and past use (last twelve months). By 1990, the rates had fallen much more sharply for the high-school graduates, particularly for past use. Differences in the declines for recent use were less marked, perhaps because this included more people who were habituated to drug use. The emerging negative correlation between education and cocaine use is consistent with the changes in cigarette use.[34]

The surveys provide mixed support for hypotheses about higher rates of drug use among African-Americans and Hispanics. The high-school senior surveys consistently show sharply higher prevalence rates among whites.[35] However, the National Household Survey shows higher rates for African-Americans; in the age group 26-34, for example, in 1990, the percentage reporting some use of an illegal drug in previous month was 13.7 percent, compared to 9.5 percent for white respondents.[36]

The broad surveys can reasonably claim to provide a valid measure of trends in the extent of drug use among the general population, though they have serious weaknesses even in that role. Increased stigmatization of drug use reduces the willingness of respondents to report that they are actually users; however, that stigmatization also reduces the extent of use. Thus, the surveys may exaggerate the downward trend in use, but it is unlikely that they misrepresent the direction.

But no one doubts that the broad population surveys miss a great deal of the most important behavior, namely frequent drug use. There are at least three reasons for this. First, the surveys do not include some critical populations in their sampling frames (for example, the homeless[37] and prisoners) who are believed to have high rates of drug abuse. Moreover, the size of these non-covered populations has risen and their composition has changed; both populations now seem to include higher percentages with drug-abuse problems than they did in 1980. Second, those who use drugs frequently, even if formally included in the sampling frame, are likely to be more difficult to reach, because they behave more erratically. Third, the response rate for the survey has declined from 83 percent in 1985 to 79 percent to 1990; this non-response increase may well be related to increased disapproval of drug use and thus lower willingness to even participate in a survey.

Moreover, the credibility of the surveys as a good representation of the nation's drug problems was undermined in the late 1980s by the dramatic discrepancy between the most publicized findings of those surveys and public perception of the changing problem. While the surveys pointed to substantial declines in drug use, it was widely believed that the drug problem was getting a great deal worse. The surveys also pointed to quite modest numbers of persons with severe drug problems; for example, the number of persons using cocaine weekly or more frequently was estimated at less than 1 million, which seemed inconsistent with the severity of cocaine-related problems.

Two official indicators supported the popular beliefs. DAWN reported data on the involvement of drugs in Emergency Room (ER) cases and in Medical Examiners' (ME) reports on deaths. DAWN, in contrast to the survey data, showed dramatic increases in cocaine mentions throughout the 1980s; the total number rose more than tenfold between 1980 and 1988. Beginning in 1988, the Drug Use Forecasting (DUF) system collected data on the prevalence of recent drug use by arrestees in twenty major cities, relying on analysis of urine specimens. It found very high rates of drug use in the arrested population and produced estimates of the number of frequent users that were very much higher than those derived from the household survey. Moreover, both DAWN and DUF pointed to a concentration of problems in the inner city. DAWN, which increasingly measures the extent of drug dependence,[38]

also suggested that whatever is happening to drug use generally, the number of cocaine dependent persons rose substantially between 1980 and 1990.[39]

Dependence

Measurement of the extent of drug dependence or frequent use is casual, almost to the point of irresponsibility. Though it is often asserted that there are 500,000-750,000 heroin addicts in the United States, it is impossible to find any systematic estimates post-1980; the number has its origins in murky and questionable manipulation of little understood data series.[40] It is, however, reasonably well-documented that heroin use increased rapidly during the period of about 1967 to 1973 and that the number of new initiates fell rapidly after that. However, if the correct figure is 750,000, then the United States, fifteen years after the end of the epidemic of heroin initiation, appears to have as high a rate of heroin dependence as any developed nation.[41]

The DAWN data suggest that the heroin-addicted population is still dominated by the cohort of inner-city minorities who first became addicted around 1970 when they were in their late teens and early twenties. The population of DAWN heroin ER cases is about 50 percent Hispanic and African-American, and getting older; whereas, 32 percent were over thirty-five in 1983, that percentage had risen to 50 percent by 1989.[42] Data on admissions to publicly funded treatment programs also point to an aging population that is dominated by minorities. Most heroin addicts have been in drug-treatment programs frequently, but heroin addictions, at least in this population, shows similarity to alcoholism; it can be characterized as a chronic, lifetime, relapsing disorder. DUF shows older arrestees to be more likely to test positive for opiates (almost exclusively heroin) but also shows surprisingly high rates among youthful arrestees, suggesting perhaps a resurgence of heroin initiation among the criminally active.[43] The new initiation may occur primarily among those who are already regular cocaine users.

More attention has been given to measuring the prevalence of frequent cocaine use. Indeed, there has even been a short-lived but vigorous controversy about this, with William Bennett and Senator Biden conducting an undignified shouting match about the number on national television.[44] The household survey produces an estimate of less than one million persons using cocaine at least once a week; indeed, for 1990, the figure was only 662,000. Using data from urine tests of arrestees in major cities, analysts have produced estimates of over two million.[45]

The urinalysis data show extremely high rates of cocaine use among arrestees. In most cities, over 50 percent of those arrested test positive for cocaine; supplemental interviews also show quite high rates of self-reported dependence among those who test positive for cocaine or heroin. What makes these figures particularly alarming is that arrest is not a rare event for young males, particularly less educated youth in large cities. Tillman,[46] reporting on the 1956 birth cohort in California, found that 34 percent of white males were arrested between the ages of 18 and 29; the figure for black males was 66 percent. The 1956 cohort came to maturity before the growth of the cocaine markets. For the 1967 cohort, Reuter, MacCoun, and Murphy found that, in the District of Columbia, perhaps one-quarter of the males were charged with at least one criminal offense, mostly a felony, between ages 18 and 21.[47] For African-American males in the Washington, D.C., cohort, the rate was approximately one-third. A majority of those charged had at least one drug offense among those charges.

The DUF data have only been collected since about 1988, so they cannot be used to describe trends over the decade of the 1980s. However, in the District of Columbia, urinalysis data have been collected since 1984. Over the period 1984-1988, there was a dramatic increase in the percent testing positive for cocaine, with little decline in the percent testing positive for other drugs. There has been a substantial drop since the peak figure of 68 percent for cocaine in May 1988, but in late 1991 the percentage testing positive for cocaine was still about 50 percent, and had been at that level for a year. DUF figures show most cities to have lower rates than the peaks of 1988 and 1989, but the declines are modest. In Chicago, the cocaine positives were down to 53 percent in the first quarter of 1991, compared to the peak of 64 percent in the fourth quarter of 1989.

In summary, these and other data suggest that the number of drug users has declined since the peak of the early to mid-1980s. However, there has been a much slighter and later decline in the numbers experiencing and causing significant problems related to their own frequent use of drugs. An increasing share of the drug-abusing population is found among the inner-city poor, as the more educated became more concerned about the health consequences of drug use. The poorer users are criminally active; their criminal activity is exacerbated by this drug use. That has enormous consequences for the politics of drug policy.

Costs

It is all very well to have estimates of the numbers of drug users and abusers. What costs, social and economic, should we attach to these figures? How significant is this problem?

The federal government has sponsored a series of four estimates of the economic cost of drug abuse.[48] For 1985, the estimated economic cost was $44 billion, compared to $70 billion for alcohol abuse and $103 billion for mental illness. It is hard to know what to make of these numbers, even if taken at face value, but the simple truth is that they are essentially irrelevant for our purposes, because they are dominated by what the government spends to control the problem and they miss major elements of the social costs associated with illicit drugs. Particularly troubling is the treatment of the cost of crime associated with drug abuse. This is estimated to be $13 billion, of which 90 percent is public expenditures on law enforcement; the loss of safety and amenity is treated as zero. Yet, in terms of dollars that individuals would be willing to spend to have lower crime rates in their community, that cost might well be much larger than the figures cited above.[49]

Estimates of the number of drug users is probably not a good metric for scaling the drug problem. After all, as even William Bennett noted in the introduction to the first *National Drug Strategy*, most drug-using careers are short, with only a few episodes involving drugs other than marijuana and are ended without requiring any treatment. Estimates that large numbers experiment with drugs or use drugs on an occasional basis does not mean that use of illicit drugs constitutes a major problem. Alternatively put, is there a credible base for the popular fears that briefly made drugs the leading social problem in 1988 and 1989?

Some drugs, such as LSD and PCP, can cause substantial and lasting damage to an individual who uses them just once; this, however, is an extremely rare event for cocaine, heroin, or marijuana. It seems likely that the vast majority of those who use these latter drugs only a few times suffer little harm as a consequence. The external costs of their use in aggregate may be high, if, for example, they provide a substantial share of the total market for illicit drugs and that market generates violence and corruption, but the costs to the individuals look modest. Moreover, it seems likely that occasional users actually account for a small share of total consumption, so that it is also unlikely that they impose high external costs through their contribution to the violence and disorder surrounding markets.

It is appropriate then to focus on those who are drug abusers, in order to obtain an understanding of the costs to individuals. The standard comparison of morbidity and mortality suggests that illicit drugs present only a moderately serious problem. Compared to alcohol or tobacco, the numbers of users, abusers, premature deaths, and disease associated with all illegal drugs together is small. Tobacco accounts for about 400,000 premature deaths annually, alcohol for about 100,000. It would be hard to sustain a figure of more than 20,000 premature deaths from the direct effects of illegal drugs; even if half of all homicides are drug-related, the figure is still barely 30,000.[50] Nor are the figures for morbidity impressive. With a base of frequent users of no more than 3 million, the health effects are tiny compared to those associated with the 50 million regular cigarette smokers and the 10 million heavy drinkers. On the grounds of the health costs, it could scarcely be claimed that use of illicit psychoactives constitutes a social problem of the first order.

That is a highly aggregative argument. Whereas alcohol and cigarettes strike all socioeconomic groups, illegal drugs bear disproportionately, in terms both of morbidity and mortality, on lower socio-economic status and minority populations. Thus, it might be that for these populations, particularly in center cities, illicit drugs are, indeed, a major health issue. However, it appears that these populations are also disproportionately affected by alcohol and cigarette-related morbidity and mortality, so that in relative terms illegal drugs may not be much more important.

Yet, there are other, distinctive, and important problems associated with illegal drugs. Alcohol is comparable to cocaine in its individual criminogenic consequences. Of those sentenced to jail terms in 1989, 29 percent reported being under the influence of alcohol (and not drugs) at the time of the offense, compared to 15 percent reporting being under the influence of drugs alone; another 12 percent reported being under the influence of both.[51] However, the high price of cocaine and the extensive illegal markets associated with it have engendered crime and violence that have sources other than the direct effect of the drugs themselves. For example, Goldstein found that the majority of drug-related homicides in New York were the result of "systemic" violence (for example, disputes over territories or contractual disagreements), rather than of the psychoactive effect of the drug or the need to obtain money to purchase drugs.[52] In some cities, it is claimed that half of all homicides are drug-related, though the criteria used to make the classification are quite murky. Moreover, the earnings from drug markets are believed to have been important in increasing the lethality of guns used in urban crime. That lethality may have contributed to the rise in killings of innocent bystanders.

The spread of HIV through needle sharing and other drug-related behaviors (such as the extreme promiscuity of crack users) is another hard-to-value consequence of drug use.[53] Over one-quarter of AIDS cases include intravenous drug use as a primary risk factor, and that percentage is rising. Curiously, though, in most of Western Europe, a concern with AIDS has been a principal influence on drug policy; in the United States, it has been treated as almost a separate policy arena.[54] In particular, it has not been given much attention in the debates with which this paper is concerned.

In the last few years, a great deal of attention has been given to the phenomenon of "crack babies," who are severely damaged by the cocaine use of their mothers during pregnancy. From an official high of 375,000 in the first *National Strategy*, the estimated number of babies annually affected by mother's drug use has fallen to 30,000 to 50,000. Moreover, it is no longer so clear that the damage suffered by most of these babies is very long-lasting. The problem is an emotionally very troubling one but may be rare in most populations.

Corruption is another cost associated with drug prohibition and its enforcement. Though there are spectacular and troubling instances of such corruption, such as that involving the homicide squad in the Miami Police Department in the mid-1980s and the more recent convictions of numerous deputies in the Los Angeles Sheriff's department, the revealed corruption seems fairly opportunistic and small-scale, certainly when compared with that surrounding the enforcement of gambling laws in the 1940s and 1950s.[55]

It is difficult, then, to say much about the real social costs of drug use and abuse. Violence, AIDS, corruption, and crack babies are all important and distinctive consequences of drug use under current conditions. There is enough of each of them to make understandable the public panic of the late 1980s. They have all become familiar enough to make equally understandable the declining concern of the last two years. That latter effect has been hastened by the fact that the most visible effects are highly concentrated in inner-city communities.

Knowing the scale of the social costs generated by drugs is important for determining what society should be willing to sacrifice in order to attain the goal of reduced use and abuse. Our inability to provide meaningful measures, along with the visibility and drama of illegal drugs, facilitates the task of those who would have the nation become harshly punitive.

The Consequences of Toughness

To what extent can it be shown that reductions in drug use have been accomplished by the general toughening of society's approach to drug control? What are other negative consequences of toughness? Unfortunately, discussion of these issues must be highly speculative, since there is little research on which to draw.

The punitive approach should reduce drug use and abuse by making drugs more expensive and/or less accessible. This will drive addicts into treatment and discourage adolescents from initiating use. Intense enforcement should also increase disapproval of drugs, which will lead current users to desist earlier. The available evidence suggests that intensified enforcement has had modest success in raising drug prices and has not reduced already limited access for the middle class. Disapproval of drug use has increased, and that may well have reduced initiation, but it is unlikely that this disapproval is a function of enforcement stringency.

It is even harder to determine the costs of heavy enforcement, in other than budgetary terms. Drug enforcement bears particularly heavily on the African-American population. Large numbers of young poorly educated males are being locked up for long periods in institutions that do little to rehabilitate them. Tough enforcement may also exacerbate various harms of drug use.

The latter brings us to the issue of harm reduction, the European term for the more pragmatic approach to drug problems that takes account of the fact that goals of drug control can conflict with other social goals. The concluding part of this section describes what that approach entails, how (and why) it has been implemented elsewhere, and its possible application in the United States.

Prices, Attitudes, and Prevalence

Price is determined by the interaction of supply and demand. If the demand for cocaine was declining in the second half of the 1980s, as suggested by the surveys, the rising numbers entering treatment and increasing imprisonment rates, then, absent tougher enforcement, prices might have been expected to fall during that period. In fact, we observe a complex pattern, with retail cocaine prices declining until 1988 and then rising for the next two years.

The failure of cocaine prices to collapse may be evidence of the effectiveness of stringent enforcement. Certainly, the margins for different actors in the trade remain high and, if 1988 District of Columbia data are any guide, provide substantial wage levels (approximately $30 per hour for low-level participants in 1988). But the price increase that has been achieved is surprisingly modest; late 1990 prices were perhaps 25 percent above their 1988 nadir and close to their levels of 1986 in nominal dollars. This may reflect a growing correlation between selling and heavy use. Adult cocaine retailers are frequent users themselves; if a significant portion of their earnings from this activity go to support their own consumption, then enforcement risks will have less effect on prices.

Marijuana seems to represent more of a success for enforcement. Its price is sharply higher than ten years ago, even after adjusting for potency increases and inflation. Interdiction may well have played a role; Colombia, the low cost producer of marijuana, no longer services the U.S. market, as a consequence of increasingly effective interdiction. The primary sources are Mexico and the United States itself, both of which are very high cost producers. Moreover, the price increase has occurred over a period, during which all the indicators point to a substantial decline in demand, making even clearer the impact of enforcement.

There is only one measure of availability which comes from the High-School Senior Survey. Respondents are asked whether it would be "easy," "very easy," etc. to get a particular drug. In 1980, 48 percent said that it was easy or very easy for them to get cocaine; by 1990, the figure was 59 percent. It declined for the first time in 1991, perhaps reflecting the falling demand among the seniors; with markedly fewer buyers in this population, the market may work less smoothly. In any case, if availability is a measure of enforcement success, then it certainly has lagged the increasing toughness by a long time. Marijuana availability, as measured in the same survey, has remained essentially unchanged since the survey began in 1975; each year 80 to 85 percent report that marijuana is readily available or available.

These data make it difficult to evaluate enforcement success. In the legal market, where cocaine is available as a local anesthetic, it sells for $4 per pure gram, compared to the $130 on the streets. It is not readily available for many segments of the population. Marijuana prices are high by historical and international standards; indeed, high enough to perhaps encourage more use of other drugs, such as alcohol and cocaine. The question is whether less rigorous enforcement, with fewer dealers incarcerated, would much reduce price or increase availability.

A striking feature of the general population surveys over the 1980s was the changing attitude toward both the dangers and perceived popularity of drug use. Whereas in 1980, only 31 percent of high-school seniors believed that using cocaine once or twice was very risky, that percentage had risen to 59 percent in 1990; for marijuana, the figures were 15 percent in 1980 and 37 percent in 1990. The responses stressed health dangers rather than legal dangers.

Fewer respondents also saw drug use as the norm. Whereas, in 1980, 76 percent disapproved of using cocaine once or twice, the 1990 figure was 92 percent. The most sophisticated analysis of the high-school senior survey data has found that it is these attitudinal changes which best explain declining drug use.[56]

As mentioned earlier, the evidence suggests that drug use has declined more sharply among those who have graduated from high school than those who have not. At the same time, it appears that enforcement risks have increased more for the less educated. It may well be that the more educated have greater sensitivity to the threat of arrest, but the evidence is against enforcement as the primary engine for reduced drug use.

Incapacitation

Toughness works through incapacitation of sellers and users, as well as through the effect of deterrence on prices. Locking up sellers should raise the price of drugs by removing those who were the most willing to be dealers. On the other hand, locking up users should lower the price. Even if they use drugs while in prison, they are likely to use less; urinalysis programs for prisoners show very low use rates generally. Thus incapacitation can have ambiguous effects on prices, depending on the composition of the imprisoned population.

We have already seen that an increasing number of drug sellers were locked up during the second half of the 1980s. There was an even larger rise in the number of drug users incarcerated.

Over the second half of the 1980s, there was a dramatic increase in the number of prison and jail inmates, continuing a trend that goes back to the mid-1970s. Between the end of 1985 and the end of 1990, that figure increased from 750,000 (including federal, state, and local correctional facilities) to 1,200,000. The incarcerated population became richer in drug users over that time; in 1988, nearly one-third of those sent to state prison were convicted of drug offenses, compared to only 23 percent in 1986. Moreover, the data from local urinalysis programs suggests that the percentage of those imprisoned on non-drug charges who were drug users also rose. Taking account of both the increasing population of prisoners and the rising share that were drug users, perhaps a total of 450,000 additional drug users were removed from the population that might be involved in regular use or selling of drugs.[57]

Table 3
Race Characteristics of Arrestees

| | Percent Black | | |
	1980	1985	1990
All Offenses	24.5	26.6	28.9
Crime Index	32.8	33.7	34.4
Drug Abuse	23.6	30.0	40.7

Source: *Uniform Crime Reports.*

What are the effects of this increase? In the context of an estimated 2 to 3 million frequent drug users, that is a substantial change and may do much to explain the decline in various indicators, including both DAWN and DUF. That is, declines in the numbers of persons showing up in emergency rooms for drug-related problems or in the percentage of arrestees testing positive for drugs may reflect not just declines in drug-using behavior but also the incapacitation of large numbers of drug users. The gains then are contingent on continued incarceration, given the lack of effective treatment in most prison facilities.

Other Consequences

A standard charge against the war on drugs is that it is racist and has led to a serious erosion of civil liberties. It is certainly true that African-Americans make up an extraordinarily high proportion of those charged with drug offenses, even when compared to their proportion in criminal offenses generally or to their share of the population of frequent drug users. That does not imply racism on the part of police or courts, but it does point to the possibility of selective enforcement.

Table 3 provides data on the high and growing fraction of drug arrestees who are categorized as black in the Uniform Crime Reports.

That share has increased dramatically over the ten years from 1980 to 1990, from less than one-fourth to more than two-fifths. The percentage has risen much faster for drug offenses than for others, including the more serious (represented by "Crime Index" offenses).

The emphasis on crack seems to have exacerbated this tendency. For example, the Minnesota legislature in 1989 raised the maximum penalty for possession of 3 grams of crack to twenty years; the same quantity of cocaine powder involved a maximum of five years. As it turned out, 96.6 percent of those charged with crack possession were African-American; for powder cocaine, the figure was about 20 percent. The Minnesota Supreme Court overturned the statute for that reason in 1991.[58]

The high and rising drug-arrest rates for African Americans represents another dilemma for drug policy. It is in poorer sections of large cities, with high percentages of young African-American males, that the problems of disorder and violence surrounding drug distribution are most acute. These are the communities that have the greatest need for active drug enforcement. Yet, that enforcement, responsive to community concerns, results in the incarceration of alarmingly high percentages of young males from the same communities.

This brings us to another concern, namely that those who are locked up are unimportant figures in the drug trades and that their sentences are too severe for the crime, particularly when prisons are regarded as more likely to worsen an inmate's behavior than to rehabilitate him. The contention about the role of those locked up is almost irrefutable because of the highly pyramided nature of the drug trade. Cocaine enters this country in 100 kilogram lots and sells in 1 gram units; under reasonable assumptions about how many others a wholesale dealer is willing to transact with, there are about 1,000 retailers for each importer. Thus, most of those who are locked up must be retailers and their support personnel. There simply aren't 100,000 significant figures in the cocaine trade; indeed, there probably aren't more than 10,000 whose removal would make the trade go somewhat slower.[59]

Those locked up receive long sentences now, particularly at the federal level. The expected time served for conviction on a drug-trafficking offense in federal court is over six years. Though federal courts confront the highest-level dealers, they also sentence numerous minor agents of these dealers, such as the Colombian sailors who transport cocaine from that country. The sentences received by these agents are not light. Indeed, a horrible irony of the existing federal sentencing guidelines is that the only mitigating circumstance for shortening of the mandatory sentences is effective cooperation with the prosecutor. Unimportant agents, such as sailors, have little to offer; whereas, the principal figures in seller networks can, if they choose, provide valuable information.

At the state level, the average sentences are not particularly long by contemporary U.S. standards, but, as we saw above, about 90,000 persons received sentences of at least one year for drug offenses in 1988. At a time of overcrowded prisons, even one uncomfortable with the level of incarceration in the United States must ask whether the space could not be allocated more sensibly for more serious offenses.

One response to this is that those sentenced for drug offenses are also involved in more serious offenses; the drug selling is merely a marker for these other crimes. Little data are available on this matter. In the District of Columbia, in a sample of drug dealers on probation in 1988, only 5 percent reported a violent offense in the previous six months. Indeed, drug selling in that sample looked very much like a substitute for other kinds of income-generating (and sometimes violent) crimes.

The issue here is that of the seriousness of the offense. Legislatures have been impressed by claims that drugs cause great harm and have consequently demanded that the criminal-justice system treat this as a serious offense. As always, it is a question of emphasis and allocation of resources, but I confess that it is not clear to me that marijuana selling, or even possession with intent to distribute cocaine, should necessarily lead to lengthy incarceration, particularly at a time when punishment capacity is stretched so thin. That so many of those being locked up in state prisons and local jails for drug offenses are African Americans makes it particularly important that we judge whether this incarceration is necessary.

Moreover, there are other harms that may be exacerbated by tough enforcement. Frequent harassment of street drug sellers increases the incentives to use violence for the maintenance of market share. More variability in the purity of heroin, resulting from occasional large seizures, may cause more overdoses. Stringent enforcement has raised marijuana potency, while head-shop laws prevent marijuana users from using water pipes; marijuana is consumed in the most harmful possible manner.

The list of conjectured harms from intense enforcement can be extended. How significant each of them is and what they amount to in the aggregate is impossible to even guess at. I believe, though, that they are troubling enough that one needs to consider whether there is an alternative approach to drug control that takes them into account.

Harm Minimization and Aggressive Owls[60]

Illicit drug use has become a prominent issue in much of Western Europe in recent years. For example, a survey of popular perceptions of the principal public health problems of the nations of the European Community found that, in almost all of them, illicit drugs was one of the top three concerns, always ahead of alcohol.[61] In four countries, it was identified as the leading health problem. Deaths from drug use, almost exclusively involving heroin, have increased rapidly in Germany, Italy, and Spain. Switzerland, the south of France, Italy, and Spain

have HIV epidemics dominated by intravenous drug users.

Despite these concerns, the reality and rhetoric of drug policy in most of Western Europe is very different from that in the United States. The crime consequences of drug use are given far less attention, though property crime is often believed to be substantially raised by drug addiction. The health consequences dominate discussion in most of Europe, though that has led to only a moderate hatching of doves. Syringe exchange schemes, scarcely permitted even on a pilot basis here, have become common in Britain, the Netherlands, Italy, and the German cantons of Switzerland. Spain and the Netherlands, with very different social policies toward drug use generally, have given the criminal law a minor role in dealing with drug users.

The discussion of drug policy in Europe, outside of Scandinavia, is dominated by debate about harm minimization, rather than minimizing the prevalence of drug use. Cannabis use, outside of Scandinavia, is almost entirely ignored. The emergence of AIDS has been the catalytic force. As the Advisory Council on the Misuse of Drugs in Great Britain said in a 1988 report, "HIV is a greater threat to public and individual health than drug misuse."[62] Policy measures that might increase the extent of drug use but lower the prevalence of HIV are likely to be endorsed under this hierarchy of values.

The policy view extends, though, to more than just AIDS-related matters. If tough enforcement lessens the likelihood of drug addicts seeking treatment, then less stringent enforcement might be preferred. Some Europeans even talk about police making harm-minimization choices in their tactics; for example, using selective enforcement to focus on heroin injectors rather than heroin smokers, since smoking poses lower risk of both HIV and hepatitis B.

My colleagues and I conjecture that the difference in policy tone between Europe and the United States is importantly affected by the much lower prevalence of violence associated with drug distribution and use in Europe. That, in turn, may reflect simply the lower level of violence in European crime generally. Without that violence, it is much easier to see health measures as the most appropriate response.

How successful have harm minimization policies been? Precisely because they are more concerned with reducing harms than drug use, they cannot be judged simply by the extent of drug use that they have engendered. The Dutch make a reasonable case that their very conscious adoption of the harm minimization approach has permitted their addicts to lead healthier and less crime ridden lives than their counterparts in the United States. However, the much more generous income support schemes available to prime age males in Holland may be more significant here than any facet of targeted drug policy.

Harm minimization is not a policy but a framework for making decisions which considers that drug policy, particularly related to application of the criminal law, has effects on other aspects of the quality of life. The one instance of the application of harm minimization in American drug policy is in the developing consensus that drug-abusing pregnant women should not be subject to criminal prosecution for the risks that they pose to their babies.[63] The belief that such prosecutions would reduce the probability of use of prenatal care seems to have played an important role in this consensus.

However, most U.S. owls currently do not take the harm minimization approach. Their acceptance of the need for vigorous enforcement, which precludes consideration of the negative consequences of that enforcement, has made their contribution to drug policy discussions of limited value so far. We now turn to the sources of their timidity.

The Political Dynamics of Drug Policy

The success of the hawks is in part a function of how the drug problem has been characterized in the United States. So long as crime is the dominant part of the public image of the problem, then law enforcement is plausibly the most appropriate response. Drugs are produced by evil syndicates (the Medellin cartel), sold by ruthless gangs who kill innocent bystanders and generate fabulous incomes for the sellers (media stories about inner-city kids earning $1,000 a day[64]) operating in settings that generate neighborhood fear and disorder (street corners and crack houses); so runs the standard version of the problem.

That growing association between crime and drug use in popular perception reflects the reality of changing patterns of drug use reported earlier. As young, poorly educated males become a larger part of the population that is heavily involved with drugs, so drugs and crime have truly become more strongly associated. In this sense we are reliving the experience of the early twentieth century United States with respect to opiates. Courtwright argues that the total number of opiate addicts declined through the first quarter of this century but that the decline was much more pronounced among the middle class, where the addiction was generally associated with medical treatment.[65] The recreational user/addict, typically less educated, and more frequently a criminally active young urban male, was less likely to drop out of opiate use as disapproval increased and more restrictions were placed on access to drugs. Thus opiate addiction came increasingly to be seen as a behavior leading to crime. That helped create a climate of opinion in which criminal prohibitions on use and strict penalties against sellers received broad support; The Harrison Act of 1914 attracted little controversy.

Table 4
Preferences for Different Drug-Control Programs

	Percent Favoring Program		
PROGRAM	White	Nonwhite	Total
Interdiction	19	42	34
Prosecution/Arrest	17	9	12
Education/Prevention	41	29	33
Treatment	23	21	22

Note: Responses to question: "Which program should receive the most money and effort in the fight against drugs?"
Source: *The District of Columbia 1990 Public Opinion Survey of Drug Abuse and Crime.*

The media reporting of the "drug crisis" has undoubtedly helped here. An analysis of prime-time network news bulletins in 1988 found that illegal drugs were the second most frequently mentioned item. Most of those news stories dealt with the drama of crime associated with drugs; few of the stories concerned drug treatment or prevention. The standard media mention of the issue is drugs and crime, rather than addiction to psychoactive substances of varying legal status.

All this has made it difficult for owls or doves to win the debate. No member of Congress has had political problems as the result of pressing for tougher penalties or expanded enforcement. The risks in arguing for more lenient punishment of drug users or dealers are clearly very serious, in face of popular opinion inflamed to believe in the need for toughness. It is depressing to note that a 1986 "Sense of Congress" resolution, demanding the additions to the federal drug-control budget be split evenly between enforcement and demand-side programs, has led only to a modest shift in the balance of funding, even as federal drug budgets have rapidly escalated.

There is not a lot of good survey research on public opinion with respect to drugs, in particular about what people perceive to constitute the drug problem. The most relevant research survey was carried out in the District of Columbia in 1990 and showed a lack of faith in local enforcement. Respondents were asked to rate four kinds of programs in terms of their importance for controlling drug abuse. Table 4 presents the results for both whites and non-whites.

Three features of these responses are striking. The first is the relatively greater faith in interdiction (stopping drugs from coming into the country), as compared to enforcement at the local level. That reverses what I take to be the growing consensus among those who analyze drug enforcement. The second is the modest support for treatment, though a majority of respondents in the survey did believe that drug treatment was the appropriate sentence for arrested drug users. Third, whites and non-whites have notably different attitudes. Non-whites are more for enforcement than whites; 51 percent of non-whites chose one of the two enforcement options, compared to 36 percent of whites. But the non-whites more strongly prefer that enforcement take the form of interdiction rather than arrest and prosecution in their own community. A higher percentage of whites show faith in education and pre-

vention. But demand-side programs do get strong support from both whites and non-whites; overall, a bare majority favor such programs. Thus, there may be more of a base of public opinion to support less punitive approaches than is currently believed.

Conclusion

A particularly disturbing aspect of the current situation is the difficulty of dismantling the punitive apparatus that has been assembled since the mid-1980s. With declines in drug involvement among American youth likely to continue for some years, the justification for the draconian sentences at the federal level, with their personal and fiscal costs, will be even harder to sustain. The problem is increasingly that of the adult drug addicts who became dependent during the heroin epidemic of 1967-1973 or the cocaine epidemic of the 1980s.

Yet, the political forces are not favorable to changing this bent in the near future. The doves are likely to be pushed back to the fringe status they held until 1987. Their appearance on center stage was fueled by the pervasive sense of despair in the late 1980s that the nation's drug problem was continuing to worsen, despite tough and intrusive control. That sense of despair has lessened, reflecting at last the great decline in initiation into drug use among the vast middle class of the nation. Notwithstanding the rhetoric of liberals and conservatives alike that it is "everybody's problem," drugs now seem to be moving to another entry on the long list of ills that emanate from the inner city and poor minority populations in particular. Hawkishness may not have been the primary cause for the diminution of the problem, but, nonetheless, the diminution occurred during the hawks' ascendancy, so that hawks find it easy to claim that "toughness worked." Those who argue that the problem also worsened during the earlier ascendancy of the hawks will find a small audience. Calls for major changes in policy, in particular for the legal availability of what have come to be seen as "devil drugs," no matter how stringent the associated regulation, will also have limited appeal.

Owls may do better than doves. The imagery of war ought to work in their favor; victory is often followed by a period of humanitarian outreach by the winning side, an effort to help the casualties of war. The continuing decline in initiation among America's youth will make ever clearer that the drug problem is mostly the dangerous behavior of a relatively small number of adults, caught in the cocaine epidemic of the 1980s. Maybe locking them up will start to look more expensive and less attractive than developing better quality health and social services aimed at reducing their drug use and at improving their social functioning. Owls, even if their message lacks the simplicity and clarity of the competing birds, may yet come to dominate the aviary.

* * *

Peter Reuter, "Hawks Ascendant: The Punitive Trend of American Drug Policy," reprinted by permission of *Daedalus,* Journal of the American Academy of Arts and Sciences, from the issue entitled, "Political Pharmacology: Thinking About Drugs," Summer 1992, Vol. 121, No. 3. Copyright © 1992 by *Daedalus*.

For Discussion

Reuter argues that current drug polices reflect the Hawk philosophy of enforcement. Why are legislators hesitant to recognize the benefits of drug treatment?

Notes

1. Punishing drug users should reduce demand; to that extent the "supply-sider" label has an element of exaggeration.

2. This debate was given its most explicit formulation in the congressional debate on the 1988 Omnibus Anti-Drug Control Act.

3. Joseph Nye, Graham Allison, and Albert Carnesale, "Analytic Conclusions: Hawks, Doves and Owls," in Allison, Nye, and Carnesale, eds., *Hawks, Doves, and Owls: An Agenda for Avoiding Nuclear War* (New York: W. W. Norton, 1985), 206-22.

4. Nye et al.'s tripartite division added owls to the conventional hawks and doves. Whereas, hawks believed that war could be avoided only if both sides have enough weapons to impose unacceptable damage on the other, and doves believed that disarmament was essential to prevention of nuclear war, owls believed in confidence-building measures and other elements of process, rather than the scale and comparability of nuclear arsenals as the key to peace.

5. The most appropriate measurement of treatment success is a vexed issue. Does one include the large number of persons who drop out early in a particular program, perhaps because they decide that other programs are more suitable? What constitutes success: abstinence or improved social functioning? The authoritative review is Dean Gerstein and Hendrick Harwood, eds., *Treating Drug Problems* (Washington, DC: National Academy Press, 1990).

6. The argument is made most explicitly in reports of the Office of National Drug Control Policy. See *National Drug Strategy*

(1989 and 1990) and *White Paper on Drug Treatment*, 1990.

7. I shall not deal with the fringe dove movement that emphasizes the positive effects of psychoactive drugs. Thomas Szaz is probably the leading intellectual evangelist of this group; see Thomas Szaz, *Ceremonial Chemistry: The Ritual Persecution of Drugs, Addicts, and Pushers* (Garden City, NY: Anchor Books, 1974).

8. Ethan Nadelmann, "America's Drug Problem," *Bulletin of the American Academy of Arts and Sciences XLV* (3) (December 1991): 24-40.

9. Most acknowledge an exception for children; criminal prohibitions for the sale to children is a staple of dove advocacy.

10. Recent statements of this pessimism include Peter Andreas, Eva Bertrand, Morris Blachman, and Kenneth Sharpe, "Dead-End Drug Wars," *Foreign Policy (85)* (Winter 1991-1992); and *The Andean Initiative: Squeezing a Balloon*, Report prepared by the staff of the House Judiciary Committee's Subcommittee on Crime and Criminal Justice, 24 February 1992.

11. Gerstein and Harwood, *Treating Drug Problems*.

12. Some colleagues have argued that the imagery is loaded; after all, owls are generally thought of as wise. My own image of owls is more mixed, being derived from childhood readings of Winnie-the-Pooh, in which Owl is, indeed, learned (he can misspell long words) but unrealistic and self-deluded. The owls of Nye, Allison, and Carnesale exhibit some of the latter qualities.

13. The most refined discussion of these matters is Mark Kleiman, *Against Excess: Drug Policy for Results* (New York: Basic Books, 1992).

14. A point made by James Q. Wilson, "Drugs and Crime," in Michael Tonry and James Q. Wilson, eds., *Drugs and Crime* (Chicago: University of Chicago Press, 1990).

15. For example, there are few cities or metropolitan areas with data on the prevalence of drug use in the general population, so that it is impossible to model the effect of policy variables on the extent of drug use. Other proxies, such as the number of deaths related to drug use, turn out to be unsatisfactory for this purpose.

16. To estimate the share of criminal-justice expenditures accounted for by drug enforcement, I separated police, courts, and corrections. The share of police expenditures on the drug "account" was measured by the ratio of drug-selling arrests to Part I arrests plus drug-selling arrests. For courts, it was the ratio of drug-felony convictions to all felony convictions. Finally, for prisons, I used the share of all commitments to prison that were for drug offenses. These are all crude estimates. The only systematic effort to measure state and local expenditures on drug enforcement by police, Gerald Godshaw, Ross Pancoast, and Russell Koppel, *Anti-Drug Law Enforcement Efforts and Their Impact* (Bala Cynwyd, PA: Wharton Econometric Forecasting Associates, 1987), showed an even higher share of the police expenditures going to that effort in 1985 and 1986.

17. It is striking just how state and local governments have succeeded in keeping the public debate focused on the federal budget allocation. State and local expenditures on treatment and prevention have been growing very slowly compared to

those of the federal government, even though these services are delivered almost exclusively by the lower levels of government.

18. See Joan Petersilia, Joyce Peterson, and Susan Turner, *Intensive Probation and Parole: Research Findings and Policy Implications* (Santa Monica, CA: RAND Corporation, 1992).

19. *New York Times*, 22 March 1992.

20. Richard Doblin and Mark Kleiman, "Marijuana as an Antiemetic Medicine: A Survey of Oncologists' Experiences and Attitudes," *Journal of Clinical Oncology 9* (July 1991).

21. "Out of Joint," *New Republic*, 15 and 22 July 1991.

22. A more detailed account is given in Reuter, "On the Consequences of Toughness," in Krauss, Melvyn, and Edward Lazear, eds., *Drug Policy in America: The Search for Alternatives* (Stanford, CA: Hoover Institution Press, 1991).

23. The Uniform Crime Reports system of the FBI combines heroin and cocaine arrests into a single category. It is generally believed that the increase in this category throughout the 1980s was dominated by an increase in cocaine-related arrests.

24. Bureau of Justice Statistics, *Felony Sentences in State Courts* (Washington, DC: 1989, 1990).

25. Since these possession charges were prosecuted as felonies, they are presumably possession with intent to distribute rather than simple possession offenses, which in most states are misdemeanors only.

26. The declining average time served probably reflects two phenomena. The first is simply prison overcrowding, which has led to a reduction in the share of sentence actually served. The second is that the rapid increase in the number of drug offenders receiving prison sentences means that some are now being imprisoned for less severe offenses.

27. All of these dispositional data, both national and Californian, bear on felonies, primarily related to distribution and/or manufacture. There are literally no published data concerning the sentences received by those arrested on simple possession charges.

28. The household survey produces an estimate of ten million current users (i.e., reporting at least one use within the prior thirty days) in 1990. Allowing for one third underreporting gives a total of fifteen million.

29. Peter Reuter and Mark Kleiman, "Risks and Prices: An Economic Analysis of Drug Enforcement," in Norval Morris and Michael Tonry, eds., *Crime and Justice: A Review of Research 7* (Chicago: University of Chicago Press, 1986).

30. Peter Reuter, Robert MacCoun, and Patrick Murphy, *Money From Crime: A Study of the Economics of Drug Dealing in Washington, D.C.*, RAND: R-3894-RF (Santa Monica, CA: June 1990).

31. Mark Kleiman sensibly notes that this kind of statement ignores the prevalence of alcohol use. It may well be that the average hours of intoxication per citizen is no higher in the United States than in nations, such as France, where alcohol is more widely abused. Without denying the relevance of that measure, there are distinctive problems arising from use of illegal substances, and it is worth considering differences among societies in the extent of that use.

32. The federal government defines the use of an illicit drug as drug "abuse." Both medicine and ordinary language make a distinction between use and abuse or dependence. Though the latter two terms have different origins and formal definitions, they will be used interchangeably here to reflect levels and patterns of drug consumption that create health and/or behavioral problems to the user. None of the existing data systems allows for accurate measurement of the prevalence of one rather than the other.

33. During the 1980s, the National Institute on Drug Abuse funded three surveys of drug use in the household population; that survey has been conducted annually since 1990. Each year since 1975, the University of Michigan has surveyed a sample of approximately 16,000 high-school seniors.

34. "Thirty years ago, smoking was not associated with social class. It is now. In 1980, a quarter of professional men smoked, a third of white-collar men, and almost half of blue-collar men. . . ." Thomas Schelling, "Addictive Drugs: The Cigarette Experience," *Science 255* (24 January 1992): 430-31.

35. Nor is this simply explained by higher drop-out rates among African Americans, which would suggest that the high-school senior population was a more select group within their age cohort when compared to the white seniors. Drop-out rates in recent years have been almost equal for the two populations.

36. That difference is particularly striking, since the percentage of incarcerated males aged 26-34 is much higher for African Americans than for the rest of the population. The incarcerated males are much more likely to be drug users than the non-incarcerated; if the two ethnic groups have the same prevalence rate overall, the non-incarcerated African-American rate should be lower than the white race. Note that these are all unadjusted rates; the differences should not be ascribed to ethnicity but may be a function of urbanness, education, employment rates, etc.

37. In 1991, the survey for the first time included homeless in shelters.

38. The DAWN reports include data on the patient's motive for using the drug. In 1983, 42 percent reported that they took cocaine for its psychic effects (i.e., for pleasure) and 47 percent reported dependence. By 1989, 63 percent of those episodes involving cocaine were classified as drug dependence, and for only 28 percent was "psychic effects" the motive for taking the drug.

39. The number of DAWN cocaine mentions flattened out in 1988 and then fell by about 25 percent between the second and third quarters of 1989. The numbers then rose over the following two years, close to their prior peak. Little effort has been made to understand these changes, which may be affected by shifts in emergency-room policies during an urban health-care financing crisis, or by alterations in the behavior of addicts rather than by their numbers.

40. For a severe criticism of those estimates, see Reuter, "The (Continued) Vitality of Mythical Numbers," *The Public Interest* (Spring 1984). A recent review of the literature leaves me with little reason to change that critique.

41. Italy may have a higher rate; there are sharply conflicting estimates of the total number of addicts. If one trusts numbers of unknown provenance from distant lands, it is possible that Pakistan and Thailand have higher rates of heroin ad-

diction. See the State Department's annual *International Control Strategy Report*.

42. The figures on age composition refer to unweighted data which are only available through 1989. For purpose of describing long-term trends, the new weighted data are not appropriate.

43. The evidence for a new heroin epidemic is presented in BOTEC Analysis Corporation, *Heroin Situation Assessment*, a Working Paper prepared for the Office of National Drug Control Policy, 10 January 1992.

44. See the MacNeil/Lehrer News Hour, September 1990; debate between ONDCP Director, William Bennett, and Senator Joseph Biden.

45. Eric Wish, "U.S. Drug Policy in the 1990s: Insights from New Data on Arrestees," *International Journal of Addictions 25* (3A) (1990-1991): 377-409. See also Senate Judiciary Committee, *Hard-Core Cocaine Addicts: Measuring and Fighting the Epidemic* (Washington, DC: 1990).

46. Robert Tillman, "The Size of the 'Criminal Population': The Prevalence and Incidence of Arrests," *Criminology 25* (3) (Fall 1987).

47. Reuter, MacCoun, and Murphy, *Money from Crime*.

48. The most recent is Dorothy Rice, Sander Kelman, Leonard Miller, and Sarah Dunmeyer, *Economic Costs of Alcohol Abuse, Drug Abuse and Mental Illness, 1985* (Rockville, MD: Alcohol, Mental Health and Drug Abuse Administration, 1990).

49. To get a sense of this, the reader should consider what would happen to the value of her house, if the crime rate in the surrounding area reached a figure comparable to that on Capitol Hill in Washington, D.C.

50. A better measure is Years of Life Lost (YLL), which takes account of how premature a death is; for example, the average YLL is higher for alcohol than cigarettes, since lung cancer typically strikes its victims in late middle age, while many alcoholics die in early middle age. DAWN data suggest a much higher average YLL (i.e., earlier age of death) for illicit drugs, but even that would not raise the significance of illegal drugs to that of either alcohol or tobacco.

51. Bureau of Justice Statistics, *Profile of Jail Inmates, 1989* (April 1991).

52. Paul Goldstein, H. H. Brownstein, P. J. Ryan, and P. A. Belluci, "Crack and Homicide in New York, 1988," *Contemporary Drug Problems* (1990).

53. Medical costs for treatment and lost wages capture only the direct costs; the increased fear associated with sexual intercourse is an instance of those indirect consequences that seem both difficult to value and potentially very important.

54. See the recent complaints by the National Commission on AIDS about lack of drug-treatment capacity, *The Twin Epidemics of Substance Use and HIV* (1991), 7-10.

55. This is discussed in more detail in Reuter, "Police Regulation of Illegal Gambling: Frustrations of Symbolic Enforcement," *Annals of the American Academy of Political Science* July 1984).

56. Jerald G. Bachman, Lloyd D. Johnston, and Patrick M. O'Malley, "Explaining the Recent Decline in Cocaine Use Among Young Adults: Further Evidence that Perceived Risks and Disapproval Lead to Reduced Drug Use," *Journal of Health and Social Behavior 31* (June 1990).

57. If 45 percent of the 1985 incarcerated population were drug users and the figure for 1990 were 65 percent, then the total number of drug users locked up rose from about 350,000 to 800,000. Both percentages seem fairly conservative.

58. *Washington Post*, 14 December 1991, A10.

59. This is not to say that the more senior figures are at low risk. Indeed, it seems unlikely that one could operate as long as five years in most American cities in the high levels of the drug market without facing substantial risk of long-term imprisonment.

60. This section draws on ongoing work being done in collaboration with James P. Kahan and Robert MacCoun.

61. Public Opinion in the European Community, *Eurobarometer*, December 1989.

62. The Advisory Council on the Misuse of Drugs, *Report: AIDS and Drug Misuse* (London: HMSO).

63. I owe this example to Douglas Besharov.

64. See, for example, the alarmist cover story in *Time*, 9 May 1988, 21-33.

65. David Courtwright, *Dark Paradise: Opiate Addiction in America Before 1940* (Cambridge: Harvard University Press, 1982). ✦

Subject Index

A

Addiction xiii, 12–40, 17, 19, 23, 25–26,
28, 30, 39, 64, 74, 189, 222, 224, 237, 299–
300, 353.
   to alcohol 12, 48, 314–317.
   biochemistry of 12–17.
   causes of 1.
   to cocaine 164, 182.
   genetic predisposition toward 17.
   to heroin 109, 111–142, 147, 149, 151,
237, 299, 309–313, 353.
   hidden 222.
   to marijuana 88, 106, 108, 329.
   medical model of 222.
   to nicotine 57–62.
   psychogenic theory of 310.
   to steroids 74–75.
   sociological theories of 23–32.
   street addicts 222.
Advertising 20, 44, 118.
AIDS 77, 81, 108, 144–146, 172–173,
259, 265–296, 299, 327, 330, 355.
   and needle exchange 284–296.
   and needle sharing 268–275.
   and prostitution 267.
Airplane glue 112.
Alcohol 3, 5–6, 43, 45–56, 80, 112, 115,
165, 238, 243, 246, 328, 330–331, 342,
355.
   biological effects of 46–47, 50–51, 53–
54, 56.
   Blood Alcohol Content 47–48.
   and health 48.
   history of xii, 45–49.
   and sexual behavior 51–52, 56.
   social role of 48–49.
   and violence 48, 53–54, 256, 326.
Alcoholics Anonymous 13, 300, 302,
314–317.
Amenorrhea 136.
Amphetamines 18–19, 80, 112, 115–116,
118, 156, 165.
Analgesics xiii.
Angel Dust see PCP
Antagonism xiv.

B

Barbiturates 112, 115, 118, 156, 165.
Benzodiazepine 63–70.

C

Caffeine 165.
Cannabis see Marijuana
Cocaine 19–20, 80, 112, 116, 159–185,
209, 229, 248–249, 272, 281, 287, 323,
329–330, 339, 342–343, 351, 353.
   biological effects of 16, 343.
   circumstantial-situational use of 167.
   compulsive use of 167.
   costs of 160.
   crack-cocaine 161, 172–176, 245–254,
248–249, 338, 355, 358.
   dosage 165–166.
   experimental use of 166.
   freebasing 160.
   Freud and 159, 163.
   hallucinations 164, 168–170.
   history of 160–162.
   inhaling of 144–146.
   stereotypes of users 178–185.
   and women 172–176.
   youth crime and 245–254.
   HIV/STD risk 175–176.
   intensified use of 167.
   intoxification effects of 167–169.
   medicinal value of 159, 327.
   multiple drug use and 165.
   and pregnancy 339, 355.
   prostitution and 180–181.
   psychosis and 164, 169.
   recreational use of 160, 162–170.
   and sexual behavior 173–174, 176, 181–
182.
   social use of 166.
   and violence 255, 257, 326.
Codeine 109.
Crack-cocaine 172–176, 245–254, 287.
Cross-addiction xiv.
Cross-tolerance xiv.

D

Depressants xiii.
"Designer drugs" 109.
Detoxification xiv.

Dopamine 343.
Drug users
    experimenters 2.
Drugs and crime 54, 123–124, 129–130,
    150, 183, 221–262, 324–326, 328, 340–
    341, 350–351.
    drug-distribution crimes 229–230.
    history of 224–234.
    self-reported 226.
    stereotypes of criminals 227–228.
Drugs and violence 255–262.
Drugs in the media 194–212, 222, 245,
    326.

E

Ecstasy (MDMA) 189–193, 327.

G

Gangs 121, 123.

H

Halcion 63, 66–67, 69.
Hallucinogens xiii, 165, 187–220, 330.
Harrison Act xiii, 88, 221.
Hashish 85–86, 94.
Hashoil 85.
Heroin 18–19, 53, 74, 109–146, 200, 229,
    237–244, 247, 254, 270, 272, 281, 287,
    323, 327, 330, 336–338, 342, 349.
    and crime 221, 237–244.
    distribution of 121–132, 229, 258.
    ethnic identity of users 115–116.
    history of in New York City 122–124.
    initial use of 111–112.
    medicinal value of 327, 349.
    nonaddictive use of 147–156.
    patterns of usage 111–120.
    and pregnancy 136–137.
    and sexual behavior 133–134.
    social use of 112, 123.
    stereotype of user 111.
    and violence 257.
    and women 133–142.
HIV 174–176, 266–267, 274, 277–280,
    282, 284–287, 295.
Hypnotics xiii.

I

Idiosyncracy xiv.

L

Legalization and decriminalization 94–
    105, 233, 320–344.

See also Public policy.
LSD 18, 20–21, 112–113, 115, 166, 187–
    188, 200, 209, 212, 214–220, 330, 354.
    chromosome damage and 217.
    dangers of 209.
    medicinal value of 214–220, 327.
    psychiatry and 214–220.
    psychosis and 217.

M

Marijuana 34–40, 85–108, 112, 115, 165–
    166, 188, 209, 246, 256, 322–323, 327,
    329, 349.
    biological effects of 106–107.
    dangers of 106–108, 209.
    Marijuana Tax Act 88.
    medicinal value of 100–105, 327, 349.
    and pleasure 34–40.
    retail markets in Amsterdam 94–99.
    and sexual behavior 107.
Mescaline 6–7, 113.
Methadone xiv, 109, 116, 128, 148, 232,
    299, 309–312, 322, 338.
Morphine xii, 23, 25–26, 30, 53, 109,
    127, 222, 327.
Mothers 138–140.

N

Narcotics 111–156.
Needle access 284–296.
Needle sharing 80–81, 266–269, 277,
    281, 286–288, 291–292.
Newborns
    and addiction 137.

O

Opiates 24.
Opium 109, 125.
    history of xii.
Over-the-counter medicines xii.

P

PCP 204–212, 230, 255–256, 340, 354.
Peer pressure 17, 20, 36, 72–73, 118,
    222, 320.
Potentiation xiv.
Prescription drugs 118.
Prohibition 49, 86, 102, 326–327, 331–
    332.
    Prohibition of drugs 322–333.
Prostitution 134, 181, 183, 242, 256,
    267, 274.
Prozac 66–67.

Psychoactive drugs xiii.
Public policy 94–99, 154, 161, 232, 270,
    284–296, 319–362.
        See also Legalization and decriminiliza-
        tion.
Pure Food and Drug Act xiii, 159.

S

Sedatives xiii, 63–70.
Shooting galleries 259, 268–282, 286–
    287 289.
Side effect xiv.
Social sanctions 153.
Steroids 43, 71–82.
        biological effects of 79.
        distribution of 76.
        personal trainers and 77–79.
Stimulants xiii.
Stress 192.
Synergism xiv.

T

Teenagers and adolescents 20–21, 57–61,
    72–74, 77, 79, 88–90, 123, 245–254, 326,
    352.
THC 85, 100, 106–107.
Therapeutic communities 300–308.
"Toad licking" 193–201.
Tobacco 43, 57–62, 322, 328, 330–331,
    355.
Tolerance xiii.

Tranquilizers 118.
Treatment 21, 109, 130, 132, 152, 155,
    231–232, 299–317, 337, 341.
        detoxification 299–300.
        outpatient 299–300.
        punitive 345–362.
        residential 299–300.
        self-help groups 299–300.
        therapeutic communities 301–308.
Twelve-step programs 314–317.

V

Valium 64.
Vietnam veterans 149, 337.
Violence 255–262.
        economic-compulsive 257.
        psycopharmalogical 256.
        systemic 257–258, 260–261.

W

War on drugs 61, 102, 189, 193, 296,
    319–320, 336.
Withdrawal xiv, 17, 24–31, 116, 119,
    128, 137, 230, 256, 299.
Women addicts 133–142, 172–176, 180–
    184.

X

Xanax 63–70, 103.